EXPLORING HEALTH

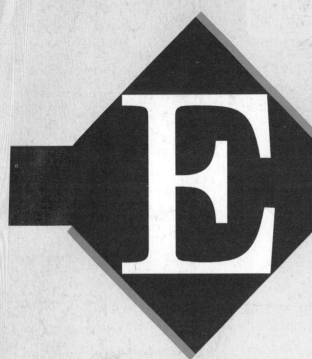

EXPLORING

Expanding the Boundaries of Wellness

Jerrold S. Greenberg
University of Maryland

George B. Dintiman
Virginia Commonwealth University

Prentice Hall
Englewood Cliffs, New Jersey 07632

HEALTH

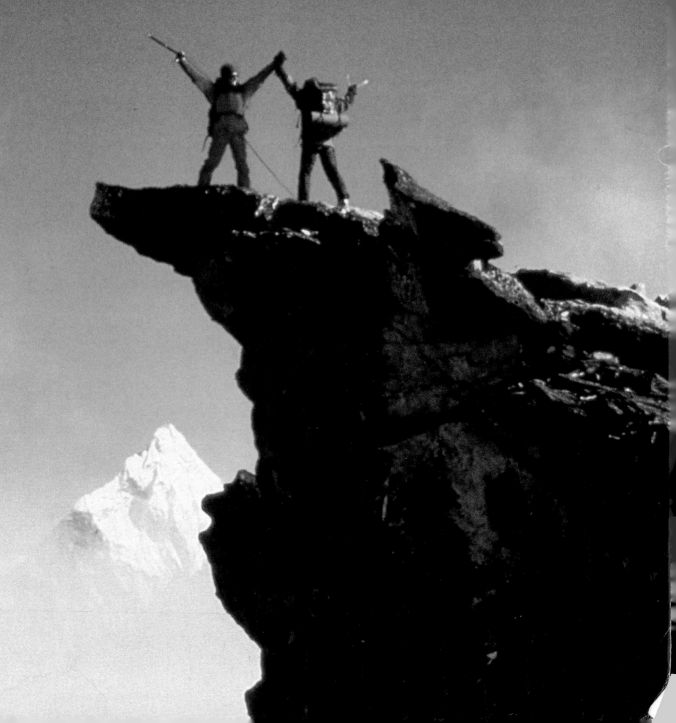

Library of Congress Cataloging-in-Publication Data

Greenberg, Jerrold S.
  Exploring health : expanding the boundaries of wellness / Jerrold
S. Greenberg, George B. Dintiman.
    p.   cm.
  Includes bibliographical references and index.
  ISBN 0-13-297151-8
  1. Health. I. Dintiman, George B. II. Title.
RA776.G7888 1992
613—dc20   91–31613
                          CIP
                          AC

*To the memory of Donald B. Rose,
Rosa Elena Chico-Garcia,
and David Greenberg*

Acquisitions editor: Ted Bolen
Editor-in-chief: Phil Miller
Development editor: Thom Moore
Editorial/production supervision: Patricia V. Amoroso
Marketing manager: Chris Freitag
Copyeditor: Stephen Hopkins
Design director: Janet Schmid
Interior design: A Good Thing, Inc.
Cover design: Aurora Graphics
Page layout: Meryl Poweski
Prepress buyer: Herb Klein
Manufacturing buyer: Patrice Fraccio
Photo research: Rona Tuccillo
Cover photograph © Alex Stewart, The Image Bank

© 1992 by Prentice-Hall, Inc.
A Simon & Schuster Company
Englewood Cliffs, New Jersey 07632

Printed in the United States of America
10 9 8 7 6 5 4 3 2 1

ISBN 0-13-297151-8

Prentice-Hall International (UK) Limited, *London*
Prentice-Hall of Australia Pty. Limited, *Sydney*
Prentice-Hall Canada Inc., *Toronto*
Prentice-Hall Hispanoamericana, S.A., *Mexico*
Prentice-Hall of India Private Limited, *New Delhi*
Prentice-Hall of Japan, Inc., *Tokyo*
Simon & Schuster Asia Pte. Ltd., *Singapore*
Editora Prentice-Hall do Brasil, Ltda., *Rio de Janeiro*

Brief Contents

Contents

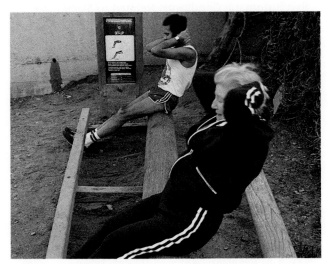
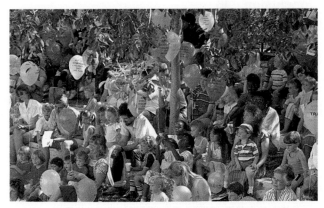

Chapter 3: Stress and Stress Management 46

What Is Stress? 48

Bodily Expressions of Emotion 48

The Stress Response Pattern 49

Distress and Eustress 50

Stress and Life Changes 50

Stress and Personality 51

Part Three   Maintaining Personal Relationships and a Healthy Sexuality

Chapter 4: Intimate Relationships: Dating, Marriage, and the Family 66

Gender Roles 68

Gender, Sex, Sexuality, and Gender Roles 68

The Development of Gender Identity 69

Our Society's Gender-Role Expectations 69

Intimacy: A Learned Process 70

The Challenge of Intimacy 71

Dating 71

Love 73

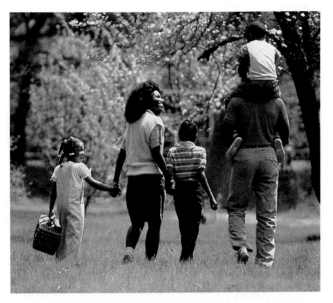

Part Four   Health and Your Body

Chapter 7:   Nutrition   156

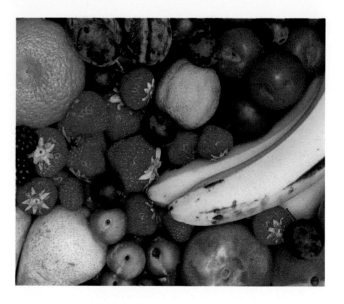

Chapter 8: Weight Control 190

Chapter 9: Fitness 216

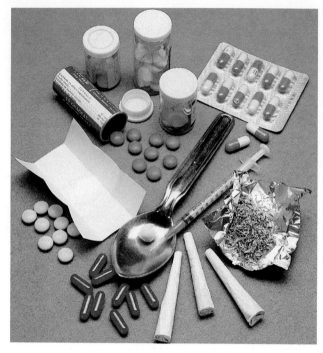

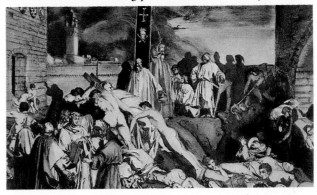

Part Six   Diseases

Chapter 13: Infectious and Noninfectious Diseases 330

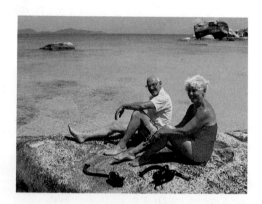

Part Seven   New Beginnings and Challenges

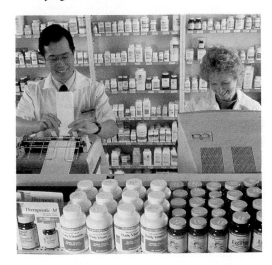

Part Eight   Health and Society

Chapter 19:   Preventive Health Care and the Consumer   482

Chapter 20:   Choosing Medical Service and Health Insurance   506

Preface

The 1980s witnessed the arrival on the scene of many new personal health textbooks, as well as revisions of many venerable older textbooks. Perhaps the most significant trend that is discernible in all of these books has been the shift in emphasis away from methods for disease prevention and detection to strategies for achieving optimum personal wellness.

We are indeed fortunate in our society to be able to strive for "wellness" rather than for "health" alone. Wellness, as we understand it in the United States, is not only a matter of health basics (surviving, eating right, and avoiding disease from day to day), it is also a matter of quality of life above and beyond the basics. We are offered lifestyle choices and opportunities that many other societies in the world do not enjoy. However, with these choices and opportunities come responsibilities.

The potential for wellness rests in large measure with each of us and the decisions we make every day of our lives. We believe that the responsibility for health and wellness rests primarily with the individual. The main title we have chosen for this book, *Exploring Health*, is intended to focus attention on the need for each person to arrive at informed conclusions about how to take responsibility for his or her personal wellness. We hope that, at the very least, we will be able to stimulate self-analysis of health-related attitudes and behaviors and that the individual will, if necessary, alter them.

Personal wellness is an admirable goal, and certainly we cannot help others achieve wellness before we have mapped out a wellness plan of action for ourselves. Yet, as we look toward the next century, we must realize that we cannot simply construct our own isolated worlds of wellness. We all live in a society that consists not only of our own family and friends, but also of the various smaller communities we live in, such as colleges, neighborhoods, and professions, as well as the larger communities we are a part of, like cities, states, countries—and the world. To ignore the influence of other people and the communities we inhabit on our own health, and the influence of our health-related decisions on the health of those people and communities, would be inappropriate. Consequently, we have developed and organized this book to include an emphasis on the individual as he or she interacts with the wider community. The subtitle we have given this book, *Expanding the Boundaries of Wellness*, is intended to focus attention on the health and wellness of other people. As students and instructors of personal health, we have the knowledge and power to go beyond the "boundaries" of personal health-related concerns and get actively involved in improving the health of the communities we live in.

To help students incorporate this understanding into their learning, we have included several unique features throughout the text:

- *Year 2000 National Health Objectives* appear in special boxes and relate chapter content to health objectives developed by the United States government in conjunction with health professionals and organizations. These objectives deal with important issues facing our whole country and its individual citizens.

- Each chapter contains two or more *Exploring Your Health* activities, whose two main objectives are self-assessment and behavior change.

- Because a prevalent theme in the book is to challenge readers to participate not only in improving their own health but also the health of other people, we have included a chapter-end set of *Get Involved!* activities. These provide specific ideas or steps the reader can take to put whatever has been discussed in the chapter to use immediately in their interactions with friends, family, and their communities.

- *A Question of Ethics* boxes in each chapter involve students in ethical decision making related to social and individual health issues.

- *Issues in Health* boxes in each chapter provide brief, thought-provoking discussions of controversial health issues that society is attempting to resolve. The reader's responsibility to be an informed citizen and to participate in the resolution of these issues is made evident in these boxes.

- Each chapter concludes with *Questions for Personal Growth*. Not merely a "chapter review," these questions encourage the reader to discuss how the chapter content pertains to his or her life.

- A *running glossary* places key terms and their definitions right there on the page for ease of study. Key terms are also listed and defined in a full glossary at the end of the book.

Teaching and Learning Aids

A valuable collection of supplementary educational and enrichment materials accompanies this book.

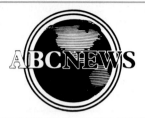

ABC News/PH Video Library for Health   The media age has established video as a dominant influence in American life. Video is one of the most dynamic and effective means of communication you can use to enhance learning in the classroom. But the quality of the video material and how well it relates to your course can make all the difference.

Prentice Hall and ABC News have brought together their talents in academic publishing and global reporting and are proud to present the most comprehensive video ancillaries available in the college market today. Prominent and respected anchors, such as David Brinkley, Ted Koppel, and Peter Jennings, bring together their insights in health into your classroom. ABC and Prentice Hall offer your students a resource of these feature and documentary-style videos, which relate directly to the issues and applications in *Exploring Health: Expanding the Boundaries of Wellness.*

The ABC News/PH Video Library pulls together critically acclaimed selections from Nightline, This Week with David Brinkley, and World News Tonight. The programs are of extremely high production quality, present substantial content, and are hosted by well-versed, well-known anchors. Carefully researched selections effectively complement and enhance the material in *Exploring Health.*

The New York Times

New York Times Contemporary View   The *New York Times* and Prentice Hall, two leading publishers in academia and world news, are proud to co-sponsor **A CONTEMPORARY VIEW,** a program designed to enhance student access to current and relevant information in the world of health.

Your students will receive a 16-page dodger—a student version of the *New York Times* containing approximately 30 articles to be used in conjunction with *Exploring Health: Expanding the Boundaries of Wellness.* The stories in the dodger are actual articles that appeared in current issues of the *New York Times* and relate specifically to the world of health. The selected articles include events and new developments in personal health, health-related services and technologies, and national and international issues in health.

Knowledge of world events is invaluable. Reading a premier news publication such as the *New York Times* establishes a practice of staying abreast of the events happening in today's society. Students who deepen their appreciation of print in the learning environment will remain devoted to the medium throughout their lives.

Instructor's Resource Manual   Offers the instructor detailed outlines, discussion questions, and in and out-of-class activities for each chapter. Includes a video guide to the ABC/Prentice Hall Video Library.

Test Item File   A compendium of over 2,000 multiple choice, matching, short answer, and essay questions.

Testing Software   The test item file on disk, available for IBM and Macintosh computers, gives the instructor the ability to edit or delete existing questions and create and edit new questions.

Prentice Hall Health Transparencies   A complete set of beautiful full-color transparency acetates produced from a wide range of illustrations from the text and from other sources. Available free to qualified adopters.

Slide Set for AIDS and Other Sexually Transmitted Diseases   This valuable resource is available free to qualified adopters. Please ask your Prentice Hall representative for details.

Study Guide and Workbook   (For Sale Item) This handy student resource offers learning objectives, self-quizzes on text material, additional self-assessment activities, and behavior change strategies.

Acknowledgments

We are grateful for the thoughtful criticism and helpful suggestions of the following reviewers for *Exploring Health.*

Judy A. Baker	East Carolina University
Rick Barnes	East Carolina University
Donald L. Calitri	Eastern Kentucky University
Vivien Carver	University of Southern Mississippi
Joseph S. Darden, Jr.	Kean College of New Jersey
Gary English	Ithaca College
Monte J. Gagliardi	University of Arkansas
Raymond Goldberg	SUNY at Cortland
Patricia A. Gordon	Arkansas Tech University
William C. Gross	Western Michigan University
Kathleen S. Hillman	Springfield College
Marsha Hoagland	Modesto Junior College
Jack A. Jordan	University of Wisconsin, LaCrosse
Judith Nelson	Burlington County College
Kim Roberts	Eastern Kentucky University
Steve Roberts	University of Toledo
Norma Jean Schira	Western Kentucky University
Sherm Sowby	California State University
Donald B. Stone	University of Illinois

Eric P. Trunnell   University of Utah
Parris R. Watts   University of Missouri
Noah Young   UCLA Drug Abuse Research Group

We also wish to thank Brenda Dintiman-Shanahan, M.D., dermatologist, for her assistance with sections on skin care and skin cancer, and Lawrence Cappiello, H.S.D., and John Rousselle, Ph.D., for writing chapter 11 on Using and Abusing Alcohol.

In addition, we owe a debt of gratitude to the people at Prentice Hall who committed themselves to the careful review, editing, and production of this book. In particular, we wish to acknowledge the help and encouragement of Ted Bolen, Phil Miller, and Diane Schaible (College Editorial), Thom Moore and Ray Mullaney (College Book Development), Patricia Amo-roso (College Book Editorial Production), Janet Schmid (College Art), and Rona Tuccillo (Photo Research). They provided us with valuable insight and guidance in all phases of the creation of this book, from the first written word to the last details of organization, design, illustration, and production. We publicly thank them.

Finally, our families provided us with the support that all authors need. They were there to bounce ideas off of, to console and to cajole (whichever happened to be needed at the time), and to provide a haven of love to which we could retreat. Although we have come to expect these things from our families, we nevertheless would like to take this opportunity to acknowledge that we probably do take them for granted too often and announce loudly for all to hear: Thanks for being there!

EXPLORING HEALTH

CHAPTER

1

Health and Wellness

CHAPTER OBJECTIVES

After reading this chapter, you should understand:

- How your current behavior may or may not be keeping you healthy.

- Why your own health behavior affects our nation's health.

- That the United States government has established an extensive set of national health objectives for the year 2000. The object of the Year 2000 National Health Objectives is to suggest specific ways to achieve the general goal of improving the nation's health.

- How, in defining health in terms of all its components, including physical, social, mental, emotional, and spiritual health, we arrive at the concept of wellness.

- Some of the many human behavior theories that have been proposed to explain why people behave as they do.

CHAPTER OUTLINE

Your Personal Health

Health Behavior Questionnaire

The Nation's Health

Defining Health

Theories of Human Behavior

Health Behavior

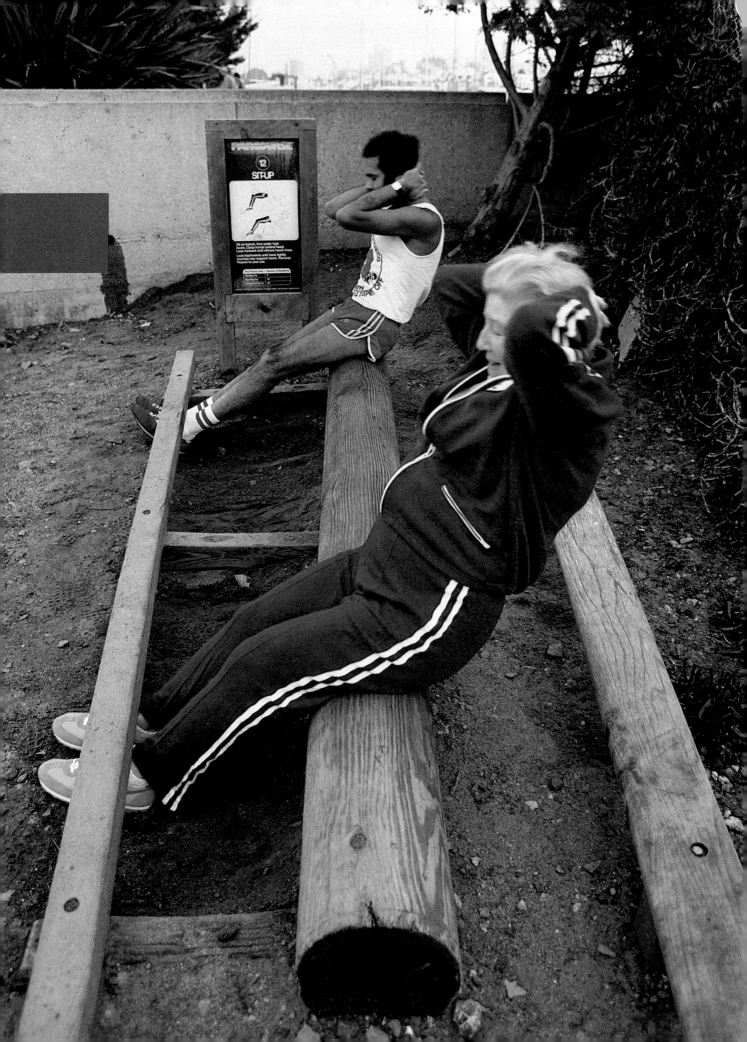

Your Personal Health

The United States government has become increasingly interested in our health-related behavior. You see, when you adopt what are called health "risk factors"—for example, smoking cigarettes, abusing drugs, or mismanaging stress—you'll need to use the medical care system more than otherwise. The more that system is used, the higher the cost of health care will be. When this cost becomes high, governmental support services are called into play: medicare, medicaid, social services. The result is that taxes increase, inflation plagues the country, and the economy is thrown into turmoil. The federal government believes that helping you to maintain your health—and prevent or postpone illness—can have beneficial financial implications for the nation as a whole. For that reason, governmental agencies have been enlisted—most notably, the Office of Disease Prevention and Health Promotion (ODPHP)—to encourage Americans to adopt healthy behaviors. ODPHP has developed an instrument that measures the degree to which people are behaving in healthy or unhealthy ways. This instrument appears here. Take a minute and complete the *Health Behavior Questionnaire*.[1] The interpretation of your scores can be found at the end of the questionnaire.

Health Behavior Questionnaire

This is not a pass-fail test. Its purpose is simply to tell you how likely your behavior is to keep you healthy. The behaviors covered in the test are recommended for most Americans. Some of them may not apply to persons with certain chronic diseases or handicaps. Such persons may require special instructions from their physicians or other health professionals.

You will find that the test has six sections: smoking, alcohol and drugs, eating habits, exercise and fitness, stress control, and safety. Complete one section at a time by circling the number corresponding to the answer that best describes your behavior (2, 3, or 4 for "Almost Always," 1 for "Sometimes," and 0 for "Almost Never"). Then add the numbers you have circled to determine your score for that section. Write the

score on the line provided at the end of each section. The highest score you can get for each section is 10.

Cigarette Smoking

If you never smoke, enter a score of 10 for this section and go to the next section, "Alcohol and Drugs."

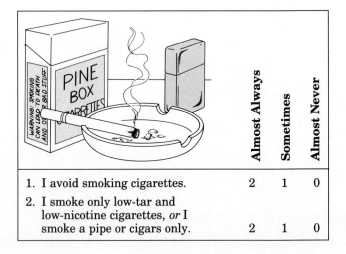

	Almost Always	Sometimes	Almost Never
1. I avoid smoking cigarettes.	2	1	0
2. I smoke only low-tar and low-nicotine cigarettes, *or* I smoke a pipe or cigars only.	2	1	0

Cigarette Smoking Score: _____

Alcohol and Drugs

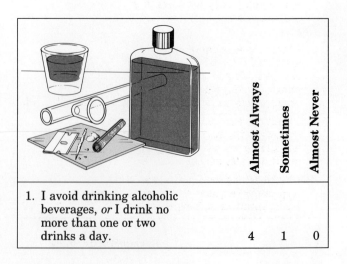

	Almost Always	Sometimes	Almost Never
1. I avoid drinking alcoholic beverages, *or* I drink no more than one or two drinks a day.	4	1	0

	Almost Always	Sometimes	Almost Never
2. I avoid using alcohol or other drugs (especially illegal drugs) as a way of handling stressful situations or the problems in my life.	2	1	0
3. I am careful not to drink alcohol when taking certain medicines (for example, medicine for sleeping, pain, colds, and allergies).	2	1	0
4. I read and follow the label directions when using prescribed and over-the-counter drugs.	2	1	0

Alcohol and Drugs Score: _____

Eating Habits

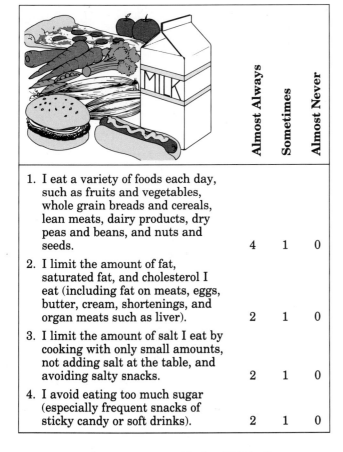

	Almost Always	Sometimes	Almost Never
1. I eat a variety of foods each day, such as fruits and vegetables, whole grain breads and cereals, lean meats, dairy products, dry peas and beans, and nuts and seeds.	4	1	0
2. I limit the amount of fat, saturated fat, and cholesterol I eat (including fat on meats, eggs, butter, cream, shortenings, and organ meats such as liver).	2	1	0
3. I limit the amount of salt I eat by cooking with only small amounts, not adding salt at the table, and avoiding salty snacks.	2	1	0
4. I avoid eating too much sugar (especially frequent snacks of sticky candy or soft drinks).	2	1	0

Eating Habits Score: _____

Exercise and Fitness

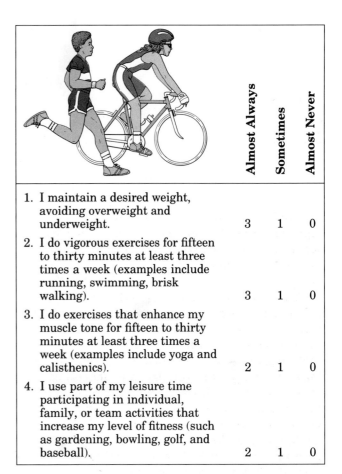

	Almost Always	Sometimes	Almost Never
1. I maintain a desired weight, avoiding overweight and underweight.	3	1	0
2. I do vigorous exercises for fifteen to thirty minutes at least three times a week (examples include running, swimming, brisk walking).	3	1	0
3. I do exercises that enhance my muscle tone for fifteen to thirty minutes at least three times a week (examples include yoga and calisthenics).	2	1	0
4. I use part of my leisure time participating in individual, family, or team activities that increase my level of fitness (such as gardening, bowling, golf, and baseball).	2	1	0

Exercise and Fitness Score: _____

Stress Control

	Almost Always	Sometimes	Almost Never
1. I have a job or do other work that I enjoy.	2	1	0
2. I find it easy to relax and express my feelings freely.	2	1	0
3. I recognize early, and prepare for, events or situations likely to be stressful for me.	2	1	0
4. I have close friends, relatives, or others whom I can talk to about personal matters and call on for help when needed.	2	1	0

asymptomatic An asymptomatic medical condition has no visible symptoms and may, therefore, be unknown to the individual.

	Almost Always	Sometimes	Almost Never
5. I participate in group activities (such as church and community organizations) or hobbies that I enjoy.	2	1	0

Stress Control Score: _____

Safety

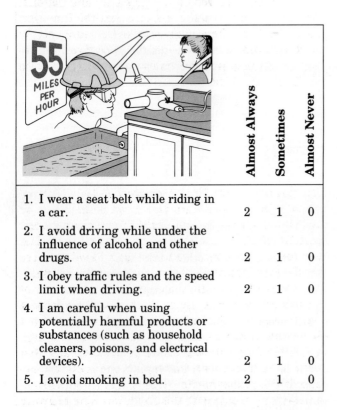

	Almost Always	Sometimes	Almost Never
1. I wear a seat belt while riding in a car.	2	1	0
2. I avoid driving while under the influence of alcohol and other drugs.	2	1	0
3. I obey traffic rules and the speed limit when driving.	2	1	0
4. I am careful when using potentially harmful products or substances (such as household cleaners, poisons, and electrical devices).	2	1	0
5. I avoid smoking in bed.	2	1	0

Safety Score: _____

Your Health Style Scores

After you have figured your score for each of the six sections, circle the number in each column that matches your score for that section of the test.

Cigarette Smoking	Alcohol and Drugs	Eating Habits	Exercise and Fitness	Stress Control	Safety
10	10	10	10	10	10
9	9	9	9	9	9
8	8	8	8	8	8
7	7	7	7	7	7
6	6	6	6	6	6
5	5	5	5	5	5
4	4	4	4	4	4
3	3	3	3	3	3
2	2	2	2	2	2
1	1	1	1	1	1
0	0	0	0	0	0

Remember, there is no total score for this test. Consider each section separately. You are trying to identify aspects of your lifestyle that you can improve in order to be healthier and to reduce the risk of illness. So let's see what your scores reveal.

What Your Scores Mean to You

Scores of 9 and 10 Excellent! Your answers show that you are aware of the importance of this area to your health. More important, you are putting your knowledge to work for you by practicing good health habits. As long as you continue to do so, this area should not pose a serious health risk. It's likely that you are setting an example for your family and friends to follow. Although you received a very high score on this part of the test, you may want to consider other areas where your scores could be improved.

Scores of 6 to 8 Your health practices in this area are good, but there is room for improvement. Look again at the items you answered with a "Sometimes" or an "Almost Never." What changes can you make to improve your score? Even a small change can often help you achieve better health.

Scores of 3 to 5 Your health risks are showing! Would you like more information about the risks you are facing and about why it is important for you to change these behaviors? Perhaps you need help in deciding how to make the changes you desire. In either case, help is available in this book.

Scores of 0 to 2 You may be taking serious and unnecessary risks with your health. Perhaps you are not aware of the risks and what to do about them. In this book you will find the information and help you need to improve your scores and, thereby, your health.

The Nation's Health

In addition to the health of each individual, the government has responsibility for the health of the nation as a whole. Because of this, the government helped in the development of health objectives for the nation, which were first designed to be attained by the year 1990. Subsequently, national health objectives have been established for the year 2000. Although the objectives are made available in U.S. government documents, they do not constitute a Federal plan. Developed by public health officials, private practitioners, health scientists, and academicians, they serve as a challenge to both public and private sectors of American society as an ideal toward which we should strive. This national initiative recognizes the contributions made to the nation's health by such public health measures as immunizations, sewage disposal, and food and water sanitation regulations, which have decreased the incidence of communicable disease. However, the initiative also recognized that the leading causes of disease and premature death in the 1990s result not from communicable diseases but from degenerative diseases such as heart disease, stroke, and cancer. Medical scientists have concluded that the risk factors for these diseases could be attributed to: heredity, 20 percent; environmental factors, 20 percent; inadequate health care delivery system, 10 percent; and unhealthy lifestyles, 50 percent. The factor that contributes most to premature illness and death is the factor over which we have the most control—our lifestyle. *Prevention* has become the key to improving the nation's health. As individuals improve their personal health through the adoption of a health-enhancing lifestyle, they reduce their chances of premature illness or death.

The History of National Health Objectives

The development of national health objectives began in 1979 with the surgeon general's report on health promotion and disease prevention entitled *Healthy People*.[2] That report established broad national goals for improving the health of Americans at the five major life stages.

The specific national health goals identified were:

1. To improve infant health, and, by 1990, reduce infant mortality by at least 35 percent, to fewer than 9 deaths per 1,000 live births.
2. To improve child health, foster optimal childhood development, and, by 1990, reduce deaths among children ages 1 to 14 years by at least 20 percent, to fewer than 34 per 100,000.
3. To improve the health and habits of adolescents and young adults, and, by 1990, to reduce deaths among people ages 15 to 24 by at least 20 percent, to fewer than 93 per 100,000.
4. To improve the health of adults, and, by 1990, to reduce deaths among people ages 25 to 64 by at least 25 percent, to fewer than 400 per 100,000.
5. To improve the health and quality of life for older adults, and, by 1990, reduce the average annual number of days of restricted activity due to acute and chronic conditions by 20 percent, to fewer than thirty days per year for people aged 65 and older.

These goals served as the target for the national initiative to improve the nation's health. However, progress toward these goals required a more specific set of measurable and well-defined objectives. Consequently, the five national goals were converted into specific health objectives in 1980.[3]

Developing the National Health Objectives: High Blood Pressure Control, an Example

The manner in which the original (1990) national health objectives were formulated can perhaps best be understood by studying one of the fifteen priority areas more closely. Let's use high blood pressure control as an example. Data indicated that high blood pressure was the most potent risk factor for coronary heart disease and stroke, as well as a contributor to diseases of the kidneys and eyes. Heart disease was the leading cause of death in the United States and stroke was not far behind. However, in spite of the danger and high incidence of high blood pressure (it was estimated that about 60 million people had high blood pressure), because it is **asymptomatic**—that is, it is without symptoms—many people with this condition were unaware of it. Given the significance of the condition and the general lack of awareness on the part of large numbers of people who suffered from it, high blood pressure control was deemed a priority in order to achieve the health goals. The next issue was how to increase high blood pressure control. That necessitated specifying measurable objectives in the areas of risk reduction, increased public and professional awareness, improved services for prevention, and improved surveillance and evaluation. Most of the objectives were based upon the status of high blood pressure control as identified by various data sources, for example, the National Center for Health Statistics; the Bureau of the Census; the Bureau of Labor Statistics; the National Heart, Lung, and Blood Institute; and other branches of the National Institutes of Health. Once the baseline status was known, achievable and realistic objectives were formulated. The result was that millions more became aware of their high blood pressure and sought treatment. Unfortunately, however, the specific objectives were not achieved. As we will soon see, these objectives were carried over into the next decade.

Year 2000 National Health Objectives

Many of the 1990 National Health Objectives were achieved; many were not. However, the coordination among health professionals was considered so positive, the focused effort nationally toward better health so valuable, and the commitment so impressive that objectives have been developed for the year 2000. In 1987, a steering committee was formed within the U.S. Public Health Service to oversee the process of developing national health objectives for the year 2000. Hearings were held around the country in which health professionals from various settings—medical care, community health departments, schools, worksites—

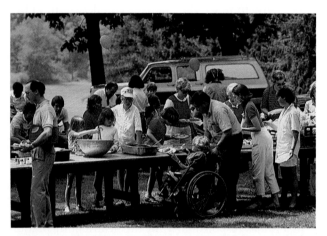

testified regarding what the health priorities ought to be, and in September 1989 a draft of the Year 2000 National Health Objectives was published for comment by other health experts. In September 1990 the Year 2000 National Health Objectives were finalized and published.[4] They are to serve as a goal for the nation's health professionals and for each of us as individuals. Working together we can improve our nation's health.

The nation's Year 2000 National Health Objectives begin with three broad goals:

1. *To Increase the Span of Healthy Life for Americans.* Data indicate that Americans had a life expectancy of 73.7 years in 1980 (it was actually 75 in 1987). However, on average, only 62 of those years were spent in a healthy state; 11.7 years included dysfunctions such as acute and chronic illnesses, impairments, and handicaps. One goal of the Year 2000 National Health Objectives is to decrease the number of dysfunctional years.

2. *To Reduce Health Disparities among Americans.* Even as average life expectancy at birth edged into the upper 70s, the expected life span for black Americans has actually declined since 1986. The average life expectancy for whites in 1988 was 75.6. For blacks it was 69.4. Furthermore, whites experience fewer years of dysfunction than do blacks or American Indians, although more years of dysfunction than experienced by Hispanics. One goal of the Year 2000 National Health Objectives is to reduce this disparity.

3. *To Achieve Access to Preventive Health Services for All Americans.* One of the reasons for the disparity

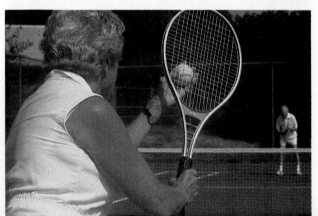

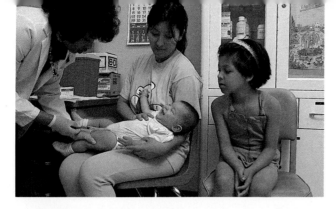

between ethnicity and life expectancy is the inequitable use of preventive health services. For example, whereas 79 percent of white pregnant women received first trimester prenatal care, only 61 percent of black pregnant women did. The result is that the infant mortality rate for black infants is 17.9 deaths per 1,000 live births, but the rate for whites is only 8.6. Another result of the inequitable use of preventive health services can be found in the death rate statistics for people age 74 and younger. In 1987, the death rate for whites was 367 per 100,000 population; whereas, for blacks it was 628 per 100,000 population. One goal of the Year 2000 National Health Objectives is to assure access to preventive services for all Americans so as to improve health and ensure years of healthy life.

The twenty-two priority areas identified in the Year 2000 National Health Objectives stem from four major areas of concern—health promotion, health protection, preventive services, and the use of surveillance and data systems. Here is a list of the 22 priorities, grouped under their four major areas of concern:

A. Health Promotion Priorities
    1. Physical activity and fitness
    2. Nutrition
    3. Tobacco
    4. Alcohol and other drugs
    5. Family planning
    6. Mental health and mental disorders
    7. Violent and abusive behavior
    8. Educational and community-based programs
B. Health Protection Priorities
    9. Unintentional injuries
    10. Occupational safety and health
    11. Environmental health
    12. Food and drug safety
    13. Oral health
C. Preventive Services Priorities
    14. Maternal and infant health
    15. Heart disease and stroke
    16. Cancer
    17. Diabetes and chronic disabling conditions
    18. HIV infection
    19. Sexually transmitted diseases
    20. Immunization and infectious diseases
    21. Clinical preventive services
D. Surveillance and Data System Priorities
    22. Surveillance and data systems

It should be evident that the achievement of the nation's health objectives depends upon the efforts of federal, state, and local governments, educational and public information institutions such as schools and the media,[5] the private sector such as large and small businesses, and each and every one of us. We can each contribute by lobbying for the government to prioritize health, insisting that our schools teach health education, arguing for the appearance of public service messages in the media, and maintaining our own good health through a beneficial lifestyle.

This Book's Focus: You and the Nation

Achieving national health objectives requires action by Americans in all walks of life, both health professionals and the lay public, governmental agencies and private businesses, schools and community health centers. Certainly, the diagnosis and treatment of disease and illness are the primary responsibilities of health professionals and organizations. However, prevention of diseases and illness is also a major individual responsibility. In this book, we will focus upon your own health. We will describe how you can maintain a high level of health and wellness by adopting a particular lifestyle. For example, we show you how to exercise to improve the health of your heart and thereby prevent the early onset of heart disease. However, we will also focus upon national health, since it is vital to all of us. We have chosen to do that by highlighting, at appropriate points in each chapter, the progress made in achieving related national health objectives. In addition, we present a boxed insert in every chapter, titled *Get Involved!*, that lists several suggested ways you can help improve society's health as it relates to the topic of that chapter. For instance, in the chapter concerned with stress, we boxed in a list of activities in which you could engage to improve the health of your community, the nation, or the world.

Remember, our goal is to help you focus upon your own health and the responsibility you have for your health, but also to help you recognize that you are part of a national community and as such you have a responsibility and a contribution to make to the status of your community, nation, and world's health.

Defining Health

Most of us assume we know what health is. Before proceeding with this chapter, write down your definition of health.

To a large extent, how we define health determines how we behave. This becomes clear when we realize that all of us want to be healthy. Whether we define health in terms of the quality of life or its quantity (length), all of our goals are related to health.

physical health Those aspects of health that concern the physical body alone and do not directly concern the social, mental, emotional, or spiritual health of the individual.

wellness Wellness is the harmonious integration of all aspects of health, physical and otherwise, by the individual at any level of that individual's own health or illness.

For example, if you define health as the absence of disease, illness, or injury, then you are probably a person who obtains regular medical examinations, drives an automobile with caution, and gets adequate sleep. If you define health as deriving satisfaction from life, then you may be a person who is willing to risk your physical health in order to achieve this satisfaction. You may, for instance, sky dive, drive fast, or ski for excitement, even though each of these activities poses some threat to your physical health. For most of us, both aspects of "health"—absence of disease *and* satisfaction from life—are important, and therefore in each situation we weigh the benefits of the risk involved against its dangers in deciding how to behave.

Look at the definition of health that you wrote. Does it pertain to physical well-being alone? When most people think of health, they think of the body,

and they usually think of preventing illness rather than of being healthy. These are concerns of **physical health,** which allows you to meet daily requirements and have energy and the capacity to respond to unforeseen events. But physical health is not the total health picture; there are other components:

- **Social health.** Ability to interact well with people and the environment. Having satisfying interpersonal relationships.
- **Mental health.** Ability to learn and intellectual capabilities.
- **Emotional health.** Ability to control emotions so that you feel comfortable expressing them when appropriate and do express them appropriately. Ability to suppress emotions when it is appropriate to do so.
- **Spiritual health.** Belief in some unifying force.

Issues in Health

Which Component of Health Is the Most Important?

There are five components of health: social health, mental health, emotional health, spiritual health, and physical health. Most people agree that all of these components of health are important, but people differ in the importance they place on each. Some people argue that social health is of utmost importance since humans are social beings. To live alone or to be ineffective in our interactions with others condemns us to a life of dissatisfaction. Others believe mental health to be the most important health component since humans need to think well to achieve a satisfactory life. They believe the essence of being human is the higher brain function that separates us from other animals.

For others, social and mental health pale compared to emotional health. They believe that people's

feelings have such a profound impact upon their individual realities and perceptions that the ability to control these feelings and use them to their advantage is the most significant component in achieving a healthy life.

Still others disagree. They believe that one's spiritual well-being is infinitely more important than one's body or mind. They argue that life on this earth is short, but one's longer existence—whether that includes an after-life or connotes being a part of nature's constantly evolving world— is forever. They argue that the achievements of this life, while important, cannot compare to one's eternal achievements.

When most people speak of health, they are referring to physical health. Therefore it is not surprising

to learn that some people believe physical health is most important. These people suggest that poor physical health will negatively affect other health components. For example, if a person has a fever, he or she will have difficulty interacting effectively with other people, will not be able to concentrate enough to learn well, will be easily angered or frustrated, and will not be able to appreciate spiritual aspects of existence. In short, a physically ill person's social, mental, emotional, and spiritual health will, of necessity, suffer. Therefore, they believe that physical health is the most important health component.

Which component of health do you believe to be the most important? Why do you believe this? How confident are you that you are correct?

For some people that will be nature, for others it will be scientific laws, for others, it will be a humanistic approach, and for others it will be a godlike force.

For example, consider the case of an overweight man who enjoys his involvement in a gourmet club and decides to maintain that involvement even though he is doing apparent harm to his physical well-being by eating foods high in saturated fats. This man has chosen to enhance his social health at the expense of his physical health.

The Health-Illness Continuum

It is important to consider health as being separate from illness. You may wonder why, for many people define illness as lack of health, and health as lack of illness. These people might depict health and illness as a straight line and call that line a "health continuum," with ill health at one end and perfect health at the other (see Figure 1.1).

Perfect health	A little health	A little illness	Ill health

FIGURE 1.1 • The Health Continuum

However, when we consider illness and health as separate entities, the continuum will not show them overlapping. That is, at some point one must stop and the other must begin. Figure 1.2 shows the model for this conceptualization. Illness occupies the right half of the continuum and ends at the midpoint; health begins there and occupies the left half of the continuum.

Perfect health	Health	Illness	Death

FIGURE 1.2 • The Health-Illness Continuum

Of course, one may argue that even if someone is ill, that person may have some degree of health. For example, a physically handicapped person who exercises regularly and participates in the Wheelchair Olympics may be healthier than a person who is not ill, but who is not physically fit. For now, though, let's withhold objection until we can explain how we intend to use the health-illness continuum.

Wellness

We'd now like you to look at the health-illness continuum under a microscope. Notice that the line isn't a line at all, but a series of dots. The continuum would then look like Figure 1.3.

Perfect health	Health	Illness	Death

FIGURE 1.3 • The Magnified Health-Illness Continuum

If we could get an even more powerful microscope and focus it on just one of the dots on the continuum, you might see something like Figure 1.4. Each dot on the continuum, then, is composed of the five components of health. When we integrate social, mental, emotional, spiritual, and physical health at any level of health or illness, we achieve what we will call **wellness.** Put another way, you can be *well* regardless of whether you are ill or healthy. Paraplegics, for example, may not be defined as healthy; but they could have achieved high-level wellness by maximizing and integrating the five components of health so that, within their physical limitations, they are living a quality life. They may interact well with family and friends (social health); they may succeed at school, on the job, or with a hobby (mental health); they may be able to express their feelings when appropriate (emotional health); they may have a sense of how they fit into the "grand scheme of things" through a set of beliefs (spiritual health); and they may exercise within the boundaries of their capabilities, for example, by finishing a marathon on crutches or in a wheelchair (physical health).

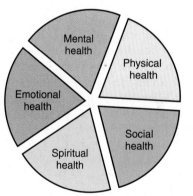

FIGURE 1.4 • A Single Health-Illness Continuum Dot

Each of us, then, has some degree of wellness. We may be ill and yet possess high-level wellness, or we may be healthy but have low-level wellness. Likewise, a person who is physically healthy may have unsatisfying interpersonal relationships, may lose control of emotions easily, and may even maintain a low level of physical fitness. And, of course, there are many points between these extremes, so that a person may have some components of health at high levels and other components at low levels.

The integration of these components is important. For example, someone may emphasize one component of health to such a degree that the other components suffer. We all know people who are so concerned with

values Those thoughts and feelings about life that the individual most strongly regards as being true.

self-actualization In Abraham Maslow's "Hierarchy of Needs" system, self-actualization is the need for the individual to achieve his or her fullest potential as a human being. It can be addressed only after all other needs have been met.

their physical health that they approach obsession; they jog, lift weights, or do calisthenics for so many hours a day they have no time for developing other sides of their total health—meaningful relationships, reading, and so forth. Others always want to have fun and socialize, and they may sacrifice adequate physical fitness or success in school. The person possessing high-level wellness can integrate each component of health into a lifestyle that includes attention to the other components of health.

High-Level Wellness Let's consider exercise as an example to understand wellness better. Remember that we understand wellness to be the integration of the five health components—social, mental, emotional, spiritual, physical—into any one life, so that one component is not improved at a significant cost to the others.

Let's first look at poor attempts at wellness. Many of us can remember the tough, unsympathetic physical education teacher we met somewhere during our schooling. We'll call that teacher A. Symmetrical. Now A believed that people—children, in particular—had to be pushed and threatened in order to tolerate the

Adjustment Theory provides one way to explain why many college students join college organizations.

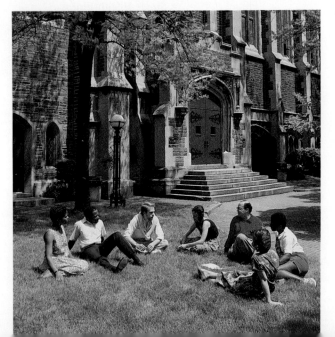

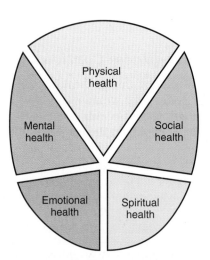

FIGURE 1.5 • The Asymmetrical Dot on the Health-Illness Continuum

pain of strenuous physical activity. Without such pain, A believed, fitness was not being improved. Left to themselves, people would not get beyond the pain and therefore would not develop high levels of physical fitness. So A. Symmetrical pushed, and A. Symmetrical threatened. If we were young, and sufficiently scared, we may even have become physically fit, while hating every minute of it. The world is full of sedentary people who were turned off to regular exercise by an A. Symmetrical. To them, physical activity is associated with pain, threats, and fear. You see, A. Symmetrical exaggerated the physical component of health to the detriment of the others, creating an asymmetrical dot on the health-illness continuum. This dot is depicted in Figure 1.5.

As you can see, the dot is no longer round. If used as a tire, it would give a bumpy ride. When our health components are organized in this manner, we too get a bumpy ride, and eventually suffer for it. One typical reaction is to deflate the large portion of the tire—in this case, physical health—while inflating the others. That is what A. Symmetrical's students are doing when they are so turned off to physical activity that they become sedentary.

The physical education teacher concerned with wellness will attempt to create a well-rounded dot—and person. Physical fitness will be stressed, but not at the expense of the other health components.

Health and Values

Health and wellness are perceived differently by different people, and these perceptions are a matter of **values**—those things about which one feels very strongly. Once again, consider the gourmet club member:

> A businessman might be 15 pounds overweight for no apparent reason other than careless eating habits, or an unawareness of the advantages of trim physique, and ignorance of the basic principles of weight control. This should be classed as a remedial health defect and one important indicator of reduced health status.
>
> However, let us compare this case with the case of another businessman, equally overweight, who happens to be a well-informed and enthusiastic amateur gourmet. His library of cookbooks includes directions for preparing many of the most popular dishes of other cultures. He spends many interesting hours in offbeat markets shopping for hard-to-get food items. The meals he prepares constitute focal points of an interesting and satisfying social life. This man realizes he is overweight; he knows how to reduce and control his weight; and he may even suspect that his coronary may arrive a year or two ahead of schedule, but he does not care. His overweight condition constitutes a health defect only in the absolute sense. When viewed in relation to his value system, it represents a logical concomitant to his particular pattern of good health.[6]

Clearly, our judgments of behavior as healthy or unhealthy depend on our values and the factors surrounding each situation. Our values contribute a great deal to our evaluation of situations.

Theories of Human Behavior

Why do people adopt certain health-related behaviors and not others? Although many theories have been proposed to explain why people behave as they do, no one knows for sure. The theories described below, however, are often cited as the most adequate explanations of why some people smoke cigarettes and others do not, why some people abuse drugs and others do not, and generally why some people behave in a healthy way and others do not. This is no magic list, though. Your instructor or other sources can provide you with additional theories of human behavior.

Hierarchy of Needs

Abraham Maslow proposed that human beings behave in ways that are designed to satisfy certain needs. Further, there exist levels of needs, and the high-level needs do not emerge until the low-level needs are satisfied (see Figure 1.6).

Until hunger and thirst (physiological needs) are satisfied, you will not be concerned with safety. In fact, if you need food badly, you might even chase a lion

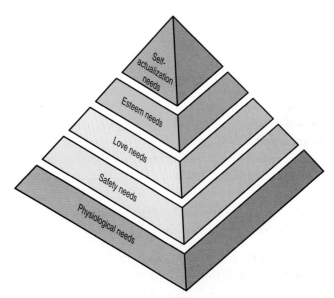

FIGURE 1.6 • Maslow's Hierarchy of Needs
Source: Abraham Maslow, *Toward a Psychology of Being.* Copyright © 1962 by D. Van Nostrand. Reprinted by permission of Brooks/Cole Publishing Company, Monterey, California 93940.

away from a felled prey. Until you feel safe and secure (safety needs), you will not be concerned with others loving you. Until you are loved (love needs), you will not be concerned about whether others respect you (esteem needs). And until you are respected by others, you will not care whether you can achieve your potential (**self-actualization** needs).

In our society, most of these needs are met to some degree. However, the degree to which they are met varies and consequently our behavior varies. Some of us might display sexual behavior that is contrary to our nature because of our need for love. Others might conform to friends' drug behavior because of the need for esteem.

Force Field Theory

According to Kurt Lewin,[7] human behavior is characterized by a constant tension between driving and restraining forces. When one set of forces becomes stronger than another, you behave one way. When the other set of forces becomes stronger, you behave another way.

For example, you might want to lose weight but you live with someone who eats high-calorie foods. If the attraction of these foods is stronger than your desire to lose weight, your diet goes down the drain.

Adjustment Theory

Others believe that human beings are constantly striving to adjust to their environments. The adjustment is

covert rehearsal Vividly imagining yourself performing some desired behavior.

covert modeling Vividly imagining someone else performing a desired behavior and then substituting yourself for that person.

covert reinforcement Rewarding yourself for being able to imagine yourself performing some desired behavior.

---

needed to maintain an equilibrium necessary for a healthy existence. When the environment places us in disequilibrium we behave in ways designed to right ourselves. Thus when a student enters college and leaves home for the first time, he or she seeks to replace the family with close friends. To acquire these friends might mean joining college organizations, taking drugs, or acquiring other behaviors designed to restore equilibrium.

The Health Belief Model ✳

One model of health behavior looks at what motivates people to behave as they do.[8] This theory states that people will adopt a health behavior if:

- They consider it likely that they will contract a disease or illness if they don't *(susceptibility)*.
- The illness or disease they may contract is severe enough to be a serious concern *(severity)*.
- The health behavior, if adopted, can prevent the contraction of the severe illness or disease *(prevention)*.
- The barriers to performing the health behavior are not too difficult to overcome *(removal of barriers)*.

Health educators have developed programs based on this model. For example, consider an exercise program. One component of the program might be describing the likelihood *(susceptibility)* that those who don't exercise regularly will contract a serious illness such as coronary heart disease *(severity)*. Exercise must then be demonstrated to be effective in *preventing* the development of coronary heart disease. Finally, any *barriers* to regular exercise must be removed or diminished. For example, exercise clothes (shorts, sneakers) should be placed on the dresser first thing in the morning to prepare for exercise after classes or work. Or arrangements can be made to exercise with a friend so that time is not taken from socializing.

Which health behaviors would you like to adopt? Why not use this health behavior model to adopt those behaviors successfully?

Health Behavior

Techniques for Changing Health Behavior

Changing such behaviors as smoking cigarettes, eating poorly, or exercising inadequately is not easy. However, behavioral researchers have found the techniques described below very helpful. Select a behavior you'd like to change and keep it in mind as you read these techniques. In this way you'll be better able to decide which of these techniques can best help you meet your behavior change goal:

- **Social support.** Get another person who is close and important to you to encourage and help you. That person should periodically ask how you're doing, congratulate or reward you if you're doing well, or work with you to adjust your goals or activities as necessary.
- **Contracting.** Make a specific agreement with yourself or others. The contract should call for a specific behavior change (for example, average only ten cigarettes a day this week), a specific deadline, and rewards for achieving the goal or punishments for not achieving it.
- **Reminder systems.** Make notes to remember your behavior goal. Leave notes on the bathroom mirror or on the refrigerator.
- **Gradual reduction.** Reduce the unhealthy behavior over a period of time. For example, rather than set a goal of complete cessation of cigarette smoking, set a goal of smoking half a pack this week, one quarter of a pack next week, and no cigarettes the next week.
- **Tailoring.** Adjust a behavior change goal to your own lifestyle, limitations, and goals. For example, if you travel a lot, an exercise program of football playing would be inappropriate. It is difficult to get people together to play football when you are in an unfamiliar town. Jogging would be a better exercise choice. Make the program fit you.
- **Professional help.** Enroll in classes, join clubs or

spas, or participate in diet clubs *conducted by professionals,* for instance, to acquire the necessary information and help in meeting your behavioral goals.

- **Chaining.** Make it difficult to perform a behavior you are trying to give up, or make it easy to participate in a behavior you are trying to adopt. Behaviors are often made up of a number of connected behaviors, like links in a chain. Thus if you add links, it becomes less likely you'll perform the behavior, and if you remove links it becomes more likely you'll perform the behavior. For example, assume you want to stop drinking beer. If you place your bottle of beer in a sock, wrap masking tape around the sock, put the sock in a locked cabinet, and keep the key to the cabinet in another room, you'd be less likely to drink that beer—especially if you had to wait to chill it. Conversely, say you want to exercise more. If you place all the necessary clothes on your bed in the morning and set aside a specific time for exercise, it will be easier for you to exercise later.

- **Covert techniques.** Think about changing behav-

ior. As surprising as it may sound, imagining yourself behaving in ways you desire has been shown to help change behavior. There are several covert techniques. **Covert rehearsal** requires you to summon up an extremely vivid image of performing the behavior—an image so vivid that you smell the atmosphere, hear the sounds, notice your surroundings, and so on. **Covert modeling** is used when the behavior is so foreign to you that you can't imagine yourself performing it (for example, if you never were physically active, you might not be able to envision yourself exercising). In this instance, you would first vividly imagine someone else you know engaging in the behavior —someone to whom this behavior is not so foreign. Then you would just substitute yourself for that other person, imagining yourself doing exactly what you imagined the other person doing. **Covert reinforcement** is rewarding yourself for being able to imagine behaving as you would like to behave. You can reward yourself by indulging in a pleasant fantasy (for example, spending a day at the beach) or a few minutes of deep muscle relaxation (see Chapter 3).

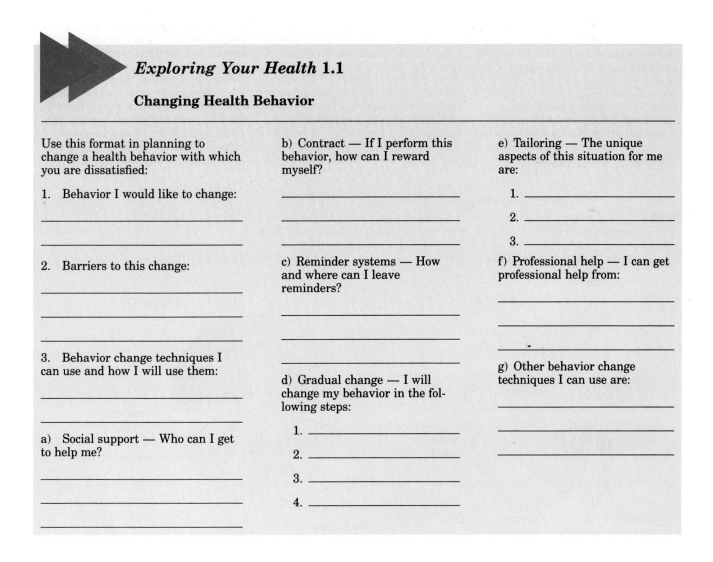

Exploring Your Health 1.1

Changing Health Behavior

Use this format in planning to change a health behavior with which you are dissatisfied:

1. Behavior I would like to change:

   _____

   _____

2. Barriers to this change:

   _____

   _____

   _____

3. Behavior change techniques I can use and how I will use them:

   _____

a) Social support — Who can I get to help me?

   _____

   _____

   _____

b) Contract — If I perform this behavior, how can I reward myself?

   _____

   _____

c) Reminder systems — How and where can I leave reminders?

   _____

   _____

   _____

d) Gradual change — I will change my behavior in the following steps:

   1. _____

   2. _____

   3. _____

   4. _____

e) Tailoring — The unique aspects of this situation for me are:

   1. _____

   2. _____

   3. _____

f) Professional help — I can get professional help from:

   _____

   _____

   _____

g) Other behavior change techniques I can use are:

   _____

   _____

   _____

A Question of Ethics

Should Educators and Health Professionals Try to Change People So Their Behavior Is More Healthy?

One point of view is that people behave in unhealthy ways because of many influences of which they are unaware. Their friends influence them, the media influence them, role models influence them, the desire to be "with it" influences them—and misinformation leads them to behave in unhealthy ways. Consequently, it is the role of the educator or health professional to counteract these influences by cunning and effective education. Educators and health professionals know what is best for people even if people do not know that themselves. To manipulate

people to give up cigarette smoking, for example, is certainly in their own best interest; and some people believe that any means used to accomplish such a worthwhile goal is justified.

Another point of view is that only the individual can decide for himself or herself how to behave. Since choosing a healthy behavior depends on our values (gaining one component of health often means giving up some of another), it is inappropriate for educators or health professionals to apply their values and decide how someone else should

behave. In addition, health scientists are often uncertain just what is healthy. (For example: Is strenuous exercise healthy or stressful? What effect does diet have on heart disease or hypertension?) If scientists are not quite sure what is healthy, then how ethical is it for educators and health professionals to manipulate people to behave in "healthy" ways?

Thus we have created an ethical dilemma. Do we allow people to behave in ways we believe harmful to them because we value freedom of choice? Or do we try to change people because we value health more?

FIGURE 1.7 • Age-Adjusted Rates for Major Causes of Death in the United States in 1900 and for Leading Causes of Death in 1989. AIDS was the eleventh major cause of death (1.0%).
Source: National Center for Health Statistics

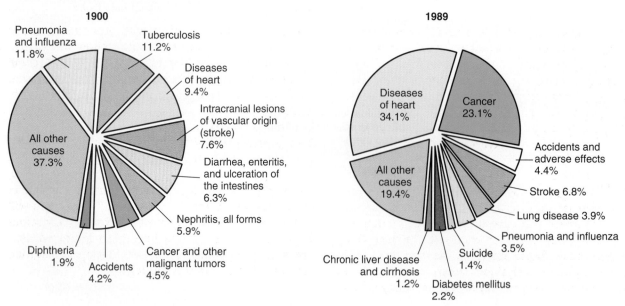

Get Involved!

Exploring Health and Wellness for Yourself and for Others

You can contribute to the health of your community, nation, and world in numerous ways. The suggestions below are merely illustrative of how you might accomplish this goal.

1. Help to improve the spiritual health of your community by volunteering to clean up nature paths and other natural "recharge" areas. You could also participate in church or synagogue programs concerning health matters (for example, AIDS education programs).
2. Clean up the neighborhood in which you live. Pick up litter, paint murals on walls of buildings that are unattractive (perhaps they are abandoned), or plant flowers in dirt-filled areas.
3. Lobby restaurant owners to include heart-healthy (low fat) foods and low salt foods on their menus and identify these with symbols. In this way you will be helping your neighbors eat more healthfully.

4. Participate in food drives for your neighborhood's homeless people, volunteer to help collect supplies for earthquake victims, or walk in patrols designed to discourage drug dealers from setting up drug markets.
5. Join an organization like Big Brothers/Sisters or the Foster Parent Program where your time can be used, and where you can also contribute financially to children in need of your help.
6. Help to collect funds, acquire supplies, or coach a team for the Special Olympics (mentally disabled children and adults).
7. Write legislators to encourage improvements that will make your world healthier. For example, write local politicians to install a traffic light at a dangerous intersection, or write your senator to support national laws that make discrimination illegal, or write the White House to insist foreign aid be provided to peoples of countries in desperate need.

Reducing the Number of Premature Deaths

The major causes of death in the United States have changed since the beginning of the century. What do you think the three major causes of death were in 1900? What are they today?

If you look at Figure 1.7, you will see how greatly things have changed. In 1900 the three leading causes of death were communicable diseases (pneumonia, influenza, and tuberculosis). As a result of legislation pertaining to quarantine, inoculation, sewage disposal, and food and water sanitation, only one of these re-

mains in the top ten today. Statistics prove that the government response was effective. But today the three leading causes of death are noncommunicable conditions that require the responses of individuals rather than governments (such as heart disease and cancer). Experts believe that if individuals exercise adequately, eat properly, have periodic medical examinations, stop smoking, drive automobiles safely and soberly, and keep medicines out of the reach of children, the number of deaths from cardiovascular diseases (heart attacks and strokes), cancer, and accidents will be dramatically affected.

Conclusion

Health relates to all aspects of our lives: from our physical well-being to our social interactions, our mental and emotional capacities, and even our spiritual lives. Defining how healthy we are at any one time involves assessing the very complex interaction of all of these facets of our health, as well as ordering them in terms of their value to us. It is meaningless, then, if not outright impossible, to assess someone else's health without involving that person in the assessment. The remainder of this book will help you evaluate how healthy you are and provide you with guidance in improving those aspects of your health that *you* decide need improvement. We have started you off in that regard by presenting behavior change techniques that researchers have found effective. As you read this book, employ these techniques when you identify a health behavior that you would like to change. You

might also want to consult with your instructor or someone at your campus health center for advice. There are plenty of resources for you to use to become even healthier than you are now and that can help you maintain that improved health status once it is obtained.

In addition to maintaining your own health, you have a responsibility to help your local community, your nation, and your world become healthier. We will make suggestions in this regard in each of the following chapters. Your role is to actually try at least one of the suggestions in the "Get Involved!" boxes. You will feel better for having behaved in a socially conscious way and your health will have been improved. For, you see, when your environment becomes healthier, your own life becomes healthier, too.

Summary

1. The United States government first developed national health objectives for the year 1990. Many of these objectives were met, but many were not. However, the effectiveness of having health objectives to strive toward resulted in the Year 2000 National Health Objectives. The year 2000 objectives pertain to twenty-two priority areas stemming from four major areas of concern: health promotion, health protection, preventive services, and surveillance and data systems.

2. The way people behave can have dramatic effects on their health. Cigarette smoking, irresponsible use of alcohol and other drugs, poor eating habits, lack of exercise and physical fitness, mismanagement of stress, and disregard for safety can all lead to premature death or disability or injury.

3. Our personal definitions of health largely determine how we behave. Those of us who define health as more than the absence of disease are concerned with the quality of our lives and not just with postponing death.

4. Advocates of a comprehensive perspective on health view emotional, mental, social, spiritual, and physical health as interdependent. Considering one component of a person's health without concurrently considering the other components is contrary to the practice of this view of health.

5. Wellness concerns the quality of life. Even if a person is not ill, he or she may not be happy or self-actualized and, therefore, may not have achieved a high level of wellness.

6. Health is a dynamic process. We move up and down the health-illness continuum depending on the status of our emotional, mental, social, spiritual, and physical health at any particular time.

7. Each person's values differ and, therefore, each person will define health somewhat differently. Some people value social health more than they do mental health, and consequently might spend more time socializing than reading or attending classes. Some people value spiritual health more than they do physical health, and therefore spend more time praying or communing with nature than they do exercising or engaging in physical activity.

8. Abraham Maslow theorized that people behave as they do in order to satisfy certain needs. In addition, Maslow hypothesized about the existence of levels of needs: high-level needs do not emerge until the low-level needs are satisfied. Maslow's hierarchy of needs consisted of physiological needs, safety needs, love needs, esteem needs, and self-actualization needs.

9. Kurt Lewin theorized that human behavior is characterized by a constant tension between driving and restraining forces. When one set of forces becomes stronger than another, a person behaves one way. When the other set of forces becomes stronger, a person behaves another way.

10. Adjustment theory states that human beings are constantly striving to adjust to their environments. When the environment places a person in disequilibrium, the person behaves in ways designed to regain balance.

11. Several effective techniques are available to help people change their health-related behavior. Among these techniques are social support, contracting with self and others, reminder systems, gradual reduction, tailoring, professional help, chaining, covert rehearsal, covert modeling, and covert reinforcement.

12. The biggest health problems of the early 1900s were communicable diseases. Government legislation, such as quarantine and sanitation laws, was enacted to prevent the spread of these diseases. Today the major causes of death are noncommunicable and largely a function of individual health behavior.

Questions for Personal Growth

1. For which of the components of health do you need the most improvement? How did you get to the point of neglecting this component more than the others? What can you do to improve that component of your health?

2. Of the four broad national health goals appearing in the Year 2000 Objectives for the Nation, which do you think is the most important? Why do you believe that to be true? Relative to these broad goals, which of the following do you consider the most valuable to help achieve these goals: health promotion, health protection, preventive services, or the use of surveillance and data systems?

3. Do you think it appropriate to place some responsibility for your community's health on you? How about your nation's health? Global health?

4. What are you willing to commit yourself to do by way of contributing to the health of your community, the nation, or the world? When will you start this action? When will you have completed this action?

5. What do you need to do to achieve better health? To achieve wellness? To achieve high-level wellness?

6. Given both your lifestyle and the causes of death as presented in Figure 1.7, of what do you think you are most likely to die? What adjustments can you make in your lifestyle that will decrease your chances of dying from this condition? Do you actually intend to make these adjustments? If you do, consult the behavior change techniques presented in this chapter. If you do not intend to make these adjustments, explore why you are unwilling to do so.

References

1. U.S. Department of Health and Human Services, *Health Style: A Self Test* (Washington, D.C.: Public Health Service, 1981).

2. Surgeon General of the United States, *Healthy People* (Washington, D.C.: U.S. Department of Health and Human Services, 1979).

3. U.S. Department of Health and Human Services, *Promoting Health/Preventing Disease: Objectives for the Nation* (Washington, D.C.: U.S. Department of Health and Human Services, 1980).

4. U.S. Department of Health and Human Services, *Promoting Health/Preventing Disease: Year 2000 Objectives for the Nation* (Washington, D.C.: U.S. Department of Health and Human Services, 1990).

5. Jerrold S. Greenberg, *Health Education: Learner-Centered Instructional Strategies* (Dubuque, Iowa: Wm. C. Brown, 1992).

6. Walter Greene, "The Search for a Meaningful Definition of Health," in *New Directions in Health Education: Some Contemporary Issues for the Emerging Age,* ed. Donald A. Read (New York: Macmillan, 1974), p. 114.

7. Kurt Lewin, *Resolving Social Conflicts* (New York: Harper, 1948).

8. Marshall H. Becker, "The Health Belief Model and Personal Behavior," *Health Education Monographs* 2 (1974): 326–473.

2

Mental Health: Health in Your Head, and Beyond

CHAPTER OBJECTIVES

After reading this chapter, you should understand:

- The characteristics of emotional health.

- The theories of Freud, Erikson, Behaviorism, Piaget, and Kohlberg regarding human personality development.

- How psychosocial factors such as self-esteem, alienation, locus of control, assertiveness, values, and peer pressure contribute to our health behavior.

- How and why we use unconscious and conscious modes of coping when faced with anxiety-producing situations and common problems.

- Several types of mental disorder.

- Where to go for help in dealing with mental disorders and some of the different types of therapy available for improving mental health.

CHAPTER OUTLINE

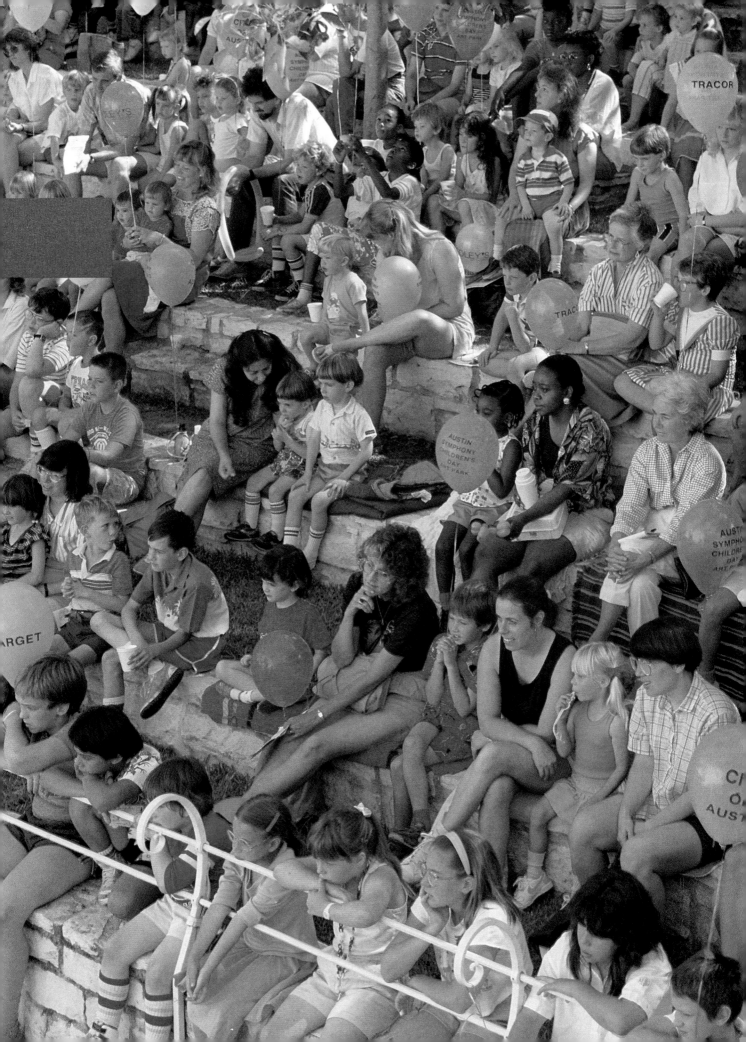

emotional health The ability to deal constructively with reality, regardless of whether the actual situation is good or bad.

socialization The influences of our home life, our experiences at school, and our interactions with other people that help determine the type of individual we become.

id In Freudian psychology, the part of our personality that seeks pleasure and gratification.

ego In Freudian psychology, the part of our personality that is in touch with reality.

superego In Freudian psychology, our conscience; our sense of right and wrong.

Mental health is a significant part of our well-being. If we feel good about ourselves, we can be expected to interact well with others, to be confident in our abilities to do meaningful work, and to derive greater satisfaction from our lives. This chapter explores mental health and recommends ways in which it can be improved.

Notice that we entitled this chapter mental *health,* not mental *illness.* Focusing upon maintaining health rather than preventing illness, we will explore such topics as characteristics of emotional health, personality development, psychosocial influences on health behavior, and modes of coping with mental stress. Because some people do have problems with their mental health and develop mental illness, however, we have included some discussion of mental disorders and their treatment.

We also present information on such problems as anxiety, shyness, jealousy, anger, and mild depression. Many of us experience these conditions and yet don't consider them to be related to our mental health. They are mental health problems, however, and we therefore include a discussion of them in this chapter.

Characteristics of Emotional Health

Think of someone you know whom you would describe as emotionally healthy. This may seem premature when emotional health hasn't even been defined yet, but having someone in mind when the characteristics of emotional health are discussed will provide you with a model of these characteristics. With this model in mind, it will be easier for you to emulate the emotionally healthy characteristics of this person so that you too can be emotionally healthy.

Emotional health includes the ability to deal constructively with reality; it is a component of mental health. If things aren't going your way and you are emotionally healthy, you are probably making the best of a bad situation. For example, suppose you meet a person with whom you would like to be friendly but who has another person as a best friend. You could mope around or act angrily toward the person with whom you would like to be friends. This behavior cer-

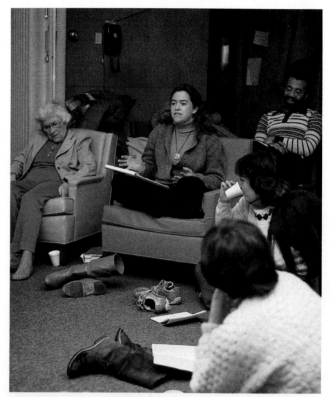

One important aspect of emotional health is the ability to accept your own emotions as well as the emotions of others.

tainly wouldn't win the friendship, but it is how many people would act when not getting what they want. An emotionally healthy person would savor the time spent with the other person, however limited, and develop other friendships.

An emotionally healthy person also adapts to change and realizes that life would be dull without it. Rather than viewing changes as threatening and always attempting to maintain the status quo, an emotionally healthy person considers change an opportunity for new experiences and new challenges. Although change is not always for the better, an emotionally healthy person will recognize when change is inevitable and adjust to it as well as possible.

An emotionally healthy person exercises a reasonable degree of independence (not overly conforming but also not overly individualistic), has the ability to make long-range choices, and can work productively.

In addition, the emotionally healthy individual can establish satisfactory relationships by showing concern and love for other people. These relationships provide companionship, love, someone with whom to share joys and sorrows, and a focus outside the self. Developing such relationships requires the ability to live with emotions. The emotionally healthy can accept their own emotions as well as those of others. Fear, anger, insecurity, and love are accepted as part of living and do not incapacitate the emotionally healthy.

Now to return to that emotionally healthy person we asked you to think about: Does the description above characterize that person? No one has *perfect* emotional health, so no one will demonstrate all of these characteristics all the time. Generally, however, emotionally healthy people function as we have described. Which behaviors of your emotionally healthy model would you benefit from emulating? Would someone use you as a model for an emotionally healthy person? If so, what are you doing right? If not, what can you change to become more emotionally healthy?

Personality Development

Our emotional health depends in large part on our **socialization,** which makes us the persons we are through such influences as our home life, our experiences at school, and our interactions with friends. To change our behaviors, we first need to understand these socializing influences on them. The theories of personality development discussed in this section offer various perspectives on socialization as it affects emotional health and styles of *coping,* which may be defined as responding to whatever threatens our emotional health.

Freud's Theory

One well-known theory of human behavior is Sigmund Freud's analysis of pyschosexual development. Freud proposed that the personality is composed of three basic elements: the id, the ego, and the superego. The **id** is the part of us that is always seeking pleasure. The **ego** is the part that is in touch with reality—the intellectual part. The ego uses defense mechanisms (discussed in the next section) to control the id. The **superego** represents our conscience—our sense of right and wrong. These three elements are constantly in conflict. We seek pleasure (id) but realize reality places limits on our pleasure seeking (ego). Our conscience (superego) then takes over and seeks the best course for that situation. The superego is like the rider pulling on the reins (ego) of the wild horse (id). For example, you might be tempted to get high on drugs (id) but realize that drug abuse is illegal and risky to your health (ego). Your conscience (superego) then decides to pull in the

reins on your desire to get high, and you pass up the drugs.

Freud believed that we always seek pleasure but are controlled by our sense of reality and our conscience. Therefore, we are constantly trying to balance these forces and sometimes engage in unpleasurable activities that we believe are right or good for us.

Have you ever done this? When you find it difficult to cope, could you understand your behavior better by considering how the id, ego, and superego interact with one another?

Erikson's Theory

Psychoanalyst Erik Erikson, a student of Freud, proposed a theory of psychosocial stages of development. According to Erikson's theory of human behavior, there are eight stages of life. In each of these stages we experience a crisis with which we must cope. Although Freud and Erikson differ on the particular tasks and crises at different stages, they agree that how the goals of each stage are handled determines a person's personality. Let's briefly go over the stage in Erikson's theory that pertains to your life right now—Stage 6, The Young Adult years—and then turn our attention to the following two stages (so that you'll know what to expect later in life!). See Table 2.1 for a portrayal of all eight Erikson stages.

Stage 6: Young Adult Years   From ages seventeen to twenty-two the crisis is *intimacy versus isolation.* Most people are forming sexual relationships during these years, but intimacy also refers to closeness with friends and relatives. If an ability to be intimate with others is not developed, you will not have anyone

TABLE 2.1

Erikson's Stages of Life

Erikson theorized that we go through eight stages in life, each of which presents a crisis needing resolution. These eight stages and their crises are:

1. Ages 0–1	Trust Versus Mistrust
2. Ages 1–3	Autonomy Versus Shame
3. Ages 3–5	Initiative Versus Guilt
4. Ages 5–12	Industry Versus Inferiority
5. Puberty and Adolescence	Identity Versus Role Confusion
6. Young Adult Years	Intimacy Versus Isolation
7. Middle Adult Years	Generativity Versus Stagnation
8. Older Adult Years	Integrity Versus Despair

behaviorism A psychological theory that postulates that behavior is caused, or conditioned, by dynamics and stimuli that are external to the individual.

heteronomous stage In Piaget's theory of the personality, at this stage of development the individual

relies upon rigid and authoritarian rules for behavioral guidance.

autonomous stage In Piaget's theory of the personality, at this stage the personality is less dependent on external authority as a guide to behavior.

Freud's Stages of Psychosexual Development

Freud described five stages of psychosexual development. He believed that sexuality was the central motivator of human behavior and that personality was determined by whether the goals of each psychosexual stage of development were achieved. These five stages are:

1. **Oral stage.** From birth to 18 months of age, sucking and other oral stimulation are extremely satisfying and important to the child. The conflict of this stage centers around receiving adequate oral gratification. Children who are weaned (taken off the breast or bottle) too early may experience frustration and become fixated (arrested) at this stage of development. Among the traits associated with an "oral" personality are dependency and excessive optimism or pessimism.

2. **Anal stage.** Beginning at approximately a year and a half and lasting until age 3, control of anal functions develops, and satisfaction shifts from the mouth to the anus. According to Freud, those who do not achieve anal control or for whom this focus is prolonged or exaggerated may develop certain personality traits. For instance, children who are anal-retentive (who did not successfully give up their feces by achieving the goal at this stage) may become stingy, obstinate, or obsessively clean adults.

3. **Phallic stage.** Beginning at age 3, the focus of attention is on the sexual organs. Pleasure is derived from handling and viewing these organs. In addition, Freud suggested, this stage is the one in which an unconscious sexual desire for the parent of the opposite

sex and jealousy of the parent of the same sex develop. The goal of this stage is to resolve this *Oedipus* (boy-father) *complex* or *Electra* (girl-mother) *complex* and identify with the parent of the same sex. Those unsuccessful during this stage may be unable to establish close relationships with other people.

4. **Latency stage.** Appearing in schoolchildren, this stage is represented by social conformity and by repression of sexuality and sex. If personality development is successful at this stage, the individual will establish friendships with members of the same sex. The adult fixated at this stage may have difficulty developing close relationships with other people of the same sex.

5. **Genital stage.** This stage begins in puberty, when sexual maturity occurs, and is characterized by a renewed focus on the genitals as a source of pleasure. The genitals remain the focus of sexual satisfaction throughout life. However, fixation at this stage can lead to sexual permissiveness, adultery, excessive flirting, and a general overemphasis on sexual gratification compared with other kinds of satisfaction in adult life.

It should be noted that Freud's theory is just that —a theory. Some people believe a major portion of it is valid, whereas others consider its emphasis on sexuality as the motivator of human behavior misplaced. The debate goes on.

with whom to share your joys and sorrows. A lack of intimate relationships is related to the onset of physical and mental illness and certainly limits the quality of life. Research clearly indicates that developing intimate relationships during this stage will give you the social support you need to cope with life's stressors and the possible consequent illnesses or diseases.

Are you working to develop close relationships with friends and relatives? If you find it difficult to achieve intimacy with other people, you might find it helpful to discuss this with your instructor or with counselors at your campus health center.

Stage 7: Middle Adult Years The crisis at this stage is *generativity versus stagnation*. This crisis involves focusing on a concern beyond oneself, such as devoting oneself to parenthood or a cause, versus satisfaction only of one's personal needs. An overemphasis on the self results in stagnation or lack of growth.

Stage 8: Older Adult Years The crisis at this stage is *integrity versus despair*. The question here is whether one comes to accept the life one has lived or despairs about what might have been. One who successfully copes with this crisis develops a feeling of continuity with those who have come before and those who will come after. The individual develops an identification with all of humanity. Failure to resolve this conflict successfully may result in a sense of futility, that is, the feeling that life has been useless.

Behavioral Theory ✳

Behaviorism is a psychological theory concerned with external dynamics rather than what goes on in the mind. Whereas Freud and Erikson focused on personality development through the stages of life and the consequences of success or failure with the tasks of each stage, behaviorists emphasize present behavior. Behaviorists believe people behave as they do because they are conditioned to do or not do certain things throughout their lives. In *conditioning,* we grow up being rewarded for some behaviors and punished or ignored for others. We repeat rewarded behaviors until they become part of our general behavior pattern. We do not adopt ignored or punished behaviors.

For example, if you are dieting to lose weight, the scale reinforces your behavior every time it records a lower weight. You therefore continue your diet. However, initial weight loss is mostly lost water, and the early stages of a diet often show a rapid loss of water. During the later stages of the diet, fat is lost, but more slowly. Consequently, the later stages of a diet are less rewarding and people often give up at that point.

Behavioral theory is more complex than it appears at first glance. For instance, you would think that a child who is repeatedly punished for interrupting conversations would stop this behavior. However, perhaps that child is really seeking attention. The attention the child gets from interrupting—the punishment—is the reward the child sought. Therefore, the interruptions will continue.

If you want to change one of your behaviors, you can use behavioral theory and increase your chances of success. The first step is to identify a reward, which can be material, such as presents, or intangible, such as recognition or attention. Once you have chosen the reward, decide what frequency or degree of changed behavior will earn the reward. For example, if you're trying to give up cigarette smoking and now smoke twenty cigarettes a day, you could reward yourself when you smoke only ten. Reserve punishments for not reaching your target behavior. Ignoring undesirable behavior has been shown to be more effective than punishing it.

Piaget's Theory ✗

Jean Piaget viewed social development somewhat differently from Freud or Erikson. In Piaget's view, maturation is a function of genetic determination. That is,

people are genetically programmed for certain traits and abilities and must wait until maturation occurs to demonstrate these traits and abilities. For example, although infants are programmed in the womb to walk, they don't jog around the delivery room when born. Instead, they must wait until they are developed enough to be able to take those first steps. Even before those first steps, however, infants work at pulling themselves up, crawling, and standing.

Similarly, Piaget theorized that intellectual and social development were genetically predetermined but had to go through patterned stages of development. One aspect of intellectual and social development particularly relevant to health issues and discussed in some detail by Piaget is morality. Piaget described two sequential stages of moral development. The first he called the **heteronomous stage.** Moral decisions at this stage are rigid and authoritarian. There are hard and fast rules by which behaviors are judged. If any behavior violates the rule, it is immoral. During this stage of development, the person is egocentric; only willing to help someone else if told to do so. Piaget believed this stage lasted until a child reached the age of 7 or 8.

Piaget believed that moral judgments become less rigid and less dependent on authority figures at about the age of 8. This stage he called the **autonomous stage.** The person is now more influenced by peers, considers other people's needs, and is capable of socially conscious and responsible behavior.

Some people have difficulty making the transition from one stage to the other. Other people develop only minor amounts of flexible thinking and are still too often governed by hard and fast rules. Where are you relative to Piaget's theory of moral development? Are you satisfied where you are? If not, how can you develop more socially conscious attitudes? Consult the social responsibility box at the end of this chapter for some ideas in this regard.

✗ Kohlberg's Theory of Moral Development

Lawrence Kohlberg was particularly concerned with the development of morals. He theorized that people go through stages of moral development as their moral thinking matures. Kohlberg argued that we initially judge morality according to concepts of punishment and obedience. That is, what we are told is "moral," we view as moral; what is punished is obviously "immoral." The next stage uses the satisfaction of our own needs as the criteria for what is moral. As we develop, however, we begin to judge our actions by whether other people think they are good or bad. As we mature further, we decide moral issues by whether the action is legal. If it is, it is moral; if it isn't, it is immoral. Moving through the stages of moral development, we next mature enough to take into account another person's

alienation The feeling of being separated from the society in which one lives.

Issues in Health

Should People Be "Socialized" to Fit into Our Society?

A high-school student, so the story goes, wrote the following poem and left it on his desk at school just before taking his own life:

He always wanted to say things.
But no one understood.
He always wanted to explain
things. But no one cared.
So he drew.

Sometimes he would just draw and it
wasn't anything. He wanted to carve
it in stone or write it in the sky.
He would lie out on the grass and look
up in the sky, and it would be only
him and the sky and the things inside
him that needed saying.

And it was after that, that he drew
the picture.
It was a beautiful picture. He kept it
under the pillow and would let no one
see it.
And he would look at it every night
and think about it. And when it was
dark, and his eyes were closed, he
could still see it. And it was all of him.
And he loved it.

When he started school, he brought it
with him. Not to show anyone, but
just to have it with him like a friend.

It was funny about school. He sat in a
square, brown desk like all the other
square, brown desks and he thought it
should be red.
And his room was a square, brown
room.
Like all the other rooms. And it was
tight and close. And stiff.

He hated to hold the pencil and the
chalk, with his arm still and his feet
flat on the floor, stiff, with the teacher
watching and watching.
And then he had to write numbers.
And they weren't anything. They were
worse than the letters that could be
something if you put them together.
And the numbers were tight and
square, and he hated the whole thing.

The teacher came and spoke to him.
She told him to wear a tie like all the
other boys. He said he didn't like
them, and she said it didn't matter.
After that they drew. And he drew all
yellow and it was the way he felt
about morning. And it was beautiful.

The teacher came and smiled at him.
"What's this?" she said, "Why don't
you draw something like Ken's draw-
ing? Isn't that beautiful?"
It was all questions.

After that his mother bought him a
tie, and he always drew airplanes and
rocket ships like everyone else. And he
threw the old picture away.
And when he lay out alone looking at
the sky, it was big and blue and all of
everything, but he wasn't anymore.

He was square inside and brown, and
his hands were stiff, and he was like
anyone else.
And the thing inside him that needed
saying didn't need saying anymore.

It had stopped pushing, it was
crushed. Stiff. Like everything else.

Pro Some would say schools are supposed to prepare people to function in society and that requires giving up some individuality.

Con Others believe society can only develop and improve if people's individualities are nurtured.

What do you think?

Source: Unknown.

rights when determining the morality or immorality of an action. Lastly, Kohlberg theorizes that we ignore society's judgments of morality and begin to use universal ethical principles in deciding moral issues—we begin to use principles such as the ideal of justice and equal rights for all.

You will need to employ moral reasoning to decide many health issues. For example, moral reasoning is required in decisions about how to behave sexually, about whether to drink alcohol or to use other drugs, and about what to regard as your responsibilities concerning the environment. See Table 2.2 for a summary of Kohlberg's stages of moral development.

Are you up to the task of reasoning at a high stage of moral development? At which stage of moral development are you now? How do you decide whether an

TABLE	2.2

Kohlberg's Stages of Moral Development

Preconventional Level

Stage 1: Punishment and Obedience Orientation

Stage 2: Self-Centered or Hedonistic Orientation

Conventional Level

Stage 3: Good Boy/Good Girl Orientation

Stage 4: Legalistic, Law-and-Order Orientation

Postconventional Level

Stage 5: Social Contract Orientation

Stage 6: Universal Ethical Principles Orientation

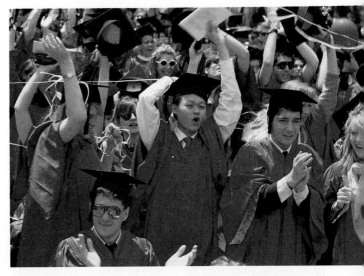

Contributing to your own self-esteem and that of other people is relatively easy. Share your achievements with friends and family and make an effort to share in their achievements, too.

action is moral or immoral? Would enrolling in a philosophy course or a course specifically dealing with morality help you advance through the stages of moral development more quickly? Would you then make more valid moral decisions about health and other issues?

Psychosocial Influences on Health Behavior

The decisions we make about health are very complex. To illustrate, consider the apparently simple decision one might make to exercise. Exercise might be viewed as a simple solution to a concern about physical health. Most likely, however, there is more to it than this. The desire to present a pleasing physical appearance, to achieve athletic goals and thereby feel more competent, and to interact socially with others via sporting activities may also be involved in the decision to exercise. This section is concerned with our psychosocial reasons for behaving as we do. Throughout, you have the opportunity to determine for yourself which psychosocial factors are influencing your own behavior.

Self-Esteem

Self-esteem refers to how highly you regard yourself. People who have low self-esteem and do not feel good about themselves or respect themselves do not regard their own opinions and decisions as worthwhile. If we lack confidence in our own opinions and decisions, we are more apt to be influenced by others. Television advertisements, behaviors of respected peers, or adult models will then unduly influence our health decisions. Thus self-esteem is a significant component of our health choices.

To increase your self-esteem, focus on your good traits and achievements, rather than on your poor traits and failures. Too often we relive situations in which we "goofed" by playing them over and over again in our minds. We remember past embarrassments and actually feel them again by recalling what we did to make ourselves embarrassed. Those things are in the past. They've already happened. Learn from them, and then forget them.

On the other hand, we should make a conscious effort to pat ourselves on the back when we have succeeded at something or when one of our positive traits has been recognized. If you do well on an exam, tell others about it. You don't need to be boastful in a negative sense. You can say, "I'm proud about something, and I'd like to share it with you." When you have a spare moment, think about how well you did on that exam, rather than thinking about those on which you "bombed." Focus on the positive, on your good side. Build yourself up; don't rely on others to do it for you. You can estimate your own level of self-esteem in Exploring Your Health 2.1.

Alienation

Alienation, or the feeling of being separated from the society in which one lives, consists of three factors:

- **Social isolation.** The lack of significant others (friends, relatives, and so forth) in whom one can confide.
- **Normlessness.** The lack of rules, regulations, and standards by which one chooses to live.
- **Powerlessness.** The feeling of not being in control of one's own destiny.

To determine your scores on each of these three factors, complete the Alienation Scale in Exploring Your Health 2.2.

When this scale was administered to male undergraduates, they averaged 36.64, with the following subscores:

Social isolation: 11.76
Normlessness: 7.62
Powerlessness: 13.65

Undergraduate women averaged 36.25, with these subscores:

Social isolation: 14.85
Normlessness: 7.63
Powerlessness: 12.73

If you scored higher than 37 you may be more alienated than the average college student. If that is the case, perhaps your mental health is being influenced by your degree of alienation, and you might decide to do something about this. To begin, inspect your subscores. Is one subscore way out of line with the average scores reported above? If so, that is the component of alienation that needs attention. If it is social isolation, you may be conforming to other people's behaviors because you're lonely. To develop friendships, you might want to join a club on campus or get involved with the student newspaper, yearbook, or student government. If you scored high on normlessness or powerlessness, joining an organized group will also help. You will have a set of standards (the group's) to guide your behavior and to which you can relate, and the sense of being unable to control your destiny may be diminished by working with others toward a common goal.

Researchers have found that alienation is related to health behavior. For instance, the use of marijuana is greater for college students who are highly alienated than for those less alienated. Further, researchers have found that suicide, the second leading cause of death among college students, is directly related to alienation. Human isolation and withdrawal appears to be the single most prevalent distinction between those who kill themselves and those who do not. People who commit suicide usually have no close friends with whom they can share their thoughts and problems and from whom they can receive psychological support.

It seems evident, finally, that if you scored high in powerlessness, for instance, you might decide not to behave in a healthy manner because you would feel that you had little control over your health anyway.

Locus of Control

Internal locus of control refers to the belief that one can influence events, whereas *external locus of control* refers to the belief that one has very little influence over events. It stands to reason that those with an internal health locus of control would be more apt to adopt positive health behaviors than those with an external health locus of control.

Each of us is in control of much more of our lives than we may realize. Experiments with biofeedback equipment (discussed in Chapter 3) suggest that people can exert some control over their own blood pressure, brain waves, body temperature, secretions of acid in the stomach, and serum cholesterol level. We may not be able to control others or our environment, but we can control our reactions to these external stimuli. For example, consider people who say, "So-and-so got me angry." No one gets you angry. You *allow* yourself to be angered by so-and-so. The anger is your own doing. To prove this point, aren't there some days when you awake in a great frame of mind, the sun is shining, you anticipate an enjoyable day, and you tell yourself, "This day is so great, nothing can bother me today"? On those days, nothing will bother you even though things might happen that would drive you up a wall on any other day. You are in control on those days.

Of course, some things are beyond our control. We don't live on an island separated from the rest of the human race. Our environment places many demands upon us, as do other people about whom we care. In a very real sense, we co-create our futures with external forces and events.

Exploring Your Health 2.1

Self-Esteem Scale

For each of the statements in the Self-Esteem Scale, check the letter that most accurately describes how you feel:

1. I feel that I'm a person of worth, at least on an equal plane with others.

    a) _____ Strongly agree

    b) _____ Agree

    c) _____ Disagree

    d) _____ Strongly disagree

2. I feel that I have a number of good qualities.

    a) _____ Strongly agree

    b) _____ Agree

    c) _____ Disagree

    d) _____ Strongly disagree

3. All in all, I am inclined to feel that I am a failure.

    a) _____ Strongly agree

    b) _____ Agree

    c) _____ Disagree

    d) _____ Strongly disagree

4. I am able to do things as well as most other people.

    a) _____ Strongly agree

    b) _____ Agree

    c) _____ Disagree

    d) _____ Strongly disagree

5. I feel I do not have much to be proud of.

    a) _____ Strongly agree

    b) _____ Agree

    c) _____ Disagree

    d) _____ Strongly disagree

6. I take a positive attitude toward myself.

    a) _____ Strongly agree

    b) _____ Agree

    c) _____ Disagree

    d) _____ Strongly disagree

7. On the whole, I am satisfied with myself.

    a) _____ Strongly agree

    b) _____ Agree

    c) _____ Disagree

    d) _____ Strongly disagree

8. I wish I could have more respect for myself.

    a) _____ Strongly agree

    b) _____ Agree

    c) _____ Disagree

    d) _____ Strongly disagree

9. I certainly feel useless at times.

    a) _____ Strongly agree

    b) _____ Agree

    c) _____ Disagree

    d) _____ Strongly disagree

10. At times I think I am no good at all.

    a) _____ Strongly agree

    b) _____ Agree

    c) _____ Disagree

    d) _____ Strongly disagree

Scoring You have just completed a self-esteem scale. To score the scale and thereby derive a measure of your self-esteem, follow these instructions.

1. The positive responses for questions 1–3 are:
   question 1: (a) or (b)
   question 2: (a) or (b)
   question 3: (c) or (d)
   If you answered two or three of these questions positively, give yourself 1 point.

2. The positive responses for questions 4 and 5 are:
   question 4: (a) or (b)
   question 5: (c) or (d)
   If you answered either one or both of these questions positively, give yourself 1 point.

3. If your answer to question 6 was (a) or (b), give yourself 1 point.

4. If your answer to question 7 was (a) or (b), give yourself 1 point.

5. If your answer to question 8 was (c) or (d), give yourself 1 point.

6. If your answer to question 9 or 10 or both was (c) or (d), give yourself 1 point.

Add up all the points you gave yourself.

The range of scores on this self-esteem scale is 0–6. The higher the score, the more positive your self-esteem.

Source: Morris Rosenberg, *Society and the Adolescent Self-Image* (Princeton, N.J.: Princeton University Press, 1965), p. 305. Copyright © 1965 by Princeton University Press; Princeton Paperback 1968. Reprinted by permission of Princeton University Press.

Unfortunately, many of us forget *our* impact on the future and on our health behavior. If we possess an external locus of control, we might decide not to work hard at giving up smoking. "After all, not everyone who smokes gets lung cancer. The air we breathe is so polluted that it doesn't matter whether we smoke or

Exploring Your Health 2.2

Alienation Scale

Below are some very general statements with which some people agree and others disagree. Indicate whether you agree or disagree with each item. Check the appropriate blank, as follows:

_____ A (Strongly agree)

_____ a (Agree)

_____ U (Undecided)

_____ d (Disagree)

_____ D (Strongly disagree)

I 1. Sometimes I feel all alone in the world.

_____ A _____ a _____ U

_____ d _____ D

P 2. I worry about the future facing today's children.

_____ A _____ a _____ U

_____ d _____ D

I 3. I don't get invited out by friends as often as I'd really like.

_____ A _____ a _____ U

_____ d _____ D

N 4. The end often justifies the means.

_____ A _____ a _____ U

_____ d _____ D

I 5. Most people today seldom feel lonely.

_____ A _____ a _____ U

_____ d _____ D

P 6. Sometimes I have the feeling that other people are using me.

_____ A _____ a _____ U

_____ d _____ D

N 7. People's ideas change so much that I wonder if we'll ever have anything to depend on.

_____ A _____ a _____ U

_____ d _____ D

I 8. Real friends are as easy as ever to find.

_____ A _____ a _____ U

_____ d _____ D

P 9. It is frightening to be responsible for the development of a little child.

_____ A _____ a _____ U

_____ d _____ D

N 10. Everything is relative, and there just aren't any definite rules to live by.

_____ A _____ a _____ U

_____ d _____ D

I 11. One can always find friends if one acts friendly.

_____ A _____ a _____ U

_____ d _____ D

N 12. I often wonder what the meaning of life really is.

_____ A _____ a _____ U

_____ d _____ D

P 13. There is little or nothing I can do toward preventing a major "shooting" war.

_____ A _____ a _____ U

_____ d _____ D

I 14. The world in which we live is basically a friendly place.

_____ A _____ a _____ U

_____ d _____ D

P 15. There are so many decisions that have to be made today that sometimes I could just "blow up."

_____ A _____ a _____ U

_____ d _____ D

N 16. The only thing one can be sure of today is that one can be sure of nothing.

_____ A _____ a _____ U

_____ d _____ D

Source: Dwight G. Dean, "Alienation: Its Meaning and Measurement," *American Sociological Review* 26 (1961): 753–758. Reprinted by permission.

not. It's a matter of luck or chance whether or not we get lung cancer." If we possess an internal locus of control, we might say, "Although I have no control over the air I breathe in, I don't have to contaminate that air further. I can give up cigarette smoking and decrease my chances of getting lung cancer. I can exercise some degree of control over my health."

Assertiveness

How assertive are you? It stands to reason that if you have difficulty asserting your own needs and desires, you will be more likely to do what others expect of you than what you think is right.

It should be noted that assertive behavior differs from aggressive behavior. You can assert yourself firmly but nicely, rather than by being argumentative or belligerent. In any case, being submissive is not conducive to making the health-related decision that is right for you.

Some definitions seem in order here:

- **Assertiveness.** Expressing yourself and satisfying your own needs. Feeling good about this and not hurting others in the process.
- **Nonassertive behavior.** Denying your own wishes to satisfy someone else's.
- **Aggressive behavior.** Seeking to dominate others or to get your own way at their expense.

I   17.   There are few dependable ties between people any more.

_____ A _____ a _____ U

_____ d _____ D

P   18.   There is little chance for promotion on the job unless a person gets a break.

_____ A _____ a _____ U

_____ d _____ D

N   19.   With so many religions around, one doesn't really know which to believe.

_____ A _____ a _____ U

_____ d _____ D

P   20.   We're so regimented today that there's not much room for choice even in personal matters.

_____ A _____ a _____ U

_____ d _____ D

P   21.   We are just so many cogs in the machinery of life.

_____ A _____ a _____ U

_____ d _____ D

I   22.   People are just naturally friendly and helpful.

_____ A _____ a _____ U

_____ d _____ D

P   23.   The future looks very dismal.

_____ A _____ a _____ U

_____ d _____ D

I   24.   I don't get to visit friends as often as I'd really like.

_____ A _____ a _____ U

_____ d _____ D

Scoring   You have just completed an alienation scale. To score this scale, award yourself the number of points indicated below for each response you made: You will notice that each question is preceded by an I, an N, or a P. All the questions designated I indicate your level of social isolation; N questions test your level of normlessness; and P questions test your level of powerlessness. The higher you score, the more strongly you possess these factors.

1.   4 A 3 a 2 U 1 d 0 D
2.   4 A 3 a 2 U 1 d 0 D
3.   4 A 3 a 2 U 1 d 0 D
4.   4 A 3 a 2 U 1 d 0 D
5.   0 A 1 a 2 U 3 d 4 D
6.   4 A 3 a 2 U 1 d 0 D
7.   4 A 3 a 2 U 1 d 0 D
8.   0 A 1 a 2 U 3 d 4 D
9.   4 A 3 a 2 U 1 d 0 D
10.   4 A 3 a 2 U 1 d 0 D
11.   0 A 1 a 2 U 3 d 4 D
12.   4 A 3 a 2 U 1 d 0 D
13.   4 A 3 a 2 U 1 d 0 D
14.   0 A 1 a 2 U 3 d 4 D
15.   4 A 3 a 2 U 1 d 0 D
16.   4 A 3 a 2 U 1 d 0 D
17.   4 A 3 a 2 U 1 d 0 D
18.   4 A 3 a 2 U 1 d 0 D
19.   4 A 3 a 2 U 1 d 0 D
20.   4 A 3 a 2 U 1 d 0 D
21.   4 A 3 a 2 U 1 d 0 D
22.   0 A 1 a 2 U 3 d 4 D
23.   4 A 3 a 2 U 1 d 0 D
24.   4 A 3 a 2 U 1 d 0 D

DESC An acronym that expresses an effective way to assert oneself verbally: *Describe, Express, Specify, Choose.*

defense mechanism The attempt by an individual to manage anxiety-provoking situations by unconsciously distorting reality.

Assertiveness is not only a matter of *what* you say but also a function of *how* you say it. Assertive body language consists of straight, steady posture and eye contact and speaking in a clear, steady, audible voice, fluently, confidently, and without hesitation. In contrast, nonassertive body language is marked by lack of eye contact (looking down or away), swaying and shifting weight from one foot to the other, and whining, hesitant speech.

Aggressive behavior can also be recognized by body language as well as words. Aggressive behavior often includes leaning forward with glaring eyes, pointing a finger at the person to whom one is speaking, shouting, clenching fists, and placing hands on hips.

If you want to act assertively, you must pay attention to your body language. Practice and adopt assertive nonverbal behavior, while concentrating on eliminating signs of nonassertive and aggressive behavior. Even if you make an assertive verbal response, you will not be believed if your body's response is nonassertive.

DESC   As to *what* you say, an effective formula in helping people express themselves assertively is the **DESC** form.[1] The verbal response is divided into four components: *Describe, Express, Specify,* and *Choose.* Figure 2.1 depicts how the DESC form of assertiveness can be used.

To demonstrate the DESC form of organizing assertive responses, let's assume Jim and Kathy are dating. Jim wants Kathy to date him exclusively. Kathy believes she's too young to eliminate other men from her love life. Jim's assertive response to this situation might be:

> [Describe] *When you go out with other men,* [Express] *I feel very jealous and have doubts about the extent of your love for me.* [Specify] *I would prefer that we only date each other.* [Choose] *If you only date me, I'll make a sincere effort to offer you a variety of experiences so that you do not feel you've missed anything. We'll go to nice restaurants, attend plays, go to concerts, and whatever else you'd like that we can afford and that is reasonable. If you do not agree to date me exclusively, I will not date you at all. The pain would be more than I'm willing to tolerate.*

Values and Peer Group Pressure

If you have ever observed the reactions of an audience at the end of a movie, play, or concert, you probably will have noticed one phenomenon: very different reactions among the people who have attended the event. One reason for this is that we all have different value systems. For instance, some people smoke cigarettes because they value the immediate pleasure it provides and are willing to risk the inherent long-term danger. Other people refrain from smoking cigarettes because they value physical fitness and abhor any impairment of physical health. One student may seek sexual liaisons with as many partners as possible because he or she values pleasure, whereas another may limit sexual behavior to marriage because he or she has great respect for religious teachings. Of course, many factors lead to any one behavior, but values are important.

For most people, peer group pressure is a very powerful force. In particular, if you possess low self-esteem, an external locus of control, and little assertiveness, you are probably greatly influenced by your friends.

Other Influences

Many psychological and sociological (or *psychosocial*) variables besides self-esteem, alienation, locus of control, assertiveness, values, and peer pressure influence health behavior. Fear of medical procedures or of becoming ill, anxiety, stress, and shyness may all be related to a person's health decisions. Certain sociological factors, such as education, age, religion, and race, have also been found to be related to health behavior and health status. Access to health care and to health information disseminated through various media also affect health behavior.

The list goes on and on. The point is that health status and health behavior are complex variables with both physiological and psychosocial components. This point will become even clearer in Chapter 3 when we discuss stress. This point will become increasingly clear throughout this book, in topics as diverse as stress, sexuality, nutrition, weight loss, and even the environment.

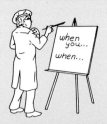

1. **Describe.** Paint a verbal picture of the other person's behavior or the situation to which you are reacting. "When you . . ."; "When . . .".

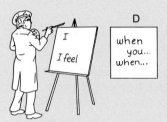

2. **Express.** Relate your feelings regarding the other person's behavior or the situation you have just described. Use "I" statements here: "I feel . . .".

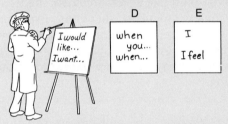

3. **Specify.** Identify several changes you would like to see in the other person's behavior or in the situation. Rather than saying, "You should . . . ," again use "I" statements: "I would prefer . . . ," "I would like . . . ," "I want . . .".

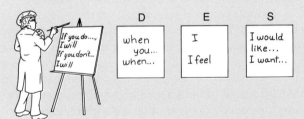

4. **Choose.** Select the consequences you have decided to apply to the behavior or situation. What will you do if the other person's behavior or the situation changes to your satisfaction? "If you do . . . , I will. . . ." What will be the consequences if nothing changes, or if the changes do not meet your needs? "If you don't . . . , I will . . .".

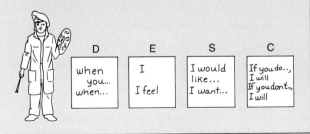

FIGURE 2.1 • How to Use DESC Assertiveness

Modes of Coping ⨉

To survive anxiety-producing situations, we usually take one of two coping actions. We can defend ourselves by taking drugs or by using some other external crutch in order not to deal directly with the anxiety-provoking stimulus. This solution is really not a solution at all, since the anxiety will return when the drugs wear off. Other, more subtle means of defending against rather than dealing with the anxiety producer are defense mechanisms.

Defense Mechanisms

Sometimes people attempt to manage anxiety-provoking situations by unconsciously distorting reality. Freud called such attempts **defense mechanisms** and said they affected only a person's perception of reality and not the actual situation. All of us could profit from perceiving some situations as less distressing. However, when the use of a defense mechanism becomes a person's predominant coping strategy, anxiety is only temporarily relieved and returns when the defense mechanism is no longer used or no longer works. In addition, the use of a defense mechanism often involves other people in the self-deception and therefore tends to have a negative effect on interpersonal relationships.

Some common defense mechanisms include:

- **Compensation.** Covering our weaknesses by emphasizing desirable traits or making up for frustration in one area by overgratification in another.
  Example: A man who feels inferior because he is short may strive to achieve a powerful position of leadership.
- **Denial.** Protecting oneself from unpleasant reality by refusing to accept something that is obviously true.
  Example: A boy whose mother has died insists that she's going to be coming home soon.
- **Displacement.** Shifting feelings, attitudes, and impulses from the original source to a different object or person.
  Example: I'm angry at my teacher, but I can't yell at her so I yell at my friend.
- **Fantasy.** Gratifying desires that have been frustrated or cannot be achieved in reality by the use of imagination.
  Example: A little girl who has no friends pretends that her dolls are companions.
- **Intellectualization.** Using logic, reason, and theory to detach oneself from an emotionally threatening situation.
  Example: A doctor treats the physical ills of his or her patients and avoids dealing with them on an emotional level.

- **Isolation.** Detaching feelings from objects and people who produce anxiety.

  Example: A man who is going to have major surgery is unaware of any feelings of fear.

- **Projection.** Attributing one's own unacceptable feelings and attitudes to others.

  Example: Sue is jealous of Joan but does not want to acknowledge this feeling in herself, so she insists that Joan is jealous of her.

- **Rationalization.** Attempting to assign rational or desirable motives to our behavior so that we seem to have acted appropriately.

  Example: John fails a test he didn't prepare for and insists, "I failed the test because I went out last night."

- **Reaction formation.** Preventing dangerous impulses from surfacing or being expressed by behaving in the opposite manner.

  Example: A man who is afraid of his sexual impulses becomes involved in a crusade against pornography.

- **Regression.** Retreating to earlier developmental levels that involve less mature responses.

  Example: When a new baby is born in the family, the older child begins to wet his or her bed.

- **Repression.** Preventing painful or undesirable feelings, memories, or impulses from entering consciousness.

Example: A man whose wife was killed in a fire cannot remember the event.

Learn to recognize your own defense mechanisms in Exploring Your Health 2.3.

Conscious Modes of Coping

Whereas defense mechanisms are usually *unconscious* modes of coping, there are several *conscious* modes of coping with anxiety-producing situations. Exploring Your Health 2.4 will help you identify the conscious modes of coping that you use.

Generally speaking, there are three conscious modes of coping.

Submission Avoiding the problem or situation. This mechanism may be appropriate when a problem is insurmountable. For example, consider the dilemma faced by a teacher who believes that rapport between student and teacher is a prerequisite to learning but who is employed in a school system that discourages teachers and their students from becoming too friendly with one another. The teacher might decide to leave that school system rather than attempt to change a central principle of its philosophy of education. In other instances, submission may be inappropriate because it is based on a fear of facing a problem or situa-

Exploring Your Health 2.3

Recognizing Defense Mechanisms

In the blank space provided after each statement, name the defense mechanism being expressed. Answers are provided below.

1. The boss made me angry at work and now you ask me for a favor! _____

2. I never wanted that promotion anyhow. _____

3. I don't care about your feelings. Let's look at this objectively. _____

4. I have no recollection of having been raped, although I know that I was. _____

5. Even though I've failed every test and haven't turned in any of the assignments, I know that somehow I'll pass this course. _____

Answers (1) displacement, (2) rationalization, (3) intellectualization, (4) repression, (5) denial.

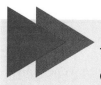

Exploring Your Health 2.4

Coping with Difficult Situations

How do you cope with difficult situations? Choose one response to each of the situations described below and circle the letter of that response:

1. If a salesclerk refuses to give me a refund on a purchase because I've lost the sales slip:
   a) I tell her, "I'm sorry—I should have been more careful," and leave without the refund.
   b) I tell her, "You're the only store in town that handles this brand of merchandise. I demand a refund, or I'll never shop here again."
   c) I say, "Look, if I can't have a refund, can I exchange it for something else?"

2. If I had irritated a teacher by questioning his theoretical position and he retaliated by giving me a D on an excellent paper:
   a) I wouldn't say anything; I would realize why it happened and be quieter in my next class.
   b) I would tell him he was dead wrong and that he couldn't get away with being so unfair.
   c) I would try to talk to him and see what can be done about it.

3. If I worked as a TV repairman and my boss ordered me to double-charge customers, I would:
   a) Go along with him; it's his business.
   b) Tell him he's a crook and that I won't go along with his dishonesty.

   c) Tell him he can overcharge on his calls, but I'm charging honestly on mine.

4. If I gave up my seat on the bus to an older woman with packages, but some teenager beat her to it:
   a) I would try to find the woman another seat.
   b) I would argue with the teenager until he moved.
   c) I would ignore it.

5. If I had been waiting in line at the supermarket for twenty minutes, then some woman rushed in front of me saying, "Thank you— I'm in such a hurry":
   a) I would smile and let her in.
   b) I would say, "Look—what do you think you're doing? Wait your turn!"
   c) I would let her in *if* she had a good reason for being in such a hurry.

6. If a friend was to meet me on a street corner at 7:00 one night and at 8:00 he still wasn't there, I would:
   a) Wait another thirty minutes.
   b) Be furious at his thoughtlessness and leave.
   c) Try to telephone him, thinking, "Boy, he'd better have a good excuse!"

7. If my wife (or husband) volunteered me for committee work with someone else she (or he) knew I disliked, I would:
   a) Work on the committee.
   b) Tell her she had no business volunteering my time . . . call

the committee chairman and tell him the same.
   c) Tell her I want her to be more thoughtful in the future, and then make a plausible excuse she can give the committee chairman.

8. If my four-year-old son "refused" to obey an order I gave him, I would:
   a) Let him do what he wanted.
   b) Say, "You do it—and you do it now!"
   c) Say, "Maybe you'll want to do it later on."

Scoring The responses provided above can be classified as either submissive, aggressive, or compromise. Give yourself 3 points for each (a) (submissive) response, 2 points for each (b) (aggressive) response, and 1 point for each (c) (compromise) response.

The range of possible scores is 8–24, with the higher scores representing a pattern of submission when conflict occurs, the lower scores representing a pattern of aggression, and scores near the middle of the range (14–18) representing a pattern of compromising. What have you learned about your style of coping?

Source: Lila Swell, *Educating for Success: Workbook* (New York: Queens College, 1972), pp. 46–47. Reprinted by permission of the author.

tion. For instance, you may yearn to date a particular person but refrain from asking that person out because you fear rejection. In this case, you are withdrawing from a situation that it would have been better to face, despite the risk of rejection.

Aggression Approaching the problem head on and working your hardest to resolve it in the way you think best. Like other coping behaviors, aggression can be adaptive (arguing or fighting for things that involve your values or ethical judgments) or maladaptive (always expecting to get your way). For instance, if you are waiting in line to enter a movie theater and some-

one slips into the line ahead of you and you punch that person in the nose, you have acted aggressively. Not only could this get you in trouble with the law, but it might also mean a fight and you might miss the movie.

Compromise Fitting in; accepting things as they are. If you and a friend can't agree on which of two restaurants to eat at, you could be submissive and agree to your friend's choice, you could be aggressive and argue until you get your way, or you could compromise and go to a third restaurant that will please both of you.

The point worth reiterating in this section is that

most coping behavior cannot be easily categorized as healthy or unhealthy. To evaluate a coping response, you need to know the specifics of the situation and the qualities of the person making the response. When you are faced with a problem or situation, stop to think of all possible actions and their consequences before de-ciding how to act.

Coping with Common Problems

All of us face many problems. Anxiety, shyness, jeal-ousy, anger, and depression are common to people of all ages, and many people cope with them successfully. This section describes these problems and discusses how you can cope with them.

Anxiety

Anxiety refers to feelings of apprehension that may stem from either real or imagined concerns. We all know the symptoms of anxiety. We feel edgy and un-comfortable (afraid), our heart races, we perspire, and our muscles feel tense. Most of us learn to deal with anxiety by trying to discover what is causing it. When the cause is obvious, for example, an upcoming test, it may be relatively easy to cope with anxious feelings. However, when the cause is more complex, we may need help understanding it. Nevertheless, there are things you can do for yourself to cope with the anxiety you experience. These strategies include environmen-tal planning, self-talk, relabeling, and systematic de-sensitization.

Environmental Planning Sometimes it is appro-priate to avoid the anxiety stimulus. Suppose you are afraid to fly in an airplane. If the quality of your life would not be diminished by never flying, it wouldn't be worth the effort to try to overcome this fear. How-ever, if your fear of flying prevents you from visiting loved ones who live in different parts of the country, the anxiety is diminishing the quality of your life and is therefore worth managing. The process of adjusting your environment to reduce anxiety that the environ-ment gives rise to is called "environmental planning." For instance, you might be able to move closer to loved ones so you don't have to fly at all or so often. How might you adjust your environment to manage your anxieties?

Self-talk Most common anxiety-causing problems are not catastrophic. Have you experienced anxiety about taking tests? One way of overcoming it is by having a **self-talk,** a dialogue with yourself. The self-talk might go something like this:

I probably won't fail since I studied well and have been con-scientious about my schoolwork. But even if I do fail, that wouldn't be the end of the world. I can always repeat the course, or make up the grade on the next test. That won't be a good situation, but it's better than being so worried that I can't function.

Take a moment right now to practice this tech-nique. Try making up a self-talk to manage the anxious feelings you might have about interviewing for a job.

Relabeling Everything has a positive and a nega-tive component to it. Even if things are terrible, you could tell yourself, "At least it can only get better from here." **Relabeling,** or changing the value or descrip-tion ascribed to something, uses this concept to man-age anxiety. For example, instead of thinking of an airplane trip as dangerous, claustrophobic, and nerve-racking, you can label it as a chance to get away from a busy schedule to a place where no one can bother you. Instead of labeling an upcoming test as a threat, you can consider it an opportunity to demonstrate how much you have learned.

Which of your anxieties can be better managed by relabeling them?

Systematic Desensitization Developed by psy-chiatrist Joseph Wolpe, this technique assumes that many forms of anxiety are learned and can therefore be unlearned. **Systematic desensitization** involves arranging anxiety-producing stimuli in a hierarchy or sequence according to the amount of fear they evoke. The anxious person proceeds very gradually through the hierarchy in an effort to face the anxiety-producing stimulus without fear. Suppose Jim is very fearful of receiving injections. His fear hierarchy might include such stimuli as a picture of a nurse holding a needle, a picture of the nurse aiming the needle toward someone's arm, and so on, with the final image being of the nurse giving the person an injection. Each time Jim looks at one of the pictures, he is encouraged to relax. When he is able to look at the picture without anxiety, the next picture is shown, until Jim is finally able to look at the slide that creates the most anxiety. Systematic desensitization has been used very successfully to help people overcome phobias—severe fears that include fear of enclosed spaces, fear of snakes, and the like. If you have a phobia, you might want to contact the school psychology department, which can refer you to a behavior therapist who uses systematic desensitization.

Shyness

All of us feel shy at times. *Shyness* is fear of people, especially people who are emotionally threatening, strangers we want to impress, people who wield power and authority, and people in whom we are sexually interested. Shyness makes it hard to think clearly and communicate effectively, to meet new people, and to assert our opinions and needs. Because it is often accompanied by feelings of depression, anxiety, and loneliness, shyness prevents significant human interaction.

Although overcoming shyness requires a good deal of hard work, Philip Zimbardo, in *Shyness: What It Is and What to Do About It,* suggests taking the following steps:

1. Recognize your strengths and weaknesses and set your goals accordingly.

2. Decide what you value, what you believe in, what you realistically would like your life to be like.

3. Determine what your roots are. By examining your past, seek out the lines of continuity and the decisions that have brought you to your present place. Try to understand and forgive those who have hurt you and not helped when they could have. Forgive yourself for mistakes, sins, failures, and past embarrassments. Permanently bury all negative self-remembrances after you have sifted out any constructive value they may provide . . .

4. Guilt and shame have limited personal value in shaping your behavior toward positive goals. Don't allow yourself to indulge in them.

5. Look for the causes of your behavior in physical, social, economic, and political aspects of your current situation and not in personality *defects* in you.

6. Remind yourself that there are alternative views

to every event. "Reality" is never more than shared agreements among people to call it the same way rather than as each one separately sees it. This enables you to be more tolerant in your interpretation of others' intentions and more generous in dismissing what might appear to be rejections or put-downs of you.

7. Never say bad things about yourself; especially, never attribute to yourself irreversible negative traits, like "stupid," "ugly," "uncreative," "a failure," "incorrigible."

8. Don't allow others to criticize *you* as a person; it is your *specific actions* that are open for evaluation and available for improvement—accept such constructive feedback graciously if it will help you.

9. Remember that sometimes failure and disappointment are blessings in disguise, telling you the goals were not right for you, the effort was not worth it, and a bigger letdown later on may be avoided.

10. Do not tolerate people, jobs, and situations that make you feel inadequate. If you can't change them or yourself enough to make you feel more worthwhile, walk on out, or pass them by. . . .

11. Give yourself the time to relax, to meditate, to listen to yourself, to enjoy hobbies and activities you can do alone. In this way, you can get in touch with yourself.

12. Practice being a social animal. Enjoy feeling the energy that other people transmit, the unique qualities and range of variability of our brothers and sisters. . . .

13. Stop being so overprotective about your ego; it is tougher and more resilient than you imagine. . . .

14. Develop long-range goals in life, with highly specific short-range subgoals. Develop realistic means to achieve these subgoals. Evaluate your progress regularly and be the first to pat yourself on the back or whisper a word of praise in your ear.[2]

Jealousy

Jealousy is a common emotion, one that almost all of us experience at some point in our lives. Most theorists agree that jealousy has two basic components: (1) a feeling of battered pride, and (2) a feeling that one's property rights have been violated. Most of us respond to jealousy in one of two ways: We use either defense mechanisms or some conscious method of coping. For example, if you feel jealous because a coworker has been given a pay raise and you haven't, you might rationalize by saying, "Taxes would eat up most of any pay raise I received anyhow," or you might try harder to get a pay raise by taking work home with you.

How can you control jealous feelings? Just as in the case of anxiety, the first step is to find out exactly

depression A psychological condition or illness characterized by feelings of sadness, despair, and lack of self-esteem.

anxiety disorders Mental disturbances in which individuals experience high levels of anxiety, including phobic disorders and obsessive-compulsive disorders.

what is making you jealous. Usually something specific about a situation is bothering you. In the example above you may be jealous not because your coworker is getting extra money, but because your coworker is considered more valuable than you are. Key questions to ask are:

- What was going on in the few moments before you started to feel this way?
- What are you afraid of?
- What rights of yours seem to have been violated?
- Why is your pride hurt?

Next try to put your jealous feelings in perspective. Is it really so awful that your coworker received a raise and you didn't? Wouldn't you want that person to be pleased if you received a pay raise? Is it of any value to feel jealous and miserable? Questions like these will help you feel less jealous.

Jealousy in intimate relationships is quite common and can be very distressing. In addition to using the suggestions above, jealousy in a love relationship can be managed by negotiating a contract—one that balances security and freedom for both partners. Counselors have also found that it is easier for couples to maintain a close but not excessively possessive love relationship if they maintain some separate friends and interests. Naturally, it's easier to have confidence in your desirability if you have an independent identity and if there are others who like and admire you. You are less likely to fear being abandoned by your partner, and it's much easier to cope if you are.

Anger

How many times have you said "So-and-so made me angry"? Well, no one *makes* you angry. You *allow* yourself to be angered by someone or something. The evidence for this assertion is in your own experience. As we previously discussed, some days you wake up, look at the sunshine, and anticipate a great day. You say to yourself, albeit not consciously, "What a great day. Nothing is going to bother me today." And nothing does—because you won't let it. Other days are more problematic. You may be anxious about a test or concerned about an argument you had with a loved one

the previous day. On these days almost anything can "set you off."

The key to coping with anger is recognizing that you give it to yourself. Once you come to grips with this realization, you then know that you *cannot* give it to yourself if you do not wish to. Unbelievable as it sounds, this realization alone can change your whole outlook and let you cope with anger much better.

It is also helpful to identify exactly what it is you're angry about. In that way you can correct the situation or talk it out with someone if that is needed.

Don't get hooked on someone else's anger. For example, if I am driving my car and cut in front of your car inadvertently, you might get angry. Let's assume you pull alongside, roll down your car window, and call me a bunch of names. You may be justified in being angry and this behavior may "let off some steam." If, on the other hand, I were to get angry back at you, it would serve no useful purpose. I would have become hooked on your anger when a more appropriate response might have been to say, "Yes, I did do a stupid thing by not looking when I cut in front of you. I'm sorry." We can all learn to be in more control of ourselves and our emotions.

Depression

All of us, at one time or another, feel down in the dumps. We say we are depressed or that we feel blue. When these feelings last a short time, they are normal. However, some people have these feelings more severely or for a long time. They have an illness we call **depression.** Depression is so widespread that it is estimated one in twenty-nine Americans are affected. Col-

Year 2000 National Health Objective

In 1982, the proportion of people with major depressive disorders who obtained treatment was only 31 percent. One of the Year 2000 National Health Objectives seeks to obtain treatment for at least 45 percent of those suffering from such disorders.

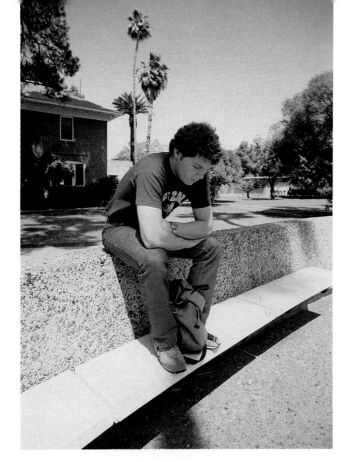

College students are especially vulnerable to depression because of the changes occurring in their lives and the impact these changes can have on their self-esteem.

lege students are especially vulnerable to depression because of the changes occurring in their lives and the impact these changes can have on their self-esteem.

Depression is a potentially serious disease, one that needs treatment. Drugs such as antidepressants, monoamine oxidase (MAO) inhibitors, and lithium carbonate may be prescribed in cases of depression; psychotherapy is recommended.

In less severe cases of depression, it is useful to talk with a close friend or a relative. In some cases, doing so will result in a whole new perspective on the situation. In other instances, comfort in knowing that someone else cares can help. Distracting activities (such as gardening or playing or listening to music) can also be helpful. And a study of female undergraduates has found that aerobic exercise and regular practice of relaxation techniques are effective in decreasing mild depression.[3]

You can analyze the way that you cope with problems in Exploring Your Health 2.5.

Mental Disorders

An individual who has severe mental problems and cannot cope effectively with them can be said to have a *mental disorder.* This section will discuss such disorders only briefly; to do so in detail would not be consistent with the theme of the chapter—mental *health.* However, a discussion of mental health is incomplete without a consideration of its counterpart—mental disorder.

Anxiety Disorders

Anxiety disorders are mental disturbances in which individuals experience high levels of anxiety. This category includes phobic disorders and obsessive-compulsive disorders. A *phobic disorder* is an abnormal fear of a particular situation or object; an *obsessive-compulsive dis-*

Exploring Your Health 2.5

Coping Analysis

The Problem

_____

_____

Possible Ways to Respond

A. _____

B. _____

C. _____

D. _____

E. _____

Things to Be Gained by Each Response Above

Response A: _____

Response B: _____

Response C: _____

Response D: _____

Response E: _____

Negative Aspects of Each Response:

Response A: _____

Response B: _____

Response C: _____

Response D: _____

Response E: _____

Assume that you could subtract the weight of the negative aspects from the weight of the gains cited above. Which response (A, B, C, D, or E) would result in the greatest plus? ___

order is a disturbance involving constant repetition of particular acts in anxiety-producing situations.

Somatoform Disorders

Somatoform disorders are mental disturbances in which individuals experience physical symptoms that have no known organic cause. Included in this category are *conversion disorders,* which are disturbances involving one relatively severe symptom (such as blindness, paralysis, or deafness).

Schizophrenic Disorders

Individuals with **schizophrenic disorders** exhibit dramatic breaks with reality and severe distortion in thought and perception. Included in this category are disorganized schizophrenia and paranoid schizophrenia. *Disorganized schizophrenia* is characterized by hallucination, delusion, strange thought and behavior patterns, and occasional violent activity and gestures. *Paranoid schizophrenia* is characterized by general suspiciousness and mistrust of people, hallucinations, inappropriate emotional expressions, and occasional hostility and violence.

Personality Disorders

Personality disorders are mental disturbances in which individuals exhibit a set of inflexible behaviors or personality traits that impair their social functioning. This category includes antisocial personality and paranoid personality. *Antisocial personality* is a disturbance characterized by chronic antisocial behavior, a lack of long-range purpose and moral sense, and feelings of anxiety or guilt. The *paranoid personality* is characterized by a pervasive and unwarranted suspiciousness and mistrust of people.

Affective Disorders

Individuals with **affective disorders** are inappropriately joyful, unrealistically sad, or both. This category includes *manic-depressive disorders,* which are character-

ized by sharp mood swings between severe depression or suicidal feelings and elation (often inappropriate).

Suicide

Approximately 300,000 people attempt suicide in the United States annually, and 30,000 of those who attempt are successful. The actual number may be as high as 80,000 because of the many deaths that are suicides but cannot be established as such.[4]

Suicide is the third (some experts say the second) leading cause of death (after accidents and homicides) on college campuses. Approximately 1,000 college students take their own lives each year, and this figure is twice as high for college students as for people the same age but not in college. The reason for these suicides is seldom difficulty with schoolwork, although the pressure to perform well is often a contributing factor. Another factor in college student suicide is the feeling of isolation that results from not being able to establish close personal relationships.

The elderly also have a high suicide rate, which is suspected to be a function of physical illness, death of loved ones, retirement and subsequent loss of purpose, and the need for dependence on children and/or medical personnel. Women attempt suicide three times more often than men, but more men actually succeed in killing themselves, probably because men choose more lethal methods.

How can you tell if someone you know is contem-

Year 2000 National Health Objective

One Year 2000 National Health Objective seeks to reduce the general population's suicide rate from the baseline of 11.7 per 100,000 people in 1987 to a rate of no more than 10.5 by the year 2000. The specific objective for college students is to reduce their suicide rate from 25.2 per 100,000 students in 1987 to a rate of 21.4 by the year 2000. Another objective seeks to reduce by 15 percent the incidence of injurious suicide attempts by young people ages 14 through 19.

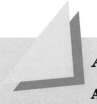

A Question of Ethics

Are We Obligated to Prevent People from Taking Their Own Lives?

It is one thing to be distanced from a suicide attempt and judge its morality from that distance. It is quite different when you are close to the attempt. For example, reading of a stranger's suicide in the newspaper may not be as disturbing as learning of a close friend's suicide. The stranger's situation as described in the article may have been quite bleak and the suicide therefore understandable. To judge that suicide as moral (right) may be reasonable. Perhaps the person was very poor, very lonely, very ill, or experiencing a great loss. However, our friend's suicide upsets us. Why didn't our friend speak with us about his or her problems? Where did *we* fail? Why didn't *we* recognize our friend's despair?

Even if we were aware of our friend's feelings, were we obligated to prevent the suicide? Are we ethically bound to do so? How about for the stranger?

One of the authors received a letter a while ago from a prisoner in the Louisiana State Penitentiary. It seems he had killed several people and had already served sixteen years in jail with no possibility of ever being paroled. He described prison as so horrible a place that he decided to take his life and was writing to seek advice about the least painful and most effective means of accomplishing this end. How he heard of the author is anyone's guess, since they were complete strangers to each other.

How would you reply to this letter? Would you describe several effective and painless ways to commit suicide? Would you attempt to change the prisoner's mind? Would you alert prison authorities to this prisoner's intentions? Would you just ignore the letter? What do you believe you are ethically bound to do in such a situation?

plating suicide? Some of the general signs include:

- Communication of feelings of hopelessness ("The world would be better off without me," "I can't see any reason to go on living," and so on)
- Actual threats to commit suicide
- A previous attempt to commit suicide
- Making sudden gifts to others, especially of the person's most valued possessions
- Exhibiting symptoms such as depression, withdrawal, weight loss, or apathy

Suppose you think your friend Mary may be suicidal. What can you do for her? First, try to talk to her. Suggest that she seek help from professionals, such as mental health counselors, and if possible, enroll in therapy with these resource personnel. You might also consider the crisis intervention technique, which can be outlined as follows:

1. Make contact at a feeling rather than a factual level; that is, show you care what happens to Mary.
2. Explore the problem.
3. Summarize the problem to Mary's satisfaction.
4. Focus on one aspect of the problem that can be improved.
5. Explore available resources in responding to this one aspect of the problem.
6. Make a contract with Mary regarding what she will do and what you will do.

The first step in crisis intervention is to accept the feelings of the suicidal person instead of evaluating or denying them. Rather than saying, "Things aren't that bad," you should say, "It must be terrible to feel so alone that you would contemplate killing yourself." This is the step most people have difficulty with, so you might want to practice giving feeling responses before actually talking with the suicidal person.

Once you have made contact at a feeling level, help the person to look at the problem in the here and now rather than talking about what might have been or might be. Then summarize the problem so the suicidal person appreciates that you really have been listening and that you understand. Now choose one part of the problem that you think the person can improve and explore resources that might help respond to this part of the problem. Obtain the suicidal person's agreement to work on that part of the problem, to meet again, and to contact you if he or she begins feeling worse. Remember, professional help is needed for a person who is suicidal, but you too can do much to help.

Seeking Help

An ancient Persian proverb states:

> That the birds of
> worry and care
> fly above your
> head, this you
> cannot change,
> But that they
>   build
> nests in your
>   hair,
> This you can
> prevent.

psychotherapy As promoted by Freud, psychotherapy is the long-term treatment of mental illness through the gradual discovery by the patient of unconscious, repressed material that affects behavior.

client-centered therapy A treatment program for mental illness developed by Carl Rogers that focuses on the positive acceptance of the patient by himself or herself.

behavior therapy A treatment program for mental illness that emphasizes behavior modification.

group therapy A treatment program for mental illness where one therapist works with several clients at the same time.

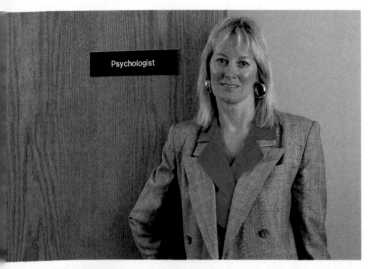

Most colleges have psychological counseling services. Would you know where to go on your campus if you or a friend needed counseling?

If you recognize the signs and symptoms of mental illness in yourself or someone else, be comforted by knowing there are resources for coping with such disorders.

Where to Get Help

A good place to start is your college campus. The medical services or psychology department probably has a

Mental Health Resources

National Self-Help Clearinghouse, 25 West 43rd Street, Room 620, New York, NY 10036. Send a self-addressed, stamped envelope for a list of local clearinghouses throughout the United States.

Recovery, Inc. For information about groups in your area, write 802 N. Dearborn Street, Chicago, IL 60610, or consult your phone book.

Emotions Anonymous. For information about groups in your area, write P.O. Box 4245, St. Paul, MN 55104.

National Alliance for the Mentally Ill. For information, write 2101 Wilson Blvd., Arlington, VA 22201.

American Schizophrenia Association. For information, write 900 N. Federal Hwy., Suite 330, Boca Raton, FL 33432.

National Self-Health Association, 1420 16th Street N.W., Washington, DC 20036.

counseling clinic or can refer you to one. Your local or state health department probably also offers counseling services. And your church or synagogue or other community organizations may be of help, too. Of course, there are many private psychiatrists, psychologists, and mental health counselors. Many clinics and some private sources of counseling offer a sliding scale of fees so that those with little money pay low fees and those who are more affluent pay higher fees.

Types of Therapy

Many different types of therapy are available according to the nature and severity of the problem and the philosophy of the patient and clinician. Psychoanalysis, for example, would not be appropriate for specific behavior disorders that could be corrected relatively quickly, and transactional analysis would not be appropriate treatment for a schizophrenic patient. The major forms of therapy are explained next.

Year 2000 National Health Objective

One of the Year 2000 National Health Objectives seeks to increase the number of people ages 18 or older with mental disorders who use community support programs by at least 30 percent. Another objective encourages the establishment of mental health mutual-help clearinghouses (self-help organizations) with the goal of having such clearinghouses in at least twenty-five states by the year 2000.

Psychotherapy Developed by Freud, **psychotherapy** is a long-term treatment (many years) requiring one or more sessions a week with the therapist. The goal is to make the client aware of repressed material that unconsciously affects his or her behavior. Once this material is brought to consciousness, the client can better understand the problem and adjust his or her behavior.

Client-centered Therapy Sometimes termed Rogerian therapy after its founder, Carl Rogers, **client-centered therapy** promotes the growth of the client by reducing destructive forces, such as anxiety. The therapist creates an atmosphere of "unconditional positive regard," empathy, and genuineness. This atmosphere of total acceptance of the patient is designed to aid patients in accepting themselves as they are. The result will then be personal growth.

Behavior Therapy Whereas psychotherapy predominantly uses interpretation and client-centered therapy uses acceptance and empathy, **behavior therapy** does not rely on one particular mode of treatment. A treatment program is tailored to the individual's needs in an effort to change behavior rather than underlying feelings. Imagine a client afraid to speak before groups of people. The psychotherapist might view this fear as a function of poor self-esteem and try to find its roots in the client's childhood. A behavior therapist, however, might have the client speak before one other person, then two, and eventually before a group, rewarding the client at each step. The behaviorist would not work on the self-esteem of that client.

The behaviorist establishes specific behavioral goals for the client and uses techniques such as systematic desensitization (discussed earlier in this chapter) to aid the client in achieving these goals. It is expected that once the behavior is changed, the feeling will change. The client who gradually learns to speak before groups of people will probably improve his or her self-esteem as a result of overcoming that fear.

Group Therapy The forms of therapy we have discussed so far have involved one therapist working with one client. **Group therapy** involves a therapist working with several clients at the same time. It was developed during World War II, when there was a shortage of therapists. Although group therapy can take many different forms, usually one therapist meets with six to ten clients, and the cost to the client is less than in individual therapy. One advantage of group therapy is that clients can learn social skills, which are often retarded in people with mental disorders. In addition, knowing that others need help too, and seeing people at various stages of mental illness (some at the latter stages of therapy) or with a shared problem, provides comfort to those greatly concerned with their own disorders. The group therapist's task is to get the members of the group to help one another by establishing an atmos-

Issues in Health

Is There Any Such Thing as Mental Illness?

Pro The notion that abnormal or socially unacceptable behavior was a result of mental illness first became popular in the middle of the nineteenth century. People exhibiting deviant behavior were considered sick, and the mental health movement developed in response to such sickness. Further refining this approach, mental health professionals classified different forms of mental illness (for example, schizophrenia) and began talking about symptoms, diagnosis, and treatment.

Con Some experts have suggested that this medical model of mental illness is inappropriate when applied to abnormal behavior. Psychiatrist Thomas Szasz even suggests that there is no such thing as mental illness. Szasz believes abnormal behavior results from an inability to manage life's stresses. If abnormal behavior is viewed as symptomatic of an illness, people cannot be held responsible for their actions but rather can blame them on their sickness. Furthermore, a particular behavior may be abnormal and unacceptable in one society but common and accepted in others. Whereas cancer is cancer, regardless of the society in which it occurs, behavior must be viewed in its cultural context to be classified as appropriate or inappropriate. How then can behavior stem from illness?

Further complicating this issue is the legal definition of mental illness. For example, when is insanity a defense for criminal or otherwise illegal behavior and when isn't it? Is Russia's incarceration of political dissidents in psychiatric hospitals a manifestation of the Russian definition of abnormal behavior (mental illness) or merely an excuse to eliminate dissent?

The debate, then, is whether there really is such a thing as mental illness.

What do you think?

family therapy Treatment for mental illness that focuses not only on the disturbed client but also on his or her family.

chemotherapy The treatment of mental illness through the use of medications, such as tranquilizers and antidepressants.

Get Involved!

Making the Mind Matter in Your Own and Other Peoples' Good Health

There are numerous possibilities for you to improve your community's and society's mental health in large and (seemingly!) small ways. For example, you might try the following suggestions.

1. Serve as a volunteer counselor at your university (usually called a "peer counselor") or at a local hospital or suicide hotline. These organizations will train you to effectively counsel people in need of help.
2. Provide companionship for a housebound person. It might be an elderly person living in a nursing home, a disabled person confined to his or her home, or a mentally ill person institutionalized in a psychiatric facility.
3. Help teach or assist another teacher to instruct in a parenthood education program. Focus your involvement in helping parents understand the developmental stages their children are presently experiencing and the stages their children will experience in the future.
4. Develop a listing of mental health facilities and services in your community. Ask the local health department about their interest in publishing this listing as a brochure to be distributed throughout the community.
5. Make a conscious effort to compliment people and point out their strengths. In this way, you will be sprinkling positive self-esteem throughout the community.
6. Volunteer as a referee or umpire for sports programs throughout the community. Athletics can serve as a release for anger and other feelings, which too often are expressed in such antisocial behaviors as child or spouse abuse.
7. Lobby local and state legislators for increased funding for mental health services. You might even contact your U.S. senator or representative to advocate increased funding for mental health on a national level.

phere of acceptance and support. In addition, the therapist tries to draw comparisons between situations and interpretations that arise in group meetings and those that the members encounter in their lives outside the group.

Family Therapy One criticism of many forms of therapy is that the therapist works with the client for a relatively short period of time, and then the client returns to a dysfunctional family unit, which counteracts the benefits of therapy. **Family therapy** is based on the premise that unless the key people in a client's life also change, the client will not improve. A family therapist usually works with individual family members at some times and with the whole family unit at other times. The goal is to help each member of the family understand his or her effect on the other members and on the unit as a whole. An important ingredient of successful family functioning is effective communication, and improving communication skills in families is a major goal of family therapy.

Chemotherapy Some people with mental disorders are treated with medication: tranquilizers, lithium, antidepressants, and antianxiety drugs. This type of treatment is called **chemotherapy.** The drugs are sometimes used in conjunction with initial therapy, but they are also often used for extended periods of time. Tranquilizing drugs were developed in the 1950s to reduce "excitement, agitation, aggressive behavior, delusions, and hallucinations."[5] Before the development of tranquilizers, seriously disturbed patients were not as able to focus on and profit from therapy. Lithium carbonate is used to treat manic-depressive disorders. It levels a person's moods and allows for more effective therapy. Antidepressant drugs are used for patients suffering from depression and are taken regularly rather than only when depression occurs, because these drugs work on a long-term, as opposed to an immediate, basis. Some therapists argue that antianxiety drugs, such as Valium, treat the symptom (anxiety)

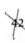

rather than the problem. Others believe anxiety must be reduced before the client can deal with its causes.

Alternative Therapies   Many other therapies are available, most of them adaptations of the ones already described. *Hypnotherapy* involves hypnotizing patients and suggesting new forms of behavior. In *psychodrama,* the patient acts out events that cause problems, and then the actions and feelings experienced by the patient are analyzed. In *transactional analysis,* interactions between people are analyzed in terms of ego—parent, child, and adult. *Rational emotive therapy* counsels the patient to adopt behaviors that will disprove his or her self-defeating thoughts. In *existential therapy,* the therapist helps the patient choose behaviors consistent with the patient's values.

Conclusion

Throughout this chapter we have emphasized that, although learning to cope with your environment is a difficult task, there are ways you can meet this challenge. However, should problems become so overwhelming that the usual coping techniques are not enough, help is available. It is unrealistic to choose to maintain a "stiff upper lip" rather than ask for help.

That sort of behavior actually increases the likelihood of problems becoming so severe that they cause illness, either mental or physical. The instructor in the course for which you are reading this book might be a good first contact. He or she may be able to refer you to someone who can help you cope. Ask for help if you need it.

Summary

1. Emotional health includes the abilities to deal constructively with reality and to adapt to change, exercising a reasonable degree of independence, establishing positive relationships with other people, and being able to live with emotions.

2. Several different theories explain personality development, including Freud's stages of psychosexual development; Erikson's stages of crises; and behavioral theory, which is more concerned with external dynamics than with what goes on in the mind.

3. Our health behavior is influenced by our level of self-esteem. If we don't think well enough of ourselves, we might not have confidence in our own health decisions, and consequently we might be inordinately influenced by other people.

4. Alienation consists of three factors: social isolation, normlessness, and powerlessness. High levels of alienation are related to such behaviors as drug abuse and suicide.

5. Our perception of the degree of control we have over our own destiny has a significant impact on our health behavior. If we view the locus of control as external, we will not expect to have much influence over our health. If we consider the locus of control to be internal, we will tend to pay attention to our health behavior in the belief that we can influence our health status.

6. If we don't know how to state our needs and

rights verbally, we are liable to behave in ways inconsistent with our real nature. Assertiveness helps us to be able to say yes and no as we desire. In this way our health behavior will be a result of our decisions.

7. Our health behavior is influenced by our values. When we choose to behave in certain ways, the choices we make reflect our values.

8. Most of us are influenced by, and exert influence upon, our friends. We hold similar values, adopt similar behaviors, and even speak and dress similarly. It is not surprising that people are more likely to smoke cigarettes, for instance, if their best friends smoke.

9. Defense mechanisms are unconscious attempts at coping with anxiety. They include compensation, denial, displacement, fantasy, intellectualization, isolation, projection, rationalization, reaction formation, regression, and repression.

10. The conscious means of coping with anxiety-provoking stimuli can be divided into three categories; submission (giving in to or withdrawing from the stimulus), aggression (fighting to overcome the situation), and compromise (fitting in).

11. Some of the problems that we all must cope with are anxiety, shyness, jealousy, anger, and depression.

12. Anxiety can be managed by environmental planning, self-talk, relabeling, and systematic desensitization.

13. Shyness is fear of people, especially those we want to impress, those who wield power and authority, and those in whom we are sexually interested.

14. Jealousy has two basic components: a feeling of battered pride, and a feeling that one's property rights have been violated.

15. Anger is a feeling we give to ourselves, and therefore we cannot give it to ourselves if we do not choose to.

16. Mild depression can be managed by sharing the feeling with a loved one, by focusing on other activities, and by exercising.

17. Mental disorders include anxiety disorders, so-matoform disorders, schizophrenic disorders, personality disorders, and affective disorders.

18. Suicide is the second or third leading cause of death among college students. Take talk of suicide seriously and seek the help of a trained professional quickly.

19. Therapy takes various forms depending on the nature of the mental disorder and the philosophy of the therapist. Forms of therapy include psychotherapy, client-centered therapy, behavior therapy, group therapy, family therapy, chemo-therapy, and such alternative therapies as hypnotherapy, psychodrama, transactional analysis, rational-emotive therapy, and existential therapy.

Questions for Personal Growth

1. How do you typically react to frustration? How do you usually express anger? Are you satisfied with these reactions? If not, how will you go about changing them?

2. When do you become shy? What is it about that situation or that person that elicits shyness in you? How can you adapt to that situation or person in order to feel less shy?

3. What experiences can you recall that have affected your self-esteem? In school? At home? With friends? How have you behaved so as to affect someone else's self-esteem?

4. In what situations do you find it exceptionally difficult to react assertively? In what situations do you find it exceptionally easy to react assertively? Try this exercise. Think of an upcoming situation in which you would like to be assertive. Develop an assertive verbal response for this situation and practice saying it in a nonverbally assertive manner.

5. Which defense mechanisms do you employ the most? Are they effective for you? Do you need to use these less and other defense mechanisms more?

6. When was the last time you were jealous? What were you afraid to lose? Was your fear realistic? How did you behave? Was that behavior appropriate given the circumstances? What will you do the next time you feel jealous?

7. What kind of situations and kinds of people make you anxious? What is it about these situations and people that provoke anxiety within you? How can you practice being in these situations and/or interacting with these people so as to be less anxious?

8. If you experienced mental health problems, would you know where to get help? On campus? Off campus? Do you know of friends or relatives who need this assistance to whom you should recommend these sources of help? Will you?

References

1. Sharon Bower and Gordon Bower, *Asserting Yourself* (Reading, Mass.: Addison-Wesley, 1976), p. 90.
2. Philip G. Zimbardo, *Shyness: What It Is and What to Do About It* (Reading, Mass.: Addison-Wesley, 1977), pp. 158–160. Copyright © 1977, Addison-Wesley, Reading, Massachusetts. Reprinted with permission.

3. "Exercising Away Depression," *Psychology Today* (December 1984): 68.

4. National Center for Health Statistics, "Births, Marriages, Divorces, and Deaths for 1989," *Monthly Vital Statistics Report* 38 (1990): 13.

5. Office of Disease Prevention and Health Promotion, *The 1990 Health Objectives for the Nation: A Midcourse Review* (Washington, D.C.: U.S. Department of Health and Human Services, 1986).

CHAPTER

3

Stress and Stress Management

CHAPTER OBJECTIVES

After reading this chapter, you should understand:

- What stress is, how our bodies express to us that we are under stress, and why positive and negative forms of stress can affect us differently under various circumstances and at different times in our lives.

- The basic physiology of stress and how constant stressful activity can lead to burnout. Your whole body is affected by stress, and each body system responds to stress in its own way.

- How stress is related to psychosomatic illnesses, such as ulcers, migraine headaches, and certain forms of mental illness.

- Several methods for coping with stress, including stress management, relaxation techniques, and physical activity.

CHAPTER OUTLINE

What Is Stress?

The Physiology of Stress

Stress and Disease

Coping with Stress

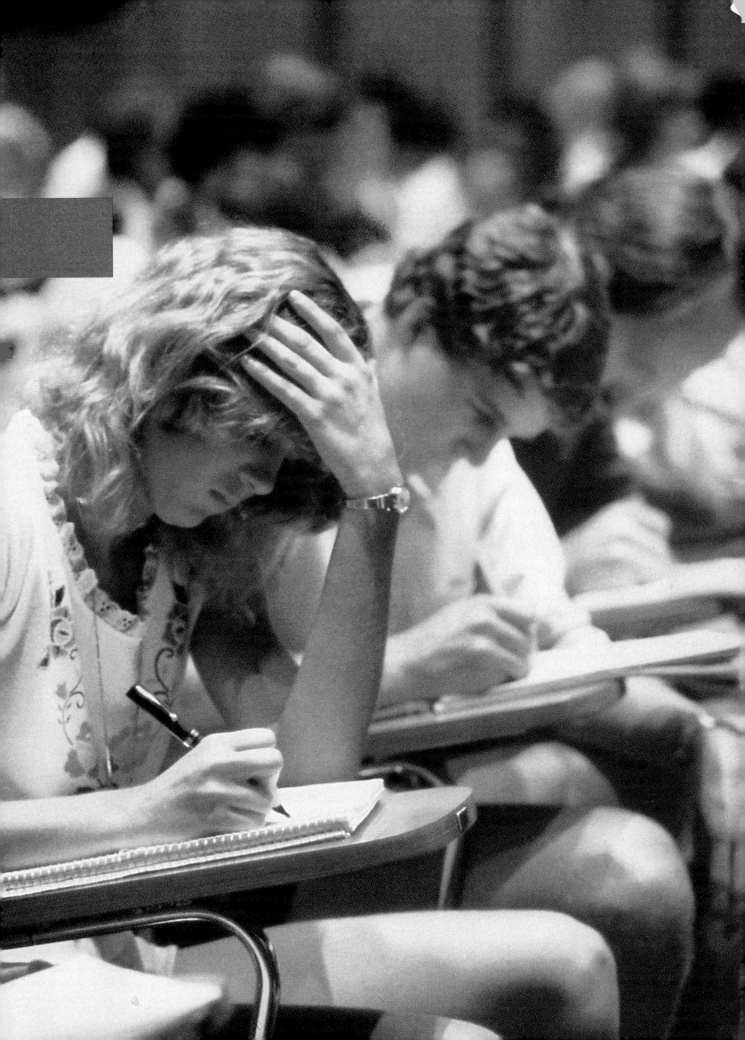

stress The nonspecific response of the body to any change and to the demands caused by that change.

stressor Any stimulus that causes stress.

It's the first week of a new semester. You meet your instructors and learn you have three term papers to do this semester, ten abstracts of journal articles to master, five big textbooks to read, five midterm examinations and five final examinations to pass, and numerous other homework assignments to complete. How will you ever manage all of that? Oh, the stress!

This chapter will help you understand these feelings of stress and show you how to better manage the stress in your life. We discuss just what stress is, its effects on your body, stress-related diseases, and methods of stress management.

What Is Stress?

There is an old saying: "A sound mind in a sound body." It is becoming increasingly evident, however, that mind and body are not as separated as this saying seems to imply. As both the functionings of the mind and the workings of the body are better understood, how the mind and body affect each other becomes more evident. Nowhere has this mind-body relationship been better demonstrated than in the area of stress. Psychological stress can have a serious impact on the body, and bodily disease can affect the health of the mind. We shall see later in this chapter that stress can be a factor in such diseases as heart disease, stroke, high blood pressure, ulcers, and even cancer. The pub-

Year 2000 National Health Objective

Reducing the level of stress for Americans is an important goal of the Year 2000 National Health Objectives. For example, one objective is to reduce to no more than 5 percent the proportion of people 18 and older who experience significant levels of stress and who do not take steps to reduce or control their stress. Another objective is to increase to at least 20 percent the proportion of people ages 18 and older who seek help in coping with personal and emotional problems.

lic, as well as health professionals, have become more and more aware of the effects of stress on people's health and have responded with many books, magazine articles, and television and radio programs concerned with recognizing and managing stress.

Bodily Expressions of Emotion

Stand before a mirror. Act out the following feelings with your face only: anger, joy, confusion. Now act out those feelings with the rest of your body as well. If you found this easy to do, it is because we do it all the time, though not always consciously. When unhappy we tend to slump our shoulders, frown, move our heads back and forth as if to say, "Why me?" and stare for-

Exploring Your Health 3.1

How We Use Body Terms to Describe Emotions

Try listing ten bodily expressions of emotion in the spaces provided at right:

1. _____
2. _____
3. _____

4. _____
5. _____
6. _____
7. _____
8. _____

9. _____
10. _____

Examples of body expressions: stiff upper lip; can't stomach it; hair-raising; no backbone; tongue-tied; catch your eye.

lornly. When confused we squint our eyes, tilt one ear in the direction of the confusion (as if to comprehend better), and scratch our heads. The next time a class of yours meets, notice that if it's an interesting class the students will be leaning bodily toward the instructor or the center of the group. If it's dull, the students will be leaning against the backs of their chairs or away from the instructor or group. In addition, look at the faces of the students in this class. Pick out three classmates and guess whether they're interested or bored, then ask them after class.

There are other ways in which the body demonstrates emotions. Individuals with low self-esteem tend to slump, don't smile much, and aren't very expressive with their arms when they talk. In contrast, individuals with high self-esteem "walk tall," talk animatedly, and smile a good deal. People exhibit hostility by a certain look, tense muscles, or an aggressive forward angle of the head, as if ready to charge.

You can probably think of other ways in which we express our emotions bodily. In fact, there are many verbal expressions that use body words to describe feelings. Examples are "no guts" and "stand on your own two feet." Exploring Your Health 3.1 gives you an opportunity to think of your own examples.

The Stress Response Pattern

Emotions, then, are manifested by the body. We will soon see that emotions are a component of the stress response and as such have implications for our health.

One of the leading researchers in the area of stress was Hans Selye. Selye defined **stress** as "the nonspecific response of the body to any demand made upon it." What this means, in effect, is that any change we encounter to which we must adapt results in stress. That change can be internal, such as the degeneration of a body organ, or external, such as having to speak in front of a large group of people. Selye found that although the stressful stimulus, or **stressor,** varies, the body's physiological response is generally the same. Thus an experience might result in feelings of joy or sorrow, but in either case the person would experience the same physiological response—stress. Exploring Your Health 3.2 helps you identify how you react to stress.

Exploring Your Health 3.2

Stress Reactivity

While seated in a comfortable position, determine how fast your heart beats at rest, using one of the following methods. (Use a watch that has a second hand.)

1. Place the first two fingers (pointer and middle finger) of one hand on the underside of your other wrist, near the thumb. Feel for your pulse and count the number of pulses for 30 seconds. (See the drawing.) Multiply your 30 second pulse count by two to determine how many times your heart beats each minute while at rest.

2. Place the first two fingers of one hand on your lower neck, just above the collar bone; move your fingers toward your shoulder until you find your pulse. Determine your heart beats per minute as before.

3. Place the first two fingers of one hand in front of your ear near your sideburn, moving your fingers until you find your pulse. Count the pulses for 30 seconds. Determine your heart beats per minute as before.

Now close your eyes and think of either someone you really dislike or some situation you experienced that really frightened you. If you are

recalling a person, think of how that person looks, smells, and what he or she does to incur your dislike. Really feel the dislike, don't just think about it. If you recall a frightening situation, try to place yourself back in that situation. Sense the fear and vividly recall the situation in all its detail. Think of the person or situation for 1 minute and then count your pulse rate for thirty seconds, as you did earlier. Multiply the rate by two and compare your first total with the second.

Most people find that their heart rate increases when experiencing the stressful memory. This increase occurs despite a lack of any physical activity; even thoughts increase heart rate. This fact demonstrates two things: the nature of stressors and the nature of stress reactivity. The stressor is a stimulus with the potential of eliciting a stress reaction (physiological arousal).

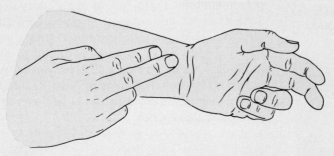

Source: Jerrold S. Greenberg, *Comprehensive Stress Management*, 3e (Dubuque, Iowa: Wm. C. Brown 1990), p. 11. © 1990 Wm. C. Brown Publishers, Dubuque, Iowa. All rights reserved. Reprinted by permission.

habituation The process of becoming used to a stimulus after experiencing it repeatedly.

Selye termed the body's response to stress the *general adaptation syndrome* (GAS). The GAS occurs in three stages, as the following shows.[1]

1. **Alarm.** The body exhibits physiological signs when it is first exposed to a stressor, such as rapid pulse, a tightening of muscles, sweaty palms, a knot in the stomach. At the same time, body resistance to the stressor is diminished, and if the stressor is sufficiently strong (severe burns or extreme temperature, for example), death may result.

2. **Resistance.** The bodily signs characteristic of the alarm reaction disappear. Now the task is to adapt to the stress and retain the normal internal state, which requires considerable energy.

3. **Exhaustion.** Following a long-continued exposure to the same stressor, to which the body has become adjusted, eventually the energy required to adapt to the stress may be exhausted. If this happens, the signs of alarm reappear. At this stage, however, they are irreversible, and the individual dies.

Of course, we usually don't get to the exhaustion stage. We learn to adapt to change after a while, and in fact are even unaware that we are adapting. For example, a family moving into a new house near an airport might at first be bothered by the sound of planes overhead, but after several weeks they no longer notice the airplanes. They have become used to the sound of the airplanes, and the noise no longer consciously bothers

Think about the last time you were "put on the spot." Maybe you had to present a paper in class? Or did you have to compete with other students for a summer internship? Did you let stress help or hinder your performance?

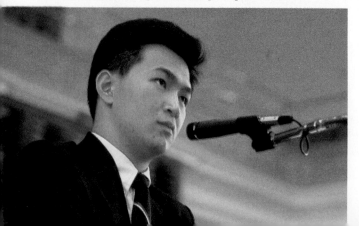

them. This process—of becoming used to a stimulus after experiencing it frequently—is called **habituation.** It should be noted here that even if habituated, you can still become ill from the stressor. However, in many cases, becoming used to a stressor is an effective means of coping with it. If you give many speeches, for example, you'll experience less stress than you did the first time you spoke to a large group.

Distress and Eustress

If you accept an invitation to give a speech before a large number of people, you might expect to feel stress. If that stress manifests itself in such anxiety that a panic reaction results and you cannot get the words out during the speech, the stress is obviously dysfunctional. However, if the stress leads you to spend a great deal of time developing the speech, making it interesting and informative, then you are using the stress productively. Thus stress can be a helper or an inhibitor. The stress associated with physical danger, for instance, can be used to place reasonable limits on the daredevil activities of a person who would otherwise get hurt. Conversely, stress could be used negatively by another person who withdraws from risk-taking activities that are stressful but that promote goal achievement and personal development.

Selye termed the negative use of stress *distress* and the positive use *eustress.* Some have described the use of stress as positive or negative by noting that the Chinese word for "stress" or "anxiety" is a combination of the symbols for the words danger and opportunity (see Figure 3.1). Certainly a stressor can cause harm to one person but offer a tremendous opportunity to another. Sometimes it's just a matter of perception. For example, you could perceive being fired from your job as highly distressing or as an opportunity to find more fulfilling work or develop a different career. We all experience stress often. Exploring Your Health 3.3 is intended to help you recognize what has been stressful to you in the past month.

Stress and Life Changes

Many things, events, or people can be stressors. Bacteria can cause stress. So can noise. So can a person

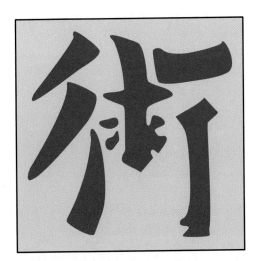

FIGURE 3.1 • The Chinese word for **stress** is a combination of two characters, one representing ''danger,'' the other, ''opportunity.''

responses they determined that some events were considerably more stressful than others, and they weighted them accordingly. The resulting scale, called the Social Readjustment Rating Scale, modified to be more appropriate for college students, appears in Table 3.1. Check those events that you have experienced in the past year.

Completing this scale should underline for you the cumulative nature of stress: the more stressors you check off, the higher your score. Studying the significance of each stressful life event, Holmes and Rahe found that a low score (below 150) indicated only a 37 percent chance of illness during the next two years, an average score (150–300) indicated a 50 percent chance of illness during the next two years, and a high score (over 300) indicated a 90 percent chance of serious illness sometime during the next two years. On the modified version of the scale, which you just completed, a score below 128 is probably low, a score between 128 and 255 is probably average, and a score above 255 is probably high. A person scoring high on this scale should make a conscious effort to avoid, whenever possible, any further life changes for the rest of the year.

What was your score? Will you make any adjustments in your lifestyle as a result of this experience?

Some researchers believe that the daily hassles we each experience are even more dangerous to our health than the major life changes that occur periodically. *Hassles* have been defined by these researchers as daily interactions with the environment that are essentially negative and, because of their chronic nature, could take a significant toll on our health. In fact, hassles have been shown to be predictive of psychological distress and related to poor mental and physical health.[2]

Stress and Personality

Some researchers believe that personality is an important indicator of whether a person will experience a

whom you dislike. The realization that there are a vast number of stressors can be disheartening when it is further recognized that these stressors combine in their effects on us. For instance, during an influenza epidemic, the people who die are usually those with chronic illnesses. People who are highly stressed are more susceptible to a number of conditions, both physical and psychological. Can you recall a time when you were stressed (for example, during final exams) and then succumbed to another stressor (maybe you caught a bad cold)?

Two researchers have determined that certain life changes, when accumulated, can become significant stressors in people's lives. Thomas Holmes and Richard Rahe, specialists in the area of stress, compiled a list of typical events that occur in people's lives. They asked people of varying ages and occupations to rate these events on a scale of 1 to 100 according to how much adjustment they felt each event required. From the

Exploring Your Health 3.3

Identifying Stressors in Your Life

List six events or stressors that you can recall having occurred in the past month:

1. _____

2. _____

3. _____

4. _____

5. _____

6. _____

Describe on a separate sheet of paper how you responded to three of the stressors you listed. Include both *positive* and *negative* responses.

Next, choose one response with which you are not completely satisfied and list other ways in which you could have responded. Do you think you'll respond differently next time? Why or why not?

Do you notice any consistencies in your reactions to stress? If so, what are they? Why not ask a friend how he or she perceives your behavior when you are under stress?

type A behavior pattern Behavior that is excessively competitive, with free-floating hostility, aggressiveness, and impatience.

type B behavior pattern Behavior that is patient, relaxed, and noncompetitive.

greater or lesser amount of stress and of the effects stress will have on the person. Drs. Meyer Friedman and Ray H. Rosenman described two personality types, Type A and Type B.[3] The **Type A behavior pattern** is a complex of personality traits that includes "excessive competitive drive, free floating hostility, aggressiveness, impatience, and a harrying sense of time urgency." Type A is a stressful pattern that has been found to be related to greater susceptibility to heart disease. **Type B behavior pattern,** by contrast, is characterized by patience, a relaxed attitude, and non-competitiveness.

If you find yourself answering yes to many of the following questions, you may possess the Type A behavior pattern:

- Do you often do two things or more at the same time (for example, eat and read the newspaper)?
- Do you speak rapidly?
- Do you walk quickly?

- Do you interrupt others?
- Do you find it difficult to wait in line?
- Do you feel guilty when you relax?
- Are you overscheduled?
- Are you often worried about being late?
- Do you drive your car too fast?
- Is it difficult for you to watch people doing things more slowly than you know you can do them?

There is some disagreement, however, as to whether all the components of the Type A behavior pattern are equally important. Many researchers have now concluded that only free-floating hostility is related to the development of coronary heart disease. If you are easily angered—you become hostile and belligerent often—you are more likely to develop coronary heart disease than if you are usually more relaxed. Type A behavior pattern is discussed further in Chapter 15 on cardiovascular disease.

Issues in Health

Should Type A's Be Changed to Type B's?

Con Some experts in the field of stress believe we are either born with or develop a pace for life. Some of us are Type A's and some of us are Type B's—period! This behavior pattern is so much a part of us that we should learn to accept it and adjust to it, rather than attempt to change it. As Hans Selye has said, you can't make a race horse into a camel, or vice versa. The animal would be terribly unhappy and probably become ill if we tried. Similarly, you can't take a Type A and change his or her pace to a Type B's. The Type A may behave as a Type B, but wouldn't be happy,

and the stress of trying to maintain Type B behavior might itself lead to illness or disease.

Pro Other experts have argued that not only should we try to change Type A's to Type B's but also that we are obligated to do so. To do otherwise would mean that these people remain susceptible to coronary heart disease. Meyer Friedman, the cardiologist who first identified the existence of Type A and Type B behavior patterns, has written a book entitled *Treating Type A Behavior and Your Heart,* in which he describes a pro-

gram that he considers effective in actually changing Type A's. Friedman advocates that this program be replicated nationwide, that we should change as many Type A's as possible, that this change can be made, and that newly created Type B's will adapt easily and with enhanced health to this change.

Do you think the Type A people you know can change to Type B and adapt to that change? If you are a Type A, could you live as a Type B?

TABLE 3.1

Modified Social Readjustment Rating Scale

Rank	Stressful Life Event (Stressor)	Value	Your Checks
1	Death of steady boy/girl friend	100	———————
2	Break up with boy/girl friend or divorce	73	———————
3	Separation with boy/girl friend (to see if you really love one another)	65	———————
4	Jail term	63	———————
5	Death of close family member	63	———————
6	Personal injury or illness	53	———————
7	Going steady, engagement, or marriage	50	———————
8	Flunk out of school or fired from work	47	———————
9	Reconciliation with boy/girl friend	45	———————
10	Change in family member's health	44	———————
11	Pregnancy	40	———————
12	Sex difficulties	39	———————
13	Change in financial status	38	———————
14	Death of a close friend	37	———————
15	Change in number of boy/girl friend arguments	30	———————
16	Loan over $10,000	31	———————
17	Change in school responsibilities	29	———————
18	Trouble with boy/girl friend's parents	29	———————
19	Outstanding personal achievement	28	———————
20	Boy/girl friend begins or stops school	26	———————
21	Starting or finishing school	26	———————
22	Change in living conditions	25	———————
23	Revision of personal habits	24	———————
24	Trouble with a faculty member	23	———————
25	Change in school hours/conditions	20	———————
26	Change in residence	20	———————
27	Change in schools	20	———————
28	Change in recreational habits	19	———————
29	Change in religious activities	19	———————
30	Change in social activities	18	———————
31	Loan less than $10,000	17	———————
32	Change in sleeping habits	16	———————
33	Change in number of family get-togethers	15	———————
34	Change in eating habits	15	———————
35	Vacation	13	———————
36	Christmas	12	———————
37	Minor violation of law	11	———————
	Add values to reveal your score: ———		———————

Source: Adapted from Thomas H. Holmes and Richard H. Rahe, "The Social Readjustment Rating Scale," *Journal of Psychosomatic Research.* Copyright © 1967, Pergamon Press, Ltd. Reprinted by permission.

hardiness Behavior that responds to stress positively, viewing stressful events as challenges rather than as threats; and being committed and exercising control over the event.

Hardiness

Researcher Suzanne Kobasa studied people who experienced a great deal of stress but never seemed to become ill as a result. Kobasa uncovered a personality trait that seems to protect people from stress. This trait was termed "hardiness." **Hardiness** consists of the three C's: commitment, control, and challenge. *Commitment* is the tendency to become involved and to feel committed to the activity. *Control* is the belief that something can be done to influence the outcome of the potentially stressful events. *Challenge* is viewing events as opportunities rather than as threats. People who possess the three C's tend to be able to manage stressors better while maintaining their health.

Intervening Variables

Although life changes and personality are important indicators of a person's chances of becoming ill from stress, a number of factors can help to reduce the chances of stress-related illness.

It has been found that social support, for instance, can act as a buffer between life change and illness. That is, people who have "significant others" (such as close friends and parents) with whom to discuss their joys, concerns, and problems are less likely to become ill when experiencing stressful life changes than are individuals without social support. Some of the variables discussed previously also affect the degree to which stress will be harmful. These include self-esteem, alienation, assertiveness, and locus of control.

Thus, stress does not *necessarily* lead directly to illness and disease. It has the potential to do so, but many factors influence this relationship. If you lack assertiveness, for example, you will not have your needs met and you will experience more stress than an assertive person. To intervene between stress and disease, you should take an assertiveness training course. If you don't feel good about yourself—if you have low self-esteem—you will find that state stressful. To intervene between stress and disease, you must work on improving the part of yourself that you hold in low esteem. Perhaps a diet will improve your physical self-esteem; maybe more reading will help you feel better about

your intellectual self; or a workshop on communication skills may improve your low opinion of your social self.

Stressors Related to College Life

For most people, college life is an experience that is both enjoyable and fondly remembered, but it can also be very stressful. Many of the stressors affecting college students are health-related. The close living quarters shared by students residing in dormitories or apartments foster the rapid spread of communicable diseases. Influenza epidemics and bouts of mononucleosis are frequent visitors to college campuses. Other stressors, such as lack of sleep, examinations, and inadequate nutrition, also contribute to the spread of such diseases.

The psychological stressors associated with college life concern changes and decisions, which are normal and part of the maturing process. Students living away from home for the first time may find it difficult to make their own decisions, independent of the family. Who will do the laundry? Who will make the bed? Who will shop for food and cook? And will there be enough time left over for studying? Separation from people whom one has seen every day of one's life can be a strain as well, and for some students, homesickness is an intense stressor.

Of course, there are substitutes for the people one misses. Friends of the same and the opposite sex often replace the absent family members. The process of making friends in itself can be stressful, however, especially for people who fear they will fail at this task.

Of course, not all college students are young people. The older college student, who may be working while going to school or returning to school after the children have left the home or after retirement, encounters stressors as well. One of the major stressors of adults returning to school is the fear of failure. However, older students do have more experience to draw on than younger students do, and this can help them understand and apply the information learned in school. College campuses are changing today, and the older student population is increasing. In an effort to help older students manage the stressors they will en-

Exploring Your Health 3.4

Stressors of College Life

List five things about college life that *you* find stressful:	For each of the five stressors you listed, state how you have tried to deal with it:	For each of the five stressors you listed, list a better way in which you might have responded:
1. _____	1. _____	1. _____
2. _____	2. _____	2. _____
3. _____	3. _____	3. _____
4. _____	4. _____	4. _____
5. _____	5. _____	5. _____

counter, many colleges offer counseling for career changes, methods of study, fear of failure, and test taking. In effect, these are stress education activities.

You have probably noticed that some responses to stress are healthier than others. For example, if you were lonely and were befriended by someone who spent a great deal of time at bars drinking alcohol, you might be tempted to drink alcohol to excess as well. The loneliness might be so unbearable that alcohol abuse would seem a small price to pay to alleviate it. A healthier response would be to join a club at which you could make friends or a social service organization where you could make friends while doing something of value for others.

The decisions college students are required to make often have long-range significance. Your decision regarding what to do for the rest of your life may be especially stressful because it involves making a major, long-term commitment. There are other decisions you must also make, which may not seem significant in themselves, but when totaled they add to the stress you must manage:

- Do I join a group? Which one? Fraternity? Sorority? Athletic team? Campus newspaper? Student government?
- Should I repair this old car or get a new one?
- What should I study for this test?
- Should I go on a vacation during spring recess or go home?
- Should I go to summer school or take some time off?
- Should I get engaged?
- Should I join the demonstration?

Whereas all of life involves decision making, college life is somewhat different. It may be the first time

that some people are required to make decisions relatively independently—decisions of real importance, that is. The fact that suicide is the second leading cause of death among college students can be better understood when the stresses of college life are considered. Some college students experience alienation and have a low sense of self-worth resulting from the pressure to make new friends and the fear of failing at this task, as well as confusion regarding important decisions that must be made. Add to this the need to succeed and the effect that failure can have on self-esteem, and the stresses of college life become clear. Exploring Your Health 3.4 will help you examine your own stressors.

Stress in the Workplace

Other aspects of life in the twentieth century create stress with which we must deal. One of these stressors is stress on the job. Occupational stress usually occurs as the result of role overload, role ambiguity, role insufficiency, or role conflict. *Role overload* occurs when too much work is required in too little time; *role ambiguity* occurs when aspects of the job are unclear. *Role insufficiency* is a situation in which a worker's background (education and training) is not adequate to accomplish the job, and *role conflict* arises when two supervisors have different conflicting expectations of a worker. If severe enough, job-related stress can result in illness or disease.

However, occupational stress is made up of more than just work-site stressors. Individuals who differ on a number of important variables—such as their self-esteem or their physical health will interpret the same work-site stressor differently. For one person, a work stressor may be so disturbing that it leads to disease. Another worker may view the stressor as less threatening and upsetting, thereby preventing the harmful stress reaction that can develop into disease.

burnout A syndrome that includes feelings of physical and mental exhaustion caused by excessive work and stress.

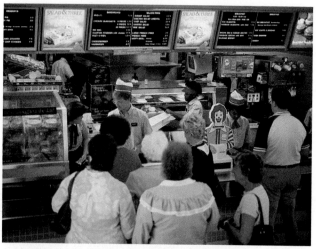

If you've ever had a job, or even a part-time job, you probably experienced occupational stress. Do you remember what caused this stress? How did you cope with it?

To complicate matters even further, stressors originating outside the workplace often affect individuals while they are at work. People do not leave their stressors from outside of work on a rack—as they would with their coats—when they enter the workplace. Instead, these stressors that seemingly have nothing to do with work are carried around throughout the work day by each and every worker. Since each worker's outside stress differs, the effects of stress from outside of work on each worker also differ.

In general, therefore, occupational stress is a function of sources of stress at work (role overload, role conflict, etc.), the unique characteristics of individual workers (self-esteem, physical health, etc.), and outside stress that affects work performance.

Year 2000 National Health Objective

Because so many people are affected by occupational stress, the federal government is attempting to get by the year 2000 at least 40 percent of those worksites that employ 50 or more people to provide programs to reduce employee stress.

Life's Other Stressors

Another stressor, which is increasingly common in our society, is the dual-career family, in which both husband and wife work. Whether the reasons are financial or related to career satisfaction, the dual-career family can create problems: how best to care for the children, how to make sure time is provided for one's spouse, and the like. Family responsibilities often conflict with job demands—for example, when a child is sick and must be cared for at home.

Urban life has its own complement of stressors. Those of you who have been stuck in rush-hour traffic, couldn't get a reservation at a restaurant, have been bothered by city noises, or feel crowded by too many people and buildings have firsthand experience with these stressors. If you're afraid for your safety or if you can't stand the smell of automobile exhaust when you're in the city, you are experiencing an urban stressor.

The physiological and psychological consequences of ignoring stress or responding to it inappropriately can be severe. However, there are ways to handle such stresses and to prepare for others that will inevitably occur. We will discuss some of these methods of stress management later in the chapter. First, let's consider what is known about how stress affects us both physically and psychologically.

Burnout

When a candle burns so long that it has very little wax or wick left, we describe it as almost burning out. Likewise, when someone has worked too hard and long and feels so frustrated that physical and mental exhaustion sets in, we describe that person as being close to burning out. **Burnout** is a syndrome made up of specific objective and subjective signs. Feelings of fatigue may develop. There may be a diminished sense of humor. Physical complaints such as muscle tension or stomach upset appear. The burned-out person may miss school or work due to illness, alcohol and other drug abuse, or feelings of depression. Some people have even begun to speak of "brownout"; that is, coming close to burning out but with some spark still remaining.

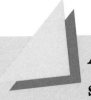

Signs of burnout are not unusual among college students. Given the extent of work required and its sometimes unrelenting nature, you should not be surprised that you sometimes feel "stressed out." Couple this with the implications of your schoolwork on your future life goals, and the potential for burnout seems very real. You might take some steps to prevent burning out during your college years. For example:

1. Enroll in some courses just for fun. For example, take a tennis class or a music class.
2. Discuss your feelings with friends and relatives. The support you receive from them will go a long way toward preventing burnout.
3. Consult with the campus health center. There are probably psychologists officed there who can help you perceive things as less frustrating and stressful.
4. Participate in intramurals or in a campus club. The camaraderie will provide both social support and a diversion from your stressors.

The Physiology of Stress

The Human Body and Stress

Stress affects various parts of your body. In order for you to see how this happens, you'll need a brief explanation of the body systems most relevant to the stress response. A more detailed description of these and other body systems appears in Appendix A.

Nervous System Consisting of the brain, spinal cord, and nerves, the nervous system coordinates body functions and helps you to be aware of situations and to react to them. For example, when you encounter a threat, your brain picks up the sight, sound, or smell of that threat and interprets it. A signal is then sent through your nerves to the parts of your body that are designed to respond to the threat. For example, your muscles may contract and heart rate increase as you prepare to run out of the path of a speeding car.

Endocrine System Glands, such as the pituitary gland, the thyroid gland, the adrenal glands, and the thymus gland, secrete fluids called hormones and are part of the endocrine system. Your hormones affect different parts of your body so that it can change to accommodate new situations. For example, when a stressor presents itself, hormones secreted by the adrenal gland increase your blood pressure so you can react physically in response to the stressor.

Digestive System All the organs concerned with the eating (ingestion) and digestion of food make up your digestive system. During a stress response, digestion is affected so you can react appropriately.

Circulatory System The body system that includes the heart, blood vessels, and blood is called the circulatory system. Blood, containing nutrients for the cells and oxygen acquired from the lungs, is pumped out of the heart through large blood vessels called arteries. It eventually reaches the cells of your body through small blood vessels called capillaries. After de-

psychosomatic illness A physical disorder that has its origin in, or is worsened by, psychological or emotional processes.

positing nutrients and oxygen in these cells so that the body can function, the blood is transported back to the heart through blood vessels called veins. When arteries that feed the heart with the nutrients and oxygen it needs to keep working become clogged—as sometimes happens because of fatty substances that accumulate on the walls of these arteries—part of the heart muscle can die and one can experience a heart attack.

Immunological System When the body encounters a foreign substance (such as some substance to which you are allergic), it marshals its forces to

FIGURE 3.2 ♦ Stress Reaction.

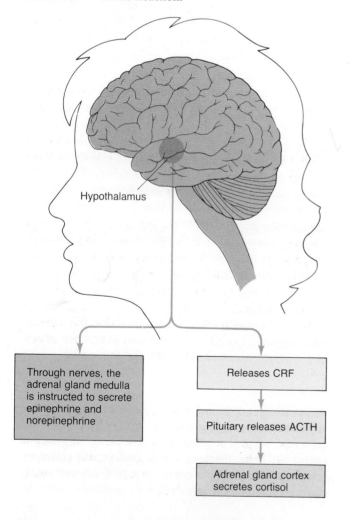

Hypothalamus

Through nerves, the adrenal gland medulla is instructed to secrete epinephrine and norepinephrine

Releases CRF

Pituitary releases ACTH

Adrenal gland cortex secretes cortisol

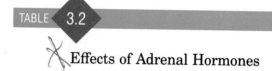

TABLE 3.2

Effects of Adrenal Hormones

Cortisol	Epinephrine and Norepinephrine
Increases glucose	Increase heart rate
Increases blood fats	Increase blood pressure
Reduces protein stores	Increase contractility of heart
Reduces white blood cell count	Increase cardiac output
Increases body-core temperature	Cause copious sweating

combat and remove the substance. The body system charged with this task is the immunological system, consisting of cells (such as T-lymphocytes and B-lymphocytes), that surround and destroy the foreign substance. Stress decreases the production of these cells and renders the immunological system less effective.

Now let's follow the path of a stressful event to see how it is processed by your body systems. As Figure 3.2 shows, when your brain perceives something as stressful, the *hypothalamus* of the brain responds by releasing a hormone called *corticotropin-releasing factor (CRF)*, which in turn activates the *pituitary gland* to secrete *adrenocorticotropic hormone (ACTH)* into the circulatory system. ACTH signals the *adrenal glands* to secrete the hormone *cortisol* from their cortex (outer section), while a direct nerve pathway from the brain to the adrenal medulla (inner section) stimulates secretion of the hormones *epinephrine* (adrenaline) and *norepinephrine* (noradrenaline). Table 3.2 lists the effects of these adrenal secretions.

As we've discussed, the endocrine system is not the only body system activated by stress. The digestive system secretes certain substances, the nervous system changes several body processes, the circulatory system and heart speed up, the brain is alerted, and the skin releases perspiration.

Exploring Your Health 3.5

Self-Test of Your Understanding of the Physiology of Stress

Match each of the following *numbered* items with the *lettered* item that most pertains to it.

Correct Letter	Numbered Item	Lettered Item	Correct Letter	Numbered Item	Lettered Item
___	1. Adrenal cortex	a) A hormone that increases glucose	___	5. Adrenal medulla	e) Stimulates the pituitary gland
g	2. Pituitary gland	b) Activates the adrenal gland	___	6. ACTH	f) Secretes cortisol
A	3. Cortisol	c) Secretes epinephrine	___	7. Epi-nephrine	g) Releases CRF
C	4. Hypo-thalamus	d) Secretes ACTH	___	8. CRF	h) Adrenaline

To test your understanding of these physiological changes, take the test in Exploring Your Health 3.5. Understanding the physiology of stress is important to your success in using the stress-reducing techniques that we will discuss later in this chapter.

Stress and Disease

Most researchers agree that stress is associated with psychosomatic diseases. A **psychosomatic illness** is a physical disorder that has its origin in or is worsened by psychological or emotional processes. In other words, in a psychosomatic illness, the mind causes or worsens an illness in the body.

Psychosomatic Conditions Related to Stress

The following psychosomatic conditions have been related to stress.

Ulcers   A fissure or open sore on the stomach lining is called a *peptic ulcer*. It is thought that the condition is associated with increased secretion of the acid juices that aid in digestion. An ulcer can result in severe stomach pain, heartburn, nausea, and a bloated-stomach sensation. Approximately 5 percent of Americans develop a peptic ulcer, and each year about 10,000 die of it. Ulcers have been produced in mice by subjecting them to psychological stress.

Ulcerative Colitis   Ulcerative colitis is characterized by a deterioration of the membrane of the colon so that it bleeds a great deal and may eventually perforate. Studies have found that people who suffer from this condition have a deep feeling of helplessness. Many believe that this feeling creates stress and contributes to the development of ulcerative colitis.

Diarrhea and Constipation   The colon is the part of the large intestine responsible for moving digested food along. When it overworks, diarrhea results. When it underworks, constipation occurs. Stress is often the culprit in either of these cases.

Allergies   Since stress affects the immunological response of the body, it has been cited as a cause of allergies. An asthmatic child, or the parent of one, does not need scientific data, however, to be convinced that emotional situations can precipitate an asthmatic reaction. Similarly, hay fever attacks often follow or immediately precede emotional excitation.

Migraine Headaches   Headaches are the cause of more than half the visits to physicians' offices in the United States. One type of severe headache is the *migraine,* in which blood vessels in the scalp are dilated. The victim feels a painful pounding in the head and experiences nausea. The patient with a migraine is usually an individual who feels a great deal of pressure to succeed and works very hard. A migraine attack generally occurs when the stress is relieved rather than during moments of stress.

Tension Headache   Another type of headache resulting from stress is termed a *tension headache.* This occurs as a result of chronic muscle tension, most often a result of stress, in the neck and scalp. Did you ever wonder where the expression "pain in the neck" came from? Have you ever had one?

hypertension Blood pressure that is abnormally high. Associated with stress, hypertension can cause coronary heart disease and stroke.

meditation A relaxation technique that focuses the individual's attention on something that is repetitive or unchanging.

Mental Illness Many researchers believe that stress can cause various forms of mental illness. One can escape a stressful existence by escaping from reality. We all know the recuperative value of vacation periods in which we "get away from it all." The mentally ill person may be unable to rejoin a world that he or she finds too stressful.

Psychosomatic Conditions over Which There Is Debate

The conditions cited above are but a few of those associated with stress, and ones about which there is little disagreement. The conditions listed below are controversial in that some experts believe stress is an important factor in their development, whereas others discount its significance.

Hypertension Perhaps as many as 33 percent of adults in the United States have **hypertension,** meaning that their blood pressure is abnormally high. Hypertension is accepted as a factor in both coronary heart disease and stroke and has been associated with stress. Some physicians are working with stress-reducing techniques as an aid to control this condition.

Coronary Heart Disease Some researchers believe that stress is a significant factor in heart attacks and in the blockage of the arteries supplying the heart. While acknowledging the importance of physical activity, levels of serum cholesterol, cigarette smoking, sex, and family history as factors in heart disease, Friedman and Rosenman, who advanced the theory of the Type A behavior pattern, regard stress as the main cause.

Stroke *Stroke* is a rupture or a blockage of a blood vessel in the brain and can result in paralysis, loss of speech, or death. Stroke is related to hypertension, and hypertension is related to stress. Thus it is logical that stroke is also related to stress.

Cancer Such factors as viruses, chemicals, and radiation are suspected of causing *cancer*, or the rapid and abnormal growth of cells. However, there is a growing belief that stress also may play a role. It is believed that cancerous cell growth occurs in all of us, but since our immunological system destroys these cells before they can multiply, most of us do not develop cancer. Likewise, it is suspected that a lowering of one's immune defenses will allow such cancerous cells to multiply. According to one theory:

> Stress helps to cause cancer because it depresses the immune response, the body's only real means of defending itself against malignant cells. It does this through the action of the adrenal cortex hormones, which particularly affect the T-lymphocytes [part of the white blood cells]. Searching out foreign substances in the body is one of the tasks of these T-lymphocytes, and significantly they measure at low levels in the tissues of most cancer patients.[4]

Further, some have theorized that the blood's increased thickness, a result of stress, causes deposits of protein to form on the walls of blood vessels which may snag passing cancer cells. The cells then take up residence and begin growing in surrounding tissues.

Diabetes Mellitus Stress has the effect of increasing sugar in the blood. Because the body is preparing to respond in some physical manner—"fight-or-flight" —when stressed, the sugar is designed to provide energy for either of these two reactions. Some researchers believe that chronically high levels of blood sugar brought about by chronic stress will diminish the

Year 2000 National Health Objective

To help Americans prevent stress-related illnesses and diseases, the government has established a Year 2000 National Health Objective that seeks to ensure that at least 50 percent of primary care physicians routinely review their patients' cognitive, emotional, and behavioral functioning as well as the resources available to deal with any problems they identify. The importance of this objective is evident in the statistic showing that between 50 and 67 percent of people who commit suicide visit a physician less than one month before taking their own lives.

ability of the pancreas to develop the insulin needed to metabolize the sugar (glucose), resulting in a permanent insulin deficiency. This condition is called *diabetes.*

Other conditions in which stress is suspected of being a factor include obesity, rheumatoid arthritis, and accidents.

Coping with Stress

Before we begin looking at ways of managing stress, let's first consider a model of the manner in which stress results in illness or disease.

How Stress Can Lead to Illness or Disease

Figure 3.3 shows a road down which a stressed individual may travel to illness or disease. The journey begins with a *situation* to which one has to adjust. As an example, let's assume that several of the major life changes discussed earlier have occurred. A couple has just moved to a new town where they both are starting new jobs. These stressors alone will not result in disease. They must first be *perceived* as distressing.

Suppose the husband is extremely concerned about how he will do in his new job. Instead of perceiving it as a challenge, he worries that he will make many mistakes and that he's not up to the demands he's going to face. He's concerned that if he loses the job, his wife's salary won't cover the mortgage payments on the new house.

If he perceives his new job as a threat, the husband has certain *emotional* reactions. He's tense, feels anxious, and is extremely insecure. These emotional reactions lead to *physiological* changes—increased heart, respiratory, and perspiration rates; increased muscle tension; increased blood pressure and a knot in the stomach. If these physiological changes occur often, are prolonged, or go unabated, he may experience an *illness* or *disease.*

FIGURE 3.3 • A Stress Consequence Model.

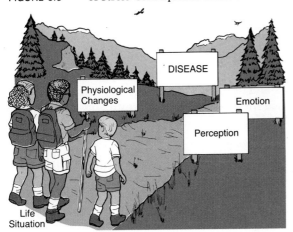

DISEASE

Physiological Changes

Emotion

Perception

Life Situation

Stress Management: Setting Up Roadblocks

The management of stress is based upon this model. Stress management entails setting up roadblocks so that the progression we have described does not reach the illness or disease level. If we could eliminate or block all potentially distressing life situations, the journey down the road would never begin. Of course, this is not only impossible, it is undesirable, because life would be extremely dull if we did not have to adapt to change.

On the other hand, there are numerous adjustments that we all could make in our lives to eliminate *unnecessary* stressors. Can you think of some stressors you could eliminate from your life?

Some stressors will sift through from the level of a new or changed situation to the next level of perception, so the stress management techniques we use will have to relate to our perceptions of these stressors. One way to perceive a stressor as less distressing is to find and focus on the positive component of the situation. Rather than focusing on the possibility of failure, the husband in our example could concentrate his attention on the positive opportunities his new job provides. This is an important approach to take toward minor stressors as well. For example, if you usually get irritated by having to wait in line, say to yourself. "Seldom in my busy day do I get a chance to do nothing. I'm going to take this opportunity to slow down. The telephone can't ring here and no one can barge in." In this manner, by not perceiving the situation as stressful, you may be able to prevent it from becoming so. You cannot control everything that happens to you, but you can certainly be in control of how you perceive those things, what you think about them, and how you behave in response to them.

Relaxation Techniques

Recognizing that some stressors will still be perceived as distressing even though you try not to view them as such, you can use various techniques to control your responses at the emotional level on our stress model. One set of techniques results in a relaxation response (for example, decreased heart rate and respiratory rate and lowered blood pressure) as opposed to the opposite, a fight-or-flight response. Relaxation techniques, as these are known, include meditation, autogenic training, progressive relaxation, and the use of biofeedback equipment.

Meditation **Meditation,** a relaxation technique that uses focused attention on something repetitive or unchanging, has been popularized in the Western world by Maharishi Mahesh Yogi's teaching of transcendental meditation (TM). This form of meditation requires forty minutes a day (twenty minutes in the

autogenic training A means of learning general body relaxation through the use of imagery and the feeling of heaviness and warmth in the body's limbs.

progressive relaxation A relaxation technique that employs the tensing and then the relaxing of muscles and muscle groups.

biofeedback The monitoring of the physiological events of the body and the instantaneous reporting of these events to the individual so that relaxation techniques may be employed.

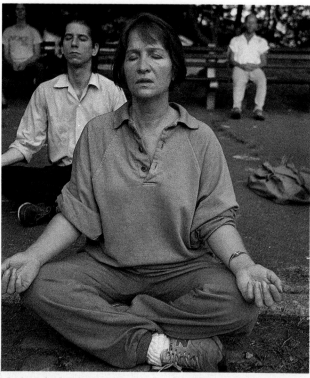

Meditation is a relaxation technique that you can begin to use right away to reduce the stress in your life. All you need is a little time each day and a quiet place.

morning and twenty minutes in the late afternoon). The meditator, who is seated in a quiet location, repeats a Sanskrit word (mantra) and when other thoughts come to mind, gently returns to the repetition of the mantra. Researchers have found that during meditation people experience a lowering of metabolic rate, respiratory rate, pulse rate, oxygen consumption, and blood pressure. This state is the opposite of the physiological condition that occurs in reaction to stress.

Dr. Herbert Benson, a heart specialist, suggests that a similar technique is just as effective in eliciting the physiological reaction to meditation. That physiological reaction is termed the *relaxation response,* and involves the following steps:

1. Sit quietly in a comfortable position.
2. Close your eyes.

3. Deeply relax all your muscles.
4. Breathe through your nose and say the word "one" each time you breathe out.
5. Do this for twenty minutes, maintaining a passive attitude; that is, don't try to bring about the desired physiological reaction.[5]

Autogenic Training   Developed by Dr. Johannes Shultz, a German psychiatrist, the **autogenic training** method of relaxation involves self-hypnosis. Using imagery and suggested feelings of heaviness and warmth in the limbs, the subject learns to recognize a relaxed state and call on it when needed. Autogenic training has been found to result in decreased respiratory and heart rates, decreased muscle tension, and an increase in alpha brain waves.

The following are typical instructions for autogenic training:

Sitting with your hands rested on your thighs (not touching each other), back straight against the chair, head hanging loosely forward, and both feet flat on the floor, close your eyes.

Imagine you've just come from a long walk and you're very tired. Your legs are most tired.

Feel the heaviness in your legs. They are very heavy. Just let your legs weigh themselves down.

Now they are feeling very warm. Just relax them, but feel how heavy and warm they are.

Enjoy this feeling. Retain it.[6]

The idea of autogenic training is similar to many of the stress-reducing (relaxation) exercises; its purpose is to provide the individual with the feeling of relaxation so that it can be called on during times of stress.

Use a tape recorder now to record the instructions for autogenic training or make up your own. Or just sit back and think of a pleasant scene. Once relaxed, try to notice the heaviness and warmth you are feeling.

Progressive Relaxation   Developed by Dr. Edmund Jacobson, a physician, the **progressive relaxation** method requires the participant first to tense and then to relax muscles in the body in order to learn to recognize tension and to learn to relax during periods of stress. It is termed progressive because it starts with muscles in one part of the body and progresses to all the other parts. Here is an example of instructions for progressive relaxation:

> *Sitting in your seat with your eyes closed, extend your right arm, with the palm upward, to the right. Now make a fist and bend your arm at the elbow and contract your biceps. After ten seconds just stop contracting all at once and the whole arm should fall to your side. Experience the muscle tension when the muscle is contracted, and the relief when it is relaxed. Learn to recognize both feelings and to be able to call upon either when desirable.*[7]

Try progressive relaxation yourself. Start with your feet and move from one muscle group to another until you relax your frontalis muscle (in your forehead). Don't rush it. Don't miss any parts of your body.

Biofeedback   Some people do not trust subjective measures of relaxation (like the ones discussed previously) and need objective measures to verify their relaxed state. **Biofeedback** is used to control functions of the body usually considered involuntary—such as brain waves, muscle tension, and skin temperature—by measuring physiological events and instantaneously reporting them back to the person. For example, electromyographic (EMG) feedback instrumentation records the amount of contraction of a particular muscle. Electrodes connected to the EMG machine are attached to the skin covering the muscle whose tension is being measured. A person hooked up to an EMG machine would have the tension of his or her frontalis (forehead) muscle measured, because this muscle gives the best indication of general body relaxation. The machine itself does not produce the relaxed state; its function is to enable the subject to recognize and control his or her own responses.

One of the advantages of biofeedback training over some of the other relaxation techniques is the speed with which the participant learns the relaxation response. The disadvantage is that it involves the use, and sometimes purchase, of sophisticated equipment that is usually available only on college campuses or in clinical settings. You might be able to locate biofeedback equipment on your campus (in the psychology, physiology, or health education department) and make arrangements for biofeedback training.

Physical Activity

Another means of diminishing stress is to engage in vigorous physical activity and use the built-up stress products, such as muscle tension and increased heart rate. Joggers and long-distance runners have reported experiencing a meditativelike state, and it is suspected that the repetition of the sound of the foot hitting the ground serves as a mantra. Many kinds of exercise and sport serve this purpose, but caution is advised. If you

are so competitive that you must win, these activities may produce stress rather than reduce it. Focus on the activity itself—not the end result of the activity. Enjoy doing it—not having won at it. If you are highly competitive and winning is important, try such noncompetitive physical activities as backpacking, hiking, cross-country skiing, or canoeing. Activities other than sports can also reduce stress. Working on a car or in a garden can serve the same purpose.

Get Involved!

Reducing Stress

College students taking a health course most frequently learn about how they can eliminate stressors from their lives and how to manage the stress they can't completely eliminate. What they don't usually learn, however, is how they can control the stressful effects they themselves may have on other people. Without realizing it, you too may be a stressor to many of the people in your life. Perhaps you are causing another student to sleep less soundly by leaving your stereo on late into the night. Maybe you compete too aggressively on an intramural volleyball team that was established more for fun and exercise than for competition. It's possible that you are pressuring someone you are dating to have sex with you. Whatever the situation, you should be aware that the stress you make for these people is just as likely to make them ill as any other form of stress.

If you can figure out when and how you create stress for other people, you can adjust your behavior to eliminate much of their stress. Imagine the total effect on our society if we all changed our behavior in such a way as to get rid of the stress we were causing others!

Here's how you can make a start at this:

1.   Ask people you interact with on a regular basis to list the ways that you make them feel stressed. You could start, for example, with friends, classmates, professors, and family.
2.   Next, ask these people to list the ways that you "stress them out" and rank them according to severity; that is, which of your behaviors creates the most stress, the next most stress, and so on.
3.   Then brainstorm at least three ways you can change your behavior to diminish or eliminate the stress for the first two items in each list.
4.   Now choose the behavior changes you think would most reduce the stress you create for the people around you. Try these behavioral changes. If it works, treat yourself to a small gift! If it doesn't, try the other changes you brainstormed until you find ones that work.

Congratulate yourself for your social consciousness. Your interest in decreasing the stress our society experiences by diminishing the stress you create for other people is to be applauded!

Which type of physical activity is best suited to your purposes? Will you do it regularly? Don't wait. Set up a schedule to begin it now.

Other Techniques

There are many other ways to relieve stress. Religion may be a source of strength to overcome stressful events. Philosophies and practices such as yoga, Sufism, and Zen can also serve the same purpose. Using imagery to relax can work, too. For example, imagining that you are at the beach or in a quiet park might help you. You probably already use some ways to relieve stress that are unique to you. What are they? Do they work? When did you last use one?

Conclusion

We have seen how our bodies manifest our emotions, how our emotions result in stress, and how stress can build up within us. Further, we have noted how stress operates physiologically and how it can cause disease. Last, and most important, we described some ways to reduce the negative effects of stress. The bottom line, however, is whether you decide to use this knowledge about stress to improve your health. You *can* eliminate some stressors in your life. You *can* perceive some stressors differently so as to make them less distressing. You *can* regularly practice a relaxation technique: meditation, autogenic training, or progressive relaxation. You *can* exercise at least every other day in order to use the built-up stress in your life. You *can* prevent illness and disease and, what's more, feel better about each day.

Summary

1. Emotions are expressed by the body. For example, individuals with low self-esteem slump and are not very expressive; individuals with high self-esteem walk tall and talk animatedly.

2. The stress response pattern has three stages: alarm, resistance, and exhaustion. This response was first identified by Hans Selye, one of the leading researchers in the area of stress.

3. Stress can be positive or negative. Positive stress is called eustress. Negative stress is called distress. The stress response is the same, regardless of the type of stress experienced.

4. Stress results from changes in life; the more changes one experiences, the more susceptible one is to illness or disease. However, certain intervening variables, such as social support, can serve as a buffer between stress and illness or disease.

5. The personality of an individual affects how he or she responds to stress. Encountering the same stressor, one person can be highly distressed while another person remains unaffected.

6. Stress is associated with college life and situations outside the school setting. College stressors include disease-causing bacteria and viruses that are spread by close contact among individuals, the pressure to get good grades, being independent, and making a new set of friends. Other stressors are urbanization, the dual-career family, and job stress.

7. Stress physiology begins with the hypothalamus, which perceives a stressor and releases CRF, which in turn signals the pituitary gland to release ACTH. The ACTH activates the adrenal gland cortex to secrete cortisol. At the same time, the hypothalamus, through nerve pathways, directly activates the adrenal gland medulla to secrete epinephrine and norepinephrine. The result of these hormonal secretions is an increase in the heartbeat, respiratory rate, mus-

cle tension, serum cholesterol, and perspiration, and a decrease in white blood cells, surface body temperature, and digestive processes.

8. Stress has been associated with such conditions as ulcers, ulcerative colitis, diarrhea and constipation, allergies, migraine and tension headaches, mental illness, hypertension, heart disease, stroke, cancer, and diabetes mellitus.

9. Stress can be depicted as beginning with a change in a life situation that is perceived as distressing. Emotional reactions to this change led to the physiological stress response. If this physiological response is chronic, prolonged, or goes unabated, illness or disease may result.

10. Stress can be managed by eliminating the stressors one encounters, perceiving stressors as less distressing, exercising to use up stress products, and regularly practicing a relaxation technique. Relaxation techniques include meditation, autogenic training, progressive relaxation, and biofeedback training.

Questions for Personal Growth

1. If one of your relatives was fired from work and needed to move, what would you advise to manage the stress of his or her significant life changes?

2. Imagine that the stress of school became overbearing. You just couldn't see how you would get through all the stress you were experiencing! What five means of coping could you employ? Which of these coping strategies do you think most fit your lifestyle and values?

3. Recognizing that hostility is the component of Type A behavior pattern most related to the development of heart disease, how would you go about being less hostile? Whose help would you seek? Are there areas of your life about which you become too hostile or angry? Are there people who you let anger you easily?

4. If you have recently experienced significant amounts of life changes—for example, you started college, or moved into a new apartment or dormitory, or switched your major, or broken up with your boyfriend or girlfriend—what strategies can you employ to make your life less stressful? That is, what can you do to routinize your life so that you have to deal with few, if any, additional changes?

5. Think of someone you know who seems to be able to manage stress well—someone who takes the attitude that things will get done, who believes life is a "bowl of cherries," and who feels relaxed much of the time. Now compare yourself —your attitudes, beliefs, behaviors—with this other person. How can you be more like this relaxed person? How can you model yourself on this person's seemingly stress-protective lifestyle? When will you begin?

References

1. Hans Selye, *Stress Without Distress* (New York: Harper & Row, 1974). Copyright © 1974 by Hans Selye, M.D. Reprinted by permission of Harper & Row, Publishers, Inc.

2. Richard S. Lazarus, "Puzzles in the Study of Daily Hassles," *Journal of Behavioral Medicine* 7 (1984): 375–389.

3. Meyer Friedman and Ray H. Rosenman, *Type A Behavior and Your Heart* (New York: Knopf, 1974).

4. Walter McQuade and Ann Aikman, *Stress* (New York: Bantam, 1975), p. 76.

5. Herbert Benson, *The Relaxation Response* (New York: Morrow, 1975), pp. 162–163.

6. Jerrold S. Greenberg, *Health Education: Learner-Centered Instructional Strategies* (Dubuque, Iowa: Wm. C. Brown, 1989).

7. Ibid.

CHAPTER

4

Intimate Relationships: Dating, Marriage, and the Family

CHAPTER OBJECTIVES

After reading this chapter, you should understand:

- The differences between gender, sex, sexuality, and gender roles, and how your gender identity develops.

- How to learn to be intimate with other people, and why and whom we date.

- Why people marry, several of the attractions of marriage, some of the things that contribute to marital success, how couples can communicate successfully, and why some couples divorce.

- How people arrive at the decision to have—or not to have—children and how individuals interact in family relationships.

- Lifestyle alternatives to marriage, including cohabitation, singlehood, and homosexual unions, and why breakups occur.

CHAPTER OUTLINE

Gender Roles

Intimacy: A Learned Process

Tradition, Innovation, and Communication in Marriage

Parenting and Family Relationships

Alternatives to Marriage

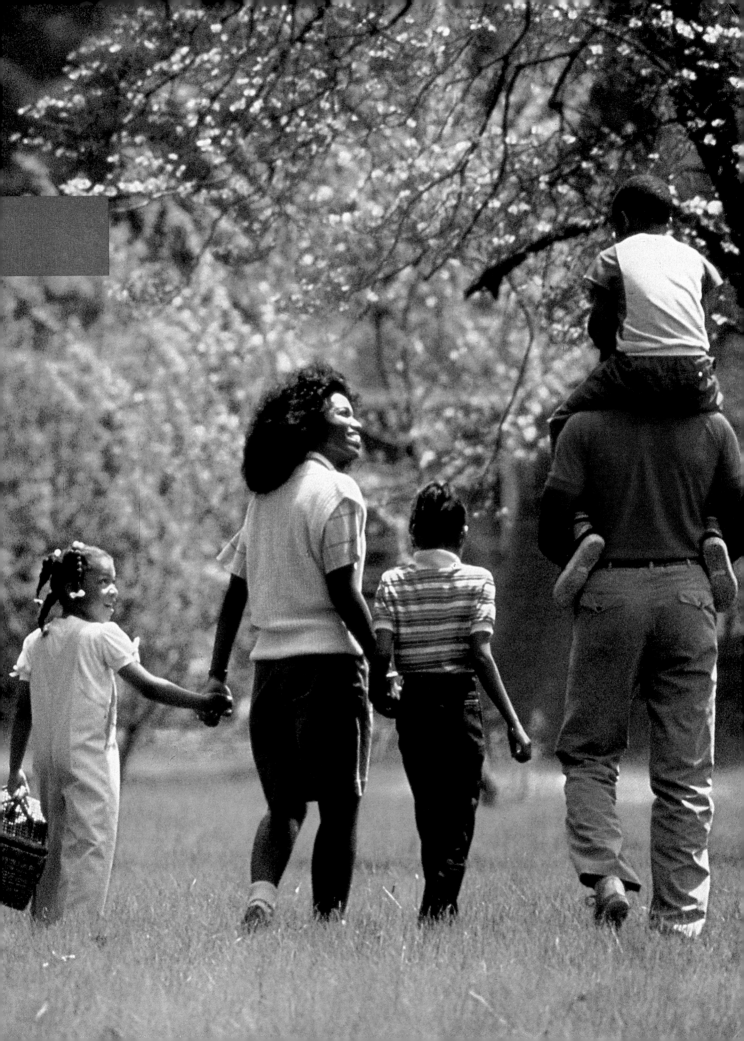

gender Gender refers to how you were born, male or female.

sex Sex refers to something you do; your lovemaking habits.

sexuality In terms of psychology, sexuality refers to an individual's socially and culturally determined gender-related behaviors.

gender roles A society's set of rules or norms that govern male and female behaviors.

gender identity The conviction about and the acceptance of being a male or a female that an individual develops as he or she matures.

sociobiology The study of the biological basis of social behavior.

sex-role or gender-role stereotyping The expectation by society that an individual should behave in particular ways because he or she is male or female.

The need for intimate relationships is central to most people's lives. Loving and being loved provide a sense of belonging, security, and well-being. We generally think of people who do not have the emotional support of relatives, friends, lovers, or spouses as being sad or isolated. In our society, most people still regard marriage as the ultimate intimate relationship, achieved through a sequential progression beginning with dating and culminating in the formation of a new family unit. Although many people experience a smooth progression, many others find the route to intimacy a difficult one. The high incidence of divorce in our society and the large number of single-parent families are testimony to this fact. In this chapter, we will focus on intimate relationships, how they form, and why they often fail. We'll also examine alternative routes to intimacy, such as cohabitation and singlehood. Finally, we'll consider some of the issues surrounding parenthood and family life. Your task will be to see how you can use what you learn in this chapter to build satisfying intimate relationships in your own life.

Gender role perceptions greatly influence the decisions men and women make about occupations, the opportunities they are afforded in society, and the roles they assume in marriage and family relationships.

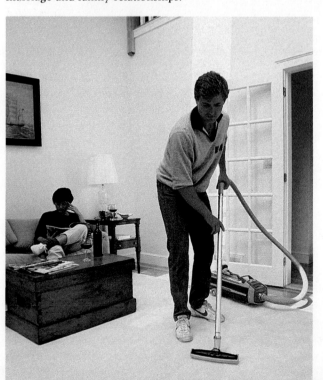

Gender Roles

Here's a riddle for you: A father and his son are involved in a car accident in which the father is killed and the son is seriously injured. The father is pronounced dead at the scene of the accident and his body taken to a local mortuary. The son is taken by ambulance to a local hospital and is immediately wheeled into an operating room. A surgeon is called. Upon seeing the patient, the attending surgeon exclaims: "Oh, my God, it's my son." Can you explain this? (Keep in mind the father who is killed in the accident is not a stepfather, nor is the attending physician the boy's stepfather.)[1]

If you are initially stumped, you are not alone. Many people have difficulty realizing that the attending surgeon is the boy's mother. That is because of the stereotypes we hold regarding males and females. We discuss the reasons for these stereotypes—that is, how they developed in our society and the effects on all of us—in this section.

Gender, Sex, Sexuality, and Gender Roles

Before we begin, we need to distinguish between sex and gender. Unfortunately, even the experts do not agree on the distinction between these terms. In some instances, *sex* is used to refer to someone's biological make-up (you are born female or male) and *gender* to the social and cultural aspects of sex (how you learn to act in the society in which you live). Yet, it is also recognized that each term has both a biological component and a social/cultural one. For example, your hormones influence your behavior, and the society in which you live influences the hormones you secrete. It is for this reason that different disciplines define these terms differently. For our purposes, we define **gender** as psychology texts do: how you were born: male or female.[2] Further, we define **sex** as something you do; your lovemaking habits. Lastly, we define **sexuality** as your socially and culturally determined gender-related behaviors. Sexuality, therefore, refers to who you are as a sexual being as well as what you do during sex. It encompasses your physical sexual characteristics and your lovemaking habits, as well as your gender.

Now into this mix we add **gender roles.** Each society has a set of rules for how its males and females should behave. These rules are called gender roles.[3] When gender role expectations—either those of society or of someone you know—are restrictive, you are likely to feel that your choices have been limited. For example, if you are expected to act sweet and cute because you are a female, you may resent not being able to be as aggressive as you would like to be. Or if you are expected to act tough and brave because you are a male, you may resent not being able to admit being frightened when you are feeling that way.

The Development of Gender Identity

Once a baby is delivered and "It's a boy!" or "It's a girl!" rings out, social influences go to work to form the baby's gender identity and mold his or her future role. Blue ribbons may adorn a boy's room and pink ones a girl's. Toys are selected that are "appropriate" for a girl or a boy. As they grow older, boys are reinforced when they act as boys "should" and girls are reinforced when they behave as girls "should." And, if behavior inappropriate to the gender role is exhibited (cross-gender behavior), negative reinforcers go to work. For instance, if a boy dresses in his mother's clothes, his friends may make fun of him and his mother may force him to change clothes immediately. Before too long, people develop a self-image as a female or a male and an attachment to the accompanying gender role. That is a process called **gender identity.** Whereas gender role is related to personality characteristics and behavior, gender identity refers to a conviction about and an acceptance of being male or female.[4]

In addition to these sociocultural influences, biological ones also affect gender development and identification. However, there is great debate over how these factors operate; that is, whether biology or learning is most important. A whole field of study and research has been developed to answer questions such as this. It is called **sociobiology,** the study of the biological basis of social behavior. Sociobiologists have tried to explain the complex biological determinants of male and female stereotypical behaviors, but have not as yet settled this debate.[5]

Our Society's Gender-Role Expectations

Gender roles differ markedly from one society to another. For example, Arapesh women do all the routine carrying, because their heads are thought to be stronger, while the men share the care of the children. Both Samoan men and women do heavy gardening

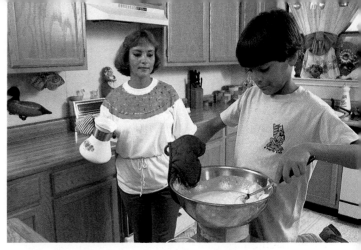

Traditionally, it has been all right for girls to participate in "boys' activities," but not vice versa.

and fishing, and both cook and do handiwork. These societies discourage any deviation from the prescribed gender roles, while others, such as ours, are now working toward flexibility and individualism in a wide variety of behaviors.

The expectation that people will exhibit certain characteristics and/or behaviors dictated by the customs and traditions of society is called stereotyping. Expecting individuals to behave in particular ways because they are males or females is referred to as **sex-role stereotyping** or **gender-role stereotyping.** There are still many rigid, unyielding traditional attitudes about gender-role behaviors that make it difficult for people to express themselves and for society to implement change. Stereotypical images of people do not take into account individual differences. Until recently, the stereotypical woman in our society was passive, quiet, and concerned primarily with home, husband, and children; and the stereotypical man was gruff, strong, unfeeling, and concerned mostly with work and money. The danger of such stereotypes is that people take them seriously and act on them, turning a blind eye to the qualities, capabilities, and interests of individuals—sometimes denying even their own interests. People too often believe that those who differ from stereotypes are not as good as those who conform to them. Thus, those who accept as true the stereotypes described might look down on a woman who cares about work or a man who chooses to stay home with his children. People become boxed in, not only by the social pressure to conform to the stereotype, but also by rigid, customary practices (such as promoting men but not women in business and professions, hiring women but not men to nurse and teach small children, or paying men more than women, regardless of their responsibilities or educational backgrounds).

Gender-role expectations greatly influence the decisions men and women make about occupations, the opportunities they are afforded in society, and the roles they assume in marriage and family relationships.

androgyny The blending of (stereotypically) "masculine" and "feminine" characteristics in one person.

intimacy The ability to form close and lasting relationships.

A Question of Ethics

Is It Ethical for Businesses to Hire Women and Not Provide Them with Childcare?

Con Those opposed to requiring businesses to provide childcare for their employees in a facility at work, or at least to reimburse employees for a portion of the cost for childcare offered outside the workplace, point to the expense involved. They argue that employees without children will be penalized because increases in salary will be less since the fringe benefit for childcare will cost the company a significant amount of money. They feel that only parents should have to pay for childcare. Further, they argue, customers will be charged more for the company's products since the cost of childcare will have to be considered in the cost of producing the products. To make matters worse, they continue, supporting childcare will only encourage more women with children to work outside the home. The result will be a generation of children that suffer the consequences of part-time parenting rather than the benefits of a steady, on-going parental presence at home. Rather than businesses being saddled with childcare payments, the government ought to encourage parents (in particular, mothers) to stay home with their young children by providing tax incentives rather than childcare tax breaks that only encourage the "depositing" of children with someone else.

Pro Advocates of requiring businesses to offer childcare point to the inequities involved in expecting large numbers of employees to produce well at work while having to worry about how their children are and whether they can afford to have them cared for well. They cite data regarding the high divorce rate, the large number of single-parent families, and the large number of women with young children working outside the home as evidence that there is a need and an obligation to help these workers with childcare. Further, a worker who has to rush home (or miss work altogether) to tend to a sick child not only costs the company that is losing his or her services, but also the worker suffers from the likelihood of withheld promotions and salary increases. In addition, since women are still the predominant nurturers, they are disproportionately affected by the lack of childcare services. In a society that is working toward more equitable gender-role expectations, the lack of childcare services acts as a barrier to this movement. Lastly, if childcare services are not provided, the workforce may lose the contribution of a significant segment of our society toward our Gross National Product (the sum of goods and services produced in this country) and our country's economic health.

What do you think?

Rapid societal change, difficult economic conditions, changing views of the roles of men and women, and more effective means of birth control are among the factors that have prompted many people to question traditional role expectations. Today, more people want to define their own roles rather than accept gender-based definitions that may not suit their individual needs. Indeed, **androgyny**—a blending of masculine and feminine characteristics in one person—represents a definite trend in our society right now. You can decide whether the roles and tasks you have assumed because of your gender are the most suitable for you or whether you wish to change them.

Intimacy: A Learned Process

The ability to form an intimate relationship that might lead to marriage does not come naturally; it is learned. **Intimacy** is the ability to form close and lasting relationships. Much of our early learning about close relationships comes from our family background. You have evolved into the person you are through inherited traits and interaction with your environment. You have inherited a physical appearance and an intellectual potential. You come from a certain socioeconomic background. You had many experiences as a boy or girl

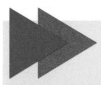

Exploring Your Health 4.1

Abilities and Aptitudes Desirable for Men and Women

For each trait listed below, indicate whether you feel it is more desirable in males (M), more desirable in females (F), or equally desirable in both sexes (B).

1. Athletic ability.
2. Social ability.
3. Mechanical ability.
4. Interpersonal understanding.
5. Leadership.
6. Art appreciation.
7. Intellectual ability.
8. Creative ability.
9. Scientific understanding.
10. Moral and spiritual understanding.
11. Theoretical ability.
12. Domestic ability.
13. Economic ability.
14. Affectional ability.
15. Observational ability.
16. Fashion sense.
17. Common sense.
18. Physical attractiveness.
19. Achievement and mastery.
20. Occupational ability.

Answers In one study, college students of both sexes were asked which abilities and aptitudes were desirable for males and females. They cited the odd-numbered items on your list and item 20 as desirable for males and the even-numbered items (except item 20) as desirable for females. How do your responses compare? Why do you think the results turned out as they did?

that shaped your perceptions of life. You had parents or other caretakers whom you observed interacting, perhaps brothers and sisters who were models, and friends with whom you shared important aspects of your life.

The Challenge of Intimacy

Intimacy doesn't just happen; it requires work. In order to be intimate with another person, we must be willing to be vulnerable and to reveal ourselves to that person. Some people are afraid to reveal themselves to others because they fear rejection. Others are afraid that if they become too close to others they might lose their individuality. Building a healthy relationship means being willing to take these risks and to find a way to balance self-revelation and closeness with the need to be one's own person. A crucial element in your ability to do this is your self-esteem. As we saw in Chapter 2, people with low self-esteem are more anxious and insecure than people with high self-esteem. They see themselves as inadequate and lack confidence in their own ideas. People with high self-esteem, in contrast, believe in themselves and accept their own feelings. They are more likely to be able to risk rejection in a relationship, because their overall perception of themselves is positive. When a relationship doesn't work out, they may be unhappy about it, but they aren't likely to retreat into themselves and never try again. Before you can expect to be happy with another person, then, you have to be happy with yourself.

Another vital component in achieving a healthy intimate relationship is communication, as we will see later in the chapter. Can you think of some other factors that contribute to building healthy relationships?

Dating

Our first intimate relationships, of course, are with our parents and siblings. As children, we also form friendships with playmates and schoolmates. At some point in adolescence, most people begin to focus their need for intimacy outside their immediate family. As they grow more independent and mature sexually, young people become increasingly interested in forming relationships with members of the opposite sex. "Dating" used to be the popular term to describe young people going out together. Today many people talk about "getting together." However, there is a distinction between the two. Dating involves a prearranged activity between a couple and is relatively formal; that is, it involves being "asked out on a date." "Getting together," however, often means not a couple but a group activity, and it is usually spontaneous rather than planned well in advance. Both have as their aim socializing and recreation. Another term associated with dating is "courtship." Not used today, courtship was the term used years ago for "serious" dating. Courtship was predominantly designed as a prelude to marriage rather than as mere socialization or recreation.

The purpose of dating, or getting together, may initially be companionship or recreation, rather than courtship, but it nevertheless serves as a training ground for future intimate relationships, including marriage. It affords people the opportunity to try out behaviors and observe how others react to them and to experience a degree of intimacy. Eventually, it helps people decide what qualities appeal to them in an intimate partner and what kinds of relationships they want to avoid. Exploring Your Health 4.2 will help you figure out what you are looking for in a date.

Exploring Your Health 4.2

Dating

To help you identify what you value in a date:

1. List five people you know personally and really like:

    a. _____

    b. _____

    c. _____

    d. _____

    e. _____

2. List five people you know personally and dislike:

    a. _____

    b. _____

    c. _____

    d. _____

    e. _____

3. List any traits (such as sense of humor) that at least three of the people you like have in common:

4. List any traits that at least three of the people you dislike have in common:

5. Of the people you dated this past year, which ones possessed the traits you identified in question 3 above, and which ones possessed the traits you identified in question 4 above:

Traits Liked	Traits Disliked

6. Why do you think you dated those people who possess traits that you don't like?

    Rank the following assigning "1" to the most valued, "2" to the next most valued, and "3" to the least valued:

    _____ Physical appearance

    _____ Intelligence

    _____ Sense of humor

    _____ Going to a show

    _____ Going to a party

    _____ Having a private conversation

    _____ Shyness

    _____ Conceit

    _____ Clumsiness

    _____ Someone you can depend upon

    _____ Someone who is unique

    _____ Someone who is experienced

    A close examination of your responses to these exercises may indicate why you date the people you do. Are there some generalizations about dating *for you* that you can now make?

Check those questions you would answer yes to:

_____ 1. Sometimes I date because I'm lonely.

_____ 2. Sometimes I date because I'm bored.

_____ 3. Sometimes I date to be popular.

_____ 4. Sometimes I date because my parents want me to.

_____ 5. Sometimes I date because a friend wants me to.

_____ 6. Sometimes I have a date but don't want to keep it.

_____ 7. Sometimes I get nervous about an upcoming date.

_____ 8. Sometimes I am embarrassed by my behavior on a date.

_____ 9. Sometimes I'm disappointed in the person I've dated.

_____ 10. Sometimes I think about why and whom I date.

Most of us could answer yes to all but question 10. Perhaps if we could say yes to question 10, we wouldn't have to answer yes to so many of the others.

Factors in Date Selection Three factors appear to be related to the selection of dating partners: prestige considerations, physical attractiveness, and personality characteristics. *Prestige considerations* are based on our understanding that, when we obtain things valued by our peers, we gain status in their eyes. Similarly, when we date someone who has characteristics valued by our peers, we gain prestige. Because prestige considerations relate to the values of a specific reference group—for example, our friends—they are not objective; that is, prestige considerations may vary according to sex, age, and region of the country. What is valued by your reference group? How does that affect your dating decisions?

The second factor related to the selection of dating partners is *physical attractiveness*. Facial attractiveness, physique, grooming, and dress all enter into the physical attractiveness equation. Although researchers have found physical attractiveness to be more important to males than it is to females, it is a factor in dating for both sexes.

The last factor related to dating is the consideration of *personality characteristics*. Although Table 4.1 supports the importance of physical attractiveness in choosing a date, the influence of personality characteristics is also evident. Men and women do not seem to differ significantly in their ranking of personality, although men tend to consider intelligence and companionship more important than women do, and women value thoughtfulness, consideration, and honesty more than men do.

Use Table 4.1 to help you identify what you value in a date.

Love

For most of us, dating serves as preparation for a deeper form of intimacy, particularly for the feelings embodied in the word "love." We all recognize that different forms of love exist; parents' love for their children is obviously different from the passionate love between a man and woman, for example.

A useful way to get at the meaning of love is to consider it in relationship to the concept of liking. Psychologist Zick Rubin tried to do this by developing self-report scales of passionate love and of liking.[6] To develop his love scale, he studied a variety of descriptions of love and concluded that the major dimensions of romantic love are *attachment*—the bond between a couple based on mutual need—and *caring*—the desire to give to the other person, such that the other's needs are perceived as just as important as one's own. Rubin determined that the major dimensions to liking are *affection*—liking based on the way another person relates to you—and *respect*—liking based on another's admirable qualities in areas apart from personal relations.

When Rubin asked couples who were dating or engaged to complete the loving and liking scales, he found that the scores on the two separate scales were not related. This supports the premise that liking and loving are essentially different. Another finding was that high scores on the love scale were related to desire for marriage, but high liking scores were not. In addition, dating partners and best friends received high liking scores, but dating partners received much higher love scores. It would seem that liking is necessary for love to occur but that a love relationship involves more than simple affection and respect.

| TABLE | 4.1 |

Qualities of a Date Most Valued by College Men and Women

Rank	Women Desired in Men	Men Desired in Women
1	Looks	Looks
2	Personality	Personality
3	Thoughtfulness, consideration	Sex appeal
4	Sense of humor	Intelligence
5	Honesty	Fun, good companionship
6	Respect	Sense of humor
7	Good conversation	Good conversation
8	Intelligence	Honesty

Source: From *The Individual, Marriage and the Family*, 3e, by Lloyd Saxon. © 1990 Wadsworth Publishing Company, Inc., Belmont, California 94002. Reprinted by permisson of the publisher.

How Love Develops Love is the result of several stages of growth in a relationship, leading to greater intimacy. As Robert Thamm describes it, this process begins by knowing and loving oneself and subsequently behaving in a manner to satisfy one's needs. Next, close relationships with others develop, which help satisfy those needs (for example, understanding, touching, emotional closeness). The next stages of learning to love are accepting other people, developing empathy for others (understanding them), and being concerned with other people's needs and security. Lastly, we learn to gratify others' needs and feel rewarded for doing so.

Love relationships, then, are the result of a growth process—a process described by one author as "an act of continuous creation." Therefore, instead of "falling in love," we usually "grow in love."

Tradition, Innovation, and Communication in Marriage

So much has been written about the difficulties of marriage and the high divorce rate that you may be surprised to learn that 96 percent of Americans will marry at some time in their lives. Despite the adjustments required by marriage, most people still believe that marriage provides the best opportunity to fulfill their psychological, sexual, and material needs.

Married couples today face some unique concerns and challenges. Whether because of economic necessity or interest in pursuing a career, more and more married women are entering the workforce. The two-earner family requires a sharing of household responsibilities (for example, cleaning, cooking, childcare, and shopping). Two incomes also permit more options regarding the use of leisure time and have led to a greater emphasis on companionship between marriage partners. Consequently, many married couples today are working out flexible arrangements that fit their needs, rather than conforming to the stereotyped view of marriage. Decisions about whether and when to have children vary greatly among married couples.

About twenty-five years ago, in his book *The Sexual Wilderness (1968)*, Vance Packard predicted a new American marriage pattern that he called "serial monogamy." *Polygamy,* the most prevalent form of marriage in the world, is the marriage of one person to two or more spouses at the same time. People in many African nations and most Moslem countries permit polygamy. Well over half a billion people are in polygamous marriages.[7] *Monogamy,* which has been traditional in the United States and other Western societies, is marriage to one spouse. Packard described *serial monogamy* as the marriage of one person to a series of spouses, one at a time, followed by divorce. As you'll see by the statistics on divorce and remarriage, presented later, his notion was not farfetched. In fact, today substantial numbers of people have sequential families or mixes of first and second families, as divorced parents marry new partners and combine their households.

Some innovations have attempted to change the nature of marriage itself, apart from broader family issues. For example, a *contractual marriage* is one in which the partners formally agree to certain conditions upon which the marriage will be based and also agree to renew the contract periodically. The woman may agree to do the cleaning and cooking, the man to earn money and do the laundry, and both to rear the children. Or a couple may specify how they will resolve conflicts between their respective jobs, decide where to live and whether to move, determine how one partner's enrollment in school will affect his or her financial responsibility, and so on. These contractual arrangements are legally binding as long as they do not contradict existing laws.

These changes have not occurred without problems. More flexibility has meant more negotiation of marital relationships, and some couples have not been capable of that task. This, plus the emphasis upon meeting individual needs, has been a factor in the increasing number of divorces.

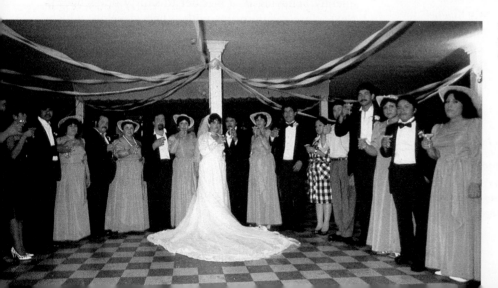

What features of marriage appeal to you the most? What features do not appeal to you?

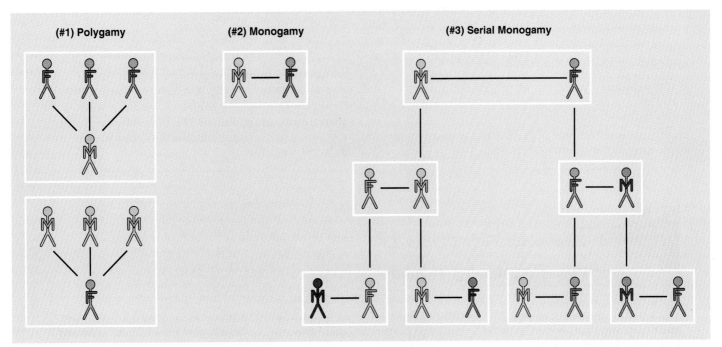

(#1) Polygamy   (#2) Monogamy   (#3) Serial Monogamy

FIGURE 4.1   •   The Three Most Common Types of Marriage in the World

The Attractions of Marriage

It appears that the attraction to marriage is the result of several factors.

- **Marriage provides companionship.** It's nice to have someone committed to spending time with you and sharing important moments in your life.
- **Marriage provides emotional security.** The intimate nature of the marital relationship can help alleviate the anxieties, fear, and insecurities you experience.
- **Marriage provides a sexual outlet.** The knowledge that your sexual needs will be satisfied in a loving, caring relationship can be quite appealing.
- **Marriage can improve your self-esteem.** Just knowing that you're "worthy enough for someone to marry" can make you believe you are an attractive, appealing, valuable person.
- **Marriage can provide financial security.** The addition of another wage earner, someone who can earn a living while you contribute to the partnership by doing chores that you would otherwise have to pay someone else to do, or vice versa, can make you more financially able to live the life you desire.
- **Marriage can legitimize reproduction.** If you want children and believe they will do best in a societally sanctioned family—a marriage—you might want to be married.

Despite the high divorce rate, marriage has numerous attractions that have led it to remain the predominant family lifestyle. However, it should be noted that not all of these attractions will be present in all marriages.

Depending on the expectations before the marriage and on other important considerations such as the personality traits of the partners and their love for each other, the absence of one or more of these advantages will either be overlooked or be deemed important enough to result in a divorce.

Factors Contributing to Marital Success

Although there is no formula for success in marriage, several elements that seem to be important have been identified. The most important factor is age at marriage. Statistically, couples who marry later (in their twenties or thirties) have a much greater chance of success than those who marry young (in their teens). Probably one reason for this is that younger couples, especially those who haven't finished high school, experience more economic difficulties than older couples. Also, many teenage women marry because they are pregnant, which creates more stress for the couple.

Another important predictor of marital success is emotional maturity. Research has shown that couples who perceive themselves as emotionally mature, as measured by such words as "fair," "rational," and "competent," tend to be self-confident and have positive self-esteem. These qualities seem to make it easier to adjust to the demands of marriage.

Similarity of ethnic, religious, social class, and educational backgrounds also seems to influence marital success. Couples whose socioeconomic backgrounds are similar apparently are better equipped to understand each other. In addition, they are less subject to external pressures, such as parental disapproval. In

self-disclosure The revealing of personal information about oneself—one's thoughts and feelings—in an intimate relationship.

confirmation The type of feedback that partners give each other in an intimate relationship.

transaction management The establishing of rules in a relationship to enhance communication and work toward common goals.

situational adaptability The flexibility needed in a relationship to ensure effective communication in different situations.

Exploring Your Health 4.3

Choosing a Marriage Partner

The following questions may help you determine whether your expectations for marriage agree with those of a potential marriage partner. Both of you should answer the questions. Compare your answers. Do you have similar expectations for marriage.

1. What are your expectations for job or career satisfactions?
2. How will you manage your income?
3. Where do you want to live? How will you make decisions about moving if one partner's career advancement calls for a change of residence?
4. How will household tasks be divided?
5. What are your expectations for your sexual relationship? How frequently do you expect to have sexual intercourse? Will extramarital relationships be permitted?
6. Who will be responsible for birth control, if any?
7. Do you want to have children? How many? How will childcare and parenting responsibilities be assigned?
8. How will you spend your leisure time and vacations?
9. What are your obligations to your respective families?
10. If you have been married before, how will you handle obligations to your former spouse or children from the previous marriage?

---

fact, studies have shown that most people choose marriage partners that do possess these similarities.

Finally, marriages are more likely to succeed when husband and wife share the same expectations about their relationship. Marriages are based on a great many assumptions regarding the rights, duties, and role obligations of the partners. When couples think about and ultimately agree on these basic assumptions, they are more likely to avoid disillusionment or disappointment. Among the issues about which partners need to reach an understanding are personal and career goals, financial matters, household arrangements, sex, children, and relationships with kin and friends. The important point is not the particular goals and responsibilities a couple decides upon, but that they are in agreement about these issues. With similar expectations, they are less likely to experience conflict and more likely to feel secure about what to expect from each other. If you have a potential marriage partner, complete Exploring Your Health 4.3 to see if you and your partner show the same expectations. If you don't have a potential marriage partner, Table 4.2 will help you decide your future mate's important characteristics.

Communication in Intimate Relationships

Earlier in the chapter, we said that communication is an essential ingredient of a satisfying intimate relationship. Research has shown that couples who are able to communicate well with each other are more satisfied with their relationships than couples who communicate poorly. In one study, marriage and family counselors reported that nine out of ten couples who sought help for marital problems said they had trouble communicating with each other.

Communicating effectively in a relationship cannot be learned overnight. It's a process that develops gradually. It depends on being aware of oneself, one's partner, and the relationship, and on wanting to nurture the relationship and help it grow.

What exactly is effective communication? One researcher suggests that, in order for a couple to communicate effectively, four components must be present: self-disclosure, confirmation, transaction management, and situational adaptability.[8]

Self-disclosure refers to revealing personal information about oneself, expressing what one is and what one feels. This need not entail telling the partner eve-

TABLE 4.2

What People Look for in a Mate

Below are thirteen characteristics that people consider important in choosing a mate. Rank these characteristics according to their importance to you in selecting your mate. After you've completed your ranking, compare that with the ranking researchers found for other women and for other men. Is your ranking similar or dissimilar to that of other women and men?

A. Adaptability
B. Creativity
C. College Graduate
D. Desire for Children
E. Exciting Personality
F. Good Earning Capacity
G. Good Health
H. Good Heredity
I. Good Housekeeper
J. Intelligence
K. Kindness and Understanding
L. Physical Attractiveness
M. Religious Orientation

Rank order obtained from females:

K, J, E, G, A, L, B, F, C, D, H, I, M

Rank order obtained from males:

K, J, L, E, G, A, B, D, C, H, F, I, M

rything one feels; rather it means expressing one's feeling while at the same time being sensitive to how the disclosure will affect the other person.

Confirmation refers to the type of feedback partners give each other, the type of responses they make. Confirming responses are those that show acceptance of the partner, as well as of what he or she is saying. A partner gives confirming feedback by being supportive and sympathetic rather than critical or judgmental.

Transaction management refers to the couple's ability to establish realistic rules for interaction and keep their communication moving toward desired goals. A couple has to decide, for example, whether it is permissible for them to shout when they are angry. If one partner is very upset by shouting, the couple should agree on another way to express anger and then stick to the agreement. Managing communication also means not allowing it to get out of hand. In some cases, this might consist simply of someone telling a partner that he or she is afraid an argument is about to begin. Once the partners are aware of the situation, they can then decide to change their pattern of interaction if necessary.

Situational adaptability refers to flexibility in communicating, knowing that what is effective communication in one situation may not be appropriate in another. Adaptability requires being aware of when to

bring up certain subjects and when not to. For example, if someone is experiencing a personal crisis, the partner will delay discussing an unrelated problem and instead offer sympathy and support.

Improving communication in a relationship isn't easy. It requires a great deal of awareness and commitment. But the effort can have very positive results. As partners learn to communicate better, their relationship has the chance to grow more intimate; as intimacy grows, communication improves.

Names and addresses of certified marriage and family therapists can be obtained from the American Association for Marriage and Family Therapy (AAMFT), 1717 K Street, N.W., Suite 407, Washington, D.C. 20006.

Managing Conflict

In all human relationships of any substance, conflict will arise from time to time; but the partners can learn to manage conflict positively. The following suggestions apply to managing conflict of all types.

- **Express emotions, but don't act out negative behavior.** It is all right to feel angry, for instance, but it is not all right to hit someone when you feel this way. Express your feelings and allow your partner to express his or hers.

- **Use reflective listening.** When conflict arises, do not argue your point of view until you understand your partner's and have let him or her know that you understand it. To do this, it is helpful to paraphrase what your partner is saying so that he or she realizes that you understand his or her point of view. A clue here is to listen to the emotions behind the words, as well as the words themselves.

- **Explain your position.** Once your partner realizes that you understand what you are being told and the feelings involved, he or she will then be ready to listen to your point of view. Describe your feelings and thoughts and the rationale behind them.

- **Explore solutions.** Mention and analyze alternative solutions to the problem and their consequences. Choose a solution.

Consider the following description of how one couple handled a conflict.

John has worked hard all day and is very tired. His wife, Mary, had a difficult day with the children. John wants to spend a quiet, relaxing evening at home. Mary wants to get out of the house.

Mary: Let's go shopping tonight.

John: Are you kidding? I had a hard day at work. I wasn't home relaxing all day, like you were. I want to stay home, plop in front of the TV, and take it easy.

Mary: I was home all day relaxing? Are you serious? It's not easy to spend the day with toddlers making constant demands. I need to get out.

John: Forget it! No way! I'm staying home.

Mary: You're being inconsiderate. I don't think you even care about me.

John: Just leave me alone.

The result of this situation might be that John goes grudgingly with Mary and complains the whole time. The shopping would not be enjoyable for either of them under these circumstances. Or Mary might go by herself but not have John's companionship. Another alternative would be for John and Mary to stay home, but Mary would complain and John would not be able to relax. Mary would also be unhappy.

Now consider how John and Mary could have responded to this conflict by employing the steps outlined above:

Mary: Let's go shopping tonight.

John: Sounds like you had a rough day and need to get out.

Mary: Rough? It was miserable. I get so keyed up having to watch the children constantly to make sure they don't get into everything or hurt themselves. I wish there was another adult I could talk to.

John: You feel pretty frustrated and keyed up. It must be hard not having some adult stimulation.

John has been paraphrasing to this point and trying to let Mary know that he understands her feelings as well as her words. They continue, and John now explains his position:

John: I had a rough day too. It seemed to be nonstop. I'm very tired and feel like a wound-up spring. I was looking forward to coming home and relaxing. Going shopping wouldn't be relaxing for me.

Mary: Gee, it sounds as though one of us will have to lose out on what we need.

John: Well, hold off a second. Let's see if there is some way we could both go out and yet make it relaxing.

Mary: Maybe we could go out for dinner or perhaps to a movie.

John: Yes, why don't we have dinner out. That way neither of us will have to cook and we can relax together. I'll call a babysitter.

The point here is that now they both get their way and feel better about the situation. In the first situation described, although at first glance it appears that one person wins, both really lose. The shopping will be miserable for Mary because of John's complaining, and staying home will not be relaxing for John because of Mary's complaining. In the second situation, although it first appears that no one wins, both really do. They neither go shopping nor stay home, but Mary gets her stimulation and John his relaxation.

This approach to responding to conflict is appropriate for all kinds of relationships. The important thing to remember is to continue your reflective listening until the other person is ready to listen to you. The other person must believe that you have been listening and that you understand the feeling being expressed before being ready to listen to you.

People in intimate relationships should be concerned with each other's feelings. They should take the time to understand them and resolve conflict positively rather than with a "no win" posture. The procedure outline here is designed to make conflict resolution a positive experience rather than a negative one, with the result being a better relationship.

Divorce

A large number of marriages end in divorce. The divorce rate peaked in 1979 at 5.3 per 1,000 population; and the highest number of divorces (1,219,000) occurred in 1981. Since that time, the rate of divorce and the actual number of divorces have declined. In 1989, there were 1,163,000 divorces and a divorce rate of 4.7 per 1,000 population. That was the lowest divorce rate

Year 2000 National Health Objective

The Year 2000 National Health Objectives recognize the need to learn conflict resolution skills, and to start to do so at a young age. Specifically, one objective seeks to increase to at least 50 percent the proportion of elementary and secondary schools that teach non-violent conflict resolution skills.

Issues in Health

Should Two People Live Together before They Decide to Marry?

Pro Some say yes. They argue that you never know people until you live with them, but once you do, their likes and dislikes, moods, and expectations become apparent. The constant association of living together serves as a trial period. It is easier to dissolve this relationship than a legal marriage, and there is less chance of having children. If such a living arrangement works out, there is good reason to believe that a marriage would be successful.

Con Others maintain that people are always changing, and there is no way of knowing if you can live with someone in the future, in spite of being able to live with that person right now. They argue that a successful living arrangement now doesn't imply a successful marriage later. They further oppose living together because sex before marriage is prohibited by religious teaching. Besides, they believe that this arrangement represents "playing at" marriage and is therefore immature.

What do you think?

since 1975. In 1984, divorcing couples had been married an average of 9.6 years.[9]

Geographically, there are some differences in the divorce rate. In 1987, there were 3.6 divorces per 1,000 population in the Northeast, 4.4 in the Midwest, 5.4 in the South, and 5.5 in the West. In 1989, the state with the highest divorce rate was Nevada, with a rate of 11.9 per 1,000 population, where there is no requirement that those being divorced be residents of that state. The lowest divorce rate was in the state of Massachusetts, with a rate of 2.6 per 1,000 population. Demographically, there are some differences too, at least between blacks and whites; blacks have a much higher divorce rate than do whites in our society at all income, educational, and occupational levels.[10]

For both races, the higher the income, the lower the divorce rate; however, as income increases, the black divorce rate does not drop as fast as the white rate. For whites, the lower the educational level, the higher the divorce rate; the black divorce rate does not correlate clearly with educational level.

Among whites, people in low-status occupations have a much higher divorce rate than those in high-status jobs such as management or the professions; occupational status does not seem to affect the rate of black divorce. For both blacks and whites, teenage first marriages are more likely to end in divorce than are older first marriages, and children whose parents divorced or deserted the household are more likely themselves to divorce when grown.

Several factors are related to today's high divorce rate:

- More wives are working outside the home, making them less economically dependent on their husbands.
- Divorce has lost the social stigma that it carried in the earlier part of this century.
- The emergence of "no-fault" divorce, whereby one partner need not prove the other to be at fault for the dissolution of the marriage, has made divorces easier to obtain.

- Some researchers believe Americans have idealistic and unrealistic expectations of what marriage should be like and are disappointed when these expectations are not met.
- A change in American values toward personal freedom and happiness and away from hard work and "stick-to-it-iveness" leads some to pursue these desires at the cost of their marriages.

When divorced people who later remarried were asked the reasons for the breakup of their first marriage, they gave both a major reason and a list of other reasons (see Table 4.3).

Perhaps now is a good time to review some of the things that keep a marriage going. Look at the statements presented in Table 4.4. Do any of these statements reflect your own thoughts about what would make a successful marriage?

Effects of Divorce on Children

In 1964, only 8.7 children per 1,000 came from families that divorced that year. In 1981, that figure was 18.7; 1.2 million children were part of families in which the parents were divorced that year. In spite of the 1987 figure retreating to 16.3 per 1,000, divorce is obviously affecting a large number of children (1,038,000 in 1987). As of 1988, there were 5.9 million children under 18 (38 percent of all children) living with a divorced parent, compared to 2.5 million in 1970.

The initial response that children have to divorce is great distress. Younger children are usually afraid that the custodial parent will leave, as well as the absent parent. They may attempt to get their parents back together again and may fantasize about the return of the absent parent. In addition, many children blame themselves for divorce, not realizing that they may have been the reason the marriage remained intact as long as it did. Physical symptoms, such as stomach aches and sleeplessness, may result, and many children of newly divorced parents experience difficulty in school.

TABLE 4.3

Reasons Given as Major for Failure of First Marriages (490 Respondents)

Reason	Number of Times Listed First	Reason	Total Number of Times Listed
Infidelity	168	Infidelity	255
No longer loved each other	103	No longer loved each other	188
Emotional problems	53	Emotional problems	185
Financial problems	30	Financial problems	135
Physical abuse	29	Sexual problems	115
Alcohol	25	Problems with in-laws	81
Sexual problems	22	Neglect of children	74
Problems with in-laws	16	Physical abuse	72
Neglect of children	11	Alcohol	47
Communication problems	10	Job conflicts	20
Married too young	9	Other	19
Job conflicts	7	Communication problems	18
Other	7	Married too young	14

Source: Stan L. Albrecht, "Correlates of Marital Happiness among the Remarried," *Journal of Marriage and the Family* 41 (November 1979): 857–867. Copyright © 1979 by the National Council on Family Relations. Reprinted by permission.

Often children will recover from the ill effects within a year of the divorce. However, some children suffer much longer than one year. Although researchers have found divorce has little effect on the child's academic achievement, it does have an effect on his or her social and emotional health. For example, one study found children of divorced parents performed worse than children of intact families on 9 of 30 measures of mental health. These children showed more dependency, more irrelevant talk, withdrawal, blaming, inattention, decreased work effort, and unhappiness. Another researcher found that girls from divorced families had a higher rate of sexual activity, substance abuse, and running away, especially when the divorce occurred before elementary school. Boys were found to hold in anger as a consequence of divorce.[11]

A key to limiting these negative effects of divorce appears to be the continued presence of the father. Children from divorced families whose fathers maintained contact with them did much better than did children whose fathers' behaviors could best be described as absent neglect.

Divorce can be traumatic for the whole family. However, large numbers of children of divorced families fare quite well. If you are from such a family or know someone who is, take heart in knowing that you can limit the potential harm—to yourself and to others who have experienced divorce—by knowing what to expect and preparing accordingly.

TABLE	4.4	

What Makes for a Successful Marriage?

When researchers asked people who were married for at least 15 years what made their marriages last, they received the following replies (listed in order of frequency):

> My spouse is my best friend.
> I like my spouse as a person.
> Marriage is a long-term commitment.
> Marriage is sacred.
> We agree on aims and goals.
> My spouse has grown more interesting.
> I want the relationship to succeed.

Perhaps your future marriage can be more satisfying and successful if you keep these points in mind when deciding whom to marry.

Parenting and Family Relationships

Today, more than at any time in the past, marriage no longer automatically means having children. Most American couples now consciously decide how many children they want to have, and a small but growing number are choosing not to have any children.

Several factors have influenced these trends. The most important is the development of effective methods of birth control, particularly the pill. Social change has had an impact too. As a consequence of the women's movement, more women are seeking careers than ever before, and although a career and parenthood need not be mutually exclusive, women who work outside the home generally find that working and having children are not an easy combination to manage. A few career women, especially those who are highly educated, are deciding not to have children. Concern about overpopulation is another factor, as are economic conditions. Today, the cost of rearing a child through the college years on a middle-class income is well over $200,000, a figure that does not include the earnings lost while a mother stays out of the work force. Economics, however, do not seem to deter couples from deciding to have at least one child. When researchers asked parents about the disadvantages of having children, parents mentioned emotional costs, such as worry and restrictions on their freedom, more often than the financial burden.

Making the Choice

The decision to have children is often made more on an emotional basis than on a practical one. Many couples have rather romantic notions about parenthood and think that being parents will be a lot of fun. Researchers suggest that these notions can lead to disappointment:

> . . . most adults come to parenthood with overromanticized fantasies and exaggerated expectations without realistic anticipation of the strain a child will bring to the marriage economically, psychologically, and sexually. There will be a decrease in the time one previously had for one's spouse. Letdown is inevitable.[12]

There is also evidence that having children can detract from, rather than contribute to, marital satisfaction. Men and women often report that, as a result of the stress and responsibilities of parenthood, their satisfaction with their marriage suffers. And, interestingly, marital satisfaction increases again when the children are grown and move out on their own. Furthermore, young parents tend to talk to each other only half as much as newly married couples and, when they do talk, the topic tends to be the children.[13]

Despite the difficulties, however, most Americans still believe there are many satisfactions in raising children. Children fulfill important social, interpersonal, and psychological needs for the parents. Among the positive values of having children that were identified in a national survey of both parents and nonparents are the following, in rank order:

- Children provide love and companionship and act as a buffer against loneliness.
- Children bring stimulation, happiness, and joy to life.
- Children help fulfill the need to find meaning and purpose in life and enable parents to attain a sense of immortality by having a part of the self live on after death.
- Being a parent brings acceptance as a mature adult.
- Having a child gives parents a feeling of creativity, and watching the child grow contributes to the parents' feelings of competence.
- Children can offer an economic contribution to the family and security in old age.
- Raising a child makes some parents feel they have become better people.[14]

Of course, it is important to point out that the values people associate with having children aren't always the same as the motives couples actually have for becoming parents. Some couples have children because they assume it is expected of them, some hope to save a troubled marriage, and others hope that children will fulfill the dreams they haven't been able to fulfill themselves. Clearly, these are not the best reasons to have children. Like other health-related decisions, the decision whether to have children should be carefully thought out. Rather than trying to live up to others' expectations, decide for yourself what is best for you. Of course, it can be helpful to seek advice from others and to discuss the issues involved. In the long run, however, it is you and your partner who will experience the benefits and disadvantages of parenthood. Are the economic burdens, the restrictions on your time, and the responsibility involved worth the joys you will derive from parenthood? To help you think about whether you are good parent material, answer the questions in Exploring Your Health 4.4.

Developing Parenting Skills

It has been suggested that parenting is too easy a job to get. Although all you need to become a parent is a problem-free reproductive system, it is becoming increasingly obvious that parenting requires skills and, further, that these skills can be learned. Parent-training courses became popular in the 1970s. The largest of these programs is Parent Effectiveness Training (PET) which in 1978 was reported to have 8,000 instructors and 250,000 students. Other such programs were the Parent Involvement Program, Responsive Parent, and the Parenthood Education program, funded by the federal government and conducted in many public schools. Today, most training for parenthood occurs in adult education classes. These classes are often given in high schools, local YMCAs, Jewish Community Centers, and other typical adult education settings.

These programs have much in common. Though employing different philosophies, they consist of approximately ten sessions in which techniques of communication and behavior modification are taught. Their goal is to improve the relationship between parent and child, while at the same time helping the child to develop and mature in a positive direction.

If you are contemplating parenthood, or have already decided that you want to be a parent, perhaps you should attend a parent education program. Many of us learn how to parent by observing the only role models we have—our own parents. Although we can learn many positive methods from our parents, we may also learn inappropriate behavior.

Family Violence

For numerous reasons, families aren't always the loving, protective, nurturing groups that we like to believe they are. Violence between family members (child abuse, sexual assault of children, and spouse abuse) is all too common. Although such cases of child abuse as the Nussbaum/Steinberg child killing of 6-year-old Lisa Steinberg acquired national attention in the late 1980s, many other cases occur daily that do not receive any notoriety at all.

Child Abuse   One of the unfortunate realities of our society is that some parents act out their frustrations by abusing their children. The U.S. House Select Committee on Children, Youth, and Families reported that each year 1.9 million children are the victims of child abuse and neglect.[15] Child abusers do not differ by race, socioeconomic status, or profession. However, they do have some common characteristics. Parents who abuse their children are more likely to have been abused when they were children than parents who do not abuse their children. It seems that we learn our parenting style from our own parents, and if they were abusers, we are more likely to be abusers ourselves. Furthermore, abusing parents tend to be lonely and isolated, to lack trust in other people, to possess a poor self-image, and to use a strict, disciplinarian style of parenting.

In addition to the characteristics of the parents, the child and the family situation also contribute to child abuse. Some children are more disobedient, more stubborn, or slower than other children. Although there is no excuse for child abuse, these traits often contribute to the parent's frustration and anger. Research has also shown that a family crisis—for example, the father losing his job or the mother finding out her husband is leaving her—often instigates the abuse.

People in professions that involve contact with children (for example, teachers) are both morally and legally required to report suspected instances of child abuse to the proper authorities.

Exploring Your Health 4.4

Am I Good Parent Material?

Does Having and Raising a Child Fit the Lifestyle I Want?

1. What do I want out of life for myself? What do I think is important?

2. Could I handle a child and a job at the same time? Would I have time and energy for both?

3. Would I be ready to give up the freedom to do what I want to do, when I want to do it?

4. Would I be willing to cut back my social life and spend more time at home? Would I miss my free time and privacy?

5. Can I afford to support a child? Do I know how much it takes to raise a child?

6. Do I want to raise a child in the neighborhood where I live now? Would I be willing and able to move?

7. How would a child interfere with my growth and development?

8. Would a child change my educational plans? Do I have the energy to go to school and raise a child at the same time?

9. Am I willing to give a great part of my life—at least 18 years—to being responsible for a child? And spend a large portion of my life being concerned about my child's well-being?

Raising a Child? What's There to Know?

1. Do I like children? When I'm around children for a while, what do I think or feel about having one around all of the time?

2. Do I enjoy teaching others?

3. Is it easy for me to tell other people what I want or need, or what I expect of them?

4. Do I want to give a child the love (s)he needs? Is loving easy for me?

5. Am I patient enough to deal with the noise and the confusion and the 24-hour-a-day responsibility? What kind of time and space do I need for myself?

6. What do I do when I get angry or upset? Would I take things out on a child if I lost my temper?

7. What does discipline mean to me? What does freedom, or setting limits, or giving space mean? What is being too strict, or not strict enough? Would I want a perfect child?

8. How do I get along with my parents? What will I do to avoid the mistakes my parents made?

9. How would I take care of my child's health and safety? How do I take care of my own?

10. What if I have a child and find out I made a wrong decision?

What's in It for Me?

1. Do I like doing things with children? Do I enjoy activities that children can do?

2. Would I want a child to be "like me"?

3. Would I try to pass on to my child my ideas and values? What if my child's ideas and values turn out to be different from mine?

4. Would I want my child to achieve things that I wish I had, but didn't?

5. Would I expect my child to keep me from being lonely in my old age? Do I do that for my parents? Do my parents do that for my grandparents?

6. Do I want a boy or a girl child? What if I don't get what I want?

7. Would having a child show others how mature I am?

8. Will I prove I am a man or woman by having a child?

9. Do I expect my child to make my life happy?

Have My Partner and I Really Talked about Becoming Parents?

1. Does my partner want to have a child? Have we talked about our reasons?

2. Could we give a child a good home? Is our relationship a happy and strong one?

3. Are we both ready to give our time and energy to raising a child?

4. Could we share our love with a child without jealousy?

5. What would happen if we separated after having a child, or if one of us should die?

6. Do my partner and I understand each other's feelings about religion, work, family, child raising, future goals? Do we feel pretty much the same way? Will children fit into these feelings, hopes, and plans?

7. Suppose one of us wants a child and the other doesn't? Who decides?

8. Which of the questions listed here do we need to really discuss before making a decision?

Source: National Alliance for Optional Parenthood (Washington, D.C. 20036). Used with permission.

A national hotline sponsored by Childhelp USA provides referral information and crisis counseling for child abuse victims, victimizers, and their families. Its toll-free number is 1-800-4-A-CHILD. Other resources are:

1. National Committee for Prevention of Child Abuse
332 South Michigan Avenue
Suite 1600
Chicago, IL 60604-4357
(312) 663-3520

2. Clearinghouse on Child Abuse and Neglect Information
P.O. Box 1182
Washington, D.C. 20013
(703) 821-2086

3. National Criminal Justice Reference Service
1600 Research Boulevard
Rockville, MD 20850
(301) 251-5500

In addition, the federal government has established the objective of reducing children's injuries and

spouse abuse When one marriage partner physically or psychologically assaults his or her spouse.

battered spouse In situations of spouse abuse, the assaulted or physically abused marriage partner is called the "battered spouse."

deaths caused by abusing parents. In 1978, the incidence of child abuse was estimated to be between 200,000 and 4,000,000 cases per year. (That's how poor the database was at that time!) In fact, the 1980 National Study of the Incidence and Severity of Child Abuse and Neglect found that only one case of maltreatment in three had been reported to a child protective agency. The reasons for the hesitancy to report child abuse cases prior to 1980 are complex. One major contributing factor was the prevalent attitude that parents can do as they like with their children, and others should not get involved.

However, the database regarding child abuse has improved dramatically since the national health objectives were first formulated for 1990. Part of this improvement resulted from a change in society's attitudes, and an increased concern about child abuse. Schoolteachers are now more likely to report suspected cases of child abuse to principals and social service agencies. Several nationally publicized cases of the physical, sexual, and psychological abuse of children have largely been responsible for this change. Furthermore, the National Center on Child Abuse and Neglect (NCCAN) and the National Institute of Mental Health (NIMH) have funded several studies of different populations to determine the extent of child abuse in the United States. The more accurate data indicated that in 1989 an estimated 2–4 million cases of child abuse and neglect were reported to child protection agencies.

Year 2000 National Health Objective

The Year 2000 National Health Objectives seek to reverse the rising incidence of the maltreatment of children from the 1986 rate of 25.2 per 1,000 population to well below that level by 2000. In particular, the objective seeks to reduce the 1986 rates for physical abuse (5.7 per 1,000), sexual abuse (2.5 per 1,000), emotional abuse (3.4 per 1,000), and neglect (15.9 per 1,000). Another objective seeks to increase to at least thirty the number of states in which at least 50 percent of children identified as physically or sexually abused receive physical and mental evaluation with appropriate follow-up.

Sexual Assault of Children Since children who have been sexually abused tend not to report this fact to others, obtaining reliable statistics on the extent of this form of family violence is difficult. However, researchers estimate that between 100,000 and 500,000 American children are molested each year. It is further estimated that 25–30 percent of all American women and 10–16 percent of American men were sexually assaulted as children and that 2–5 million American women have had incestuous relationships. The sum total, then, is that 40 million Americans—1 in 6—may have been sexually victimized as children.[16]

The abuser is most often a member of the child's family, male, young, quite respectable in appearance, and likely to have been abused himself as a child. In more cases than not, the abuse occurs between a stepfather and stepdaughter, with the child afraid to report the abuse because of threats from the stepfather, fear that she will not be believed, or fear that the marriage will dissolve. Unfortunately, the child often blames himself or herself for the abuse and lives with shame and guilt well into adulthood.

Recognizing the enormity of the problem, several of society's institutions have responded. School districts have adopted curricula on sexual assault of children, the courts are believing the children's testimonies more often, counseling programs have been developed to help abused children, and both correctional institutions and hospitals are offering therapy for abusers.

Children are now being taught:

- That it's all right to say no to an adult. Although children need to learn to respect adults and to be disciplined, they also need to learn that there are some things even adults have no right to expect them to do.
- To trust their instincts. If they feel something is wrong, it probably is, or at least may be.
- To run away or yell if they are being treated in a harmful way.
- Not to keep abuse secret. Children need to tell others about attempted or actual sexual abuse. In this way, they can be helped and subsequent abuse prevented.
- Not to blame themselves. It is not the victim's fault

if abuse occurs. Children need to give up any guilt, shame, or self-blame they have about the abuse.

If you were sexually abused as a child, perhaps you now want to speak with a trained professional about that experience and your feelings about it and about yourself. Your instructor can probably refer you to a counseling clinic. Or you might want to inquire about such services at your campus health center. This is a problem that is all too common; you are not alone. Fortunately, counseling programs are geared to help.

If you have not been a victim of sexual abuse, perhaps knowledge of its prevalence will help you to identify a child who needs help, and you may better appreciate the need to support education on this topic in your community.

Spouse Abuse   When one married partner physically assaults the other, it is referred to as **spouse abuse,** and the one assaulted is referred to as a **battered spouse.** Usually the husband assaults the wife (about 2–4 million a year), but there are also instances of the wife assaulting the husband.

Spouse abuse may be caused by a number of factors. Men may be trying to prove their "manliness" by demonstrating they have physical power and control over the relationship. Sometimes the family—the male, in particular—has a high degree of normlessness. As we discussed in Chapter 2, normlessness is an indifference to or rejection of society's rules and regulations. Someone with a strong level of normlessness does not acknowledge any social or moral controls over his or her actions but instead physically, often violently, acts out anger and frustration. The wife may also contribute to her own abuse. For example, her acceptance of family violence may help to establish a family style of resolving conflict. Or she may have such a low opinion of herself (poor self-esteem) that she believes she deserves to be abused. Or she may have grown up in a family in which spouse abuse was common, therefore accepting it as an inevitable component of marriage.

To complicate this situation, the woman often remains in the home with the man in spite of continued abuse. This may be due to her lack of finances, to her desire to preserve the marriage for the sake of the children, or to her having nowhere else to go. Consequently, counseling and education programs have been developed to advise women in the face of spouse abuse. Twenty-four-hour hotlines and emergency shelters now offer assistance to battered spouses. And support groups for battered spouses have sprung up to help their members deal with legal matters, find a new place to live, and acquire employment.

No one needs to accept physical abuse. Rather, abusers need to be separated from their victims by being jailed or forced to leave the home until the danger of abuse has passed. During this separation,

counseling should be obtained by both the abuser and the abused spouse, and often by the children as well. You can locate support groups and services by telephoning either your state's district attorney's office or your local health department.

Single-Parent Families

In 1988, 27.3 percent of all families with children under 18 years of age were single-parent families. The U.S. Census Bureau reports that 15.3 million children live with only one parent, while another 1.9 million live with neither parent. A full 59.4 percent of all black children live with only one parent. From 1980 to 1988, the proportion of white children under 18 living in one-parent households increased from 17.1 to 21.7

In addition to having sole responsibility for both emotional and financial support, single parents must also try to provide role models for their opposite-sex children.

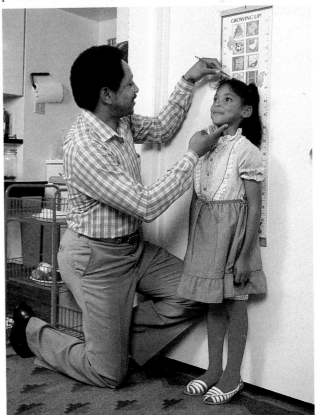

binuclear family A family arrangement in which a man and a woman no longer married, and living in separate households, still share in the care of their children, providing space in each household for the children.

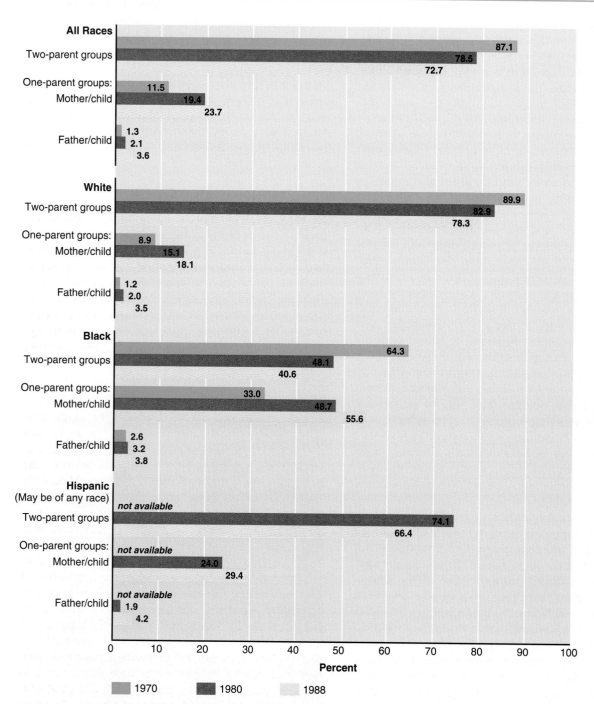

FIGURE 4.2 • Change in Composition of Family Groups with Children, by Race and Hispanic Origin: 1970, 1980, and 1988 (In percent)

Source: U.S. Bureau of the Census, Current Population Reports, Series P-23, No. 163, *Changes in American Families* (Washington, D.C.: U.S. Government Printing Office, 1989), p. 13.

percent. Among blacks, during the same period, that proportion increased from 51.9 to 59.4 percent. And among Hispanics, it increased from 25.9 to 33.6 percent. These figures are probably somewhat surprising to many Americans accustomed to the idea of a two-parent family. It is certainly surprising to see how the percentage of one-parent families has grown since 1960, when only 7 percent of white children and 22 percent of black children lived in one-parent families (data relative to Hispanic children were not computed separately in 1960). Figure 4.2 depicts the increase in single-parent families.

Note that the great majority of the single-parent families (87 percent), depicted in Figure 4.2, are headed by women, but men also head single-parent families (13 percent). The U.S. Bureau of the Census reports that in 1988 there were a total of 34.3 million families with children. Of these, approximately 25 million lived with both parents, and approximately 9.4 million lived with only one parent (8.1 million with the mother and 1.2 million with the father).

Single-parent families have particular financial, psychological, custodial, and other needs that are often more acute than the needs of two-parent families. The single parent must provide both financial and emotional support for the children single-handedly. Many single parents have the added responsibility of trying to provide role models for their opposite-sex children.

Research suggests that children in a single-parent family may have some problems during their formative years. A study by the Charles F. Kettering Foundation and the National Association of Elementary School Principals concluded that children from single-parent homes cause more disciplinary problems in schools and do not do as well academically as children from two-parent homes. The study showed that three one-parent children were disciplined by teachers for every two two-parent children disciplined. For every five two-parent children dropping out of school, nine one-parent children dropped out. And for every two-parent child expelled from school, eight one-parent children were expelled.

Such research findings might seem discouraging, especially to those who are single parents themselves. We hasten to add that these findings refer to trends in groups. Children from one-parent families often adjust very well. Nevertheless, single parenthood does present special problems requiring care and consideration. Perhaps most important, the special needs of one-parent families should be understood both by family members themselves and by those with whom they interact (for example, teachers and employers). To meet this need for understanding, a group called Parents Without Partners serves as a sounding board and a source of counsel for single parents. In addition, many books and pamphlets are available to help people cope with marital separation and divorce. Consult your local library or local health department for this literature.

Father-Headed Families When we think of single-parent families, we usually think of them as headed by women. Although this is usually the case, the number of men heading such families is rising dramatically. In 1970, only 345,000 single-parent families were headed by men. In 1981, that number had doubled to 692,000. By 1988, of the more than 9.4 million single-parent families in the United States, 1.2 million (slightly over 13 percent) were headed by men.

Father-headed one-parent families often place the father in a new role. We say "often" because nowadays men in two-earner families are sharing more of what had previously been regarded as the wife's household chores and responsibilities. For these husbands, the adjustment to heading a one-parent family may be less drastic; they are more used to cooking, cleaning, nurturing, and changing diapers. For the more traditional husband, however, undertaking these necessary chores and responsibilities, added to the financial and emotional burden of the loss of his wife, requires a greater adjustment.

Binuclear Families According to social worker Constance Ahrons, another kind of family has emerged from and survived divorce. Ahrons calls it the **binuclear family:** "a man and woman, no longer married, living in separate households with a place in each for their children."[17] In this light, divorce can be said to break up *homes*, because it splits marriages and creates new living arrangements, but not necessarily *families*. Instead, the family has changed its form, with its members now living in a two-house household. "Marriage has been separated from the family," Ahrons writes, "and the family has become a unit that can survive even divorce."[18]

Dual-Career Families Increasingly, both husband and wife are pursuing careers at the same time they are raising a family. As of 1987, 51 percent of women with children under a year old were in the labor force (see Figure 4.3). In the early 1960s, only approximately 17 percent of such women were employed. Whereas in 1965 only 45 percent of women worked during their first pregnancy, twenty years later 65 percent of such women worked (54 percent full-time and 11 percent part-time). In 1965, 52 percent of pregnant women worked during the last trimester of their pregnancy. In 1985, 78 percent of pregnant women worked during the last trimester of their pregnancy. The dual-career family is not only here to stay but is increasing in both number and proportion of total families. Although single mothers have increased their participation in the labor force (62 percent in 1976 compared to 69 percent in 1987), the most dramatic increase has been for married women. The proportion of married-couple families with both partners working increased from 37 percent in 1976 to 49 percent in 1987. Figure 4.4 depicts this trend.

latchkey children In dual-career families, children of school age who are literally given a house key so that they can come home and care for themselves.

cohabitation Living together in a sexual relationship without being married.

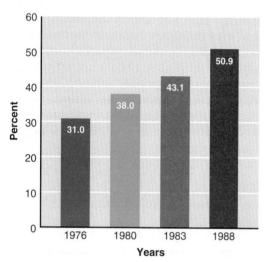

FIGURE 4.3 • Women 18 to 44 Years Old in the Labor Force Who Had a Child in the Preceding 12 Months: 1976 to 1988 (In percent)
Source: U.S. Bureau of the Census, Current Population Reports, Series P-23, No. 163, *Changes in American Families* (Washington, D.C.: U.S. Government Printing Office, 1989), p 17.

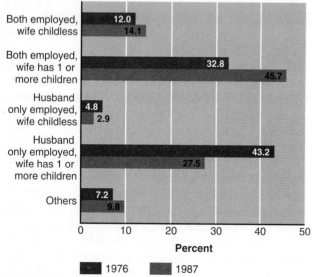

FIGURE 4.4 • Distribution of Married Couples by Employment Status and Fertility: June 1976 and 1987 (In percent)
Source: U.S. Bureau of the Census, Current Population Reports, Series P-23, No. 163, *Changes in American Families* (Washington, D.C.: U.S. Government Printing Office, 1989), p. 18.

Dual-career families present some unique advantages and disadvantages. The extra income can improve the family's lifestyle. This could mean a better education for the children, because the family can more easily afford to live in areas with good schools. Furthermore, many people value the independence developed by children who learn to spend time away from parents at an early age. And the opportunity to apply their training or education in the pursuit of a career has gone a long way toward improving the self-esteem and self-actualization of women heretofore frustrated by confining domestic roles.

On the other hand, dual-career marriages result in more divorces and extramarital affairs. It is hypothesized that this is a function of women's expanding contacts and financial independence. In the past, women may have remained at home in an unhappy marriage. Now they work outside the home, meet other men, and are better able to support themselves, both financially and psychologically.

Another problem for these families is the household division of labor. Studies indicate that a working wife still carries the major burden of housework, since other family members do not usually take on enough of the household chores. In one study, working wives spent 30 hours per week doing housework whereas their husbands spent only 4 to 6 hours per week on such chores.[19]

Furthermore, women who pursue careers tend to postpone having children. When conception is postponed until the woman is in her late thirties or beyond, the possibility of some form of birth defect is increased. Even if the child is born healthy, there remains the question of how much energy and commitment parents in their mid-fifties will have for raising a teenager.

Last, families with working mothers must find supervision for their children. Since 51 percent of working mothers with children under one year of age were in the labor force in 1987, this is no small problem. Among the solutions posed have been:

- Increase childcare by fathers whose jobs are flexible enough to allow it.
- Work only part-time and share childcare responsibilities with a neighbor who also works part-time.

- Work alternate shifts with the husband.
- Find a relative or friend to care for the child.
- Find paid work to do at home (for example, free-lance editing for a publisher).
- When children are old enough to attend school, provide them with a key so they can come home and care for themselves (these children are called **latchkey children**).
- Hire someone to care for the children at home.
- Work "flextime"—for example, ten hours a day for four days, or evening hours some days and morning hours other days.
- Place children in a day-care facility.

One of these solutions, day-care facilities, deserves special mention. Instances of sexual abuse of children in day-care facilities have been reported throughout the United States. Therefore, when placing children in day-care, parents should thoroughly investigate the program: the qualifications of the staff, the nature of the activities, the cleanliness of the facility, and other parents' recommendations. This will limit, though not eliminate, the chance of a bad experience.

Dual-career families can and do work. In order for them to be successful, however, attention must be paid to the unique problems they present—*as do all types of families.*

The Government's Response to Dual-Career and Single-Parent Families Recognizing the problems of the large numbers of single-parent families and working mothers, the federal government has passed legislation to protect their rights. Among this legislation has been:

1. Flexible and compressed work schedules were made available to some federal workers on an experimental basis in 1978 and to all federal employees in 1982. Such work schedules are still options for government workers today.
2. The Pregnancy Discrimination Act of 1978 required that employers treat pregnancy-related problems as they treat any other health condition.
3. Pension reform in 1982 encouraged states to treat pensions as community property at the time of divorce.
4. Latchkey legislation, passed in 1984, provided funds for local communities to design, establish, and conduct childcare programs for school-aged children in their public schools or community centers.

In addition, groups and individuals continue to lobby Congress for more legislation. For example, in 1987, Representatives Patricia Schroeder and William Clay introduced the Family and Medical Leave Act which originally provided unpaid family leave for up to four months of the birth, adoption, or serious illness of a child or parent. As a part of this legislation, workers would be guaranteed the right to return to their jobs and would retain continuation of their health benefits and pension and seniority rights. In 1990, a form of this legislation passed Congress but was vetoed by President Bush. His rationale was that government shouldn't interfere with businesses.

In a case before the Supreme Court (*California Savings and Loan Association* vs. *Guerra*) in 1987, the court upheld a California law ensuring that women who are medically disabled due to pregnancy are entitled to four months of unpaid leave. Furthermore, their jobs are guaranteed for them should they want to return. The business community was generally opposed to this law, arguing that it was discriminatory against men who could not get pregnant. Eleanor Smeal, then the president of the National Organization of Women (NOW), pointed out that such policies were widespread throughout the world: "More than 100 countries, including nearly every other industrialized nation, guarantee women leave for childbirth and job protection."[20]

Alternatives to Marriage

Cohabitation

In the liberal sense of the word, cohabitation means inhabiting, or living in, the same place as others. However, in the context of this book, we define **cohabitation** as living together in a sexual relationship without being married. In the last two decades, this living arrangement has become more common. According to the 1980 census, in 1970, 1.1 million adults were cohabiting. By 1985, the number had risen to almost 2 million. And, in 1988, the federal government reported that approximately a third of women aged 15–44 had lived with a boyfriend or partner at some time without being married to him.[21] By the age of 24, 60 percent of women have left single life; 30 percent by marriage and another 30 percent by cohabitation. By contrast, by age 24, 45 percent of men have left single life; 14 percent by marriage and 31 percent by cohabitation. Stated another way, half of the women and two-thirds of the men who live with someone of the opposite sex, before age 24, do so through cohabitation rather than through marriage. Overall, 33 percent of the women and 40 percent of the men who marry by age 24 have cohabited prior to that marriage. Of their first cohabiting relationships, 63 percent of the men's and 60 percent of the women's terminate within two years.[22]

Divorced or separated adults also make up a large percentage of cohabitants, and one out of ten cohabiting couples includes a partner sixty-five or over.

Issues in Health

Should Parents Place Their Children in Day-Care?

Research on the effects on children of day-care and having a mother that works outside the home provides contradictory conclusions.

Pro On the one hand, there are reports that:

1. Children with working mothers are no more likely to get sick and stay home from school than children whose mothers do not work outside the home.

2. The National Institute of Education reported that children whose mothers worked scored about the same on school achievement tests as children whose mothers did not work outside the home.

3. Older children of working mothers seem to develop just as well socially and intellectually as older children of nonworking mothers.

4. For disadvantaged children, day-care may, in some instances, offer more enrichment than home care.

Con On the other hand, there have been these findings:

1. For infants, day-care results in babies being more insecurely attached to their mothers, thereby not being as explorative as they might otherwise be.

2. The U.S. Department of Education reports that children of mothers who work outside the home score up to 9 percentile points lower on school achievement tests than do children whose mothers do not work outside the home.

3. Edward Zigler, a psychologist at Yale University, called infant day-care "the psychological thalidomide of the '80s," referring to the drug that resulted in large numbers of birth-defected babies.

The reasons for these contradictory conclusions relate to the difficulty in conducting social science research. For example, such variables as the age of the child, the time spent by the parent with the child and the nature of that time (referred to as quality of time), the nature of the day-care setting and the qualifications of the staff, and the stimulation available to the child in the home all effect the benefits or lack thereof attributable to day-care. Consequently, unless all these and other variables are controlled, different studies and researchers may be unable to agree on the effects of day-care.

How do you feel about day-care for children? At what age do you think it appropriate? Should the day-care consist of an organized program offered for many children who interact with each other or should children be individually supervised in their own homes?

Sources: Jerrold S. Greenberg et al., *Sexuality: Insights and Issues,* 2e (Dubuque, Iowa: Wm. C. Brown, 1989); "Working Mother's Kids No Less Healthy," *HE-XTRA* 12 (1986): 7; Dennis Meredith, "Day Care: The Nine-To-Five Dilemma," *Psychology Today* (February 1986): 36–44; and Charles R. Babcock, "Children of Working Mothers Suffer in School," *Washington Post* (June 26, 1983): A5.

Until the early 1960s, cohabitation was practiced primarily by celebrities, such as movie stars, and lower-class couples. In the 1960s, however, young, unmarried middle-class couples began to set up households. The availability of effective, easy-to-use contraceptives contributed to the trend by reducing the fear of pregnancy among couples who wished to live together without starting a family. In addition, the social climate of the time, which rejected many traditional standards, was an important factor.

People choose to cohabit for a variety of personal reasons. According to Macklin, some college students cite sexual fulfillment as their reason for living with their partners.[23] Often the couple began by having sex together once or twice a week, then increased the time they spent together in a more regular pattern, and finally decided that they might as well live together. Other reasons for cohabiting cited by Macklin's subjects were that they found dating laborious, they found that a large university could be very lonely, they sought a more meaningful and fulfilling relationship, they felt a need for security, and they had begun to question the institution of marriage. Although many respondents wanted to test their suitability for each other, marriage was not their initial objective in embarking on this lifestyle. Almost all Macklin's subjects reported that they were deeply involved with their mates emotionally, but none was ready or willing to make the total commitment to a permanent relationship.

Couples who live together cite several advantages. First, they claim that partners need not follow the traditional roles of husband and wife, although research suggests that roles in cohabitant relationships tend to be divided conventionally. Second, if the relationship breaks up, they do not have to go through the trauma of divorce. This does not mean that ending such a relationship is easy; indeed, breaking up can be a very difficult experience, married or not. Third, it is more convenient and less expensive to cohabit than to maintain a conventional two-residence love affair.

Most of the negative aspects of cohabitation are related to society's disapproval of this lifestyle. Even though living together is more acceptable today than it was even twenty years ago, it still meets with some objections. Parents may object to the living arrangement. Clearly, a person faced with parental rejection experiences considerable stress. Employers may disapprove, especially in conservative corporations where marriage is the norm. Cohabitors also sometimes have problems in renting or buying a residence.

Singlehood

For some people who have never been married, singlehood is just a phase of their lives that they hope will culminate in marriage. For others who have been married but no longer are, singlehood may be an interlude that will end with remarriage. However, there are also those for whom singlehood is the preferred lifestyle or who never marry because they never meet someone whom they want to marry. About 20 percent of divorced individuals never remarry. In 1988, 66 million (37 percent) of American adults were single compared to 38 million (28 percent) in 1970.

Our society has traditionally disapproved of the single lifestyle. The agrarian society that characterized eighteenth- and nineteenth-century America valued families and, in particular, children because of the pressing need for more workers. Singlehood, of course, ran counter to this need. Today, however, singlehood is becoming a more acceptable choice.

Research suggests that several factors lead people toward singlehood and other factors lead them away from a relationship with a partner. Peter Stein has described these as "pushes" to leave permanent relationships and "pulls" to remain single or return to being single (see Table 4.5).

In studies comparing single and married individuals, single men tend to score lower on intelligence tests than married men and to achieve less occupationally. Single men tend to come from authoritarian,

TABLE ◆ 4.5	

Pushes and Pulls Toward Singlehood

Pushes (to Leave Permanent Relationships)	Pulls (to Remain Single or Return to Singlehood)
Lack of friends, isolation, loneliness.	Career opportunities and development.
Restricted availability of new experiences.	Availability of sexual experiences.
Suffocating one-to-one relationship, feeling trapped.	Exciting lifestyle, variety of experiences, freedom to change.
Obstacles to self-development.	Psychological and social autonomy, self-sufficiency.
Boredom, unhappiness, and anger.	Support structures: sustaining friendships, women's and men's groups, political groups, therapeutic groups, collegial groups.
Role playing and conformity to expectations.	
Poor communication with mate.	
Sexual frustration.	

Source: Peter Stein, "The Lifestyles and Life-Chances of the Never-Married," *Marriage and Family Review* 1 (July 1978): 4. © 1978 by The Haworth Press, Inc. All rights reserved.

stressful homes where they had poor relationships with their mothers. Single women, on the other hand, tend to be better educated and more career-oriented than married women. People who have never married come from single-parent homes more frequently than those who do marry.

It is important to note in this discussion of singlehood that people who choose this lifestyle are not always unhappy or envious of their married friends. There are many happy, well-adjusted, productive people who simply prefer more independence than marriage allows.

Homosexual Couples

Although heterosexual or "straight" unions are most common in our society, homosexual or "gay" unions are also quite common. Male and female homosexuals —the latter often specifically referred to as *lesbians*— sometimes go through a formal marriage ceremony, even though such ceremonies are not sanctioned legally. However, it is more likely that they will live together without that formality. Data specific to gay relationships are difficult to obtain because many homosexuals are not willing to acknowledge their sexual preference. They may be fearful of job prejudice, of landlords who consider their lifestyle immoral, or of

homophobia An irrational fear of homosexuality.

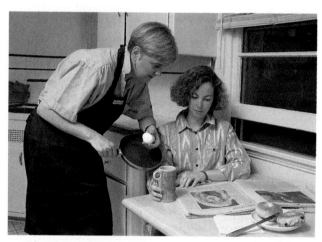

Gay couples usually blend male and female aspects of the traditional straight relationship into an equal sharing of responsibilities.

some other kind of **homophobia,** which is any irrational fear of homosexuality. This means that whatever data we have about homosexuals is probably valid for only a limited population.

Nevertheless, the data we do have indicates that homosexual unions appear to be quite similar to heterosexual ones. Like straight couples, gay couples share household chores, often enjoy sexual activity in a monogamous relationship with each other, and occasionally argue and break up. However, homosexual couples also face several problems that, while not necessarily unique, seem to occur more frequently in gay than in straight lives. The social stigma associated with being gay often creates stress for the relationship. The lack of legal validation for the relationship means that it is often easier—at least legally and financially—for homosexuals to break up. Finally, it appears that fewer gay relationships than straight relationships are sexually monogamous, and this means that the threat of AIDS and other sexually transmitted diseases (STDs) may be of particular concern to gays who, like straights, need and seek affection, acceptance, love, companionship, and committed relationships.

Despite these and other problems, gay male and lesbian relationships can be very satisfying. Reports of people in these unions reveal a great deal of sexual satisfaction; people of the same gender know exactly how it feels to be touched in certain ways. Gay relationships

Get Involved!

Intimate Relationships: Doing the Right Thing

There are several ways you can improve your society relative to intimate relationships. Some of these are listed below, but you can probably think of a number of other things to do.

1. Refrain from and try to help other people resist sex-role stereotyping, which limits people's options and forces them to adhere to a set of guidelines that may not be consistent with their natures. In this way, people around you will be more fulfilled and less likely to extend these stereotypes to other people.

2. Do not be manipulative in your personal relationships. This means: Do not attempt to coerce people to engage in sexual activities in which they are not initially willing to participate, be honest with people about your motivations in various aspects of your life, and do not withhold your beliefs and values from potential lovers or marriage partners in an attempt to convince them you are desirable as a mate. Following this prescription will result in less sexually transmitted disease, fewer divorces, and more satisfying personal relationships for people in your immediate society and in our nation.

3. Volunteer at a hospital or counseling center that treats victims of child or spouse abuse. Anything you can do to help will free up time for the professionals so they can treat more victims.

4. Do not marry until you are convinced, as best you can be beforehand, that the marriage will last. Discuss whether you will have children and how they will be reared. Several of the Year 2000 National Health Objectives speak to the improvement in the world of our children's lives. Decreasing the incidence of divorce and child abuse and neglect can be accomplished if we are more careful about whom we marry.

5. Report all suspected cases of child or spouse abuse to the appropriate authorities. If you are mistaken in your suspicions, that will soon be determined. However, if you are correct, you may have saved a life.

are also usually characterized by a sharing of chores and roles so that neither person feels "put upon." Contrary to the popular notion, gay couples do not divide themselves into "male" and "female" roles. Instead, male and female aspects of the traditional straight relationship are blended into an equal sharing of responsibilities.

As with other unions, homosexual couples can and do have fulfilling, meaningful relationships. As with other unions, they also may find themselves in relationships that are unsatisfying and need to be dissolved. Given the discrimination and other stressors that gay male and lesbian couples face, it seems especially difficult for their unions to last. And yet many do, and for many years.

Breaking Up

When a relationship becomes troubled, a decision must be made about whether it is worth spending the time and effort to repair it. Some relationships either cannot be repaired or are best left unrepaired. When college students' breakups were studied, professor Ronna Kabatznick[24] found that ending relationships led to a long period of recovery. In fact, it took men 1.6 years to recover and women 1.4 years. These relationships usually don't end immediately either, thereby prolonging the initial pain of breaking up and delaying the recovery period. It took Kabatznick's students an average of three months to break off their relationships.

You can recognize a troubled relationship in several ways. When the relationship is going sour, communication suffers, conflicts may become more prevalent, and expressions of anger and frustration may become obvious. Psychological withdrawal may occur with people not sharing their feelings as they once did. In some relationships there might even be physical abuse.

If the relationship is deemed worth saving, help is available. University health centers often have counselors who can work with students experiencing troubled relationships. Local health departments may provide similar services for residents—students or otherwise. Of course, there are also private practice psychologists and counselors whom you can approach for assistance.

If the use of these services do not improve the relationship, you might try a trial separation to determine how you feel while apart. The trial separation might result in the realization that being apart is unbearable and, therefore, encourage changes to improve the relationship. On the other hand, the separation might reveal that being apart feels better and life is more fulfilling. If so, the relationship should be permanently severed. If the breakup is to be permanent, research indicates it will have the least negative impact if the partners discuss and resolve it together. The type of breakup that is most likely to require a longer adjustment and to wreak havoc on the jilted party is one that ends abruptly without any resolution or explanation.

When you have ended an intimate relationship, it is time for you to assess the relationship and learn from it. What were the aspects of the relationship that you want to make sure will exist in a future relationship? What are those aspects you want to make sure will not be present in a future relationship? How did you act to affect the relationship negatively? How can you act more appropriately the next time? What are you willing to compromise about and what are you not? Allow some time to recover emotionally before exploring these and similar questions, but make sure that when it is time, you do so. Your future relationships and happiness may depend on such an analysis.

Conclusion

We must all make decisions concerning dating, marriage, parenthood, and family life. In this chapter, we have presented information to help you make these decisions. We have observed that the divorce rate is high, that many parents don't enter their roles with enough consideration of the tremendous responsibilities involved, and that some families' reactions to social influences have caused them to be referred to as "families in crisis." Rather than an academic study of these topics, what is needed is for people to give some thought to their personal involvement in them. Analyze what you want *from* a family and what you are capable of giving *to* a family. What is right for *you?* Marriage or remaining unmarried? Parenthood or nonparenthood? There are choices to be made, and we all must choose according to our own needs and values. The commonality of our decisions should not be in the end results, but rather in the rational process by which we come to them.

Summary

1. The stereotypes of male and female abilities and traits do not necessarily hold up under investigation. Traits such as physical strength and aggressiveness have been found to be more prevalent in males, and sociability and verbal skills have been found to be more prevalent in females. However, no difference has been demonstrated between the sexes with regard to such traits as intelligence, creativeness, and emotionality.

2. Learning plays a vital role in shaping masculine and feminine behavior. Parents, teachers, peers, toys, books, and other media are all influential in teaching children the conduct and qualities deemed appropriate for their sex.

3. There is a trend toward androgyny—a blending of masculine and feminine characteristics in one person—in today's society. In addition, a greater choice of lifestyles is available today than ever before for men as well as for women.

4. Whether the initial purpose of dating is companionship, recreation, or courtship, it serves as a training ground for future intimate relationships, including marriage.

5. Dating decisions are related to three factors: prestige considerations, physical attractiveness, and personality considerations.

6. Men and women value similar personality characteristics in their dates, although men tend to value intelligence and companionship more than women do, and women tend to value thoughtfulness, consideration, and honesty more than men do.

7. Romantic love—total absorption of two partners with each other—usually characterizes the beginning of love relationships. In long-term love, a domestic, calm, comforting relationship develops over time.

8. Love is the result of several stages of growth: knowing and loving oneself, satisfying one's own needs, developing close relationships with others, accepting and developing empathy for others, being concerned with others' needs, learning to gratify them, and feeling rewarded for doing so.

9. Successful marriages depend upon several factors, including age (couples who marry in their twenties and thirties have more successful marriages than those who marry in their teens), emotional maturity, self-confidence, and positive self-esteem.

10. Among the factors contributing to the high divorce rate are women's increased economic independence, the loss of social stigma previously associated with divorce, the emergence of "no-fault" divorce, and a change in American values toward personal freedom and happiness and away from hard work and "stick-to-it-iveness."

11. Divorce has some negative effects on children, especially during the first year following the divorce, but, with good communication between parents and children, adjustment usually takes place.

12. There are many reasons why people decide to have children (for example, for love and companionship, to find meaning in life, or to feel creative), as well as many reasons why people decide not to have children (for example, children limit one's freedom, add to one's responsibilities, and take time away from careers).

13. Family violence can come in several forms: child abuse, sexual assault of children, or spouse abuse. Usually, though not always, it is the male who engages in the violent behavior. Violence should be reported to the proper authorities so that help can be obtained.

14. Different family structures have developed to meet various needs of people in our society. We have more single-parent families, father-headed families, binuclear families, and dual-career families than ever before.

15. Cohabitation and singlehood are two alternatives to marriage that have become increasingly popular. Many people choose to cohabit or remain single for some portion of their lives rather than form permanent relationships. Both options offer a chance to redefine oneself and one's relationships.

16. Homosexual unions are quite common in our society. Homosexual couples experience many of the same stressors experienced by heterosexual couples: they argue, share household chores, and sometimes break up. However, they also experience some unique stressors that relate to the social stigma associated with being gay and the inability to legalize their relationship.

17. It often takes college students about a year and a half to recover from the breakup of a relationship. Troubled relationships can be recognized by poor communication, increasing conflicts, and expressions of anger and frustration. Trial separations are useful to determine how you feel apart when you are having doubts about continuing the relationship. University health services can be of assistance if you wish to work on improving the relationship rather than having a breakup.

Questions for Personal Growth

1. How are you similar to the stereotype of your gender? Do you believe that you possess traits stereotypical of the opposite gender? What are they?

2. How did you develop your gender role? What experiences have you had that led you to this gender role? Who was the most influential person in your life in terms of your gender role? Have your school experiences and friends influenced your gender-role development? How?

3. Can you be intimate with another person? What people and experiences in your life have helped make you able to be intimate or hindered this ability in you? Are you satisfied with your ability to be intimate? If not, what do you intend to do about it?

4. What do you look for in a date? What do your dates look for in you? How do you feel when you don't meet your date's expectations? How do you think your dates feel when they don't meet your expectations? How can these feelings be made less bothersome?

5. How do you know when you're in love? What feelings do you experience? What behaviors do you exhibit? How does "loving" differ from just "liking" someone a great deal? Can other people recognize when you're in love? What are the signs they would see?

6. If you were a matchmaker charged with matching you with several potential candidates, what kind of people would you consider? What traits and characteristics would they have to possess? What would you say about yourself to get other people interested in matching up with you? What about yourself would you hide because it would interfere with other people being interested in you?

7. Would you make a good husband or wife? Why? Why not?

References

1. Jerrold S. Greenberg, *Comprehensive Stress Management*, 3e (Dubuque, Iowa: Wm. C. Brown, 1990), p. 320.

2. Joyce McCarl Nielson, *Gender and Sex in Society: Perspectives on Stratification* (Prospect Heights, Ill.: Waveland, 1990), pp. 22–23.

3. Jerrold S. Greenberg, Clint E. Bruess, Kathleen D. Mullen, and Doris W. Sands, *Sexuality: Insights and Issues*, 2e (Dubuque, Iowa: Wm. C. Brown, 1989), p. 373.

4. Ihsan Al-Issa, "Gender Role," in *Male and Female Homosexuality: Psychological Perspectives,* ed. Louis Diamant (New York: Hemisphere, 1987), p. 155.

5. Roger D. Masters, "Explaining 'Male Chauvinism' and 'Feminism': Cultural Differences in Male and Female Reproductive Strategies," in *Biopolitics and Gender,* ed. Meredith W. Watts (New York: The Haworth Press, 1984), pp. 165–210.

6. Zick Rubin, "Measurement of Romantic Love," *Journal of Personality and Social Psychology* 16 (1970): 265–273.

7. Adelaide Haas and Kurt Haas, *Understanding Sexuality* (St. Louis: Times Mirror, 1990), p. 322.

8. Barbara M. Montgomery, "The Form and Function of Quality Communication in Marriages," *Family Relations* 30 (1981): 21–30.

9. National Center for Health Statistics, "Annual Summary of Births, Marriages, Divorces, and Deaths: United States, 1989," *Monthly Vital Statistics Report* 38 (August 30, 1990).

10. National Center for Health Statistics, "Cohabitation, Marriage, Marital Dissolution, and Remarriage: United States, 1988: Data from the National Survey of Family Growth," *Advance Data,* No. 194 (January 4, 1991).

11. Paul Taylor, "Therapists Rethink Attitudes on Divorce," *Washington Post* (January 29, 1991): A1.

12. David J. Anspaugh and Vava Cook, "Nonparenthood," *Health Education* 8 (1977): 21.

13. David Schultz and Stanley Rodgers, *Marriage, the Family and Personal Fulfillment*, 3e (Englewood Cliffs, N.J.: Prentice Hall, 1985), p. 290.

14. L. W. Hoffman and J. D. Manis, "The Value of Children in the United States: A New Approach to the Study of Fertility," *Journal of Marriage and the Family* 41 (August 1979): 583–596.

15. "A Hidden Epidemic," *Newsweek* (May 14, 1984): 30.

16. Alfie Kohn, "Shattered Innocence: Childhood Sexual Abuse Is Yielding Its Dark Secrets to the Cold Light of Research," *Psychology Today* (February 1987): 54–58.

17. Paul Bohannon, "The Binuclear Family," *Science* 2 (November 1981): 28.

18. Ibid.

19. "The Housework Gap," *Psychology Today* 22 (January 1988): 8.

20. Eleanor Smeal, "How About Paid Leave for Being a Parent?" *Washington Post, Health* (January 20, 1987): 6.

21. National Center for Health Statistics, "Cohabitation, Marriage, Marital Dissolution, and Remarriage: United States, 1988: Data from the National Survey of Family Growth," *Advance Data,* No. 194 (January 4, 1991).

22. Ibid.

23. Eleanor Macklin, "Unmarried Heterosexual Cohabitation on the University Campus," in *The Social Psychology of Sex,* ed. J. Wiseman (New York: Harper & Row, 1976).

24. National Center for Health Statistics, "Cohabitation, Marriage, Marital Dissolution, and Remarriage: United States, 1988: Data from the National Survey of Family Growth," *Advance Data,* No. 194 (January 4, 1991).

CHAPTER
5

Sexuality

CHAPTER OBJECTIVES

After reading this chapter, you should understand:

- The anatomy and function of the male and female reproductive systems.

- The sexual response cycle, including the similarities and the dissimilarities of the male and the female sexual response.

- Various forms of human sexual behavior, including masturbation, petting, oral sex, and sexual intercourse.

- Sexual problems in males and females and how these problems may be dealt with.

- Some reasons for and myths about homosexuality, as well as several variations of human sexuality that fall outside the realm of what many people consider to be "normal" behavior.

- The crimes and implications of rape and incest.

- Some ways to decide for yourself how to use your sexuality.

CHAPTER OUTLINE

The Reproductive Systems

Sexual Response

Forms of Sexual Expression

Sexual Dysfunction

Sexual Diversity

Sexuality and the Law

Sexual Behavior: Deciding for Yourself

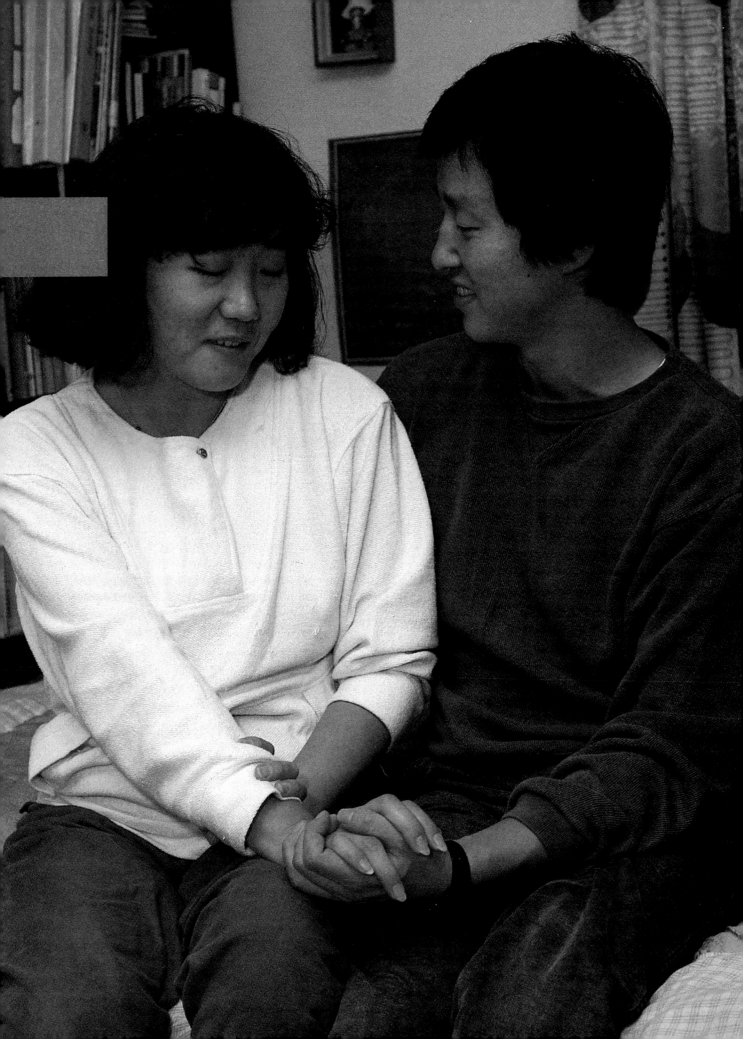

An important part of your life is your sexuality. Your sexuality is part of who you are. It includes your reproductive anatomy, the roles you play, and the societal expectations you adopt. Sex, on the other hand, is something you do: kissing, petting, having intercourse, and the like. We might say that sexuality is at your essence, your being, you, whereas sex is concerned only with sexual behavior. Sexuality is an implicit theme of this chapter. And we do deal with sexual behavior and response from both the physiological and social viewpoints.

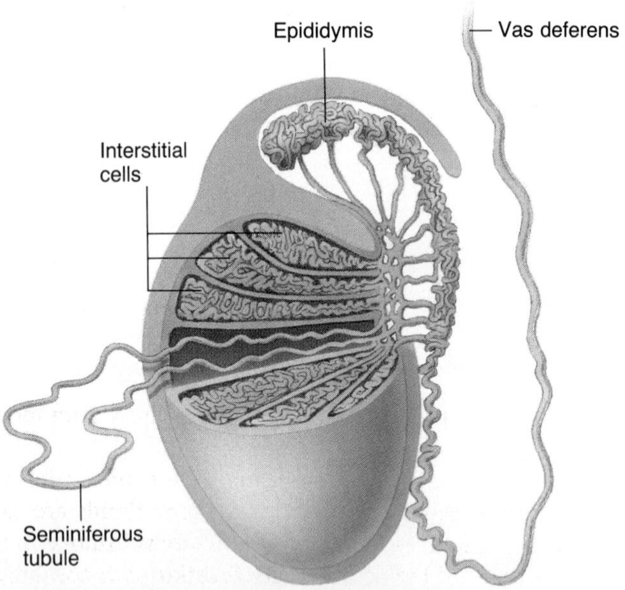

The Reproductive Systems

The Male Reproductive System

Figures 5.1, 5.2, and 5.3 depict the male reproductive system. The external male reproductive structures include the scrotum and the penis. The *scrotum* is a baglike structure containing the two *testes,* which produce *sperm* and the male sex hormone *testosterone* (see Figure 5.1). Each testis consists of several parts. The sperm is produced by cells in the part of the testes called the *seminiferous tubules.* Each testis contains approximately 1,000 seminiferous tubules, and some 50,000 sperm cells are produced each minute (150 million daily). Once produced, the sperm are carried through the *vasa*

Epididymis — Vas deferens

Interstitial cells

Seminiferous tubule

FIGURE 5.1 • The Testis (plural: *testes*).

FIGURE 5.2 • Cross-section of the male genitalia.

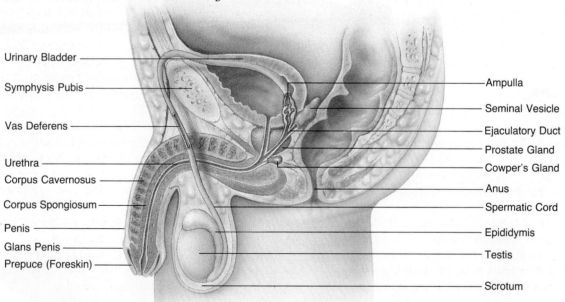

Urinary Bladder

Symphysis Pubis

Vas Deferens

Urethra
Corpus Cavernosus

Corpus Spongiosum

Penis

Glans Penis

Prepuce (Foreskin)

Ampulla

Seminal Vesicle

Ejaculatory Duct

Prostate Gland

Cowper's Gland

Anus

Spermatic Cord

Epididymis

Testis

Scrotum

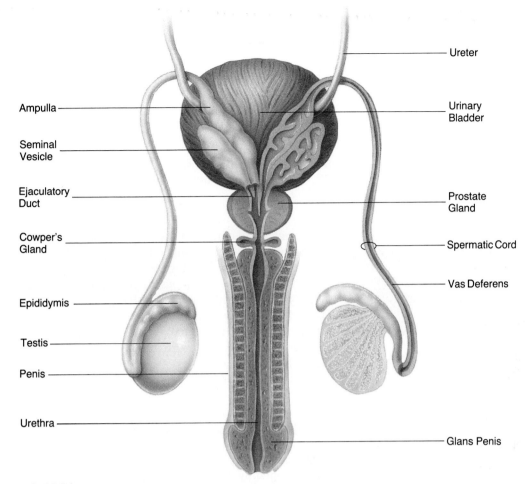

Ampulla

Seminal
Vesicle

Ejaculatory
Duct

Cowper's
Gland

Epididymis

Testis

Penis

Urethra

Ureter

Urinary
Bladder

Prostate
Gland

Spermatic Cord

Vas Deferens

Glans Penis

FIGURE 5.3 • Posterior view of the male reproductive organs.

efferentia, out of the testes to the *epididymis,* where the sperm are stored and nourished. Some of the sperm then proceed to the *ampulla,* by way of the *vas deferens,* and accumulate there until expelled at some later time. The vas deferens is encased in the *spermatic cord. Seminal vesicles* located nearby provide nutrients for the sperm's further maturation. When *ejaculation* (forceful exit of *semen* during *orgasm*) is about to occur, the seminal vesicles empty into the ejaculatory duct, and the sperm pass through this duct into the *urethra.* As shown in Figures 5.2 and 5.3, the urethra passes through the *prostrate,* which secretes a substance that helps increase sperm life. Next, the sperm pass through the urethra, which has been lubricated by the secretion of the *Cowper's gland.* This secretion neutralizes any acidity remaining in the urethra from urine. Any *preejaculatory fluid* that may be noticed is really secretion from the Cowper's gland, but it may also contain some sperm. The sperm next pass into the *penis,* which has become erect due to sexual stimulation, causing the arterioles leading to the *corpora cavernosa* to dilate. This dilation results in the corpora cavernosa becoming engorged with blood and thereby erect.

The head of the penis is called the *glans penis* and is covered by a foreskin called the *prepuce.* For hygienic, cultural, or religious reasons, the foreskin is sometimes surgically removed. Removal of the foreskin—called *circumcision*—is more usual in the United States than it

is in other countries. Figure 5.4 shows how circumcision is performed.

The rationale of circumcision, other than cultural or religious reasons, is medical. Several glands are located in the foreskin that secrete an oily substance that if not removed from under the foreskin can combine with dead skin cells to form a cheesy substance called *smegma.* If not removed it can irritate the glans penis, causing discomfort and possibly infection. However, if a man washes daily and removes the smegma, there will be no irritation. The only verifiable health-related reason for circumcision pertains to recent studies indicating that circumcised male infants experience fewer urinary tract infections than noncircumcised ones. Still, these studies need to be verified before medical practitioners are justified in recommending circumcision as a routine procedure.

Ejaculation is the result of contractions of muscles in the glands and ducts of the male reproductive system. The ampulla and seminal vesicles contract, as does the *bulbocavernosa muscle,* which surround the *corpora spongiosa* of the penis. The semen, or ejaculate, consists of fluids from the seminal vesicles, prostate, and Cowper's gland, as well as sperm. Each ejaculate contains, on the average, 300 million sperm.

Male hormone production in the male reproductive system is accomplished by the interstitial cells, which lie between the seminiferous tubules.

external genitalia Those parts of the female genitalia that can be clearly seen.

internal genitalia Those parts of the genitalia that are within the body and are not directly observable.

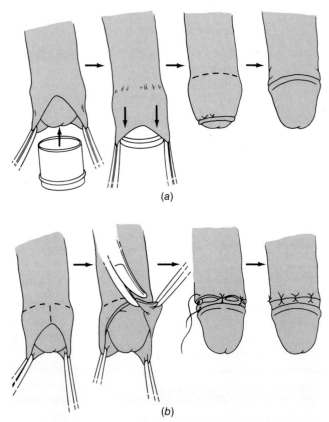

FIGURE 5.4 • Methods of performing circumcision. *(a)* In this method, a piece of plastic is placed over the glans and the foreskin is stretched over the plastic and trimmed off. *(b)* In this method, the foreskin is carefully cut "freehand" and then stitched.

Use Exploring Your Health 5.1 to test your knowledge of the male reproductive system.

The Female Reproductive System

The female reproductive system includes structures on the outside of the body that can be readily seen. These are called the **external genitalia.** The structures not easily observable are those located within the body. These are called the **internal genitalia.**

External Structures   The external structures of the female reproductive system are known collectively as the *vulva* and consist of the mons veneris, labia majora, labia minora, vestibule, clitoris, and hymen. Figure 5.5 provides a view of the external female genitals.

The *mons veneris,* or *mons pubis,* is a fleshy pad, usually covered with pubic hair, that extends back and divides to form the *labia majora,* the two large outer lips of the vulva. During sexual excitement, the labia majora become engorged with blood and pull back to open the vulva.

Just inside the labia majora lie two folds of tissue called the *labia minora.* Loaded with blood vessels and nerve receptors, the labia minora are very sensitive to stimulation. During sexual excitement, the blood vessels fill with blood, spreading the labia minora to reveal the shallow cavity called the *vestibule,* in which the vaginal opening, urethral (urinary) opening, and clitoris are located.

The upper part of the labia minora forms a hood for the small, sensitive *clitoris.* Similar (homologous) to the penis in the male, the clitoris contains a large number of nerve cells and has a corpora cavernosa (like the penis), but not a corpora spongiosa. During sexual excitement, the corpora cavernosa becomes engorged with blood and erect (like the penis).

The last external structure is the *hymen,* a thin membrane that separates the vestibule from the vagina. Although its function is uncertain, the hymen may protect the internal genitals from infection early in life. Most women find that the hymen stretches or breaks with relative ease when they masturbate, insert tampons, exercise, or experience their first sexual intercourse. However, a physician may have to remove the hymen surgically if the membrane is very thick.

Figure 5.5 also depicts a section of skin that extends from the bottom of the vulva to the anus. During childbirth, this piece of skin, called the *perineum,* is sometimes surgically cut to prevent tearing when the baby's head exits the vagina. This procedure is called an *episiotomy.*

Internal Structures   Figure 5.6 depicts the relationship of the external and internal structures in the female reproductive system. The *vagina* is the tubular passageway that leads from the vaginal opening on the outside of the body to the uterus or "womb" on the inside. The vagina is an elastic organ whose walls con-

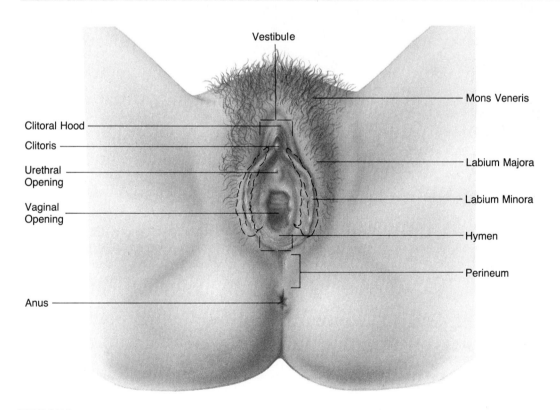

FIGURE 5.5 • Female external reproductive organs.

tain muscular membranes that stretch during sexual arousal to accommodate the penis and that expand during childbirth to let the baby pass through. The walls of the vagina are also covered with tissues that secrete a lubricant that is the first physical sign of female sexual arousal. The female's menstrual flow also leaves the body through the vagina.

Figure 5.7 offers a more detailed look at the female's internal reproductive organs. The *uterus* is a thick-walled muscular organ the size and shape of a pear. The mouth of the uterus, termed the *cervix,* extends into the vagina. The other end of the uterus is termed the *fundus.* It consists of three layers. The outermost layer is the *perimetrium,* which is very elastic and

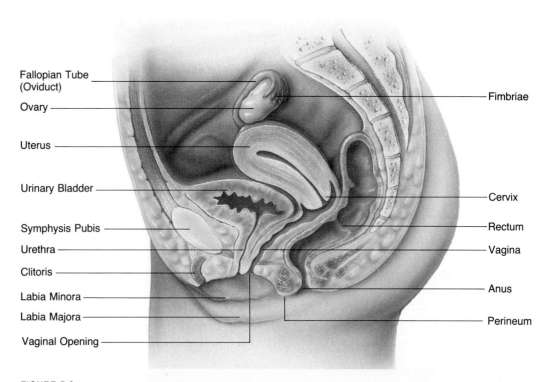

Fallopian Tube (Oviduct)

Ovary

Uterus

Urinary Bladder

Symphysis Pubis

Urethra

Clitoris

Labia Minora

Labia Majora

Vaginal Opening

Fimbriae

Cervix

Rectum

Vagina

Anus

Perineum

FIGURE 5.6 • Organs of the female reproductive system.

allows the uterus to expand during pregnancy. The middle layer, the *myometrium,* is muscular (smooth muscle) and can contract to push the newborn out through the cervix and into the birth canal (vagina). The inner layer is the *endometrium,* which is abundant in blood vessels and is partly discharged during menstruation. It is in the uterus that the fertilized *ovum* (egg) is implanted and develops into an *embryo* (to twelve weeks) and then a *fetus* (after twelve weeks).

Leading from the uterus back toward the ovaries are the *Fallopian tubes,* also called *oviducts,* which are hollow and have muscular walls. The sperm usually fertilizes the ovum in one tube or the other. Once fertilized, the ovum passes down the Fallopian tube toward the uterus.

When a female is born, she already has a supply of about half a million immature eggs (ova) in each of the two almond-shaped ovaries. Each egg (ovum) is covered by a thin tissue called the *follicle.* When the female reaches puberty, the eggs begin to mature and their follicles burst open, releasing the eggs. Normally, only

one egg is released each month. The ovum is caught by one of the *fimbria,* the fingerlike projections that jut out from the end of the Fallopian tubes. The ovaries are also responsible for the production of the female hormones estrogen and progesterone.

Sexual Response

In this section, we describe the typical human sexual response and then discuss both the similarities and the differences in this response between males and females.

The Sexual Response Cycle

The most significant research in the area of human sexual response was conducted by William Masters and Virginia Johnson.[1] They found that the human

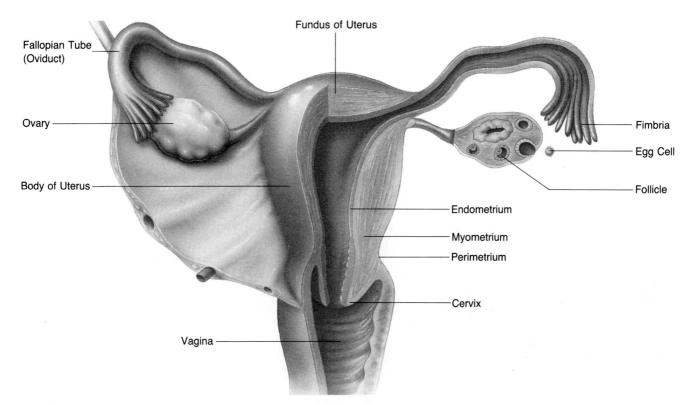

FIGURE 5.7 • An anterior view of the female reproductive organs showing the relationship of the ovaries, uterine tubes, uterus, cervix, and vagina.

Exploring Your Health 5.2

The Female Reproductive System

To test your understanding of the female reproductive system, see if you can match the following numbered items with the lettered items that most pertain to them.

Correct Letter	Numbered Item	Lettered Item
_____	1. Labia majora	a. Labia majora, labia minora, clitoris, hymen, and vestibule
_____	2. Vulva	b. Two thin folds of tissue loaded with blood vessels and nerve receptors
_____	3. Labia minora	c. Two large folds of tissue surrounding the external genitalia
_____	4. Clitoris	d. A thin connective tissue
_____	5. Vestibule	e. The birth canal
_____	6. Hymen	f. Contains the vaginal and urethral openings
_____	7. Vagina	g. Homologous to the penis
_____	8. Uterus	h. Where ova are stored prior to being discharged
_____	9. Ovary	i. Where the egg is usually fertilized
_____	10. Fallopian tubes	j. Where the fertilized egg is implanted and nourished

sexual response could be divided into four distinct phases:

1. **Excitement phase.** This phase begins with sexual stimulation of some sort, whether physical, psychological (thoughts), or both. Sexual arousal in males is indicated by erection of the penis and in females in vaginal lubrication.

2. **Plateau phase.** If the excitement phase is not interrupted, sexual tension is intensified. In the male, preejaculatory fluid is emitted at this point; in the female, the clitoris retracts under its hood.

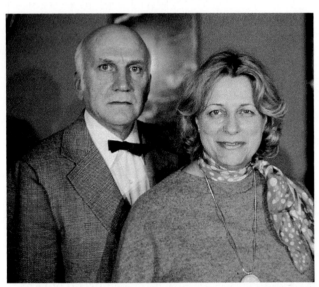

William Masters and Virginia Johnson are the researchers who have done the most to help us understand how our bodies respond to sexual stimulation. They have also been influential in encouraging sexual counseling for people with sexual dysfunctions.

3. **Orgasmic phase.** This phase consists of an *orgasm,* the involuntary muscular contraction concentrated in the clitoris, vagina, and uterus in the female and in the penis, prostate, and seminal vesicles in the male. It is in this phase that the male ejaculates.

4. **Resolution phase.** After orgasm, sexual tension is dissipated and the person returns to the pre-excitement state. Although the female can return to the orgasmic phase if sexually stimulated during resolution, the male enters a refractory period during which sexual stimulation cannot produce another full erection. In other words, females are capable of multiple orgasms, or orgasms close in time to one another, whereas males are not.

Similarities in Male and Female Response

Masters and Johnson found a number of similarities in the sexual response of males and females.

- **Nipples.** Erection of the nipples is evident in both sexes. In an early study, Masters and Johnson found nipple erection in 30 percent of men; however, they later upgraded that figure to 50 to 60 percent on the basis of further research. Not only do the nipples become erect in both sexes, they also increase in diameter.

- **Sex flush.** During high levels of sexual tension, due to *vasocongestion* (a lot of blood accumulating in an area), both sexes experience a darkening of the skin. This sex flush occurs on the neck, face, and forehead on both males and females, as well as on the chest.

- **Muscle tension.** Medically termed *myotonia,* muscle tension in both sexes first develops during the plateau phase and involves the legs, arms, abdomen, neck, and face. In addition, both sexes contract the gluteal (buttocks) muscles before orgasm. During orgasm both sexes contract the muscles of the abdomen, chest, and face. Finally, muscle tension is released by both sexes during the resolution phase. No difference has been observed between the sexes in rapidity of muscle tension release.[2]

- **Deep and rapid breathing.** Termed *hyperventilation,* deep and rapid breathing occurs in both sexes.

- **Increased heart rate.** Both sexes experience *tachycardia* (increased heart rate). During the orgasmic phase, Masters and Johnson found heart rates to increase up to 180-plus beats per minute.

Males and females respond to sexual stimulation in both similar and dissimilar ways. Still, female responses tend to be more varied than male responses.

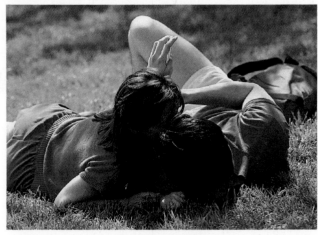

- **Increased blood pressure.** Blood pressure is elevated significantly in both males and females during sexual excitement.
- **Perspiration.** Approximately 32 percent of both sexes will develop involuntary sweating immediately following orgasm.
- **Vasocongestion.** Increased blood flow to the pelvic area occurs in both sexes, causing penile erection in the male and vaginal lubrication in the female. In addition, vasocongestion results in elevation of the male scrotal sac, and elevation of the labia majora in females who have never given birth and a thickening and separation of the labia in females who have borne children.

Differences in Male and Female Response

The differences between males and females in their physiological and anatomical sexual responses include the following:

- **Nipples.** Though both sexes experience nipple erection during sexual stimulation, females more often experience their erection during the excitement phase. Males also experience nipple erection during the excitement phase but are more apt to have it delayed until the plateau phase than are females. In addition, female nipple erection disappears rapidly after orgasm, whereas male nipple erection may be prolonged after ejaculation.
- **Sex flush.** Though both exhibit a sex flush, the female experiences it late in the excitement phase or early in the plateau phase, whereas the male sex flush occurs only in the plateau phase. The neck, face, forehead, and chest of both sexes become flushed, but the flush is also evident on the lower abdomen, thighs, lower back, and buttocks of females only.
- **Muscle tension.** Myotonia results in an increase in the length of the vagina and expansion of the

diameter of the cervix in females. In males, elevation of the testes occurs.

- **Deep and rapid breathing.** Both sexes experience hyperventilation before orgasm. Once orgasm has occurred, the male must wait for hyperventilation to subside during the resolution phase before he can be orgasmic again. However, the female can move from one orgasm to the next (can be multiorgasmic) without waiting for hyperventilation to subside.
- **Blood pressure.** Whereas blood pressure increases for both sexes, the range of increase differs. The increase in males is slightly higher than in females.
- **Perspiration.** In males, sweating after orgasm is predominantly confined to the soles of the feet and the palms of the hands. In females, it is more likely to occur on the back, thighs, and chest, and sometimes on the trunk, head, and neck.
- **Patterns of response and orgasm.** As shown in Figure 5.8a, males have an orgasm with a refractory period as part of their response cycle. Figure 5.8b shows that the female sexual response and orgasm can take several forms. Pattern A most closely resembles the male pattern, except that it shows the potential of the female for additional orgasms without the refractory period necessary for males. In Pattern B, the woman reaches the plateau level but does not have an orgasm, and in Pattern C she experiences a rapid rise to orgasm, followed by a quick resolution. Another important difference, as noted previously, is that multiple orgasms are within the capacity of most women, whereas men always experience a refractory period after orgasm. The fact that not nearly as many women actually have multiple orgasms as are capable of them may be related to the source of stimulation used to achieve orgasm. Masters and Johnson found that repeated orgasms are more often possible through manual, oral, or mechanical stimulation than through penile thrusting.

FIGURE 5.8a • The male sexual response cycle.

Source: W. H. Masters and V. E. Johnson, *Human Sexual Response* (Boston: Little, Brown and Company, 1966), p. 5. Courtesy W. H. Masters and V. E. Johnson.

FIGURE 5.8b • The female sexual response cycle.

Source: W. H. Masters and V. E. Johnson, *Human Sexual Response* (Boston: Little, Brown and Company, 1966), p. 5. Courtesy W. H. Masters and V. E. Johnson.

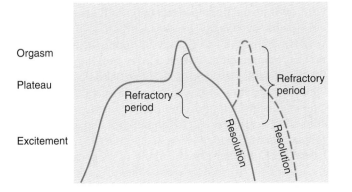

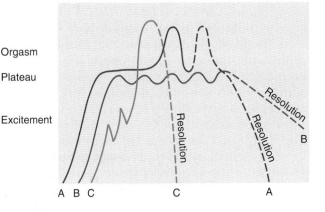

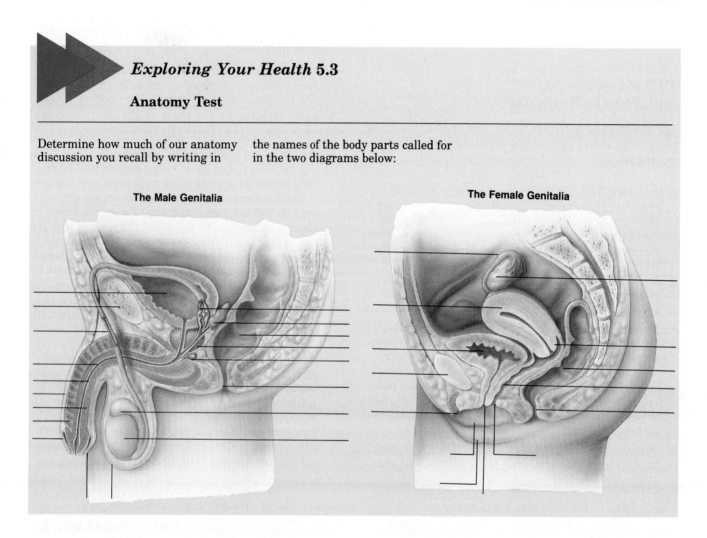
Forms of Sexual Expression

Until recently, our society imposed many restrictions on the forms of sexual expression that were considered appropriate. Today, however, a much wider range of behaviors is regarded as acceptable. Sexual intercourse is only one of many sexual choices. Indeed, people may choose different forms of sexual expression under different circumstances or at different times in their lives. Our sexual attitudes and behavior are influenced by what we think others regard as appropriate. As you read the following sections, consider to what degree your own sexual behavior has been influenced by what your peers are doing.

The most extensive study of human sexual behavior was conducted by Alfred Kinsey and his colleagues in the 1940s and 1950s.[3] These researchers interviewed thousands of people of various socioeconomic status, educational attainment, marital status, and sex education experiences. Although published in 1948 *(Sexual Behavior in the Human Male)* and 1953 *(Sexual Behavior in the Human Female)*, their studies are still con-

Issues in Health

Frequently Asked Questions and Controversies About Sex

Presented below are some of the more frequently asked questions about sex and sexuality and some of the controversial issues related to sex.

1. Does the size of the penis affect the female's sexual satisfaction?
Because the vagina is replete with nerve endings in its outer third and contains very few nerve endings in its inner two-thirds, and because the vagina is capable of grasping an object of any diameter, penis length or width is physiologically irrelevant to female sexual satisfaction. However, as different-sized and -shaped breasts appeal to different males, so too may different-sized penises appeal to different females.

2. What is the G spot?
The *G spot* is an area on the anterior wall of the vagina that when stimulated elicits sexual excitement in some females. Its erotic potential was discovered by obstetrician Ernest Grafenberg in 1950, and its existence has become increasingly popularized. Not all women feel erotic sensation when the G spot is stimulated, and some sexuality experts even disagree as to the existence of a unique area in the vagina that differs from other areas nearby.

3. Is there such a thing as a female ejaculation?
There are some sexuality researchers who believe women possess glands similar to the male prostate glands called Skene's glands. They argue that many women expel a fluid from the vagina during orgasm that comes from these glands. However, other experts disagree. Some have even tested this fluid to determine if it is similar or dissimilar to prostatic fluid. Some have reported it to be like urine, and others have reported it to be like fluid of the prostate. Whether women ejaculate is still a matter of much debate.

4. Do women have different kinds of orgasms?
Masters and Johnson reported that an orgasm was an orgasm was an orgasm, regardless of whether it resulted from stimulation of the vagina or the clitoris. However, Shere Hite surveyed women and found many reported that a clitoral orgasm was much more intense than a vaginal one. Sexual therapist Helen Singer Kaplan's experience leads her to agree with Hite. However, even if different types of orgasms are felt differently, the physiological process is the same.

5. Is it alright to engage in sexual intercourse during the time when a woman is menstruating?
There is no reason—other than their own preferences—why people cannot engage in sexual intercourse during menstruation . For those who object to the sight of blood or who view this as unclean, or for those for whom sexual intercourse at this time is religiously proscribed—for example, Orthodox Jews—refraining during menstruation may be necessary. For others, it is no problem. However, some precautions may be required. For example, so as not to irritate his glans penis with the blood products, the male might want to wear a condom. In addition, the woman might consider inserting a diaphragm to hold back the flow.

sidered the landmark research in American sexual behavior. In our discussion of forms of sexual expression, we will refer to some of the Kinsey findings, as well as to more recent studies.

Masturbation

Masturbation refers to erotic self-stimulation, usually to the point of orgasm. It has been practiced in all societies since ancient times. Even infants explore their genitals and receive pleasure from touching them. Often self-stimulation continues throughout life, whether or not the individual is a partner in a permanent intimate relationship.

Gender apparently has a substantial effect on the practice of masturbation, with males more likely to masturbate than females. This is probably the result of differences in socialization between males and females. A 1972 study of the masturbatory behavior of college students found that 80 percent of freshman males but only 33 percent of freshman females had engaged in masturbation (see Table 5.1). However, the incidence for males and females in their senior year was nearly the same (about 75 percent).[4] Other researchers have found that approximately 90 percent of adult males and slightly over 60 percent of adult females report that they have masturbated.

Even though masturbation is quite widespread, many men and women still feel somewhat ashamed of the practice. This is probably a carryover from their upbringing and from folklore that stamped masturbation as sinful, evil, and even physically and mentally harmful. Such ideas are entirely false, and today sex therapists and other experts believe that masturbation can be beneficial. It serves as a sexual outlet, a way to become more comfortable with one's own body in heterosexual lovemaking, and an alternative form of sexual expression when no partner is available.

cunnilingus The act of sucking or licking the vulva.

fellatio The act of sucking or licking the penis or scrotum.

coitus Sexual intercourse, specifically penile-vaginal intercourse.

premature ejaculation The inability to control the timing of ejaculation by the male during coitus, often resulting in a lack of sexual satisfaction on the part of the female.

TABLE 5.1

College Students' Sexual Behavior

Independent Variable	Number	Incidence of Masturbation (%)	Frequency of Masturbation*	Incidence of Sexual Intercourse (%)
Sex				
Male	52	84.62	6.73	76.93
Female	75	52.00	1.82	69.33
Marital status				
Married	21	61.90	2.81	100.00
Not married	106	66.04	4.04	72.45
Class in school				
Freshman				
Male		80.00		
Female		33.33		
Total	27	51.85	4.07	51.85
Sophomore				
Male		100.00		
Female		50.00		
Total	29	55.17	1.62	72.41
Junior				
Male		90.48		
Female		57.14		
Total	42	73.81	3.86	76.19
Senior				
Male		75.00		
Female		76.92		
Total	29	75.86	5.79	86.21
Race				
Negro	7	33.33	0.57	55.56
Caucasian	111	76.24	4.17	80.20
Other	9	42.86	2.22	85.71

* Number of times per month.

Source: Jerrold S. Greenberg, "The Masturbatory Behavior of College Students," *Psychology in the Schools* 9(1972): 427–432. Reprinted with permission.

Petting and Oral Sex

Petting is defined as erotic stimulation of a person by a sexual partner, without actual sexual intercourse. It can include kisses, genital caresses, and oral-genital contact, and may culminate in orgasm. During adolescence, petting is often a way for young people to experience intense sexual excitement without actually engaging in intercourse. Petting is carried over into adult sexual relationships as foreplay or for sexual variety.

Oral-genital stimulation takes two basic forms. **Cunnilingus** is the act of sucking or licking the vulva, and **fellatio** is the act of sucking or licking the penis and scrotum. Until recently, oral sex was viewed negatively by many people in the United States. Some have objected for religious reasons (because oral sex does not lead to procreation), others for sanitary reasons, and others because they feel uncomfortable about engaging in it. In Kinsey's surveys, only 15 percent of high school-educated married men reported engaging in cunnilingus. However, more recent surveys suggest that oral-genital sex is becoming increasingly widespread. In a study conducted by Hunt in the 1970s, a majority of both male and female respondents under the age of 25 reported engaging in cunnilingus and fellatio. Other researchers have reported that 80 percent of college students[5] and virtually 100 percent of adults in general have experienced oral-genital sex.[6]

Sexual Intercourse

Sexual intercourse, or **coitus,** is penile-vaginal intercourse. It usually begins with petting, and when the partners are sufficiently aroused, the penis is guided into the vagina. Almost all men have an orgasm with every intercourse, but this is not true of all women. A survey of 26,000 people conducted by *Redbook* magazine and published in 1987 found that 60 percent of women had an orgasm every time or almost every time they had intercourse.[7] A major reason that women do not have a high rate of orgasm during intercourse is that intercourse alone may not provide sufficient clitoral stimulation. For many women, manual stimulation of the clitoris during intercourse or choosing a position that permits effective penile stimulation of the clitoris are effective means of reaching climax.

The incidence of young people engaging in sexual intercourse has been rising in recent years. In a study of college students conducted by Parcel in the mid-1970s, 40 percent of freshmen, 55 percent of sophomores, 73 percent of juniors, and 85 percent of seniors reported having engaged in sexual intercourse.[8] Other researchers have found that two-thirds of college students had experienced sexual intercourse.[9] The most profound change in incidence has occurred among women. Only 33 percent in Kinsey's sample of female subjects under 25 years of age reported engaging in

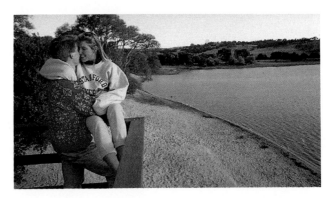

Humans are sexual beings. It is quite natural to have sexual desires. However, just because someone has an interest in sex does not mean they are ready to engage in all forms of sexual activity. Level of maturity, commitment, or concern for health may dictate restraint.

sexual intercourse, compared to 75 percent of Hunt's sample. In 1988, the National Center for Health Statistics reported that 83 percent of married women had experienced sexual intercourse before age 25.[10] The incidence for males has not increased significantly since Kinsey's study, so it appears that women are now "catching up" to men in terms of their sexual experience. Recent studies have also shown that both males and females are having their first experience of intercourse at an earlier age, many by age 14 or 15.

Sexual Dysfunction

Although occasionally an individual may not be able to function sexually—for example, after drinking a lot of alcohol—these infrequent occurrences need not cause alarm. But if such occasions are the rule rather than the exception, there may be a problem requiring expert attention.

Sexual Problems in Males

The two most prevalent sexual problems in males are premature ejaculation and erectile dysfunction, although these are certainly not the only sexual problems that males experience.

Premature Ejaculation   **Premature ejaculation** is the inability to control timing of the ejaculate, resulting in a lack of sexual satisfaction for one's partner. The difficulty in defining this condition lies in one's perception about what is "premature." For example, Masters and Johnson described it premature if the male could not "control his ejaculatory process for a sufficient length of time during intravaginal containment to satisfy his partner in at least 50 percent of their coital connections".[11] However, another definition defines ejaculation as premature only if the man or his partner considers it premature. If they do not, regardless of the time before ejaculation, it is not premature. We choose to adopt this latter definition because

impotence The inability of the male to maintain an erection long enough to have sexual intercourse.

erectile dysfunction The correct term for describing difficulty in achieving and maintaining a penile erection; popularly known as "impotence."

ejaculatory incompetence The inability of a man to ejaculate into the vagina during coitus.

dyspareunia Painful sexual intercourse.

orgasmic dysfunction Inability to achieve orgasm.

sexual unresponsiveness The inability of a woman to experience erotic pleasure from sexual contact, popularly known as "frigidity."

vaginismus The involuntary tightening of the muscles of the vagina so that the penis cannot enter or so that dyspareunia results.

---

coitus is a shared act, with different couples having different expectations and seeking to meet different needs through the sexual connection.

However, when one or both sexual partners believe that premature ejaculation is a problem in their sexual encounters, the effects of ejaculating prematurely can be harmful to the relationship and to the psychological health of the man. Men may feel less than "manly" and may have a lowered self-esteem. Not wanting to reveal their problem, premature ejaculators may refrain from sexual intercourse, thereby disappointing their partners and making them wonder about the viability of the relationship. Because premature ejaculation is estimated to affect approximately 25 percent of college students,[12] the number affected—men and women—is not insignificant.

Dealing with Premature Ejaculation   Other than the rare cases caused by surgery, trauma, or disease, premature ejaculation is a function of the psyche; that is, the mind is not able to control the body's need to ejaculate. Several self-help techniques for overcoming rapid ejaculation have been proposed. Some men will drink an alcoholic beverage to decrease the rapidity of their sexual response. Others will allow themselves an orgasm rapidly, or a small orgasm, knowing that the next one will be longer in arriving. Waiting for sufficient vaginal lubrication may help prolong ejaculation. It seems that the glans penis may experience too much friction in the presence of insufficient lubrication of the vagina, causing increased sensitivity and rapid ejaculation. A condom reduces the direct stimulation to the glans penis and may help delay the ejaculatory response. Relaxing or switching positions so as to decrease muscle tension is another recommended control technique. Too much muscular tension encourages rapid ejaculation. Lastly, creams designed to decrease sensitivity can be purchased and placed on the glans penis. Whether the benefit of controlling the ejaculate is worth the price of deadened sensations during coitus is a decision that only the sexual partners can make.

Fortunately, there is a proven, effective treatment for premature ejaculation. Developed by Masters and Johnson and described in detail in their book, *Human Sexual Inadequacy,* the "squeeze" technique is easily applied, effective, and well publicized so that sexual counselors and therapists are aware of it. The technique involves squeezing the glans penis by the man's partner when ejaculation is approaching. Repetition of this technique in several subsequent lovemaking sessions usually helps the man "learn" to delay his ejaculation.

Erectile Dysfunction   Men's difficulty in achieving and maintaining an erection is popularly known as **impotence.** The derivation of the term impotence is from Latin and means "without power." The word impotence is used to connote that a man has lost power—is no longer "manly"—when he cannot achieve or maintain an erection. Furthermore, he has lost power as a lover and has lost his reproductive capacity. The more professional, sensitive, and accurate term is **erectile dysfunction.** Men who have never had an erection sufficient for sexual intercourse are said to have *primary erectile dysfunction.* Men who have previously been able to maintain an erection long enough to have intercourse but subsequently developed an erection problem are said to have *secondary erectile dysfunction.* Secondary erectile dysfunction is approximately ten times more prevalent than primary erectile dysfunction.

Erectile dysfunction can be caused by a myriad of factors. While it was previously believed that most erectile dysfunctions were caused by psychological factors, more recent information suggests that 50 to 60 percent of such cases are at least partially the result of physiological factors.[13] Among these factors are diabetes infections; the use of drugs or medications; alcoholism; spinal cord injury; injuries to the penis, testes, urethra, or prostate; and any conditions that interfere with the flow of blood to the erectile tissue of the penis.[14] In addition, kidney disease, nerve damage (for example, from surgery), endocrine abnormalities, and neurological problems can also cause erectile dysfunction.

Among the nonorganic causes are fear of sexual performance—"Will I be an adequate sexual partner or show my ineptitude?" This fear can result in a self-fulfilling prophecy; that is, fear may make the man so anxious that he *is* unable to achieve and maintain an erection and his worst fears are realized. The result could be a lowered self-esteem that contributes to the original fear. Thus a cycle of erectile dysfunction develops. In addition, guilt about sex or shame regarding one's involvement in sex can interfere with an erection.

Ejaculatory Incompetence   For some men, the problem is not ejaculating too soon but, rather, not being able to ejaculate in the vagina at all. This condition is known as **ejaculatory incompetence,** sometimes referred to as *retarded ejaculation.* When a man has never ejaculated in the vagina and is incapable of doing so, he is classified as having *primary ejaculatory incompetence.* When he has previously been able to ejaculate in the vagina but can no longer do so, he is classified as having *secondary ejaculatory incompetence.* Men with these problems may still be able to maintain an erection and stay sexually aroused, but they can't ejaculate in the vagina. Nevertheless, they may be able to ejaculate by masturbating or through oral-genital stimulation. Treatment involves counseling to identify and respond to the causes of ejaculatory dysfunction.

Dyspareunia   Painful sexual intercourse is called **dyspareunia.** During sexual intercourse, men may feel pain in the penis, testes, or some other internal part of their bodies. Infections of the penis, foreskin, testes, urethra, or the prostate can cause such pain, as can allergic reactions to a spermicidal cream or foam that may be used as a contraceptive. When intrauterine devices (IUDs) were more available, some men reported irritation of the glans penis from the string attached to the IUD which extended out of the uterus into the vagina.

There are still other causes of dyspareunia in men. A foreskin that is too tight can cause pain when an erection develops; smegma that has not been washed away from the glans penis can develop into an infection and irritate the glans; and Peyronie's disease, where fibrous tissue and calcium deposits develop in the area around the cavernous bodies of the penis, may also create pain during sexual intercourse. Treatment involves identifying the cause and eliminating it through surgery or behavioral changes.

Sexual Problems in Females

The most common causes of sexual dysfunction in females are orgasmic dysfunction, sexual unresponsiveness, dyspareunia, and vaginismus.

Orgasmic Dysfunction   Although they may enjoy sexual intercourse, some females are *anorgasmic;* that is, they cannot or can at best rarely achieve an orgasm.

Orgasmic dysfunction may be caused by such psychological factors as anger, guilt, fear, embarrassment concerning one's body, or hostility. It may also be caused by factors external to the woman; for example, an inexperienced partner, inappropriate setting (such as the uncomfortable back seat of a car), or alcohol. Lack of orgasm in young women is usually caused by one of these external factors.

Other causes of orgasmic dysfunction are anatomical defects in the female reproductive system, hormonal deficiency or imbalance, disorders of the nervous system, drugs, and alcohol. Note the similarity between the causes of female orgasmic dysfunction and the causes of male erectile dysfunction.

Therapy for orgasmic dysfunction that is psychological in nature usually involves both partners because communication between the partners is often at the core of the problem. A knowledgeable, understanding, and aware sexual partner is an important part of the therapy for orgasmic dysfunction.

Sexual Unresponsiveness   This disorder used to be called *frigidity,* but therapists have dropped this value-laden term. **Sexual unresponsiveness** is defined as the inability to experience erotic pleasure from sexual contact. Some women with this problem are difficult to treat because they show evidence of personality disorders. Unhealthy socialization may contribute to the attitude that sex is sinful or that men are exploiters. Contrary to popular belief, however, rape does not seem to be a cause of this sexual dysfunction, although women who are raped may temporarily not want to engage in sexual relations.

Dyspareunia   In females, **dyspareunia** (painful intercourse) can stem from physical or psychological causes. Painful intercourse might result from irritation of the vaginal barrel by the glans of the penis or insufficient lubrication of the vagina resulting from physical causes. Dyspareunia can also result from too frequent intercourse or from insufficient vaginal lubrication due to insufficient sexual stimulation. Psychological reasons can also cause painful intercourse. For example, feelings of shame, guilt, or embarrassment can result in such tension that vaginal muscles will not widen enough when the penis is inserted, making intercourse painful (one such condition is *vaginismus,* described below). Because dyspareunia makes sexual intercourse unenjoyable, coitally active women should seek medical examination as soon as possible.

Vaginismus   In **vaginismus,** the muscles in the vagina involuntarily tighten so that the penis either cannot enter or causes a good deal of pain when it does enter. This condition is primarily psychological in origin; therefore, the treatment is psychological in na-

inhibited sexual desire (ISD) A lack of sexual appetite or a disinterest in sexual activity.

Exploring Your Health 5.4

Sex Knowledge Inventory

Circle the correct answer for each statement.

	True	False
1. The most satisfying position is with the male on top of the female.	T	F
2. Sex during menstruation is unclean and harmful.	T	F
3. Sex should be avoided during pregnancy.	T	F
4. A small penis is less satisfying to a woman than a large one.	T	F
5. Prostitutes are either frigid or homosexual or both.	T	F
6. It's good to sublimate the sex drive for long periods.	T	F
7. An excessively amorous woman is a nymphomaniac.	T	F

	True	False
8. Advancing age means the end of sex.	T	F
9. Any person who can't have sexual relations with a partner is suffering from severe psychiatric problems.	T	F

Answers. These statements are all untrue. Here are the correct answers:

1. The most satisfying sexual position varies with the individuals and the situation.
2. Coitus during menstruation is safe and healthy and depends only upon the personal preferences of the individuals involved.
3. Sex during pregnancy is safe except for women who have a history of miscarriage or other serious difficulties in their pregnancies.
4. The vagina expands to the size of the penis, and contracts around it; therefore the size of the penis is not related to either partner's satisfaction during coitus.

5. Women become prostitutes for many reasons. Their private sexual lives are often similar to other people's sexual lives.
6. There is no benefit in sublimating the sex drive for long periods, since the only result will be frustration.
7. An "excessively" amorous woman may be just that—amorous. There is no reason to believe that women who enjoy a lot of sexual activity are abnormal.
8. Old age requires some adjustments to sexual activity—for example, lubrication of the vagina with jelly may be necessary and penile erection may take longer—but not an end.
9. Although the predominant causes of sexual dysfunction are psychological, there are other reasons for sexual dysfunction—for example, a medical condition.

ture. Conditions found to be related to vaginismus include a sexual relationship with an impotent man, religious guilt, a traumatic sexual experience, or dyspareunia.

Inhibited Sexual Desire

Sexual therapist Helen Singer Kaplan described **inhibited sexual desire (ISD)** as a lack of sexual appetite.[15]

It is characterized by a disinterest in sexual activity. Both males and females experience ISD. The definition of ISD is difficult, as are the definitions of several of the other sexual dysfunctions. Since each person's interest in sex varies, when is little interest really too little? When the disinterest is specific to a sexual partner, is it the partner's fault or ISD? One attempt to define ISD is based on a number of orgasms experienced in a certain time period. For example, Schover diagnoses ISD when

Issues in Health

Does Sexual Dysfunction Exist if the Couple Doesn't Perceive There to Be a Problem?

Some people argue that the purpose of sex is to experience pleasure and demonstrate love for another person. If those purposes are met, regardless of the actual physiological sexual response, the sexual union has been effective. In this case, no sexual dysfunction is present. For example, if a man can't maintain penile insertion without ejaculating immediately, or if a woman can't experience an orgasm during coitus, but nevertheless they are sexually satisfied and their relationship is healthy, then no problem exists. Furthermore, to tell this couple that they have a sexual problem when they were unaware of one in the first place is to do them a dis-

service. This couple should be left alone rather than made to feel that they are abnormal and their relationship is in need of repair.

Others argue that mere ignorance of the potential of a couple's sexual relationship is no excuse for not responding to abnormal sexual patterns. Men who don't have control of their ejaculate and women who aren't able to have an orgasm during sexual intercourse can have their conditions remedied with sex therapy. Given the effectiveness of sexual therapy for most sexual disorders, it would be unfortunate not to help people whose sexual lives could be even more fulfilling than they are

now. Consequently, it is the ethical responsibility of the sexual therapist to point out to the couple the potential sexual satisfaction they are unaware of and to guide them into a therapeutic setting. Ignorance is not necessarily bliss; and in this circumstance, it definitely isn't.

If you were a sexual therapist and were made aware of a couple that could respond better sexually but were happy with their sexual lives as they were, would you point out to them ways in which they could be even more sexually functional? Or would you leave them in their present state of sexual ignorance and sexual satisfaction?

Source: Jerrold S. Greenberg, Clint E. Bruess, Kathy Mullen, and Doris W. Sands, *Sexuality: Insights and Issues* (Dubuque, Iowa: Wm. C. Brown, 1989).

the person experiences less than one orgasm every two weeks from masturbation or sexual activity with a partner.[16] This definition ignores the fact that some women may be interested in sex but are anorgasmic. However, in spite of this oversight, and as with several other dysfunctions discussed in this chapter, if the person or the couple does not perceive a sexual problem to exist, perhaps one doesn't. If the degree of interest in sex is similar between two people in a relationship, and the relationship is otherwise a healthy one, should therapists be advising the couple that they have a problem? Should they be attempting to change the couple's degree of interest in sex? What if the couple accommodates one person's lack of interest in sex by adopting sexual behaviors to meet the interested person's needs; for example, if the disinterested person engages in oral-genital sex to satisfy the interest of the partner? Does this situation need correcting? These are not easy questions to answer as one of this chapter's Issues in Health boxes discusses.

The causes of ISD are, for the most part, psychogenic. The majority of these cases are the result of such factors as poor self-esteem, a poor relationship, embarrassment regarding one's body, or a history of sexual abuse. ISD can also develop in response to another sexual dysfunction. For example, a man who has erectile dysfunction may develop a lack of interest in sex. When the thought of or opportunity for sex is presented, rather than becoming excited, this man may only envision a threat to his self-image and, quite naturally, lack interest.

It should be emphasized that a temporary sexual dysfunction upon occasion is not unusual, but a frequently recurring or permanent dysfunction should be of concern. There are effective means of helping both males and females to overcome these problems. If you feel that you have a sexual problem, you should seek counseling. Perhaps the place to start is with your own physician. If your physician determines that no physical problem exists, he or she can refer you to a reputable sexual or psychological counselor.

Sexual Diversity

Homosexuality

We briefly discussed homosexual lifestyles in the last chapter. As we learned there, *lesbianism* in women and *homosexuality* in men (both herein termed "homosexuality") refer to a sexual preference for persons of the same sex. People in the homosexual community often refer to themselves as "gay" and to heterosexuals as "straight."

There are many reasons for homosexual behavior. People who would judge homosexual behavior harshly should realize that one need not be homosexual to have had a homosexual experience. For instance, 37 percent of the males and 13 percent of the females studied by Kinsey et al. reported at least some overt homosexual experience resulting in orgasm. Some people are isolated from the opposite sex (for example,

bisexual Describes persons who engage in sexual behavior with males on some occasions and with females on other occasions.

rape The sexual penetration of an individual (usually female) against that individual's will.

statutory rape Unlawful sexual intercourse with a minor.

those in prisons, all-male or all-female schools, or the military), and their only opportunity for sexual activity (other than masturbation) is with someone of the same sex. These situational homosexuals usually are heterosexual when given the choice. Others experiment with homosexual behavior during adolescence but soon behave exclusively heterosexually. A small percentage of people are **bisexual;** that is, they engage in sexual behavior with males on some occasions and with females on others. It has been estimated that 4 percent of males and 2 percent of females are exclusively homosexual,[17] although homosexual groups cite 10 percent of the total population as gay.

Sexual activities in which homosexuals engage are both similar and dissimilar to those engaged in by heterosexuals. Obviously, penile-vaginal intercourse is not possible. However, as with straights, gay partners kiss and caress, and stimulate erogenous and genital areas by hand and mouth.[18] Anal intercourse also used to be prevalent among gay men. However, with an extensive

Homosexuality is prevalent in our society, so much so that elected officials of some of our largest cities believe they cannot be elected without the support of the local gay community.

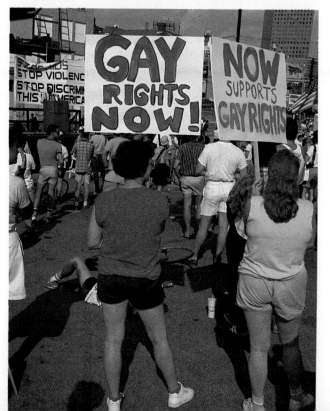

educational campaign in the gay community identifying anal intercourse as a high risk behavior for the contraction of AIDS, fewer gay men are engaging in anal intercourse. It is interesting to note that homosexual men and women sometimes report more satisfying sexual relationships than do heterosexual couples.[19] It seems that in such cases, gay men and women communicate their desires and feelings to their sexual partners more effectively than do straights. Still, this is not universally true. There are noncommunicative homosexuals as there are noncommunicative heterosexuals.

Myths about Homosexuality Many myths have been perpetuated about homosexuality. Perhaps one reason for this is that most of the early researchers who studied homosexuality used the only sample available to them—homosexuals who sought psychological counseling or therapy or homosexuals in psychiatric institutions. Encouraged by the current trend toward acceptance of the gay lifestyle and aided by the political activities of homosexuals themselves, many homosexuals who function well and are productive members of society have "come out of the closet"—that is, they no longer hide their sexual preference. Research using this new sample of homosexuals suggests that many of the earlier findings were inaccurate. Here are some of the popular myths that have been dispelled by research:

- **Homosexuals are more promiscuous than heterosexuals.** Some are and some aren't. Gay relationships are similar to straight ones. Some homosexuals maintain a single long-term relation ship, whereas others seek out sexual variety. This is equally true of heterosexuals.
- **Homosexuals are likely to seduce young children.** The data just does not support this myth.
- **Homosexuality is abnormal.** The term "abnormal" is a relative one. What is abnormal in one society or culture may be normal behavior in another. Homosexuality has been acceptable in many cultures throughout history.
- **It is easy to recognize homosexuals by how they walk or talk.** Only a small percentage of homosexuals walk with a "swish" or talk in an effeminate or (in the case of lesbians) "butch"

manner. Most are indistinguishable from heterosexuals.

- **Homosexuals can be "cured" by having sexual relationships with the "right" persons of the opposite sex.** There is no known, effective, and agreed-upon manner to change one's sexual preference. How our sexual preference develops remains unclear and, therefore, how to change it is also unclear.
- **There are more female homosexuals than male homosexuals.** As we've stated earlier, there are apparently double the number of male homosexuals as female homosexuals.
- **Homosexuals have more psychological problems than heterosexuals.** Several studies have found that there is no difference between the mental health of homosexuals and heterosexuals.[20]

Homosexuality and Society Until recently, homosexuality was considered a psychiatric illness. In 1973, however, the American Psychiatric Association reclassified homosexuality so that it is no longer considered a mental disorder. In the past, homosexuals were considered poor security risks, sometimes treated as criminals, and generally rejected by American society. More recently, homosexuals have become a powerful, organized political force. For example, it is said that a person who does not have the support of homosexuals cannot be elected mayor of San Francisco, where the homosexual population is large and well organized.

With research findings showing that most homosexuals are mentally healthy, productive members of society and have sexual lifestyles that are similar to heterosexual couples, homosexuality is becoming more acceptable and homosexuals are generally experiencing less prejudice and homophobia.

However, in spite of these more accepting attitudes, the fear of AIDS and the recognition that it has spread through the homosexual community first and then to the heterosexual community has led to a resurfacing of homophobic attitudes on the part of some people. In addition, homosexuals argue that discriminatory practices still exist, and they point to the fact that health insurance companies screen potential new insurees to eliminate suspected homosexuals that they fear may become AIDS victims.

Sexual Variations

Sexual variations refer to a category of behavior characterized by sexual interest in objects rather than people or by coitis performed under bizarre circumstances. People who engage in certain variant sexual behaviors are often assumed to have a personality disorder. The following behaviors are among the sexual variations

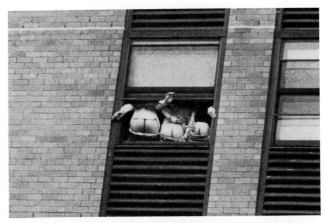

Sexual assault takes many different forms, one of which is exposing oneself to others who do not wish to be confronted in this way. Is "mooning" a sexual assault? Have you ever engaged in that activity?

that usually come to the attention of psychiatrists and psychologists:

- **Fetishism.** A compulsion in which sexual arousal is brought about only by a specific object (for example, articles of clothing) or a specific part of the body (for example, the feet).
- **Exhibitionism.** Exposure of one's genitals to involuntary observers.
- **Necrophilia.** Sexual relations with a dead body.
- **Bestiality.** Sexual relations with an animal.
- **Voyeurism.** Watching others engage in sexual behaviors as one's primary means of sexual arousal. A voyeur is a "Peeping Tom."
- **Transvestism.** Dressing up in the clothing of the opposite sex—usually, males who dress as females.
- **Transsexualism.** Gender identification with the opposite sex. For example, a person with male genitalia feeling closer gender identity with females and feeling trapped in a male's body. Sometimes, a person who identifies very strongly with the opposite sex undergoes a series of hormone treatments and a surgical procedure ("a sex-change operation") to try to assume characteristics of the opposite sex.
- **Pedophilia.** Sexual relations between a child and an adult.

Sexuality and the Law

In recent years, sex-related crimes— particularly rape and incest—have been the subject of growing concern.

Rape

Rape is defined as sexual penetration of an individual (usually female) against her will. **Statutory rape** is a

date rape Forcible sexual intercourse by one's date.

acquaintance rape Forcible sexual intercourse by anyone known to the victim.

incest Sexual intercourse or coercive sexual contact between close blood relatives.

special category referring to unlawful sexual intercourse with a female minor. The "age of consent" varies from twelve to twenty-one years, depending on the state one lives in. If a male participates in sexual intercourse with a minor, he is committing statutory rape in spite of the female's willingness, assistance, or initiation of the intercourse. In 1981, the Supreme Court upheld the constitutionality of the statutory rape laws, stating that, because female minors are in jeopardy of pregnancy, they should be uniquely protected by such laws.

Many popular misconceptions contribute to the problems of women who are raped. For example, many people still believe that rape victims "ask for it" or that women secretly enjoy being raped. Until recently, it was permissible to reveal a rape victim's past sexual history at a rape trial as a means of discrediting her testimony. As a result of pressure from women's advocates, many states now prohibit this practice. Even so, much needs to be done to erase the myths surrounding rape.

What do we know about rape? Although many people believe that the rapist and victim are usually of different races, in fact in 90 to 95 percent of cases, they are of the same race. According to the Uniform Crime Reports, over half of those arrested for rape were under 25 years of age, and half the victims were under 21. Although young women may be more frequent victims, females of all ages, from children to elderly, have been rape victims.

Men are occasionally the victims of rape by women or other men. Many cases of male rape occur in prison, in the military, and in other situations where heterosexual opportunities are restricted. Rape counselors report that male rape victims suffer physical and psychological injuries that are very similar to those experienced by female victims. However, male rape victims are generally less willing than female victims to report that they have been raped, for fear of social stigma.[21]

Date Rape and Acquaintance Rape

Two forms of rape that have been in the news a great deal in the last few years are date rape and acquaintance rape. It has been estimated that 70 to 80 percent of all rapes

are committed by men the victim knows.[22] However, more and more women are speaking out about male dates and acquaintances who assume that a woman they take to dinner or share some other activity with are simply "ready and willing" to have sex.

Date rape is forcible sexual intercourse by one's date. One researcher of date rape concluded:[23]

1. Although 25 percent of women say they have been coerced into having sexual intercourse, only 15 percent meet the legal definition of rape.

2. Only 29 percent of men denied any form of sexually aggressive behavior, and 15 percent admitted having coitus against the woman's will.

3. Sixty-one percent of men admitted that they fondled a woman against her will, 42 percent had removed clothing, and 37 percent had touched a woman's genitals against her will.

4. Thirty-five percent of men had ignored a woman's protest, 11 percent had used physical restraint, 6 percent had used threats, and 3 percent had used physical violence to coerce sex.

Acquaintance rape is forcible sexual intercourse by anyone known to the victim. Date rape is thus actually a kind of acquaintance rape. However, many women have reported being raped by men they were not dating—men who were even supposedly "friends" with whom the women would occasionally get together or see in apartment or dormitory hallways.

How should we deal with date and acquaintance rape? Many colleges and universities have sponsored programs to educate men about rape and the pain and suffering rape causes. Every man must realize and respect (1) that when a date says "No," she means "NO!," and (2) that casual conversation or other contact with a particular woman does not at all mean that she is interested in sex with that man. Unfortunately, in our society, the way we typically communicate about sex is by cues and innuendo. Consequently, when a woman says "No," the man might think that she just wants to be talked into it. This is hopefully changing now, particularly in view of the sexual openness and compassion that the threat of infections with AIDS and other sexually transmitted diseases demands.

Even one rape is a serious problem, but when we realize that every hour sixteen women confront rap-

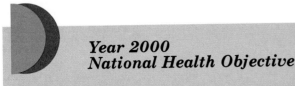
ists; that a woman is raped every six minutes; that the United States has a rape rate thirteen times higher than Britain's, nearly four times higher than Germany's, and more than twenty times higher than Japan's,[24] the magnitude of the problem takes on a new dimension.

Why Men Commit Rape There are two main theories about why men commit rape. One hypothesis connects rape with personality disturbance, such as the inability to control impulsive behaviors. The other hypothesis is that rapists are more likely than nonrapists to accept the unsupported myths about rape that are prevalent in our society. For example, they may be more likely to believe that women unconsciously wish to be raped, that women who are raped are sexually provocative, or that women enjoy violent sex. The research on these theories has not yet yielded clear results, and more study is needed.

Rape on college campuses has recently become a problem, and many colleges are now taking precautions against rape. These include better lighting, security gates, locking dormitories after a certain hour, escort services during evening hours, rape counseling and education programs, campus police patrolling the most likely rape locations, and even the distribution of rape whistles. What is your campus doing in this regard? How could you help?

Figure 5.9 illustrates self-defense techniques that can be employed against a potential rapist. Although there is still controversy about whether a rape victim should resist her attacker, most experts believe that if you can resist without risking serious harm, you should do so; however, if the attacker has a gun, knife, or other lethal weapon, the best course of action may be to submit and then seek an opportunity to escape.

Some experts argue that women should not attempt self-defense tactics when raped. Since most rapists are young men, they will probably be much stronger than their victims. In such cases, the following actions may help:

1. Speak calmly and try to give the impression of assuredness. Although it will be difficult, try not to be flustered.

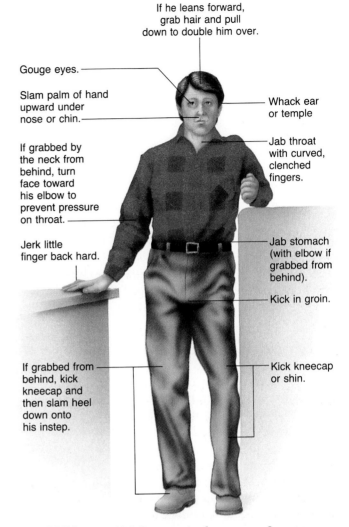

FIGURE 5.9 • Self-defense tactics for women. Some women learn "street fighting" tactics like these to ward off a sexual assault. If a woman chooses to use such tactics when she is attacked, speed, vigor, and a feeling of being in control of the situation are crucial to her ability to escape. If she struggles unsuccessfully, her attacker may become more violent.

Source: From *Sexual Choices*, 2e, by G. D. Nass, R. W. Libby, and M. P. Fisher, p. 397. Copyright © 1981, 1984 by Wadsworth, Inc. Reprinted by permission of Wadsworth Health Sciences Division, Monterey, Calif. 93940.

2. Try flattery. Make the rapist feel as though he is the best thing since sliced bread.

3. Bargain to cooperate if he doesn't harm you. Ask him to place down his weapon.

4. Tell the rapist that you sympathize with his feelings, desires, and situation, and ask him if he can sympathize with yours.

5. At all costs, try not to make the rapist angry. Do not threaten him or state how you will later retaliate.

Incest

Incest technically refers to sexual intercourse between close blood relatives. However, many therapists and researchers now define incest as any form of coercive sexual contact (not only intercourse) between a child and a relative, including stepparents and adoptive parents. Incest often engenders feelings of helplessness, guilt, shame, and anger in both parties. People (teachers, pediatricians) whose occupations bring them in contact with children are often the ones who report these incestuous relationships once the child opens up to them.

The most common form of reported incest is between father and daughter. The incestuous father is typically aggressive and domineering and may be a heavy drinker. In many cases, the mother is passive or submissive and frequently suffers from such problems as depression, alcoholism, or major illness. Because the mother's disabilities interfere with her maternal re-

sponsibilities, most tasks are shifted to the oldest daughter, to whom the father turns for emotional and sexual satisfaction.

Various community organizations offer help to incest victims and their families. These include child-protection agencies, rape crisis centers, women's centers, and organizations offering parents help to manage stressors that they associate with their children. In addition, programs to prevent incest have been developed and conducted in schools and elsewhere in communities.

When a case of incest is identified, the initial focus is upon stopping the sexual abuse and establishing a safe environment in the family. It is controversial as to whether or not the child should be temporarily re-

A Question of Ethics

Should College Students Maintain Monogamous Relationships?

Pro Some people believe college students should not engage in sexual activities at all, and certainly not sexual intercourse. However, if they insist on doing so, supporters of this view argue that college students should limit their activities to a steady boyfriend or girlfriend. Not to do so, they insist, is to act immorally. Furthermore, if college students become promiscuous—that is, have sex with several different partners, although not necessarily all at the same time—they increase the chance of contracting a sexually transmitted disease. Given society's concentrated effort to limit the spread of AIDS, and the fact that AIDS is incurable and fatal, it seems prudent to encourage monogamous relationships on college campuses. The dramatic recent increase in the incidence of syphilis is also cited as a rationale for sexual abstinence or, at the very

least, monogamy among college students. Lastly, many adults consider college to be a "training ground" for students, preparing them for entry into our society—entry as competent, moral, contributing members. To accept, or even expect, infidelity is to teach the wrong lesson; one that will not serve our society's future well.

Con Others believe advocates of monogamy on the part of college students are misguided. They argue that when students limit themselves to just one partner, they lose the advantages that varied sexual experiences afford—advantages such as learning how to interact and be intimate with different people. Varied sexual experiences, they argue, can enhance the self-esteem of college students by developing the knowledge that they are desirable. The opportunity to try out different sexual

techniques, thereby learning how to be a sexually satisfying partner, is also seen as an advantage of varied sexual behavior. Opponents of monogamy insist that if one of the purposes of college is to prepare students for the roles they will play after they graduate, then surely preparation for a sexual future should not be ignored. As regards the potential for contracting a sexually transmitted disease, students should be encouraged to practice "safe sex" rather than encouraged to be abstinent or monogamous. The use of condoms should be recommended, and "risky" behaviors, such as anal intercourse, discouraged. With these precautions, they claim, there is no reason to be concerned about contacting an STD.

What do you think? Should monogamy be encouraged on your campus? Will you make it a part of your life?

moved from the home. This might be destructive to the child by encouraging the feeling that she has done something wrong, that she is being punished, and that both parents are against her. Yet, if removal from the home is the only way to stop the abuse, it should be done.

The adult person committing incest can be treated by placing him in jail, by psychiatric counseling, by medication to decrease his urge for sex, or by a combination of these approaches. However, given the present state of knowledge, no one can claim to "cure" incest; rather, the behavior can be brought under control.[25]

Sexual Behavior: Deciding for Yourself

People engage in sexual activity for many reasons, some of which are more acceptable in our society than others. For example, sex for having babies or as an expression of intimacy and love tends to be more acceptable than sex for fun or as a remedy for loneliness. Each individual evaluates sexual behavior according to his or her own values and morals. Thus it is difficult to decide objectively which expressions of sexual activity and which purposes are "right" and which are "wrong."

How do you use sexual behavior? You have probably used sex for many reasons: perhaps to show your love, to relieve boredom, for excitement, or because it was expected of you. Analyze how you use sexual behavior. In this manner, you will be making more sense out of your sexual lifestyle.

Sex and the College Student

Though sexual behavior is important throughout one's life, it seems especially important during the college years. We have already noted one study in which it was found that 52 percent of freshmen had experienced sexual intercourse, and by the time they were seniors, 86 percent had. Another study found that 40 percent of freshman and 85 percent of seniors had experienced sexual intercourse. It seems obvious that, at least concerning sexual intercourse, colleges truly are institutions for learning. This is understandable when several factors are considered. First, many students are away from home for the first time and are experimenting with a new-found freedom. This experimentation is manifested in their sexual behavior as well as in other areas of their lives. Related to this is the need to find new friends and achieve a new status among peers on the campus, a process that took years to accomplish back home. Sexual behavior might seem to be an easy

solution to some. A female might think about how popular she could be if she were more sexually active. A male might want to become a bigshot by bragging about "sexual conquests." Some students do use sex this way.

Some people cite the availability of contraception as another reason for increased sexual activity during

Get Involved!

Sexual Health and Sexual Responsibility

You can contribute to the sexual health of your society while responding to your own sexual needs. Listed subsequently are several things you can do to achieve this goal:

1. Do not manipulate or coerce other people into having sex with you. Remember that psychological coercion is just as bad as physical coercion.

2. If you are a man or woman thinking about having sexual intercourse or a man thinking about having oral or anal sex with another man, be prepared to use a condom. Although there is no such thing as "safe sex," there is "safer sex." Your use of a condom will help prevent the spread of AIDS and other sexually transmitted diseases (STDs). Of course, if you are not considering a committed, monogamous relationship, you may do best to avoid sexual intercourse for now—that is, remain *abstinent*.

3. Refrain from prejudicial behaviors toward people whose sexual orientation is different from yours. Although, for example, no one has the right to require you to view homosexuality as "moral" if your religious beliefs dictate otherwise, you do not have the right to violate the basic human rights of gay people.

4. Sex and humor often mix well, but seldom in the case of sexual dysfunctions. If you become aware of a friend's or relative's sexual dysfunction, try to help by keeping others from ridiculing that person. Use good judgment about whether you should approach that person to let him or her know that you care. If it seems wise, tell that person that effective treatment is available, and that you are willing to help him or her find such treatment.

5. Report sexual crimes immediately. You might consider a "Peeping Tom" (voyeur) or an exhibitionist merely a nuisance rather than a threat. However, people with these tendencies sometimes commit more violent sexual crimes, such as rape and child molestation. By reporting these people to the proper authorities, you may help prevent a neighbor from being the victim of such a crime or a worse crime in the future.

As you can see, sexual responsibility begins in your own bedroom, but there are other ways you can be socially responsible with sexuality. Can you think of some other ways that you can help improve the sexual health of your society?

sexual harassment The threatening sexual advances made by someone in authority or in a position of power toward subordinates.

the college years. Students reach legal age during college and are offered sexual counseling or health services on campus. Thus contraceptives are more available to college students than ever before. This is another reason why sexual behavior during the college years deserves special consideration.

Sex and AIDS

A new factor to consider in sexual decision making is the concern for contracting Acquired Immune Deficiency Syndrome (AIDS). We discuss AIDS in detail in Chapter 14, so our presentation here is limited. Suffice it to say that AIDS is a sexually transmitted disease that has no known cure and is invariably fatal. It is transmitted by contact with bodily fluids such as semen and blood. Consequently, having sex with someone who has been exposed to the AIDS-causing virus places you in danger of also developing AIDS. Although people speak of "safe sex," there really is no such thing. Although you can decrease your chances of contracting AIDS by wearing a condom and by keeping your sexual partners to a minimum, any sexual contact is liable to transmit the AIDS virus. Some suggest the answer is abstinence; others argue for more monogamous relationships; and still others believe everyone should be tested for AIDS. The problem with testing people for AIDS is that the antibodies to the AIDS virus (which is what the test actually identifies) may take up to a year

to develop. Therefore, someone declared AIDS-free may not actually be so. Sounds complicated, doesn't it? Well, you're right; it is. Nonetheless, you should consider all of these issues before deciding on your sexual behavior.

Sex Beyond College

Obviously, sexual decision making is also necessary beyond the college years. Married couples must decide how often they should engage in sexual relations and in what form: that is, which sexual activities are acceptable to them and which are not. They must also decide whether to limit their sexual activity to their mate or engage in extramarital sex. Single adults must also decide how sexually active to be. AIDS is also a consideration in these decisions.

Whether single or married, adults who work outside the home must often decide whether a sexual advance constitutes **sexual harassment**—sexual advances made by someone of power or authority who threatens firing, lack of promotion, or some other sanction if sex is declined—and if so what to do about it.

Sexual decision making is a part of living. It is inescapable. The best we can do for ourselves is to make these decisions as logically and rationally as we can after we have gathered the pertinent information.

Conclusion

Although there are differences between males and females, there are also many similarities. Both males and females have external and internal genitalia, many of their sexual responses are similar, and the forms of sexual expression they use are the same. Both males and females may also experience sexual dysfunction, and either can be homosexual. We too often forget the sameness of people and exaggerate the differences. We have learned in this chapter to be aware of both.

We strongly urge that you consider your sexual

behavior as seriously as you consider any other important aspect of your life. Make decisions regarding your sexual behavior after consideration of your values, needs, desires, alternative choices, the consequences of these choices, and the realization that your choice need not be etched in stone. If you are unhappy with your sexual behavior after considering these factors, a change of behavior may be in order. That change requires some careful thought as well.

Summary

1. Sexuality is part of who you are: the roles you play, the societal expectations you adopt. Sex, on the other hand, is something you do: kissing, petting, having intercourse.

2. The male reproductive system consists of external structures—the scrotum and the penis—and internal structures—the urethra, testes, vas deferens, seminal vesicle, prostate and Cowper's glands, and the ampulla.

3. The female reproductive system consists of external structures—the labia majora, labia minora, and clitoris—and internal structures—the vagina, uterus, Fallopian tubes, and ovaries.

4. The human sexual response cycle consists of four phases: the excitement phase, the plateau phase, the orgasmic phase, and the resolution phase.

5. In some respects, females and males are similar in their sexual responses. For example, when sexually aroused, they both experience nipple erection, sex flush, muscle tension, deep and rapid breathing, and increases in heart rate and blood pressure.

6. In other respects, females and males differ in their sexual responses. For example, when sexually aroused, male blood pressure increases more, female perspiration is more widespread, and females can be multiorgasmic, whereas males experience a refractory period.

7. Sexual expression takes many forms. Masturbation—experienced by about 75 percent of college seniors—is one form of sexual expression; others are petting, oral sex, and intercourse.

8. Cunnilingus is the oral stimulation of the vulva, and fellatio is the oral stimulation of the penis and scrotum. Oral-genital sexual behavior is more prevalent today than it was when Kinsey conducted his landmark studies.

9. Male sexual dysfunctions include premature ejaculation, erectile dysfunction (previously termed impotence), ejaculatory incompetence, and dyspareunia. Female sexual dysfunctions include orgasmic dysfunction, sexual unresponsiveness (previously termed frigidity), dyspareunia, and vaginismus.

10. Inhibited sexual desire (ISD) is a lack of sexual appetite; a lack of interest in sexual activity. ISD may be experienced by males or females and is usually a function of some environmental or psychological factor such as shame, guilt, or embarrassment about sex.

11. Homosexuals have become more politically active and better organized in recent years. Consequently, homosexuality is accepted more by society as an alternative lifestyle. That acceptance has been tempered somewhat by the recent societal fear of AIDS.

12. Some of the more common forms of sexual variations, often referred to as deviant behavior, are fetishism, exhibitionism, necrophilia, bestiality, voyeurism, transvestism, transsexualism and pedophilia.

13. Rape is forcible sexual intercourse and occurs more often than most people realize. Date rape is of particular significance for college students since they frequently date people whom they do not know very well. Date rape and acquaintance rape can best be prevented by communicating openly and honestly about sex.

14. Incest is any form of coercive sexual contact between a child and a relative, including stepparents and adoptive parents. It most often occurs between father and daughter, with the incestuous father frequently being aggressive, domineering, and alcoholic. Treatment programs for both parents and children have been established to deal with incest and the problems it entails.

Questions for Personal Growth

1. We regularly care for our automobiles. We make sure they have the right fuel, that they are tuned up, that they are checked periodically for worn fan belts or loose wires, and that they are clean in appearance. Now that you've learned about your sexuality, what will you do regularly to care for your sexual self?

2. Which sexual response described in this chapter most surprises you? Do you think other people you know would also be surprised to learn of this sexual response?

3. How did you feel when you learned that females have more variety relative to their sexual response cycles than do males? How do you think people of the opposite gender feel when they learn this fact?

4. Which sexual misconceptions and myths did you believe to be true before reading this chapter? How prevalent do you think these misconceptions and myths are? Where do you think they usually originate?

5. Are there any forms of sexual expression that you

believe are inappropriate? Immoral? Why do you believe this? How do you think you developed these beliefs? How pervasive do you think these beliefs are in the United States? In other countries?

6. If you were experiencing a sexual dysfunction, what would you do? Would you be embarrassed to discuss your dysfunction with your friends? With your family? If so, why? Would you feel comfortable discussing your dysfunction with your physician or a sexual therapist?

7. How do you think you would feel if your sexual partner experienced a sexual dysfunction? Would you be supportive? Would your ego be threatened? Would you feel comfortable discussing your partner's dysfunction with him or her and offering advice about what to do to treat the dysfunction? Or would you be too embarrassed to discuss the matter at all?

References

1. William H. Masters and Virginia Johnson, *Human Sexual Response* (Boston: Little, Brown, 1966).

2. Ibid., p. 277.

3. Alfred C. Kinsey et al., *Sexual Behavior in the Human Female* (Philadelphia: W. B. Saunders, 1953), and Alfred C. Kinsey et al., *Sexual Behavior in the Human Male* (Philadelphia: W. B. Saunders, 1948).

4. Jerrold S. Greenberg, "The Masturbatory Behavior of College Students," *Psychology in the Schools* 9 (1972): 427–432.

5. Morton Hunt, *Sexual Behavior in the 1970s* (Chicago: Playboy Press, 1974).

6. M. D. Story, "A Comparison of University Experience with Various Sexual Outlets in 1974 and 1984," *Journal of Sex Education and Therapy* 11 (1985): 35–41.

7. Carin Rubinstein and Carol Tavris, "Special Survey Results," *Redbook* (September 1987): 147–149.

8. Guy S. Parcel, "A Study of the Relationship Between Contraceptive Attitudes and Behavior in a Group of Unmarried University Students," doctoral dissertation (Pennsylvania State University, 1974).

9. M. Hildebrand and S. Abramowitz, "Sexuality on Campus: Changes in Attitudes and Behaviors During the 1970s," *Journal of College Student Personnel* 25 (1984): 534–538, and D. Daher, C. Greaves, and A. Supton, "Sexuality in the College Years," *Journal of College Student Psychotherapy* 2 (1988): 115–126.

10. Christine A. Bachrach and Marjorie C. Horn, "Sexual Activity Among U.S. Women of Reproductive Age," *American Journal of Public Health* 78 (1988): 320–321.

11. William H. Masters and Virginia Johnson, *Human Sexual Inadequacy* (Boston: Little, Brown, 1970), p. 92.

12. Robert Crooks and Karla Baur, *Our Sexuality,* 3e (Menlo Park, Calif.: Benjamin Cummings, 1987), p. 542.

13. T. Crenshaw, "Medical Causes of Sexual Dysfunction," paper presented at the American AASECT 1984 Regional Conference (Las Vegas, October 1984).

14. David Stipp, "Better Prognosis: Research on Impotence Upsets Idea That It Is Usually Psychological," *The Wall Street Journal* (April 14, 1987): 1, 25.

15. Helen Singer Kaplan, *Disorder of Sexual Desire* (New York: Simon & Schuster, 1979).

16. L. Schover, J. Friedman, S. Weiler, J. Heiman, and J. Piccolo, "Multiaxial Problem-Oriented System for Sexual Dysfunctions," *Archives of General Psychiatry* 39 (1982): 614–619.

17. P. W. Blumstein and P. Schwartz, *American Couples* (New York: William Morrow, 1983).

18. Adelaide Haas and Kurt Haas, *Understanding Sexuality* (St. Louis: Times Mirror/Mosby, 1990), p. 348.

19. D. K. Sakheim, D. H. Barlow, J. G. Beck, and D. J. Abramson, "A Comparison of Male Heterosexual and Male Homosexual Patterns of Arousal," *Journal of Sex Research* 21 (1985): 183–198.

20. Judd Marmor, "Homosexuality: Nature Versus Nur-

ture," *The Harvard Medical School Mental Health Letter* 2 (1985): 5–6.

21. Nancy Gibbs, "When Is It Rape?," *Time* (June 3, 1991): 48–55.

22. Andrea Parrot, *Coping with Date Rape and Acquaintance Rape* (New York: Rosen, 1988), pp. 4–5.

23. "Date Rape Is Occurring Too Often, AU Professor Says," *Birmingham News* (March 23, 1987): 3B.

24. "Women Under Assault: Sex Crimes Finally Get the Nation's Attention," *Newsweek* (July 16, 1990): 23–24.

25. Judith Herman, "Father-Daughter Incest," in *Rape and Sexual Assault,* ed. Ann Wolbert Burgess (New York: Garland, 1985).

Fertility Control, Pregnancy, and Birth

CHAPTER OBJECTIVES

After reading this chapter, you should understand:

- How sex hormones work to regulate the male and female reproductive systems and, in particular, the female menstrual cycle.

- The types and uses of some of the many methods of contraception, including abstinence, the rhythm method, the condom, the diaphragm, the birth control pill, and other various new contraceptive technologies.

- Abortion methods for the first and second trimester of pregnancy and some of the issues surrounding the abortion controversy in the United States.

- How to determine pregnancy, as well as what to do and expect during gestation (the time from conception to birth).

- The childbirth process, including various kinds of delivery methods and what choices are available in terms of birthing environments and infant care.

- What causes infertility and how it can be treated.

CHAPTER OUTLINE

The Influence of Hormones

Conception Control

Abortion

Pregnancy

Childbirth

Infertility and Its Treatment

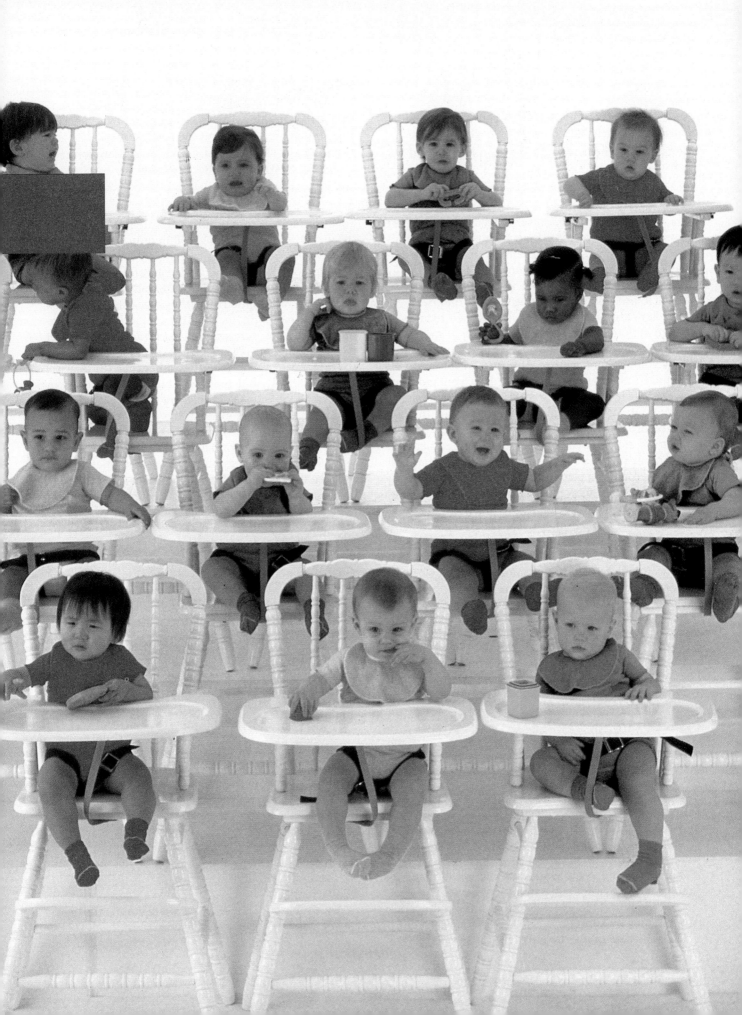

menstruation The "monthly" discharge of the endometrium and unfertilized ovum through the vagina.

menses The proper term for the monthly "period" of menstruation.

menarche The advent of menstruation in women, normally occurring between the ages of 9 and 14.

ovulation The release of one egg by an ovary, occurring in most women about once a month.

menopause The cessation in menstruation, normally occurring between the ages of 45 and 55.

As a college student, you have probably already come to several sexual crossroads: masturbation, a serious boy- or girlfriend, and perhaps even sexual intercourse. As a responsible person, you have probably also made some choices about what methods of birth control to use. You will continue to encounter new sexual crossroads, and the new decisions they require. A change in your sexual life—cohabitation or marriage, for example—may leave you feeling uncomfortable about your present method of birth control, and you will have to decide how to change it. If you and your partner decide to conceive a child, you must both make decisions about what and what not to include in your lives before, during, and after the pregnancy. Should you drink alcohol or take other drugs and, at least in the mother's case, possibly harm the fetus? What will be the method and place of delivery? Should you consent to the use of pain relievers? What will be the nature of the postdelivery phase?

Decisions about contraception and pregnancy are obviously very personal and are related to religious beliefs, value systems, and societal attitudes. These decisions can have an enormous impact on both physical and mental health, as well as on intimate relationships. This chapter offers some basic information about contraception, pregnancy, and birth so that you will be better prepared to make the decisions that are right for you in these areas of your life.

The Influence of Hormones

How Sex Hormones Work

When we previously discussed stress, we described the endocrine system. If you'll recall, we said that numerous body mechanisms, such as heart rate, blood pressure, and even the reproductive system are affected by the chemicals (hormones) secreted by endocrine glands. These glands are called "ductless" because they secrete their hormones directly into the bloodstream. Examples of endocrine glands are the pituitary, adrenal, thymus, thyroid, and parathyroid glands.

Once hormones are deposited into the bloodstream, they travel to their "target" organs where they affect that part of the body. The pituitary gland is a good example. The pituitary is located at the base of the brain and secretes eight different hormones. At least two of the hormones secreted by the pituitary affect reproduction: *follicle-stimulating hormone (FSH)* and *luteinizing hormone (LH)*. When FSH and LH are secreted they travel in the blood until they reach the female sex organs, stimulating the ovaries to produce still two other hormones; *estrogen* and *progesterone*. In males, LH is called *interstitial-cell stimulating hormone (ICSH)* since the target organs are the testes rather than the ovaries. If you'll recall from our description of the testes in Chapter 5, the interstitial cells are located between the seminiferous tubules in the testes and are responsible for manufacturing *testosterone* (male sex hormone), hence the term *interstitial-cell stimulating hormone* is used. This hormone stimulates the interstitial cells to produce testosterone. You may also hear people speak of the *gonadotropins*. Gonadotropins are hormones that have ovaries and testes (gonads) as their target organs. Therefore, FSH and LH (or ICSH) are sometimes referred to as gonadotropins.

During puberty, sex hormones are responsible for the development of secondary sexual characteristics. In females, estrogen triggers the developing of pubic hair, breasts, and fat deposits. In males, testosterone triggers the growth of pubic, facial, and chest hair; deepening of the voice; and muscle enlargement. The sex hormones also stimulate menstruation and ovulation in females and sperm production in males.

The Menstrual Cycle

Menstruation is a word derived from the Latin *menis,* meaning "month." Though considered to occur monthly, or about every 28 days, the **menses** (period) may be quite unpredictable. Beginning at **menarche** (from nine to fourteen or fifteen years of age) and ceasing at menopause (between forty-five and fifty-five years of age), menstruation is a normal physiological response to hormonal changes occurring in the female.

Several hormones are involved in menstruation. The menstrual cycle begins when the anterior portion of the pituitary gland secretes FSH, signaling the ovary to ripen one egg. The anterior portion of the pituitary gland also secretes LH, which aids in **ovulation** (the release of one egg by the ovary). Once the egg is released by the ovary, the area from which it was released, called the *Graafian follicle,* converts into a yellow body called the *corpus luteum.* The Graafian follicle secretes estrogen, and the corpus luteum secretes progesterone. Progesterone causes the endometrium (the inner layer) of the uterus to thicken and store nutrients in preparation to receive, implant, and nourish a fertilized egg. If the egg is not fertilized, the corpus luteum degenerates and is no longer able to secrete progesterone. The lack of progesterone is a signal to expel the unneeded nutrient-full endometrium, and menstrual flow, which empties the uterus, begins. The cycle is then ready to begin anew. Figure 6.1 depicts the phases of the menstrual cycle.

Menopause

Between the ages of forty-five and fifty-five, women usually begin **menopause.** Menopause is the end of the cyclical expulsion of the nourished endometrium. Menopause is the result of hormonal changes. Immediately preceding menopause, there is an increase in the secretion of gonadotropic hormones (FSH and LH). As a consequence, the feedback mechanism of estrogen and progesterone production upon the pituitary gland

FIGURE 6.1 • The 28-day menstrual cycle. In the ovaries: The pituitary gland secretes the gonadotropic hormones FSH and LH, which cause the follicle to develop and release a mature ovum (ovulation). After ovulation, the follicle degenerates into the corpus luteum. In the uterus: The developing follicle (mentioned previously) produces and releases the hormones estrogen and progesterone, which ready the endometrium (uterine lining) to receive the fertilized ovum. After about day 4 in the cycle, the endometrium begins to build up. After about day 28, if no fertilized ovum is present, the endometrium rapidly degenerates and menstruation occurs. Note the changes in basal body temperature during this cycle.

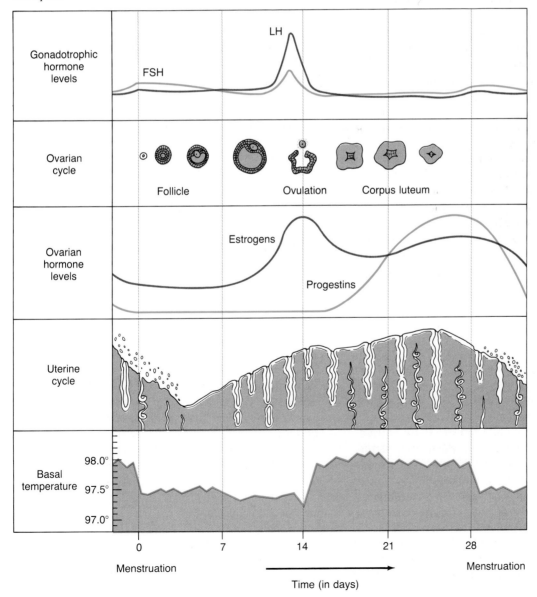

hot flashes Commonly experienced symptoms of menopause, hot flashes are sensations of heat caused by the irregular dilation of blood vessels, often in the face.

estrogen replacement therapy (ERT) Through medication, the artificial replacement of estrogen in menopausal women in order to alleviate the unpleasant symptoms of menopause.

osteoporosis The weakening of bones as a result of decalcification; found in most postmenopausal women.

contraception The prevention of fertilization of the ovum by the sperm.

is disturbed, resulting in the cessation of both ovulation and menstrual flow. Several physiological changes take place during menopause: thinning of the vaginal walls, narrowing and shortening of the vagina, and shrinking of the labia majora. In addition, there is less vaginal lubrication during sexual arousal, and uterine contractions during orgasm become stronger. These changes may make intercourse painful for a small number of women. Diminished vaginal lubrication may also increase the risk of vaginal infections. However, an extended period of foreplay may allow for enough lubrication to avoid pain and infection. The most commonly experienced menopausal symptom is **hot flashes,** sensations of heat caused by irregular dilation of the blood vessels, often in the face.

Estrogen Replacement Therapy (ERT)   Some physicians view menopause as a deficiency condition caused by insufficient amounts of estrogen. As a result, many women take prescription estrogen pills aimed at restoring the appropriate hormonal balance and thereby relieving symptoms. However, **estrogen replacement therapy (ERT)** is a controversial treatment, because studies have linked it to uterine cancer. Women taking estrogen pills were found to be six times more likely to develop cancer of the endometrium than women not taking estrogen. Consequently, some physicians recommend that women avoid estrogen replacement therapy. Instead, they recommend that menopausal symptoms be treated with relatively safe medications such as aspirin, tranquilizers, and antidepressants. However, nowadays, in addition to estrogen, progestin is administered for about ten days during the cycle. This appears to have significantly decreased the risk of endometrial cancer since the endometrial lining is sloughed off when progestin is used. This issue, however, has not been adequately determined to the satisfaction of all in the medical community. In addition, another concern about ERT was liver damage. The newer versions of ERT can be administered via a skin patch which facilitates the passage of estrogen directly into the blood, bypassing the liver and thereby decreasing the chances of damage to it. Because these newer ERT methods utilize estrogen more efficiently, they require smaller doses. With less

estrogen, there is less concern about unhealthy side effects.

ERT and Osteoporosis   Another important consideration regarding the appropriateness of ERT is the incidence of osteoporosis in postmenopausal women. **Osteoporosis** is the weakening of the bones as a result of decalcification. *Decalcification* (the loss of calcium) is a direct result of diminishing levels of estrogen; consequently, postmenopausal women are susceptible to developing osteoporosis. ERT can prevent osteoporosis, and many experts estimate that the changes of developing debilitating forms of osteoporosis without ERT are greater than the chances of developing cancer with ERT. As a result, many medical experts are now recommending that postmenopausal women, especially those experiencing disturbing symptoms of osteoporosis, be administered estrogen in combination with progestin. It should be remembered, however, that the long-term effects of ERT are unknown, and for that reason, the scientific community is not in total agreement on this recommendation. A report[1] of an increased risk of breast disease in women receiving ERT is also causing concern among medical experts. Research is presently being conducted to determine the extent of this risk.

Menopause: A Trauma?   Contrary to the notion that menopause is a major life trauma, most women make the transition smoothly. Many report increased interest in and enjoyment of sexual intercourse because the fear of pregnancy has been eliminated.[2] Eighty percent of menopausal women report mild menopausal symptoms or no symptoms at all. With understanding and patience, family members and friends can help menopausal women who may experience uncomfortable symptoms.

Do you know someone going through menopause? If you do, it might be useful to discuss with this person the changes she is experiencing. Too often menopause is considered inappropriate for discussion, and consequently some menopausal women who might need support from family and friends do not get it. Such support can be enormously useful in helping a woman cope with this life change.

Exploring Your Health 6.1

Menstruation

To test your understanding of the menstrual cycle, fill in the blanks in the following sentences:

1. The gonadotropic hormones produced by the pituitary gland are

_____ and _____.

2. FSH stimulates the production of the _____ from which the egg is released.

3. LH stimulates the development of the _____.

4. The place from which the egg is released from the ovary (answer to question 2 above) secretes the hormone _____. This hormone tells the pituitary gland to increase production of the hormone _____.

5. After 14 days of a 28-day menstrual cycle, the place from which the egg was released from the ovary secretes the hormone _____. This hormone tells the pituitary gland to slow down production of the hormone

_____ if the egg is not fertilized by a sperm.

6. During a 28-day menstrual cycle, ovulation occurs around day _____.

7. The menstrual flow continues for about _____ days during a 28-day cycle.

Consult Figure 6.1 *only* after filling in the blanks above, if you are unsure of your answers.

The Male Climacteric

There is evidence that men experience some physiological changes related to their reproductive system when they reach middle age, but these changes are not as obvious and rapid as the changes that occur in women. There is a gradual decline in production of testosterone, which causes a decrease in the frequency of erection, amount of ejaculate, and force of ejaculation. The testicles decrease slightly in size and the prostate gland enlarges. Some middle-aged men find that they require longer to achieve an erection than they did in their younger years. However, many men remain fertile throughout life.

Some men report physical symptoms related to the *male climacteric,* including erectile dysfunction, frequent urination, headaches, and even hot flashes. Changes in hormone levels may be related to some of these symptoms, but certain common aspects of middle age, such

as stress at work and reevaluation of life goals, also seem to play a large role. The psychological impact of the male climacteric is often referred to as the "midlife crisis," which is discussed in detail in Chapter 17.

Conception Control

Contraception is the prevention of the sperm from fertilizing the ovum, or of the ovum from successfully implanting on and being nourished by the endometrial lining of the uterus. In recent years, there have been great strides in contraceptive technology. Information on birth control is widely available. Such organizations as Planned Parenthood/World Population offer advice and information, as well as contraceptive devices, regardless of age or marital status.

There are many effective means to prevent pregnancy. Consequently, some experts argue that anyone who engages in sexual intercourse and doesn't plan to prevent conception is acting irresponsibly.

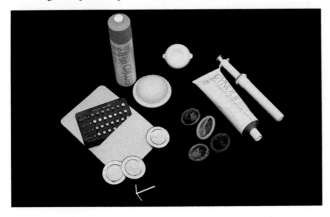

Year 2000 National Health Objective

A Year 2000 National Health Objective seeks to reduce pregnancies among girls age 17 and younger to no more than 50 per 1,000 adolescents. In 1985, that rate was 71.1 per 1,000 adolescents for girls age 15 through 17. This objective also specifically targets black and adolescent teenage girls age 15 to 19, since in 1985 their rates of pregnancy were 186 and 158 per 1,000 respectively. The year 2000 objectives seek to reduce those rates to 120 for blacks and 105 for Hispanic teenagers age 15 to 19.

abstinence Abstaining from sexual intercourse.

Nevertheless, the rate of adolescent pregnancy has increased dramatically in recent years. Research indicates that in the United States 109 out of 1,000 women between the ages of 15 and 19 become pregnant. Concern about the number of teenage pregnancies prompted the development of a national health objective to reduce this rate.

However, it's not only teenagers whose pregnancy rate is of concern to the government. The rate of pregnancies of unmarried women continues to be higher than Public Health Service officials would like.

Obviously, these young people either are not using contraception or are using it sporadically or incorrectly. In fact, studies show only one in three coitally active teenagers uses contraceptives consistently.[3] What are some of the factors that may influence people against using contraception?

The most obvious reasons are religious. Catholics, for example, have been taught that natural family planning is the only permissible contraceptive method. Nevertheless, a recent poll indicates that nearly the same percentage of Catholics are using other contraception as are non-Catholics. Because rhythm is not as effective as some other means of contraception, Catholics who want to adhere to their religious beliefs and at the same time want to limit the size of their families face a real dilemma. Some choose rhythm, whereas others opt for more effective methods.

Some of the reasons most frequently given for not using contraception are:

1. It (pregnancy) couldn't happen to me.
2. I feel guilty (immoral) if I plan in advance.
3. I'm too embarrassed to buy contraceptives.
4. Someone (for instance, parents) may find out I'm using contraceptives.
5. If I start using contraceptives, I won't be able to stop myself from participating more.
6. It wasn't a planned experience.
7. It hasn't happened yet (pregnancy or sexual intercourse), so it won't.
8. It's not natural to use contraceptives.
9. It ruins the fun.
10. I'm too lazy.
11. I could not imagine myself having a child.
12. I have intercourse too infrequently to be concerned with contraception.

In a recent study, female students seeking pregnancy tests at the University of Maryland were asked why they didn't use some method of birth control. Their answers are shown in Table 6.1. These students seem to be risk takers. They knew it was risky to engage in sexual intercourse without using some method of contraception, but they decided to take the chance anyhow. Would you make the same decision? A lack of planning seems to be another concern with college students using contraception. They just didn't think they would engage in sexual intercourse and, therefore, were not prepared with a method of contraception.

TABLE 6.1

Reasons Given by Female College Students for Not Using Birth Control at the Time of a Possible Pregnancy

	Percent Who Said:		
	Yes	No	Maybe
Wanted to become pregnant	0.0	100	0.0
Didn't think I'd have sex at the time	56.3	39.1	4.7
I'm not really very sexually active	45.9	47.5	6.6
Didn't think I'd get pregnant	35.5	50.0	14.5
Partner didn't want to use a method	20.0	73.3	6.7
Partner didn't want *me* to use a method	10.2	83.1	6.8
Knew it was risky, but took a chance	62.3	18.0	19.7
Don't believe in birth control for moral or religious reasons	1.7	98.3	0.0
Think birth control is too messy and unromantic	6.9	86.2	6.9
Didn't know how birth control works	1.7	94.9	3.4
Didn't know where to get birth control	8.3	91.7	0.0
Didn't want to see a doctor to obtain birth control	19.7	78.7	1.6
Would seem like I was planning to have sex	10.3	86.2	3.4
I was too embarrassed to get birth control	6.8	88.1	5.1
I was drinking/using drugs at the time	15.0	83.3	1.7
I am concerned with the health risks of the methods	34.5	56.9	8.6
Was forced to have sex against my will	1.7	96.6	1.7
I cannot afford to use birth control regularly	5.2	89.7	5.2

Source: Robin Sawyer and Kenneth H. Beck, "Predicting Pregnancy and Contraceptive Usage Among College Women," *Health Education* 19 (1988): 42–47.

Given the pregnancy rates on college campuses, the lack of contraceptive use (some studies show 57 percent of students engaging in sexual intercourse use no method of contraception) is especially disturbing. Campus pregnancy rates have been estimated at between 6 to 10 percent, and one university found that 22 percent of its unmarried female students became pregnant.

To encourage contraceptive use among coitally active college students, some universities are replacing cigarette vending machines with condom vending machines. This has occurred at the University of Virginia, where dormitories have machines that sell boxes containing three condoms for $1.25. Other campuses sell condoms in university bookstores.

Evaluating Contraceptive Effectiveness

One of the things you need to know before deciding on a birth control method is how well is works. The effectiveness of contraceptives is measured in terms of how successfully they work to prevent pregnancy during one year in one hundred sexually active women. When discussing effectiveness rates for methods of contraception, a differentiation is made between theoretical effectiveness and actual user effectiveness. *Theoretical effectiveness* refers to how effective the method is if used perfectly—the maximum possible effectiveness. *Actual user effectiveness* is always lower because people do not use contraceptives perfectly. Table 6.2 lists the rates of theoretical and actual user effectiveness for the methods we'll discuss. Our intent is not to influence you toward any particular method but rather to provide you with the necessary information you might need to make an informed decision if you are sexually active and plan to use contraception.

Methods of Contraception

Abstinence One way to prevent conception is **abstinence**—abstaining from sexual intercourse. Obviously, if the penis does not come near or enter the vagina, there is no chance of pregnancy. Abstinence is

coitus interruptus During coitus, the withdrawal of the penis from the vagina prior to ejaculation; a method of contraception, but not very effective.

rhythm method The timing of coitus so that it does not occur during the time of the month when the woman is most likely to conceive; only partially effective as a contraceptive method.

basal body temperature (BBT) The body's core

temperature; in women, it usually decreases before ovulation and increases during ovulation.

ovulation method A contraceptive method that involves determining the onset of a woman's ovulation by interpreting her cervical mucus pattern.

condom A sheath of latex rubber or animal skin placed on the erect penis to prevent sperm from entering the vagina.

TABLE 6.2

Contraceptive Effectiveness

Method	Theoretical Effectiveness %	Actual User Effectiveness %
Abstinence	100	?
Withdrawal	91	75–80
Rhythm	87	60–86
Ovulation method	98	75
Condoms	97	90
Diaphragm (with spermicide)	97	83
Cervical cap	97	83
IUD	97–99	95
Hormonal implants	99.7	99.7
Spermicidal foam	97	78
Spermicidal suppositories	97	75–80
Spermicidal sponge	95	80
Oral contraceptives	99.7	96

also the most effective way to prevent contracting AIDS. We discuss AIDS in Chapter 14.

People abstain from sexual intercourse for various reasons. Among unmarried couples, a common reason is religious or moral objection to nonmarital sexual intercourse. Another factor for many unmarried people is their concern about contracting sexually transmitted diseases. We know, however, that approximately two-thirds of all unmarried men and women are sexually active by age 19. Abstinence, then, is clearly not for most people. Those who are sexually active and do not want to become pregnant or (in the case of men) cause a pregnancy need some effective means of preventing conception. Let's consider the methods that are available.

Withdrawal Also called **coitus interruptus,** the withdrawal method requires the male to withdraw his penis from the vagina prior to ejaculation. In theory, it makes sense that withdrawal will prevent sperm from entering the female. However, in practice, coitus interruptus isn't very effective because it requires considerable self-control. Often the male is not able to identify the imminence of ejaculation quickly enough. The first drops of the ejaculate contain a higher concentration of sperm than later ones, therefore not withdrawing soon enough can lead to pregnancy. Moreover, pre-ejaculatory fluid (secreted from the Cowper's gland) may contain some sperm and can lead to impregnation. Consequently, a penis near or in a vagina can deposit sperm even before ejaculating.

Withdrawal is not a popular method of birth control among married couples in the United States. Unfortunately, however, it is widespread among teenagers.

Rhythm Method Fertility control by the **rhythm method** is based upon an understanding of the female menstrual cycle. As described earlier in this chapter, an egg is released by a female approximately once a month. The object of the rhythm method is not to have a sperm meet that egg while it is still viable. Though an egg begins to degenerate 24 hours after ovulation if not fertilized, sperm and the egg can remain alive up to 72 hours. The task, then, is to identify the day of ovulation and abstain from intercourse 72 hours before (so that no sperm will remain alive in the female) and after the day of ovulation. However, during a 28-day menstrual cycle, ovulation may occur anywhere from the seventeenth to the thirteenth day before the next menstruation begins. As a result, to employ the rhythm method, abstinence should be practiced from day 10 through day 17 of a 28-day cycle.

The rhythm method requires considerable commitment and presents some difficulties. Many women have irregular menstrual cycles, making it difficult for them to pinpoint the time of ovulation. It is recommended that women keep exact records of the length of their menstrual cycles for one year.

The most common way to determine the time of ovulation is to identify a shift in the body's core temperature, which is known as the **basal body temperature (BBT).** The BBT can be determined by inserting a thermometer into the mouth or the rectum. Ovulation can be recognized by a decrease of approximately 0.3 degree just before ovulation and an increase of approximately 0.5 to 0.6 degree during ovulation. To be effective in identifying time of ovulation, BBT readings should be taken each morning before getting out of bed. A BBT thermometer can be purchased in a drugstore.

If the BBT reading is usually 97.9 (it is usually lower in the morning than during the day), it will decrease to 97.6 just prior to ovulation, increase to 98.4 or 98.5 during ovulation, and remain there for three days after ovulation (the time it takes the egg to disintegrate). After the three days of a 0.5 to 0.6 degree rise in BBT, the safe days begin.

One problem with this means of identifying ovulation is that illness or activity may change the BBT. To diminish the chance of incorrectly identifying the time of ovulation, it is recommended that the thermometer and calendar be used hand in hand, the calendar helping to identify shifts in BBT resulting from sources other than ovulation, and the thermometer helping to identify an early or late ovulation.

Couples using the rhythm method of fertility were found to be more effective in preventing conception if they viewed their successes or failures as a result of their own behavior (internal locus of control) than if they possessed an external locus of control. Despite the fact that the rhythm method is somewhat difficult, it has the advantage of permitting a couple to *plan* as well as prevent a pregnancy, and it is acceptable to the Roman Catholic Church.

Ovulation Method

Use of the **ovulation method** entails identifying the onset of ovulation by interpreting the woman's cervical mucus pattern. Developed by Dr. John Billings, the ovulation method requires keeping records of the days on which mucus is secreted through the vagina and recognizing the characteristics of this mucus. After menstruation there is little or no mucus secretion—the "dry days." Soon the mucus secretions begin to change, signaling the start of the fertile period. It starts out as a yellow or white sticky discharge. When the secretion changes to a clear, stringy, and stretchy consistency, the "peak days" have occurred and fertility is at its height (that is, ovulation has occurred). During this ovulation period, the mucus may look like egg white and can actually be stretched between two fingers. Several days afterward, a cloudy discharge resumes and intercourse is considered safe once again. The fertile days in a 28-day menstrual cycle are typically days 9 to 15.

This method has several advantages. It is relatively easy to teach a women how to "read" her cervical mucus pattern, and this method is more reliable than basal body temperature. Like rhythm, the ovulation method has no side effects, is acceptable to those religions advocating the rhythm method, and can be used to plan a pregnancy as well as prevent one.

One disadvantage of the ovulation method is the possibility of misinterpreting the mucus discharge. About 30 percent of women do not have a recognizable mucus pattern. In addition, this method requires abstinence during the woman's fertile period of each menstrual cycle.

Condoms

Also called a "rubber," a **condom** is a sheath of latex rubber placed on the erect penis to prevent sperm from entering the vagina. Condoms come in various shapes and colors, and are about 7.5 inches long when unrolled (see Figure 6.2).

The condom is most effective if the male removes

FIGURE 6.2 • How to Use a Condom

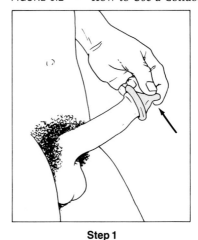

Step 1

Hold the tip of the condom to squeeze out the air. This leaves some room for the semen when you come (ejaculate). Put the condom on the end of your erect penis.

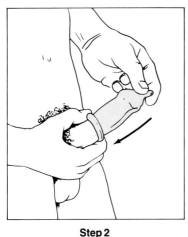

Step 2

Keep holding the tip of the condom. Unroll it onto your erect penis . . .

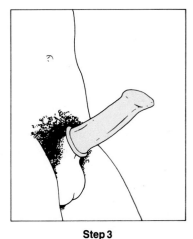

Step 3

. . . all the way down to the hair. After you come, and before you lose your erection, hold the rim of the condom tightly against your body and withdraw your penis. Never reuse a condom!

diaphragm A latex rubber cap around a collapsible metal ring, designed to fit over the cervix and prevent sperm from entering the uterus; best used in conjunction with a spermicidal cream or jelly.

cervical cap A rubber, plastic, or metal cap that covers the cervix, creating a barrier to sperm; unlike the diaphragm, it may remain in place for two days.

birth control pill Any of a variety of hormone-containing pills that women ingest on specific schedules in order to prevent conception.

---

the penis from the vagina shortly after ejaculation to avoid the possibility of semen leakage into the vagina. Breakage of the condom is rare but possible. Condoms should never be reused and should not be kept in a wallet near the body, because they can deteriorate with heat. Oil-based lubricants such as petroleum jelly, cocoa butter, or mineral or vegetable oils will also deteriorate latex condoms and should not be used with them. Water-based lubricating jelly, like K-Y jelly, may be used with latex condoms. Though the condom is criticized by some couples because putting it on requires an interruption in foreplay, other couples incorporate the use of the condom into their foreplay. An advantage of the condom is that it does not have the side effects that accompany some of the other techniques. In addition, condoms are inexpensive and easily obtained in drugstores, by mail, and from some public bathroom vending machines. No prescription is needed to purchase them, and they are very effective if used correctly.

Another important advantage of the condom is the protection latex condoms provide against sexually transmitted diseases (in particular, AIDS) and infection (animal skin condoms do *not* offer the same protection).

Condom use has grown tremendously as a result of the AIDS scare. Today, condoms represent a $200 million industry and the industry continues to grow by 10 percent annually. Traditionally marketed to men only, condoms are now marketed to women, using such names as Condom Mate. In fact, women now purchase 30 to 40 percent of condoms bought in the United States. There is even a woman's condom being tested that is inserted in the vagina rather than placed on the penis. Other condom developments include the Microcondom, a condom that covers only the glans penis, and the printing of expiration dates on condom packages. If you are interested in the effectiveness of a particular condom you might want to consult the August 1989 issue of *Glamour* magazine, which summarizes several studies of condom effectiveness.

Diaphragm Another means of preventing conception is to create a barrier that sperm cannot penetrate. The **diaphragm,** a latex rubber cap around a collapsible metal ring, is designed to cover the cervix and prevent sperm from traveling through the uterus and up the Fallopian tubes, where the egg might be fertilized. To perform its function well, the diaphragm must be fitted by a physician and should be refitted after a pregnancy or weight gain or loss of ten pounds or more. To further assure that live sperm will not enter the uterus, the diaphragm is lubricated with a spermicidal cream or jelly (discussed below) that will kill sperm on contact. The cream is placed around the edge and inside the cup of the diaphragm before putting it in place. Figure 6.3 shows how the diaphragm is used.

The diaphragm can be inserted any time before intercourse but must be left in place at least six hours afterward. Additional cream or jelly must be applied before each act of intercourse. It is recommended that the diaphragm not be left in place more than twenty-four hours. The disadvantages to the use of a diaphragm include the need to plan intercourse and the possibility of improper insertion.

If properly cared for, the diaphragm can be used effectively and comfortably for several years. Couples report that its presence does not hinder sexual enjoyment for either the male or the female.

It is recommended that the diaphragm be washed with warm water and mild soap, rinsed, and air dried. It should be dusted with cornstarch (scented talcs or petroleum jelly will weaken the rubber). Periodically check the diaphragm for wear, looking for thin spots or holes.

Cervical Cap The device known as the **cervical cap** is a latex rubber, plastic, or metal cap covering the cervix. Like the diaphragm, the cap is designed for use

Year 2000 National Health Objective

One of the national health objectives encourages the use of latex condoms; specifically, to increase to at least 50 percent the proportion of sexually active, unmarried people who used a condom during their last sexual intercourse. In 1988, that figure was 19 percent.

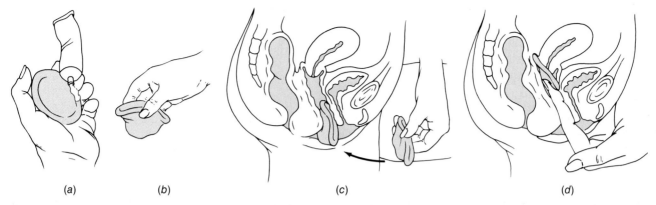

FIGURE 6.3 • Insertion of the diaphragm. (a) Spermicide is applied around the rim and in the dome. (b) The diaphragm ready for insertion. (c) Insertion before intercourse. (d) Placement with dome covering cervix for correct positioning during and following intercourse.

with a spermicidal cream or jelly, creating a formidable barrier to the sperm. It is more popular in Europe than in the United States. However, with concern over side effects of other methods of contraception, the cervical cap is gaining popularity in this country as well. About 70,000 women use the cap. The cervical cap appears to be both safe and effective when fitted properly and when the user inserts it correctly. Its failure rate is about the same as for the diaphragm. It should be left in place at least 8 hours after intercourse. In addition, the cervical cap can be left in place for two days. It is more difficult to insert properly than the diaphragm.

Some studies have found slightly higher than expected precancerous cervical abnormalities in cap users. Some other studies have not been able to verify this finding. As a result, the Food and Drug Administration, the governmental agency approving the use of the cervical cap, requires labeling that instructs women planning to use the device to obtain a Pap

FIGURE 6.4 • The Cervical Cap

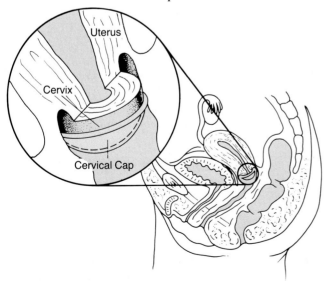

smear before being fitted for the cervical cap. Women who have had an abnormal Pap smear or who have cervical cancer should not use the cap.

As with latex condoms, oil-based lubricants should not be used with the latex rubber cervical cap because they tend to deteriorate the latex rubber in the cap. Figure 6.4 shows the positioning of the cervical cap.

The Pill   Some form of **birth control pill** is used by 10 to 15 million women in the United States. To understand how the pill functions as a contraceptive, you must understand the hormonal involvement in the menstrual cycle, described earlier. Estrogen in the pill works on the hypothalamus of the brain to prevent the pituitary gland from producing FSH and LH. The result of this action is the prevention of ovulation, and with no egg to fertilize, pregnancy can't occur. In simple terms, the body is fooled into believing it is pregnant, thereby not having to ovulate any longer. The progestins in the pill serve to prepare the endometrium for implantation and to maintain pregnancy. When provided before ovulation, however, progestins are thought to inhibit implantation. Progestin also creates a cervical mucus that results in decreased sperm transport and penetration.

The pill is really many pills. Some contain estrogen and progestin in combination, some only progestin. In addition, the amount of the hormone or hormones contained in the pill varies greatly from one brand to the next. A physician is the person best qualified to recommend which pill to take, but it is suggested that a woman starting on the pill take one with 35 micrograms or less of estrogen to minimize the possibility of blood-clotting complications. In fact, one of the Year 1990 National Health Objectives was to reduce the sale of oral contraceptives with more than 50 micrograms of estrogen to 15 percent of total sales by 1985. In 1978, 23.9 percent of sales of oral contraceptives contained estrogen above the 50 microgram level.

intrauterine device (IUD) A small object of metal or plastic that is placed into the uterus to prevent conception.

spermicide Any of several contraceptive foams, creams, jellies, or other medications that immobilize and kill or block sperm from entering the cervix.

However, by 1981 this objective was achieved; and in 1983 only 9 percent of sales of oral contraceptives contained more than 50 micrograms of estrogen.

Some varieties of the pill are taken each day for 21 days and then not taken for the next 7 days to allow for menstruation. Others are taken every day. It is suggested that during the first month on the pill another means of contraception (such as a condom) be used to allow time for the pill to become effective.

One type of pill is the "minipill," which is taken every day (even during menstruation) and contains only progestin. The advantage of this pill is that it is thought to cause fewer side effects than pills contain-

ing estrogen. A disadvantage is that it is slightly less effective than combined pills, although about as effective as the IUD.

The pill is extremely effective in preventing pregnancy. Other advantages of the pill are that it doesn't require an interruption of lovemaking and, unlike the IUD, it serves to regulate the menstrual period.

The main disadvantage of the pill is its side effects, ranging from nausea, weight gain, headaches, and yeast infections to gall-bladder disease, hypertension, and blood clots. The American College of Obstetricians and Gynecologists found that among approximately 10 million users of oral contraceptives, 500 women die

Issues in Health

Should Physicians Be Allowed to Prescribe Oral Contraceptives to Females under 18 Years of Age without Having to Obtain Their Parents' Consent?

Pro Those arguing that physicians should be allowed to prescribe the birth control pill to girls under eighteen years old without their parents' consent believe these girls will engage in sexual intercourse whether or not the pill is made available to them. It's better that they use the pill than not use it. Furthermore, many young women cannot discuss sex with their parents and would never ask for their permission to obtain an oral contraceptive. These girls would still be as coitally active, but sans contraception. Given the alarming teenage out-of-wedlock pregnancy rate, the likelihood the teenage mother will never finish her schooling, the burden society will most likely have to assume to financially support the child and the mother, and the psychological effects upon the girl and her family, providing her with a means of preventing conception seems the prudent thing

to do. Lastly, the physician-patient relationship is a private one. Without that assurance, the girl would not consult the physician in the first place. The effect of damaging the confidentiality of this relationship would be disastrous, not only regarding sexuality but also as it pertains to other health matters that women share with their physicians.

Con Those not willing to allow physicians to prescribe birth control pills to minors without their parents' approval believe such a practice would encourage or, at the least, make it easy for young female patients to engage in sexual intercourse. Given the concern about AIDS and the pervasive negative effects of a teenage out-of-wedlock pregnancy, encouraging such behavior is irresponsible. In addition, since oral contraceptives

contain hormones and can be considered as medication, parental approval for such treatment should be standard practice. Other medications cannot be dispensed to minors without parental approval; why should the pill be any different? Lastly, the physician has the responsibility to the patient to prescribe behavior that is healthy—physically and mentally—and to act in ways consistent with that advice. To advocate abstinence (as these opponents of physicians dispensing the pill without parental approval would argue doctors ought to do) and then to make available a safe means to avoid that advice is the height of hypocrisy.

If you were a physician, would you dispense oral contraceptives to girls under 18 years of age without their parents' approval?

Source: Jerrold S. Greenberg, Clint E. Bruess, Kathy Mullen, and Doris Sands, *Sexuality: Insights and Issues,* 2e (Dubuque, Iowa: Wm. C. Brown, 1989).

each year. However, if women who were over 40 years old or who smoked cigarettes were removed from these 500 deaths, the number would drop to 70 deaths annually.[4] That is about ten times lower than a woman's chances of death from an automobile accident or from childbirth. It is for this reason that the pill is not recommended for women who are over 40 (some physicians say over 35) or who smoke. In addition, women with liver function problems, hypertension, circulatory problems, sickle-cell disease, asthma, varicose veins, epilepsy, or migraine headaches should avoid using oral contraceptives as well. On the other hand, the pill seems to prevent some other conditions. For example, the incidence of rheumatoid arthritis and certain cancers (ovarian and endometrial) are reported to be lower in users of oral contraceptives.[5]

Intrauterine Device The **intrauterine device (IUD)** is a small object made of plastic and metal that is inserted by a physician into the uterus to prevent pregnancy (see Figure 6.5). Some contain copper, and some contain the hormone progesterone. Although it is not known for sure how IUDs work, they are believed to do one of several things to prevent pregnancy:

- Prevent the fertilized ovum from implanting itself on the endometrium of the uterus so that it cannot be nourished.
- Immobilize the sperm.
- In the case of copper-treated devices, alter the chemical environment needed or the hormonal secretions necessary for the development of the fertilized ovum.

Severe complications from using IUDs have been reported, including pelvic infection and uterine perforation. Another complication associated with IUD use is the possibility of expulsion without the user's knowledge. When this happens, the woman is unprotected and pregnancy may result. For this reason, women wearing an IUD should check often to see that it is still in place by feeling for the string that leads from the IUD through the cervix into the vagina. Figure 6.5 depicts the IUD in place, with its descending string.

Other complications can arise if pregnancy occurs while the IUD is in the uterus. If the IUD is removed during pregnancy, there is a 25 percent chance of spontaneous abortion, whereas if it is kept in place, infection, blood poisoning, bleeding, or premature labor may result. Finally, IUDs may lead to heavier-than-usual menstrual bleeding and a more painful menstrual period, particularly for three months or so after first being inserted.

The advantages of IUD use are its effectiveness and its constantly being in place. Couples not wanting to interrupt intercourse to insert a diaphragm or use a condom, for example, may find the IUD appealing.

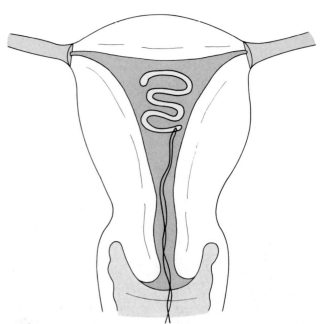

FIGURE 6.5 • IUD in position in the uterus. The thread projecting from the cervix enables the woman to check at intervals to ensure that the IUD has not been ejected from the uterus.

And users are always prepared for unplanned intercourse.

In 1986, the manufacturer of the most widely used IUDs in the United States (G.D. Searle and Company) removed them from the market due to concern over pending lawsuits. By 1985, one manufacturer of IUDs (A.H. Robbins) had paid out over $520 million in lawsuits pertaining to damage done to women's health by its Dalkon Shield IUD. As a result, by 1985 IUD sales accounted for a mere 2 percent of the $1 billion contraceptive industry.[6] When G.D. Searle removed its IUDs from the market, the availability of IUDS was virtually eliminated in the United States. However, in 1988 a new IUD (the T380A or the Copper T) was marketed in the United States. This IUD is accompanied by an informed consent form patients are expected to sign that relates known risks of IUD use.

Spermicides Spermicidal preparations offer another form of contraception. The **spermicide** is applied so as to be placed against the cervix (see Figure 6.6). The spermicide blocks the sperm from entering the cervix, as well as immobilizing and killing them. Spermicidal jellies and creams are not very effective unless used with a diaphragm. Spermicidal foam offers much better protection because it is more evenly distributed. To be effective, the foam must be inserted just before intercourse, and a new application is required with each act of intercourse. The effectiveness of foam is greatly increased when it is used in combination with a condom. Spermicides are available without a prescription.

Norplant The brand name of a new contraceptive implant which is placed just under the skin of a woman's upper arm and is effective for up to five years.

Gossypol A substance derived from cottonseed oil

that shows promise as an oral contraceptive for males, though there are some side effects.

vasectomy The most effective method of contraception for males, vasectomy involves minor surgery that severs the vas deferens.

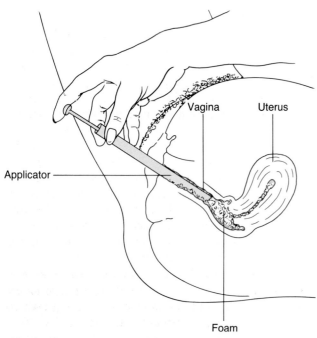

FIGURE 6.6 • Application of a Spermicidal Foam

Since the spermicide nonoxynol-9 helps to immobilize the AIDS virus, any brand of spermicide used for contraceptive purposes should contain nonoxynol-9.

Spermicidal suppositories are also available. When one is inserted in the vagina, the moisture and warmth effervesces or dissolves the suppository into a sperm-killing barrier. The suppository should be inserted at least 10 to 15 minutes before intercourse, and it remains effective for approximately one hour. A new suppository should be inserted for each act of intercourse.

Spermicidal suppositories are free of serious side effects. However, they are less effective than spermicidal foam, because they do not distribute the spermicide as evenly.

Spermicidal Sponge   In April 1983, the United States Food and Drug Administration approved the marketing of a *spermicidal sponge*, a vaginal contraceptive sponge containing a spermicidal agent—brand named "Today." The sponge, which feels like a powder puff, is made of a special polyurethane material and

contains the spermicide nonoxynol-9. It is placed in front of the cervix after being dampened with two tablespoons of water and is believed to act in several ways: Its spermicide kills sperm, the sponge itself absorbs the ejaculate (thereby preventing sperm from entering the uterus), and it acts as a mechanical barrier to block the cervical opening.

The sponge can be purchased without a prescription, can remain in place and be effective for 24 hours, does not need to be fitted by a physician, is easier to insert than a diaphragm, and is not as messy as the other spermicidal forms (for example, foams, jellies, or creams).

However, the sponge is relatively expensive (more than $1 per sponge), it is less effective than some other forms of contraception (for example, the pill, the IUD, the diaphragm), and there are no long-term studies of the use of the sponge (for example, the effect of absorption of the spermicide through the vaginal walls). The manufacturer of the sponge (VLI Corporation) has established a toll-free telephone number to answer questions about this method of contraception. The number is 800-223-2329.

Douching   *Douching* refers to squirting a special solution into the vagina after sexual intercourse in an effort to flush all the semen out of the vagina. This method is extremely ineffective, because sperm can reach the cervical canal as quickly as 90 seconds after ejaculation. Some experts contend that douching may actually facilitate the passage of sperm to the cervical opening, because the douche is squirted under pressure. In addition, frequent douching may irritate the tissues of the vagina. Although some women douche for sanitary reasons, there is no evidence that this practice is necessary or beneficial.

New Contraceptive Technology   Research to develop more effective and safer methods of contraception has resulted in several new leads:

1. **Implants.** A time-released capsule of oral contraceptives can be placed just beneath the skin, eliminating the need to remember to take the pill daily. The implant can be removed any time the

woman wants to become pregnant. Otherwise it is effective for up to five years. Presently, some forty countries allow implant use.

On December 10, 1990, the U.S. government gave approval to a contraceptive implant sold under the brand name Norplant. **Norplant** contains a synthetic progesterone called levonorgestrel and is effective for up to five years. The implants are placed just under the skin of a woman's upper arm by a physician and can be removed at any time. Side effects of Norplant include headaches, mood changes, and nausea in some women, and it may cause irregular menstrual bleeding in others. The advantages of implants are their effectiveness (as effective as oral contraceptives), and they do not rely on the user's behavior (thereby eliminating any errors in use that would diminish its effectiveness). Contraceptive implants are recommended for women who are interested in long-term contraception, are unable to take estrogen-based oral contraceptives, are dissatisfied with barrier methods because of their ineffectiveness or inconvenience, or are older than 35 and are concerned about taking the pill beyond that age.[7]

2. **Ovulation predictors.** Equipment that can determine the time of ovulation is available but not accurate enough to be used for contraception, although it is being used to enhance conception.

3. **Spermicidal agents.** New ways of using spermicides are being researched; for example, the penile cap which releases a spermicide during coitus, the spermicidal diaphragm which enlarges as it absorbs fluid and then releases a spermicidal agent, and the vaginal ring which is inserted over the cervix and is designed to release either a spermicide or a hormone.

4. **Male contraceptives.** The difficulty of developing a male contraceptive relates to finding a substance that would decrease sperm production while not affecting production of testosterone (male sex hormone) and sexual libido (interest in sex). One substance being experimented with is **Gossypol.** Taken from cottonseed oil, Gossypol seems to sufficiently decrease sperm production and doesn't negatively affect libido. However,

once it is no longer taken, sperm production does not revert to normal in approximately 25 percent of men. In addition, it can reduce blood potassium; cause paralysis; affect the heart, liver, and gastrointestinal system; and cause fatigue or dizziness.

Testosterone enanthate (TE) is another male contraceptive being experimented with. TE treatment involves injections that lower sperm production while providing synthetic testosterone.

Sterilization

Sterilization is a usually permanent form of birth control that can be applied to either the male or the female. In the case of the male, the vas deferens is cut and tied by a physician so that the sperm cannot be transported out of the penis. Termed a **vasectomy,** this procedure is performed on an outpatient basis, and the patient can return home shortly after the procedure. Only a small incision in each side of the scrotum, to reach the vas, is necessary (see Figure 6.7). At present the procedure is generally considered irreversible, although use of microsurgery has become increasingly effective in reversing vasectomies. Clips and plugs can also be used to interfere with the vas deferens passageway, but the most widely used technique involves cutting the vas and sealing off its ends (by suturing or cauterizing).

The female sterilization procedure can take several forms: *minilaparotomy, laparotomy,* or *laparoscopy.* The "minlap" involves a small incision, through which the Fallopian tubes are brought and blocked by either cutting them—*tubal ligation*—or using clips or rings. Figure 6.8 depicts a typical tubal ligation procedure. Laparotomy involves making a larger incision, inserting medical instruments into the incision (rather than bringing the tubes through the incision), and blocking the tubes. Since a general or spinal anesthesia is required, laparotomy is only used if the minlap or laparoscopy cannot be performed. The laparoscopy entails making one or two small incisions, inserting a viewing instrument (laparoscope) and medical instruments through this incision, and blocking the tubes by liga-

FIGURE 6.7 • Vasectomy

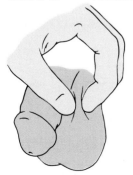
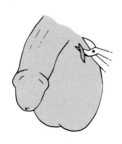
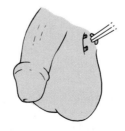
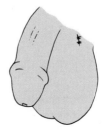
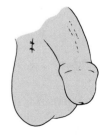

1. Locating vas deferens

2. Vas deferens exposed by small incision in scrotum

3. A small section of vas deferens removed and ends tied and/or cauterized

4. Incision in scrotum closed

5. Steps 1–4 repeated on right side

abortion The termination of a pregnancy.

abortifacients Chemical substances that cause abortion or terminate pregnancy.

DES DES (Diethystilbestrol) is a synthetic estrogen used in emergency cases of rape or incest to terminate pregnancies.

RU 486 A French-manufactured pharmaceutical used to terminate unwanted pregnancies.

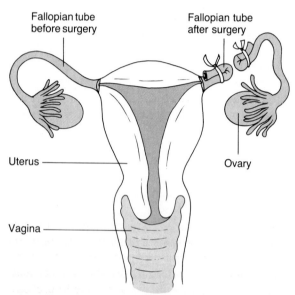

FIGURE 6.8 • Tubal ligation. This is a relatively safe surgical procedure, which is generally irreversible. In sterilization, the procedure is performed on both tubes.

tion, clips, or rings. There are other less commonly used female sterilization procedures as well, for example, open laparoscopy where a tube (cannula) is inserted through an incision and around which the skin is sutured. Instruments are then passed through the cannula. In addition, the tubes can be approached through the vagina in a procedure called *culpotomy.*

Sterilization is becoming increasingly popular in the United States. In 1988, 28 percent of women using some method of birth control were sterilized, and, when male and female sterilization are combined, 39 percent of contracepting couples were employing sterilization.[8] Sterilization is the leading method of contraception in the United States.[9]

Abortion

Abortion is the termination of pregnancy. If the pregnancy is not terminated intentionally, the abortion is said to be *spontaneous.* If the abortion is intentional, it is said to be *induced.* There are several methods of induced

abortion, with the stage of pregnancy usually determining the method of choice.

First Trimester Abortion Methods

During the first trimester of pregnancy (see our discussion of trimesters under "Gestation," below), either *dilation and curettage* or *suction curettage* are the methods of choice.

Dilation and Curettage Commonly known as a *D and C,* this method employs two instruments: a *speculum* that dilates the cervix and a *curette* that scrapes out the products of conception (see Figure 6.9).

Suction Curettage Rather than scraping out the products of conception, sometimes a vacuum is used to suction them out. This method is called *suction curettage.*

Second Trimester Abortion Methods

When the fetus is larger, other abortion methods are used.

FIGURE 6.9 • Dilation and curettage method of abortion. The cervix is opened with a speculum and the curette scrapes the uterine lining.

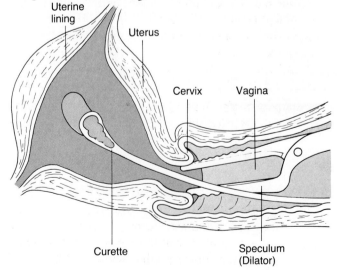

Exploring Your Health 6.2

Contraceptive Decision Making

Evacuation and Curettage When the products of conception are too large to be sucked out through the vacuum tube, they need to be scraped into smaller parts with a curette. Once small enough, they are then suctioned out with a vacuum. This method is called *evacuation and curettage.*

Induced Labor One of the most frequently used methods of abortion during the second trimester is called *induced labor.* A saline solution is injected into the amniotic fluid surrounding the fetus to induce labor. Sometimes prostaglandins (synthetic hormones) are used instead of the saline solution.

Hysterotomy Another second trimester method that is used, albeit rarely, involves making an incision in the abdomen and through the uterus to remove the fetus. This procedure is called a hysterotomy.

Morning-After-Pills

In addition to the methods described above, there are two chemicals that are used as **abortifacients** (substances that cause abortions). These chemicals can be taken shortly after sexual intercourse to terminate a suspected pregnancy.

Diethylstilbestrol (DES) **DES** is a synthetic estrogen that was administered to pregnant women in the 1950s with a history of miscarriages (spontaneous abortions). Unfortunately, the female offspring of these women were more likely to develop reproductive tract cancers, and the male offspring were more likely to develop testicular cancer and become infertile more frequently than would normally occur. To make matters worse, DES was found to be ineffective in preventing miscarriages! However, it was discovered that DES would prevent a fertilized egg from implanting on the endometrium lining of the uterus. Without implantation the egg would be sloughed off with the menstrual flow. Yet, because of its health hazards, DES is now only used in emergency cases, such as rape or incest, to prevent pregnancy.

RU 486 Another chemical has also been found to prevent a fertilized egg from remaining implanted on the endometrium lining of the uterus. Named after Roussel-Uclaf, the French pharmaceutical company that developed it, **RU 486** can be taken within three weeks of a missed period. Within 48 hours of its being taken, a small dose of prostaglandin is administered through an injection or a suppository. Soon the woman begins menstruating with a heavier than usual flow. However, RU 486 has created a great deal of controversy, particularly in the United States. Women's groups have been especially vocal in their advocacy for the approval and marketing of RU 486. They argue that women should have available to them yet another option to terminate a pregnancy—an option that requires no surgery and is safe and effective. However, those opposed to abortion disagree. They believe RU 486 would just encourage irresponsible sex, since all one need to do is take a pill the morning after. At the

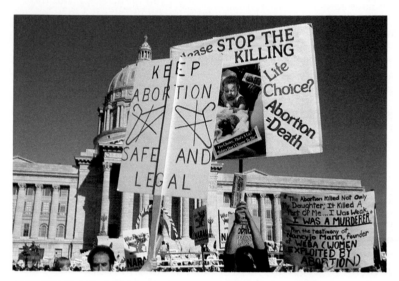

Both those in favor of giving women a choice to abort and those opposed have found similar vehicles for expressing their opinions. Marches are not uncommon, and efforts to lobby for legislators favoring their positions is a common strategy as well.

time of this writing, RU 486 is not being marketed in the United States, and the antiabortion lobby has threatened to boycott other products of any company that does market RU 486. That threat, coupled with the threat of costly lawsuits, has led to its unavailability.

The Abortion Controversy

Currently, abortion is being vehemently debated in the public sector. Although in vitro fertilization, contraception, and sterilization all have their controversial aspects, none of them generates the political, religious, and emotional heat that abortion does. Some people believe induced abortion to be murder of a living being, whereas others see it as a medical intervention in a biological process. Some people feel that the question of when life begins is central to this debate: Is it at conception, or at some point when the unborn could (with help) exist outside the uterus, or at birth? But a person's view of when life begins is only one factor in shaping his or her attitudes on whether induced abortion is morally acceptable. Another central issue is whether the individual woman has the right to make a decision so basic to her own life or whether the government has that right and power. Other attitudes also enter into the debate—for instance, attitudes regard-

ing world population, religious issues, women's roles, political power, poverty, public and private child care, and the degree of responsibility people should assume for their sexual behavior.

Political groups generally called "pro-life" are actively supporting candidates who are totally opposed to abortion. Their goal is to pass legislation making abortion illegal or even to pass a constitutional amendment prohibiting abortion in the United States. Groups labeled "pro-choice," on the other hand, believe women should have the right to decide for themselves what they will do with their bodies. Consequently, they oppose legislative restrictions on the availability of abortion to women who choose that option and they wish to uphold the Supreme Court decision of the 1973 *Roe* v. *Wade* case, which established the current legal status of abortion in the United States. The Court ruled that abortion should be available to women during the first trimester (the first three months) of pregnancy. The decision whether to take this option is made by the pregnant woman and her physician, preferably also in consultation with her sexual partner. Regarding abortions during the second trimester, the Court ruled that the states can develop the regulations they deem necessary to maintain the pregnant woman's health. In the third trimester, the states can actually prohibit abortions even if the mother's health is not in jeopardy.

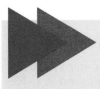

Exploring Your Health 6.3

Should Abortions Be Permitted?

1. Should abortions ever be allowed?

        yes   no

2. If yes, under what circumstances?

   (a) Only if conception is a result of rape or incest.

        yes   no

   (b) If the pregnancy will cause economic hardship.

        yes   no

   (c) If the pregnancy will harm the woman's physical health.

        yes   no

   (d) If the pregnancy will harm the woman's mental health.

        yes   no

   (e) Only during the first trimester.

        yes   no

   (f) During the first and second trimesters.

        yes   no

   (g) If the woman is unmarried.

        yes   no

   (h) If the woman is a teenager.

        yes   no

   (i) If the woman is over 40.

        yes   no

   (j) If amniocentesis determines that the fetus is defective.

        yes   no

   (k) Only if the woman undergoes counseling first.

        yes   no

3. Should government funds be used for abortions for poor women?

        yes   no

4. Should the father's agreement be required before an abortion can be performed?

        yes   no

5. Should the father be held financially responsible for the cost of the abortion?

        yes   no

In 1983, the Supreme Court reaffirmed its 1973 decision and stated that the government could not interfere with abortion unless such interference was clearly justified by "accepted medical practice." In effect, this ruling prohibited governmental interference even in the second trimester and invalidated state laws that required abortions during the second trimester to be performed in a hospital.

However, by 1989, with several replacements of justices making up the Supreme Court, the environment changed and was less protective of the *Roe* v. *Wade* decision. For example, in 1989 the Court ruled in *Webster* v. *Reproductive Health Service* that the Missouri law requiring doctors to test fetuses prior to abortions to determine if they can live outside the womb was constitutional. In 1990, the Court overturned a Minnesota law requiring both parents of pregnant teenagers be notified of a pending abortion. However, the rationale used by the Court was not that states couldn't interfere with abortions in the early trimesters, but rather that there needed to be an option for the courts to be notified in the case of abusive or absent parents. It appears that the Supreme Court is now receptive to states regulating abortions—even first trimester ones. It is possible in this climate for the passage of various regulations making abortions more difficult to obtain. In fact, the Louisiana legislature passed a law prohibiting abortions for any reasons other than if the woman's life was in danger. Abortions under that law were illegal even if they were the result of rape or incest. That Louisiana law was never activated because it was vetoed by the governor, but it is an example of the kind of legislation that might be proposed to prevent abortions or make them more difficult to obtain.

In 1977, the Court made a decision that has profoundly affected the availability of legal abortions. It ruled that the federal government could refuse to fund abortions even though it funded other health care for the poor (the Hyde Amendment). The result of this action is to prohibit poor women from obtaining safe abortions with Medicaid funds; affluent women can still receive abortions by paying for them. People who oppose abortion acknowledge that an inequity exists between poor and affluent women regarding the availability of abortion, but they view this circumstance as leaving the unborn of more wealthy women unprotected by law.

Exploring Your Health 6.3 gives you an opportunity to examine your views on abortion.

Pregnancy

Although pregnancy may be indicated by such symptoms as morning sickness, swollen breasts, and frequent urination, these can all be signs of other bodily processes. Even a missed menstrual period is not a sure sign of pregnancy, because many women do not ovulate every month during their menstruating life.

early pregnancy tests (EPTs) Do-it-yourself kits of varying accuracy that women can use on their own for determining pregnancy.

fetal alcohol syndrome Central nervous system dysfunctions and growth deficiencies found in babies whose mothers drank alcoholic beverages during pregnancy.

gestation The period of time from conception to birth.

Pregnancy can be determined most accurately by examination of the urine. The most frequently used urine test looks for the presence of the hormone *human chorionic gonadotropin (HGC),* a hormone produced by the uterus once the fertilized ovum is implanted in it. This test for pregnancy is highly accurate when the menstrual period is two weeks overdue. Because early identification of pregnancy is necessary for proper prenatal care, it is wise not to postpone diagnosis by a physician or medical laboratory. If six weeks have passed since your last menstrual period and you have participated in sexual intercourse, you should have a pregnancy test. Results can be obtained about two minutes after the urine is analyzed.

Early Pregnancy Tests

You may have seen **early pregnancy tests (EPTs)** sold at a neighborhood drugstore. These do-it-yourself kits test for the presence of human chorionic gonadotropin (HCG) hormone in the urine. If HCG is present, the antibodies in the pregnancy test kits, which are added to the urine, turn a specific color, thereby indicating a positive result.

Consumers Union reports these tests to be very accurate when the result is positive. However, up to 25 percent of women receiving negative results may be pregnant. These are termed "false negatives." In fact, the earlier in the pregnancy the kit is used, the more likely a false negative will occur. Because the kits are usually used before consulting a physician and obtaining a laboratory test, Consumers Union recommends having only one test, the laboratory test. If a self-test is made, it is suggested it be done no sooner than fourteen days after a missed period, and if the result is negative, a second self-test should be administered a few days later.

Our advice: Save your money and peace of mind by having the test done at a physician's office, a clinic (for example, Planned Parenthood), or a county or state health department office.

Prenatal Care

The embryo (conceptus before twelve weeks) and fetus (conceptus after twelve weeks) are nourished through the blood of the mother. The blood carries nutrients

Year 2000 National Health Objective

In 1978, the infant mortality rate was 13.8 per 1,000 live births. Public health officials felt that this rate was too high and addressed the problem in a Year 1990 National Health Objective that aimed for an infant mortality rate of 9 per 1,000 live births. This objective was not met. Consequently, a Year 2000 National Health Objective seeks to reduce infant mortality from the 1987 rate of 10.1 per 1,000 live births to no more than 7 per 1,000 live births. This objective also specifically targets blacks, American Indians/Alaska Natives, and Puerto Ricans because their 1987 rates were 17.9, 12.5, and 12.9 respectively, compared to a rate of 8.6 for whites. The national health objective seeks to reduce these rates to 11 for blacks, 8.5 for American Indians/Alaska Natives, and 8 for Puerto Ricans.

and oxygen necessary for the baby's development in the uterus and is passed to the baby through the *placenta.* The placental membrane prevents certain substances or organisms from passing from the mother to the fetus. Other substances, however, some harmful, can pass through this placental barrier. For this reason, it is highly important that a pregnant woman obtain prenatal care as soon as she knows she is pregnant.

The most crucial phase of development in utero is the first three months. This is the time when the mother's lifestyle is most important. What she eats, whether she smokes or drinks alcohol—all of these decisions should be made with medical assistance. At the very least, medication, alcohol, and cigarettes should be discontinued until medical advice is obtained.

The need for early medical advice cannot be overemphasized. Inadequate prenatal care has been found to contribute to infant mortality and low-birth-weight babies. The factors contributing to the high infant mortality rate are late entry into prenatal care, teenage pregnancy, unintended pregnancy, older maternal age, and poor health habits such as smoking, alcohol consumption, and drug abuse.

To help make wise decisions, pregnant women should be aware of the following findings:

- Although past practice had suggested that pregnant women limit their weight gain to 20 pounds, a woman of average weight is now usually advised to gain between 25 and 35 pounds during pregnancy.

- Smoking during pregnancy is associated with lower birth weight, shorter gestation period, higher rates of spontaneous abortion, more frequent complications of pregnancy and delivery, and higher rates of infant mortality.

- Research with monkeys demonstrates that tetrahydrocannabinol (THC), the primary psychoactive agent in marijuana, can pass through the placental barrier and concentrate in the fatty tissue of the fetus.

- Even moderate consumption of alcohol while pregnant is related to central nervous system dysfunction and growth deficiency in babies. **Fetal alcohol syndrome** is the name given to the physical and psychological characteristics present in babies of mothers who drank heavily when pregnant.

- Aspirin taken by the mother is suspected of being associated with physical defects, blood-clotting problems and central nervous system dysfunction in the baby.

- Mothers addicted to heroin will give birth to babies addicted to heroin. The newborn must then go through withdrawal. Other narcotic drugs (such as cocaine) will lead to similar addictions.

- Pregnant women need to eat foods that are high in protein to aid fetal tissue growth and high in calcium to aid bone growth.

- Several complications of pregnancy can occur and should be recognized. *Toxemia* is pregnancy-induced hypertension, with swelling caused by fluid retention and the possibility of coma or convulsion. At the first signs of these symptoms, a physician should be consulted.

- Some pregnant women have an Rh negative blood factor that destroys the baby's Rh positive red blood cells. This combination is usually dangerous in second and subsequent pregnancies, where, if untreated, the baby could die. The method of

Year 2000 National Health Objective

One objective seeks to reduce the incidence of fetal alcohol syndrome from the 1987 rate of 0.22 per 1,000 live births to no more than 0.12 by the year 2000. Specifically targeted in this objectives are American Indians/Alaska Natives and blacks because their rates in 1987 were 4 and 0.8 respectively. These rates were 33 and 7 times higher than the rate for whites. The objective is to reduce these rates to 2 for American Indians and Alaska Natives and to 0.4 for blacks.

Determining the Due Date

You should know that even experts are not adept at specifying the date on which a pregnant woman will deliver. There are just too many variables involved. Everyone has probably heard of an obstetrician who, just one week before the baby was born, guessed incorrectly. What can be provided, however, is an approximation of the Expected Due Date (EDC).

Using Nägele's rule, named after the developer of this method, take the first day of the last menstrual period, subtract three months, add seven days, and then add a year. By way of example, if the first day of the last menstrual period was November 20, 1990, you would subtract three months (August 20, 1990), add seven days (August 27, 1990), and then add one year. In this case, the EDC would be August 27, 1991.

Nägele's rule works fairly well. When studied, 39 percent of newborns were delivered within five days of the predicted EDC and 55 percent were delivered within ten days of it.

Source: L. M. Hellman and J. A. Pritchard, *Williams Obstetrics* (New York: Appleton-Century-Crofts, 1971).

treatment is to give the newborn a transfusion with Rh negative blood. In time, the baby will replace this Rh negative blood with the Rh positive blood it produces.

It is clear that pregnant women have responsibility to maintain their health for the sake of their unborn babies. Given the importance of this responsibility, encouraging behaviors conducive to healthy births was a priority area of the national health objectives.

Educational campaigns aimed at pregnant women have been effective. There is data to indicate that when the diagnosis of pregnancy is made, smoking and drinking are reduced. The National Center for Health Statistics' 1980 National Natality Survey and 1980 National Fetal Mortality Survey reported that, before pregnancy, 30.9 percent of mothers smoked and 55 percent drank. During pregnancy, these figures were reduced to 25.5 percent who smoked and 39.2 percent who drank. In addition, numerous state and local governments have adopted programs to educate pregnant women about nutrition, smoking, alcohol, and drug abuse. It is anticipated that these programs will have a beneficial effect upon pregnant women's knowledge regarding means of enhancing their babies' health.

Gestation

Gestation is the period of time from conception to birth. The term of pregnancy is usually divided into three time periods, called *trimesters,* each of which is three months long.

labor The birth process.

cesarean section (C-section) A fetal delivery proce-

dure that involves cutting through the abdominal wall into the uterus, performed when a vaginal delivery would place the mother or the baby at risk.

The First Trimester At the end of the first month of pregnancy, the embryo is approximately one-quarter inch long. During this month, three cell layers are formed: the *ectoderm,* or outer layer, from which the skin, sense organs, and nervous system will form; the *mesoderm,* or middle layer, from which the muscular, circulatory, and excretory systems will form; and the *endoderm,* or inner layer, from which the digestive and glandular systems and the lungs will form.

At the conclusion of the second month, the embryo is approximately one and a quarter inches long and weighs one-thirtieth of an ounce. At this point, the embryo slightly resembles a small human, although its head is half its bulk and the forehead is very large. Also noticeable at this stage of development are the eyes, nose, lips, and tongue.

At the end of the first trimester, the fetus is three inches long and weighs one ounce. The fetus can move now but this movement is not noticeable or felt by the mother. At this stage, nails have grown on the fingers and toes, and the genitalia can be identified as male or female.

During the first trimester, the pregnant woman may experience a range of emotions and physical symptoms. It is interesting to note that the same woman may experience different feelings—psychologically and physically—in different pregnancies. Hormonal changes elicit many of the sensations pregnant women encounter. However, numerous factors influence the effects of these hormonal secretions. For example, women who are financially stable, who have a loving relationship with the father, and have high self-esteem can be expected to react differently from women who are less advantaged.

Among the physical changes pregnant women can expect are a cessation of the menses, an increase in size and tenderness in the breasts, a darkening of the nipples, and occasional nausea (commonly referred to as "morning sickness").

The Second Trimester The fourth month is characterized by great growth. The fetus grows to six inches in length, with the head now only one-third the body length. The fetus demonstrates an ability to suck, predominantly by sucking on its thumb. Usually, by the end of this month, the fetal movements can be felt by the mother. This movement is called *quickening.*

The conclusion of the fifth month finds the fetus twelve inches long and weighing one pound. The fetus now has all its essential structures.

At the end of the sixth month, the fetus is about fourteen inches long and weighs about two pounds. The eyes have formed, and the fetus is sensitive to light. The fetus can also hear uterine sounds.

During the second trimester, women typically experience a need to urinate frequently due to the pressure on the bladder from the enlarging fetus. The waistline becomes wider and the belly begins to protrude. The good news is that "morning sickness" disappears during the second trimester.

The Third Trimester During the last trimester, the fetus develops a layer of fat, making it appear more babylike. By the seventh month, the fetus generally has a good chance of survival if born prematurely. By the end of the eighth month, the fetus weighs about five pounds, four ounces, and is twenty inches long. During the last month of pregnancy, the baby's head moves into position in the pelvis. Figure 6.10 shows the development of the fetus at several stages.

During the last trimester, the uterus and abdomen enlarge, producing pressure on the stomach, intestines, and bladder. The result may be some discomfort, indigestion, and frequent urination.

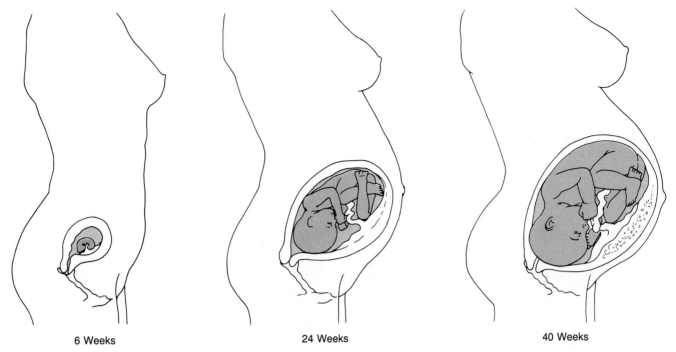

| 6 Weeks | 24 Weeks | 40 Weeks |

FIGURE 6.10 • Development of the fetus at 6 weeks, 24 weeks, and term. The relationship between changes in the fetus and changes in the mother is shown.

Childbirth

The Birth Process

First Stage The birth process, or **labor,** begins with rhythmic contraction of the uterine muscles.

The first stage of labor lasts an average of ten and a half hours for the first pregnancy and six and a half hours for subsequent pregnancies. The task of the first stage of labor is to open the neck of the cervix wide enough (ten centimeters) for the fetus to exit.

Second Stage The second stage of labor, consisting of pushing by the abdominal muscles, lasts about one-half to two hours. As the head of the fetus appears in the vaginal opening, an incision, known as an *episiotomy,* may be made by the physician to prevent the vaginal tissue from tearing. We mentioned the episiotomy procedure in the previous chapter. Episiotomies used to be common practice; now they are often deemed unnecessary.

Third Stage The third stage of labor results in the discharge of the placenta and occurs from two to twenty minutes after birth. When the umbilical cord stops pulsating, it is clamped and then cut. The baby is then checked for vital body functions and drops are deposited in its eyes to prevent gonorrheal infection.

Of course, this routine birth process can vary. If the fetus is positioned in the uterus for a *breech birth*— that is, with the buttocks rather than the head first—or if the pressure on the head of the fetus becomes too great, thereby decreasing its oxygen supply, other procedures are employed. The fetus may be delivered with the aid of forceps to pull it out gently or removed through an incision in the woman's abdomen.

Cesarean Section Delivery of the fetus by incision through the abdominal wall into the uterus is called a **cesarean section (C-section).** This procedure is performed when a delivery through the vagina would be a risk to the mother or baby. The baby's head may be too large, the baby may be in stress, labor may be prolonged, or labor contractions may not be strong enough for a vaginal delivery.

The number of C-sections has been increasing at a very high rate in the past decade (from 6 to 24 percent of births). One reason for this increase may be the use of the electronic fetal monitor, which checks uterine

Year 2000 National Health Objective

A Year 2000 National Health Objective now calls for reducing cesarean deliveries to no more than 15 per 100 deliveries. In 1987, that rate was 24.4 per 100 deliveries. More specifically, the objective seeks to reduce the 1987 first-time cesarean delivery rate of 17.4 to 12, and to reduce the repeat cesarean rate (women who have had a previous C-section) of 91.2 to 65.

bonding The attachment that develops between mother and newborn soon after birth.

Four scenes from childbirth

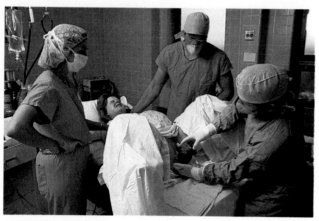

After nine months of gestation and hours of birth labor, the baby emerges.

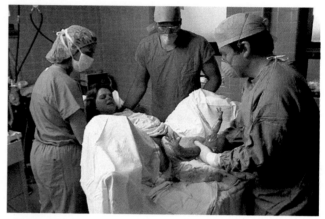

The baby is now nearly out; only the feet remain inside.

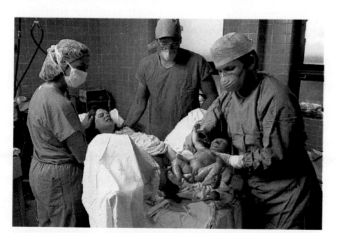

It's a new baby girl, seconds after her delivery (with the umbilical cord still attached).

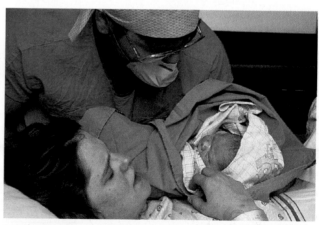

Let the bonding begin!

contractions and fetal heart beat during labor and can reveal problems physicians might otherwise miss. However, some physicians may misinterpret a labor variation as "fetal distress" and overreact by performing a C-section. Consequently, it has been suggested that the fetal monitor be used only in cases where there is a special need to watch the fetus.

There are other reasons for the large number of cesarean sections. For example, women who delivered by C-sections used to be told they would have to deliver other children in the same manner. This was because of concern that the incision would not be able to withstand the strains of subsequent pregnancies. In the past, women had C-sections with the incision running vertically. More recently, women have started to have C-sections with the incision running horizontally. The effect is that this horizontal incision is less likely to tear as a result of subsequent pregnancies. Consequently, a cesarean in one delivery doesn't necessarily require a cesarean in subsequent deliveries.

Making Decisions about Birthing

As a result of the increasing evidence that drugs used to decrease pain during childbirth remain in the baby's system long after birth, many women are choosing to give birth without drugs. Prepared childbirth consists of classes that teach the prospective parents what to expect and how to behave during delivery. Women are taught to relax through breathing exercises. Men are taught to coach. An important decision regarding birth, then, is whether to give birth without drugs.

Another decision being made more frequently in recent years is to deliver in the home rather than in the hospital. Gilbert D. Nass and G. W. McDonald summarize the pros and cons of home birth as follows:

> *Home birth offers a number of advantages, including the familiar surroundings, the presence and often the active participation of family and friends, the ability to make decisions about delivery with a doctor who is sympathetic to the couple's particular needs, the reduced expense, and the assurance that the couple will not be separated from their newborn for any length of time. The major drawback is the lack of immediate emergency equipment should complications arise.*
>
> *Home births require careful planning. Couples are screened for possible risks, they generally attend classes designed especially for those planning home births, and they often employ the services of a midwife who monitors the course of the pregnancy and is present at the birth along with a doctor. Women who are under twenty to over thirty and are giving birth for the first time are considered at higher risk and are usually discouraged from home birth. And women who experience problems during a first pregnancy or have a history of pregnancy-related problems are advised to give birth in a hospital.*[10]

Another decision relates to the ideas of French obstetrician Frederick Leboyer. Leboyer believed that birth was traumatic for the baby and should be made as comfortable as possible. He argued that the delivery room should be dimly lit, quiet, and warm. Further, the baby should not be turned upside down and spanked to encourage breathing but rather placed gently on the mother's abdomen and permitted to begin breathing gradually. Next the baby should be placed in water warmed to body temperature. Some physicians worry that babies will not begin to breathe properly if handled as recommended by Leboyer; others see no special advantage in the Leboyer method.

Still another decision in hospital births is whether to have the baby kept in the mother's room *(rooming-in)* or in a nursery area of the hospital, from which it is brought periodically to the mother for feeding and attention. Though the mother obtains valuable rest when the baby is kept in the nursery, there is evidence to suggest that mothers of first children who choose rooming-in feel more confident in themselves as mothers than those who do not choose rooming-in.

Bonding

There is evidence that **bonding,** or attachment between mother and newborn, develops quickly and can be delayed by extended separation just after birth. The initial contact between mother and child—fondling, holding, gazing, talking—somehow seems to enhance attachment of the mother to the newborn. Studies have shown a higher incidence of child abuse and a greater number of deaths in infants separated from their mothers at birth, compared to infants not separated from their mothers at birth. Premature infants are often separated from their parents, and the greater attention they require may cause stress for the parents.

The importance of bonding between father and child should also be recognized. Father-child attachment can be enhanced through home birth or natural childbirth, because in both types of birth the father is present and involved during the birth process.

Breast and Bottle Feeding

During pregnancy, secretions of estrogen, progesterone, and lactogen lead to an increase in breast tissue and glandular ducts. After delivery, a pituitary hormone named *prolactin* activates the mammary glands to produce milk. For three to four days after delivery, a

Some experts believe it is best for both the baby and the mother to breastfeed. The mother recovers from the delivery process more rapidly and the baby is afforded the protection of some antibodies.

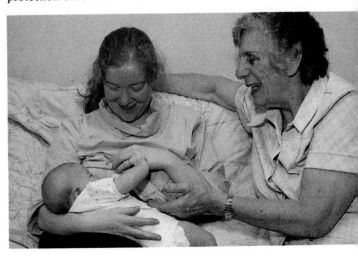

infertility Generally defined as the inability to conceive after a year or more of sexual relations without contraception.

artificial insemination The impregnation of a woman with the aid of medical techniques, using semen gathered from her husband or from another donor if the husband is sterile.

thin, yellowish liquid called *colostrum* is secreted; mature milk production begins four to seven days after delivery.

Breast feeding has distinct advantages over using infant formula. Breast milk contains antibodies that provides the infant with immunity to several diseases. In addition, the psychological attachment between mother and baby is enhanced by breast feeding.

However, not all women are able to breast feed, and many find bottle feeding more convenient. Although infant formula cannot supply the antibodies breast milk does, it provides all the nourishment a baby needs in order to thrive. Some couples prefer bottle feeding because it enables the father to participate in feeding the baby. Breast feeding for some meals and bottle feeding for others is another way of ensuring that the father is able to enjoy this aspect of baby care.

Infertility and Its Treatment

Infertility is generally defined as the inability to conceive after a year or more of sexual relations without contraception. Some experts report that 10 to 15 percent of American couples who want a child are infertile.[11] In about 30 percent of cases, both partners have a fertility problem. In the remaining 70 percent, about half of the problem can be traced to the woman and half to the man.

Causes of Infertility

Infertility, sometimes referred to as *sterility,* can have psychological or physiological causes. In men, infertility usually results from insufficient production of sperm or low *motility* (ability of the sperm to swim). This, in turn, can be a result of damage to the reproductive organs, mumps that caused injury to the seminiferous tubules, gonorrhea that caused scar tissue to form in the vas deferens, ingestion of drugs (heavy use of marijuana, for example), or psychological problems that create sexual dysfunction.

In women, infertility can be caused by pelvic infection, blockage of the Fallopian tubes, *endometriosis* (a condition in which tissue that normally grows in the uterus grows on various other abdominal structures), or several other factors. For example, women wearing intrauterine devices for more than two years without replacing them increase their susceptibility to pelvic infections that can lead to infertility. In addition, such factors as anemia, vitamin deficiency, malnutrition, and psychological stress can result in a failure to ovulate.

Treatment of Infertility

The success rate of treatment for infertility has been rising in recent years, and it is estimated that 50 to 70 percent of all childless couples are eventually able to have a baby.

Fertility may be enhanced with some simple education. For example, instructing women to lie on their backs for an hour after coitus so as to aid sperm in traveling up, rather than out of, the vagina, or even recommending more frequent intercourse, especially near the time of ovulation, may enable some couples to conceive. In addition, the use of the man-on-top coital position will increase the chances of conception. For many couples, however, these simple instructions are not enough.

Other procedures have been developed to enhance fertility. In all cases, however, the first step is an examination to determine why a couple is unable to conceive. Once the cause or causes have been determined, treatment can be prescribed. Checked ovulation can be restarted through hormone therapy or increasing body fat through nutritional therapy; and blocked Fallopian tubes can be cleared through new microsurgical techniques. Other techniques to treat infertility are described below.

Artificial Insemination About 20,000 babies yearly are produced by **artificial insemination.** There are two types of artificial insemination: AID (artificial insemination by a donor) and AIH (artificial insemination by the husband). Artificial insemination by the husband is generally attempted in couples where the husband has one of a number of problems such as a misplaced urinary meatus (that is, the opening in the glans penis is not where it should be), impotence, or low sperm count. The semen is collected from the husband by masturbation or immediately after coitus. Either the specimen is collected by the couple and brought to the clinic or the man masturbates at the clinic. The sperm are then introduced into the woman's uterus by means of a syringe or by placing the semen in a cervical cap fitted against the cervix.

Artificial insemination by a donor is done when there is no husband or where the husband produces no sperm, has a sperm count too low to ensure fertilization, has sperm that are not viable enough for insemination, or a combination of the last two. The donor is screened for health factors and matched to the husband in physical appearance and genetic background, though generally his identity is unknown by the receivers. For legal reasons, if the husband can produce even a minimal amount of sperm, some physicians mix his semen with that of the donor before inseminating the woman. Because in some states the question of legal paternity arises where AID is used, mixing of

Get Involved!

Fertility Control, Pregnancy, and Birth

After learning the information in this chapter, you will be able to make suggestions to people with whom you interact to help them improve their sexual lives. For example, if you have a postmenopausal woman in your family, you might suggest she consult with her physician regarding estrogen replacement therapy to ward off osteoporosis. If you know someone who is experiencing difficulty conceiving a child, you can let her know of the many options available and advise her to consult with her gynecologist. If you know an unmarried, coitally active individual, you can discuss contraceptive effectiveness and the pros and cons of various methods of birth control. In this way you will be helping others and improving the health of your society.

There are other things you can do for your community, nation, and world to enhance its health relative to fertility control, pregnancy, and birth. For example:

1. Be an informed citizen and vote for politicians whose views are consistent with yours on such issues as abortions, availability of contraceptive services, and funding for alternative methods of conceiving.

2. If concerned about the growth in world population, you can write your legislator(s) to support financial assistance to Third World countries attempting to limit the population growth that drains their own national resources. This assistance might take the form of making various methods of contraception available in those countries.

3. If coitally active, use some method of contraception to decrease the chance of bringing an unplanned child into this world. The method of contraception chosen should be consistent with your religious beliefs, values, and other considerations.

You can be more socially responsible if you really want to be!

sperm can help ensure the husband's status as father. In states that have no legal guidelines or statutes regarding paternity in such cases, lawyers encourage husbands to legally adopt children produced through AID. Given new methods of genetically analyzing cells and thereby determining the father of the baby, it is probably advisable for the husband legally to adopt an AID-produced baby as a precaution.

Artificial insemination allows people to experience natural parenthood even when they are unable to conceive through intercourse. And with AID, mothers at least are the biological parents of their offspring. Furthermore, many single women who are physically, emotionally, and economically capable of being

in vitro fertilization The fertilization of a human egg (ovum) by a sperm cell outside the body in a sterile, medically controlled environment. The fertilized egg is then placed within the mother-to-be's body for gestation and eventual birth.

A Question of Ethics

Is Surrogate Mothering Ethical and Should It Be Allowed?

As a result of developments in medical science and changing social mores—as well as a general void in legislation—women need not carry their babies in utero. Instead, they can hire another woman to be impregnated via artificial insemination by the husband's sperm. This impregnated woman—the surrogate mother—carries the baby to term and then turns it over to the couple when it is born. For "incubating" the child in this way, the surrogate mother is usually paid in excess of $20,000. And, to expedite this process, John Stehura published *Surrogate Mother* directory, which included photographs of surrogate mothers and suggested prices.

Some people are outraged by this practice. They feel that the bond between mother and child will be negatively affected; that our society is headed toward a cold, noncaring, futuristic world; and that surrogate

mothering is contrary to nature's and a supreme being's laws. Further, they argue, what if the surrogate becomes attached to the baby and refuses to give it up? This actually occurred in the celebrated "Baby M" case. In that case, a surrogate mother from New Jersey decided to keep the newborn and challenge her surrogacy contract with the biological father. Her decision created a good deal of animosity between herself and her family on the one side and the biological father and his family on the other. The courts ruled in 1987 that the father should have custody of the baby and the surrogate mother was only entitled to visiting rights. Or what if the baby is born with a serious birth defect and the couple refuses to accept possession of the child? Who is responsible for supporting the child under such circumstances?

Advocates of surrogate mothering say that laws can be passed to govern such situations. Blood tests can determine who the actual father was, and legal contracts can be drawn to govern all possibilities. Beside these legal issues, however, these advocates argue that pregnancy would actually threaten the lives of certain women; surrogate mothering allows these women to have children too.

This is certainly a difficult issue to resolve, but if you were required to vote for or against surrogate mothering, how would you vote?

mothers are unwilling to be impregnated through intercourse but are willing to be artificially inseminated. Obviously, while artificial insemination offers the option of parenthood to many to whom it was formerly barred, it also raises many questions of a moral nature, for example, whether it is fair to a child to intentionally bring it into the world with no known biological father.

"Test-Tube Babies"   While there is some artificiality to artificial insemination, there is even more to a newer procedure, **in vitro fertilization.** This fertilization technique allows conception to occur outside a woman's body, in the laboratory. The child of such a union is popularly called a "test-tube" baby.

To start the process, the physician inserts a laparoscope (a viewing instrument) into a woman's abdominal cavity through her umbilicus and looks for ripe follicles on the ovary indicating that eggs are ready to be released. The doctor inserts a needle through the laparoscope to break through the follicle and suck out several eggs. Timing, of course, is of critical importance in capturing ripe ova. Once eggs are isolated, they are put in a Petri dish (not really a test tube) and covered with some of the man's sperm—there, one hopes, to be fertilized. If the eggs are fertilized and successfully divides to the eight-cell stage, they are placed in the woman's uterus, where, if timing is right, they implant. Several eggs are used at one time due to the high rate of failure.

The first baby born by in vitro fertilization was born in England as a result of the efforts of Dr. Patrick Steptoe and Dr. Robert G. Edwards. Named Louise Brown, this historic baby was born on July 25, 1978. Since then many, many other children have been born as a result of in vitro fertilization. The first birth of an in vitro fertilization baby conceived in the United States occurred on December 28, 1981. The first test-tube twins were born in 1981 in Australia. The first American test-tube twins entered this world on the morning of March 24, 1983, in New York State.

In 1975, Joseph Califano, then Secretary of Health, Education and Welfare, created a thirteen-member advisory board of lawyers, doctors, and ethicists called the Ethics Advisory Board of the Department of Health, Education and Welfare. The board researched test-tube baby-making and approved the procedure in 1979. Currently, the potential for laboratory-created parenthood is phenomenal. Along with the ability to make families, however, this procedure too raises moral, ethical, social, and legal questions.

Embryo Transplant Embryo transplant, another alternative method of conception, involves a collection of women's eggs (usually sold to clinics by women for approximately $200). Then when a woman wants to have a child and cannot otherwise, an egg is selected, fertilized by her husband's sperm, and implanted in her uterus. The charge for each pregnancy is in the range of $10,000. The technology allowing for this procedure also provides for transplanting an ovum that has been fertilized in one woman to the uterus of another. Consequently, a couple seeking to conceive a child can have the male artificially inseminate another woman. Then approximately five days after conception, just before it is due to implant on the wall of the uterus, the egg is flushed out into a catheter and inserted by syringe into the uterus of the male's intended partner. The first successful embryo transfer resulted in a birth in 1984.

Conclusion

Many decisions must be made about contraception, pregnancy, and birth. Unmarried people must decide if they should participate in sexual intercourse; if so, whether to use contraceptives; if pregnancy occurs, whether to abort or deliver the unborn; and if the latter, if they should raise the baby, give it up for adoption, or abandon the child. Married people make similar decisions.

Additional decisions that must be made concern where to give birth, what method of delivery to use, and whether to breast feed.

The information and issues discussed in this chapter should help you make informed decisions about contraception, pregnancy, and birth.

Summary

1. Hormones are chemical substances produced by endocrine glands and affect organs throughout the body. The hormones that affect sexual development are estrogen and progesterone in females and testosterone in males.

2. The menstrual cycle is governed by the hormones FSH, LH, estrogen, and progesterone.

3. There is some evidence supporting the existence of a male menopause; for example, testosterone levels diminish over time. However, the changes in males are not as traumatic as those in females, and some men remain fertile throughout life.

4. There are many reasons why people choose not to use conception control even though they do not wish to conceive a child: they believe pregnancy couldn't happen to them, they feel guilty or immoral planning for coitus, they're too embarrassed to purchase contraceptives, or they believe they experience coitus too infrequently to be concerned with contraception.

5. Contraceptive effectiveness is evaluated in terms of failure rates. Theoretical or ideal failure rate refers to how effective the method is when used perfectly; actual user failure rate refers to how effective the method is when used by people outside controlled laboratory situations.

6. Conception control can be obtained in several ways: abstinence, withdrawal, rhythm, natural family planning, condoms, diaphragm, cervical cap, intrauterine devices, spermicides, the birth control pill, hormonal implants, and sterilization.

7. Abortion is termination of a pregnancy. Abortions that are not intentionally caused are called

spontaneous. Abortions performed intentionally are called induced. Methods of abortion include dilation and curettage, suction curettage, evacuation and curettage, hysterotomy, and induced labor by injection of saline solution. The choice of method depends on the stage of pregnancy.

8. Pregnancy is usually determined by a laboratory test for the hormone human chronic gonadotropin in the urine. Results can be obtained about two minutes after the urine is analyzed.

9. Prenatal care is recommended as soon as pregnancy is determined. Good prenatal care and nutrition are related to fewer birth defects and lower infant mortality.

10. Cigarette smoking, use of drugs, consumption of alcoholic beverages, and poor nutrition are related to spontaneous abortion, birth defects, and infant mortality. Therefore, pregnant women should adjust their behavior in these respects during the gestation period.

11. Childbirth consists of three stages of labor. In the first stage the neck of the cervix opens wide enough for the fetus to exit, in the second stage the baby is delivered, and in the third stage the placenta is discharged.

12. Among the decisions regarding childbirth are where to have the delivery, whether to use drugs or deliver without medication, whether to have rooming-in, and whether to subsequently breast feed.

13. Infertility is a problem for some 10 to 15 percent of couples in the United States who want a child. The success rate for treatment of infertility has been rising in recent years. When the male is infertile, many couples choose artificial insemination, in which sperm from an anonymous donor is introduced into the vagina of the female partner with a syringe.

Questions for Personal Growth

1. If you were a parent, which method of contraception would you recommend to your daughter? Which would you recommend to your son? Which recommendation would you feel more confident about? Why?

2. Which of your behaviors or feelings do you think are related to the hormones in your body? Can you identify any behaviors or feelings that result from hormonal secretions in someone of the opposite gender that you know well?

3. What feelings do you think women experience when they go through menopause? Do you think men have similar feelings when they reach a comparable age? How do you think they can help each other?

4. What do you think someone should say to a sexual partner who refuses to use a condom? Would you feel comfortable speaking in this way?

5. How are relationships affected by the AIDS crisis? How are sexual relationships affected by the AIDS crisis?

6. Should RU 486 be made available to American women? If not, why not? If so, what strategies would you suggest to encourage its marketing in the United States?

7. When, if ever, should an abortion be allowed? What restrictions would you place on legal abortions? (For example, would you place restrictions on where it is to be done, by whom it is to be done, or when during the pregnancy it is to be done?)

8. Is a politician's views on abortion important enough to you for you to vote for him or her solely on that criterion? What would be other criteria you would consider?

9. What will you do to make your society better in relation to fertility control, pregnancy, or birth? By when will you do it? Who else will you involve?

References

1. J. L. Berkowitz et al., "Estrogen Replacement Therapy and Fibrocystic Disease in Postmenopausal Women," *American Journal of Epidemiology* 121 (1985): 238–245.

2. Juanita H. Williams, *Psychology of Women: Behavior in a Biosocial Context,* 3e (New York: W. W. Norton & Co., 1987), p. 480.

3. J. Trussel, "Teenage Pregnancy in the U.S.," *Family Planning Perspectives* 20 (1988): 262–272.

4. Christine Russell, "Doctors Say Fear of Pill Exaggerated," *Washington Post* (March 6, 1985): C5.

5. Robert A. Hatcher et al., *Contraceptive Technology, 1986-87* (New York: Irvington, 1988).

6. Richard Hantula, "IUDs," *Spotlight on Health* 1 (1986): 7.

7. Jane Patterson, "The Contraceptive Implant," *Shape* (August 1990): 30–31.

8. William D. Mosher and William F. Pratt, "Use of Contraception and Family Planning Services in the United States, 1988," *American Journal of Public Health* 90 (1990): 1132–1133.

9. William D. Mosher and William F. Pratt, "Contraceptive Use in the United States, 1973–1988," *Advance Data* 182 (March 20, 1990): 2.

10. Gilbert D. Nass and G. W. McDonald, *Marriage and the Family,* 2e (Reading, Mass.: Addison-Wesley, 1982), pp. 321–322.

11. William H. Masters, Virginia E. Johnson, and Robert C. Kolodny, *Human Sexuality,* 3e (Glenview, Ill.: Scott Foresman and Company, 1988), p. 142.

CHAPTER
7

Nutrition

CHAPTER OBJECTIVES

After reading this chapter, you should understand:

- The six different kinds of nutrients, the recommended dietary allowances (RDAs) of certain nutrients, and the basic four food groups.

- The three kinds of energy nutrients—carbohydrates, fats, and proteins—and how they provide the body with energy, which is measured in calories.

- The three kinds of non-energy nutrients—vitamins, minerals, and water—and why they too are essential for the body's proper functioning.

- How to eat a variety of healthy foods while regulating dietary intake of foods with too much fat, sugar, and sodium.

- How the United States government regulates food additives and food labeling and how you can read a food label.

- Several nutritional myths.

- The special nutritional needs of athletes and active individuals.

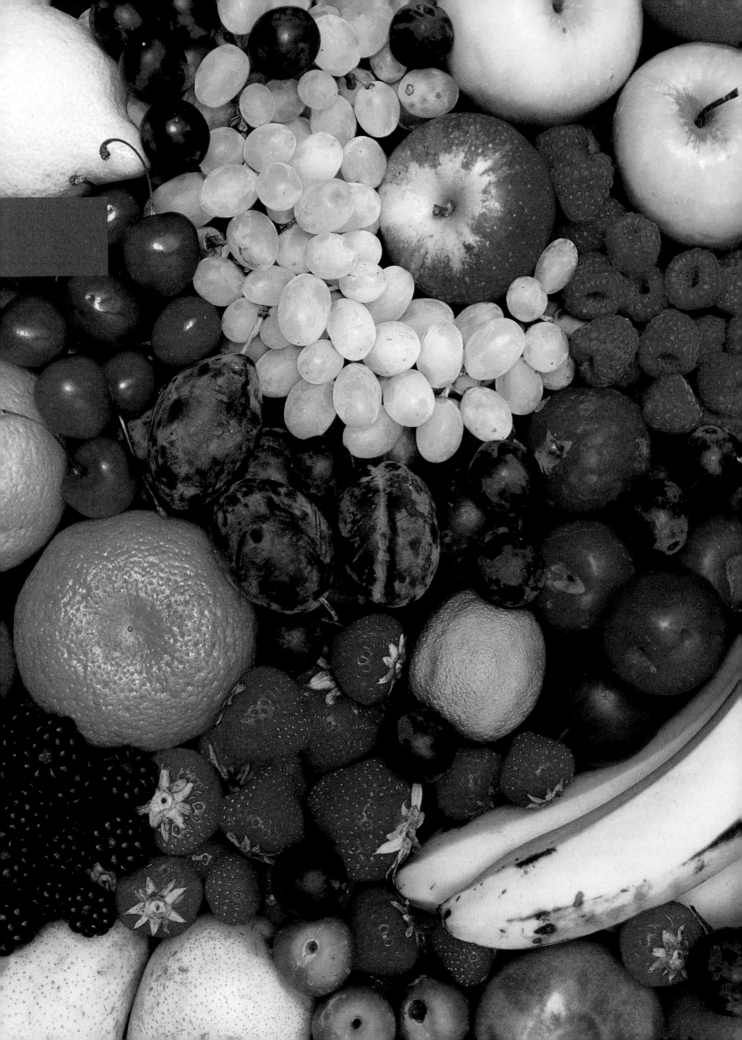

What is the relationship between nutrition, health, and performance? The old cliché "you are what you eat" is taking on new meaning as evidence mounts associating dietary practices with health and longevity. The volume of information available on nutrition is almost overwhelming. As a result, it is often difficult for individuals to determine what constitutes a healthy diet for their particular needs. This chapter offers enough basic information to help you make appropriate choices.

Basic Food Components

Kinds of Nutrients

Six categories of nutrients—carbohydrates, fats, and proteins (the energy nutrients), and vitamins, minerals, and water (the non-energy nutrients)—satisfy the basic body needs:

- Energy for muscle contraction
- Conduction of nerve impulses
- Growth
- Formation of new tissue and tissue repair
- Chemical regulation of metabolic functions
- Reproduction

The body's use of these nutrients for conversion into body tissue, muscle contraction, and maintenance of chemical machinery is called *metabolism*.

Recommended Dietary Allowances

Every five years, the Food and Nutritional Board of the National Academy of Sciences' National Research Council reviews for possible revision the recommended dietary allowances (RDAs) of certain essential nutrients.[1] RDAs are recommendations, not the minimum requirements, of essential nutrients and represent generous intake levels of essential nutrients considered to meet adequately the known nutritional needs of practically all healthy persons in the United States. The margin of safety of these recommendations is substantial, and it is estimated that two-thirds of the

recommended amounts is adequate for most healthy people. Failing to meet recommended dietary allowances for one day does not mean you have a deficient diet; however, RDAs should average out over a 5- to 8-day period. Separate RDAs are provided for infants, children, males, females, and pregnant and lactating women. You can use Table 7.1 to determine whether your basic nutritional needs are being met.

The **U.S. RDA** is nothing more than a simplified RDA appearing on the labels of food products (see the food labeling section of this chapter), which shows the percentage of each nutrient's RDA provided by one serving of the food.

The Basic Four Food Groups

Foods of similar nutrient value have been placed into four categories, referred to as the basic four food groups. Table 7.2 lists some common foods found in each group and the recommended number of servings daily for children, teenagers, adults, and pregnant and lactating women. There are also some foods that do not fall naturally into one of the four food groups, such as fats, sweets, non-juice beverages, and condiments, which are commonly listed as "others or miscellaneous."

The Four Food Group Plan offers an alternative to

The Basic Four Food Groups and the recommended number of servings for the various groups.

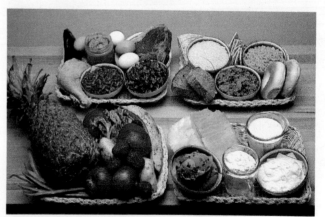

TABLE 7.1

Food and Nutrition Board, National Academy of Sciences—National Research Council Recommended Dietary Allowances,[a] Revised 1989. *Designed for the maintenance of good nutrition of practically all healthy people in the United States*

Category or Condition	Age (years)	Weight[b] (kg)	Weight[b] (lb)	Height[b] (cm)	Height[b] (in)	Protein (g)	Vitamin A (µg RE)[c]	Vitamin D (µg)[d]	Vitamin E (mg α-TE)[e]	Vitamin K (µg)
Infants	0.0–0.5	6	13	60	24	13	375	7.5	3	5
	0.5–1.0	9	20	71	28	14	375	10	4	10
Children	1–3	13	29	90	35	16	400	10	6	15
	4–6	20	44	112	44	24	500	10	7	20
	7–10	28	62	132	52	28	700	10	7	30
Males	11–14	45	99	157	62	45	1,000	10	10	45
	15–18	66	145	176	69	59	1,000	10	10	65
	19–24	72	160	177	70	58	1,000	10	10	70
	25–50	79	174	176	70	63	1,000	5	10	80
	51+	77	170	173	68	63	1,000	5	10	80
Females	11–14	46	101	157	62	46	800	10	8	45
	15–18	55	120	163	64	44	800	10	8	55
	19–24	58	128	164	65	46	800	10	8	60
	25–50	63	138	163	64	50	800	5	8	65
	51+	65	143	160	63	50	800	5	8	65
Pregnant						60	800	10	10	65
Lactating	1st 6 months					65	1,300	10	12	65
	2nd 6 months					62	1,200	10	11	65

Vitamin C (mg)	Thiamin (mg)	Riboflavin (mg)	Niacin (mg NE)[f]	Vitamin B6 (mg)	Folate (µg)	Vitamin B12 (µg)	Calcium (mg)	Phosphorus (mg)	Magnesium (mg)	Iron (mg)	Zinc (mg)	Iodine (µg)	Selenium (µg)
30	0.3	0.4	5	0.3	25	0.3	400	300	40	6	5	40	10
35	0.4	0.5	6	0.6	35	0.5	600	500	60	10	5	50	15
40	0.7	0.8	9	1.0	50	0.7	800	800	80	10	10	70	20
45	0.9	1.1	12	1.1	75	1.0	800	800	120	10	10	90	20
45	1.0	1.2	13	1.4	100	1.4	800	800	170	10	10	120	30
50	1.3	1.5	17	1.7	150	2.0	1,200	1,200	270	12	15	150	40
60	1.5	1.8	20	2.0	200	2.0	1,200	1,200	400	12	15	150	50
60	1.5	1.7	19	2.0	200	2.0	1,200	1,200	350	10	15	150	70
60	1.5	1.7	19	2.0	200	2.0	800	800	350	10	15	150	70
60	1.2	1.4	15	2.0	200	2.0	800	800	350	10	15	150	70
50	1.1	1.3	15	1.4	150	2.0	1,200	1,200	280	15	12	150	45
60	1.1	1.3	15	1.5	180	2.0	1,200	1,200	300	15	12	150	50
60	1.1	1.3	15	1.6	180	2.0	1,200	1,200	280	15	12	150	55
60	1.1	1.3	15	1.6	180	2.0	800	800	280	15	12	150	55
60	1.0	1.2	13	1.6	180	2.0	800	800	280	10	12	150	55
70	1.5	1.6	17	2.2	400	2.2	1,200	1,200	320	30	15	175	65
95	1.6	1.8	20	2.1	280	2.6	1,200	1,200	355	15	19	200	75
90	1.6	1.7	20	2.1	260	2.6	1,200	1,200	340	15	16	200	75

[a] The allowances, expressed as average daily intakes over time, are intended to provide for individual variations among most normal persons as they live in the United States under usual environmental stresses. Diets should be based on a variety of common foods in order to provide other nutrients for which human requirements have been less well defined. . . .

[b] Weights and heights of Reference Adults are actual medians for the U.S. population of the designated age, as reported by NHANES II. The median weights and heights of those under 19 years of age were taken from Hamill et al. (1979). . . . The use of these figures does not imply that the height-to-weight ratios are ideal.

[c] Retinol equivalents. 1 retinol equivalent = 1 µg retinol or 6 µg β-carotene. . . .

[d] As cholecalciferol. 10 µg cholecalciferol = 400 IU of vitamin D.

[e] α-Tocopherol equivalents. 1 mg d-α tocopherol = 1 α-TE. . . .

[f] 1 NE (niacin equivalent) is equal to 1 mg of niacin or 60 mg of dietary trypotphan.

Source: Subcommittee on the Tenth Edition of the RDAs Food and Nutrition Board, Commission on Life Sciences, National Research Council. *Recommended Dietary Allowances,* 10e. (Washington, D.C.: National Academy Press, 1989).

calories A unit of measurement indicating the amount of energy contained in a given amount of food.

basal metabolism or metabolic rate The number of calories burned by a person while at rest but not while sleeping.

TABLE 7.2

A Recommended Daily Pattern

Food Group	Recommended Number of Servings				
	Child	Teenager	Adult	Pregnant Woman	Lactating Woman
Milk	3	4	2	4	4
1 cup milk, yogurt, or calcium equivalent:					
1½ slices (1½ oz) cheddar cheese*					
1 cup pudding					
1¾ cups ice cream					
2 cups cottage cheese*					
Meat	2	2	2	3	2
2 oz cooked, lean meat, fish, poultry or protein equivalent:					
2 eggs					
2 slices (2 oz) cheddar cheese*					
½ cup cottage cheese*					
1 cup dried beans, peas					
4 tbsp. peanut butter					
Fruit-Vegetable	4	4	4	4	4
½ cup cooked or juice					
1 cup raw portion commonly served such as a medium-sized apple or banana					
Grain, whole grain, fortified, enriched	4	4	4	4	4
1 slice bread					
1 cup ready-to-eat cereal					
½ cup cooked cereal, pasta, grits					

Note: Others complement but do not replace foods from the four food groups. Amounts should be determined by individual caloric needs. The recommended daily pattern provides the foundation for a nutritious, healthful diet. The recommended servings from the four food groups for adults supply about 1200 calories. The chart gives recommendations for the number and size of servings for several categories of people.

* Count cheese as serving of milk *or* meat, but not simultaneously.

the complicated RDA tables as a means of determining whether you are obtaining an adequate diet. If you consume the proper number of servings from each food group on a regular basis, you can assume that you are meeting the RDAs discussed previously.

The Energy Nutrients: Carbohydrates, Fats, and Proteins

Carbohydrates and fat provide the body with its two main sources of energy to perform work. Only under semistarvation conditions is protein utilized for energy. All food has energy potential, which is measured in **calories.** Since one calorie is too small a unit to be convenient, nutritionists use a large, or "kilocalorie" (kcalorie), as a measure. One kilocalorie is equal to one thousand small calories. In most of today's literature, the term calorie is used when reference is really being made to the larger calorie, or kilocalorie. One *calorie (kilocalorie)* is the amount of heat required to raise the temperature of one kilogram (approximately one quart) of water one degree Celsius. As an example, the energy in one peanut can add one degree of heat to two gallons of water. Only carbohydrates, fats, and protein contain calories; vitamins, minerals, and water contain no calories.

Carbohydrates	4 calories per gram
Protein	4 calories per gram
Fats	9 calories per gram
Alcohol	7 calories per gram

1 gram = approximately $\frac{1}{5}$ level teaspoon

100 grams = $\frac{1}{2}$ cup

1 milligram = $\frac{1}{1000}$ of a gram

As you can see, carbohydrates contain only 4 calories per gram, the same as protein. Fats and alcohol, on the other hand, possess nearly twice as many calories per gram.

Your **basal metabolism,** or **metabolic rate,** is the number of calories burned while at rest but not sleeping. Your body is in a state of caloric balance when food intake in calories is exactly equal to food expenditure and elimination through basal metabolism, activity, and calories lost in excreta. In this state, no weight gain or loss will occur.

Caloric needs depend on age, height and weight, metabolism, and activity patterns (work and play). We will discuss how to estimate your caloric needs and achieve caloric balance in Chapter 8.

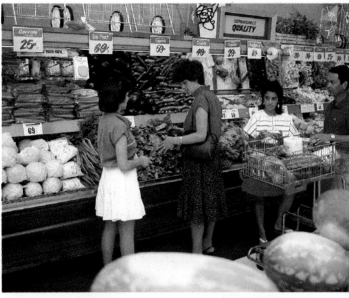

The average adult consumes less than one-half of the recommended amount of complex carbohydrates daily, yet they are the most important group of foods in our diet and our only source of dietary fiber.

Carbohydrates

Carbohydrates are organic components of various elements that provide a continuous supply of energy in the form of *glucose* (sugar) to trillions of body cells. There are three types of carbohydrates: *simple carbohydrates,* sugars that occur naturally in such foods as vegetables and fruits; *concentrated carbohydrates,* such as refined sugar made from cane or beet sugar; and naturally occurring *complex carbohydrates.* The complex carbohydrates are chains of sugar molecules that are linked. The most important of these is starch, found in vegetables, fruits, and whole grains. About 50 percent of the American diet is composed of carbohydrates.

Carbohydrates are broken down into six simple carbon sugar molecules to permit absorption into the bloodstream. After food is eaten, the blood sugar level is elevated and there is an increase in glucose transported to the cells. Excess sugar is converted to glycogen and stored for future use. Once maximum storage capacity is reached, excess sugars are converted to body fat and stored as adipose tissue.

In the past seventy-five years, starch intake in the American diet has decreased by 30 percent and sugar intake as risen by about the same amount. Unlike sugars, starches are the body's chief source of fuel. Their reputation as being fattening is due to the fact that they are normally eaten with fat, such as butter on bread or potatoes. Sugar, on the other hand, provides empty calories and contributes to weight gain, tooth decay, and the development of some diseases.

Complex carbohydrates such as fruits, vegetables,

dietary fiber The undigested portion of complex carbohydrates, a nonnutritive substance that comes from plant sources.

cholesterol One of the sterols or fatlike chemical substances manufactured by the body and also consumed in foods of animal origin. Excess cholesterol is associated with coronary heart and artery disease.

and grains are our major source of vitamins, an important long-term energy source, and the only source of roughage or fiber. Only vitamin B_{12} is not found in carbohydrates. Complex carbohydrates burn efficiently, leave no toxic waste in the body and do not tax the liver or raise blood triglyceride levels. Fruits, vegetables, and grains also have high nutritional density, providing many nutrients and few calories.

Complex carbohydrates should make up approximately 48 percent of the American diet. The intake of simple carbohydrates, currently 24 percent of the American diet, should be reduced to 10 percent.

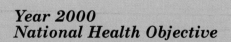 **Fiber** **Dietary fiber,** the undigested portion of complex carbohydrates, is a nonnutritive substance that comes from plant sources. Fiber cannot be digested by the enzymes in the human body, although intestinal bacteria can break down some of the fiber. Six of the seven types of fiber are carbohydrate. Only lignin, found in fruit and vegetable skins and the woody portions of plants, is a noncarbohydrate.

Table 7.3 provides an overview of key information on fiber, including *water-soluble* and *water-insoluble* fiber, *dietary fiber* and *crude fiber,* recommended daily fiber intake, the nutritional advantages of adequate dietary fiber, the dangers of too much fiber, and the food sources of both water-soluble and water-insolable fiber. Although an extra portion or so of fiber will cause no problems, the key to sound fiber intake is using moderation and variation when choosing foods from among the four food groups and avoiding fiber supplements or exceeding 35 grams daily. Use Exploring Your Health 7.1 to determine whether or not your diet includes enough fiber.

Fats

Fat is critical to the human body. Fat provides energy for the body and stores and transports vitamins A, D, E, and K. The fat in our food is a concentrated source of energy. It carrys linoleic acid (an essential fatty acid), increases the flavor and palatability of foods, provides sustained relief from hunger, and spares protein from being used as energy. The fatty tissue in our body supports organs, cushions them from injury, and aids in the prevention of heat loss. Fat is present in most body tissue, with bone marrow containing 96 percent, liver 2.5 percent, and blood 0.5 percent. Unfortunately, too much fat on the body and high blood fat levels can shorten life and increase the vulnerability to numerous chronic and degenerative diseases, such as cardiovascular disease and cancer.

The fat in our food is classified as *saturated* (fats derived from animal sources, such as meat, milk, butter, and cheese, and chocolate, coconut, lard, palm oil, poultry, vegetable shortening); *polyunsaturated* (liquid vegetable oils, such as corn, soybean, safflower, cottonseed, and sunflower oils, almonds, pecans, walnuts, filberts, fish, soft margarine); *monounsaturated* (avocados, cashews, peanut and olive oils). **Cholesterol,** one of the sterols or fatlike chemical substances manufactured in the body and consumed from food of animal origin, is used in the synthesis of sex hormones, vitamin D, and bile salts. It is also associated with artery clogging and heart disease (see Chapter 15). Blood cholesterol consists of the cholesterol in our diet and that produced by the body. The average American consumes over 55 pounds of *visible fat* (butter, lard, margarine, shortening, and cooking and salad oils) and over 130 pounds of *invisible fat* (dairy products, eggs, meat, poultry, fish, beans, nuts, soy products, cocoa, fruits, vegetables, grain products) each year. Dietary fat contributes approximately 42 percent of the total calories

TABLE 7.3

All About Fiber

Types	
Water-Insoluble	Cellulose, forming the cell walls of many plants, is the most abundant insoluble fiber. Cellulose and lignin (from the woody portion of plants, parts of fruit and vegetable skins, and whole grains) cannot be broken down, digested, or made to provide calories for the body.
Water-Soluble	The fiber in food that can be broken down and digested to provide calories for the body is referred to as water-soluble. Dried beans and peas (8 grams per $\frac{1}{2}$ cup), oat bran, and the flesh of fruits and vegetables are excellent sources of water-soluble fiber.
Label Reference	
Dietary fiber	Undigested residue after the action of the body's enzymes; much more concentrated than crude fiber. (1 gram of crude fiber = 2–3 grams of dietary fiber.) Dietary fiber is reported on most labels that list fiber content.
Crude fiber	Remaining portion of food that cannot be dissolved or broken down into a liquid when exposed to acids and alkalies in the laboratory. This fiber, consisting of cellulose and lignin, was reported on product labels and tables for many years. Due to inaccurate measurement, the crude fiber was reported at levels two to three times lower than dietary fiber.
Daily Needs	25–35 grams. It is important to increase your daily intake slowly if you are unaccustomed to adequate fiber to avoid frequent bowel movements and diarrhea. Add several grams daily over a period of a few weeks to give your system a chance to adjust.
Nutritional Advantages of Consuming Adequate Fiber	*Insoluble* fiber increases transit time (digestion and elimination of food) and decreases the amount of time the bacteria in the food has to act on intestinal walls. It helps prevent colon and rectal cancer and *diverticulosis* (outpouchings in the wall of the large intestine), provides bulk to the stools, helps eliminate constipation, helps maintain normal bowel movement, and helps to control and maintain normal body weight and fat. *Water-soluble* fiber is associated with lower cardiovascular disease, lower blood cholesterol, and lower blood pressure.
Dangers of Excess Fiber	Excess fiber binds to some trace minerals and causes excretion prior to the absorption of these minerals. Excessive fiber intake causes poor absorption of nutrients, interferes with the absorption of some drugs, reduces the ability to digest and absorb food by speeding up digestive time, and causes irritation of the intestinal wall. The high phosphorus content of high-fiber foods may create special problems for some individuals, such as those with kidney problems.
Food Sources	Complex carbohydrates (fruits, vegetables, and grains) are the sole source of fiber. Both water-insoluble and water-soluble fiber are contained in some food sources, such as in the skin of fruits and vegetables (insoluble) and in the flesh of fruits and vegetables (soluble). Raw fruits and vegetables are a major source of insoluble fiber, dried beans and peas (8 grams per $\frac{1}{2}$ cup). Oat bran and grains are a major source of soluble fiber.
	Many hot and cold cereals (unprocessed bran, 100 percent bran, shredded wheat, oatmeal) contain 2–5 grams of fiber per serving. Legumes provide about 8 grams per portion ($\frac{1}{2}$ cup of garbanzo beans, kidney beans, or baked beans). Fruits provide about 2 grams per serving (one small apple, banana, orange; two small plums, a medium peach, $\frac{1}{2}$ cup strawberries, ten large cherries). Vegetables also provide about 2 grams per serving (broccoli, brussels sprouts, two stalks of celery, small corn cob, lettuce, green beans, small potato, tomato), and 1 gram of fiber is provided by ten peanuts, $\frac{1}{4}$ cup walnuts, $2\frac{1}{2}$ teaspoons of peanut butter, and a pickle. Additional foods with fiber are breads (whole wheat, whole grain), crackers, and flours (wheat germ, wild rice, cornmeal, buckwheat, millet, rice, raisin, and popcorn). Cooking does not significantly reduce the fiber content of foods.

nonessential amino acids Those amino acids that can be manufactured by the body if not obtained from the diet.

essential amino acids Those amino acids that cannot be manufactured by the body and must be obtained from food.

Exploring Your Health 7.1

Does Your Diet Contain Enough Fiber?

Record the foods you eat on three consecutive days from the time you awake until you go to bed. Using the chart below, determine whether you are obtaining sufficient fiber daily.

Food	Amount	High Fiber	Low Fiber
Day 1			
Day 2			
Day 3			

High-fiber foods: breads (whole-wheat and whole-grain breads and crackers), cereals (bran-type cereals such as unprocessed and concentrated bran, 100 percent bran, shredded wheat, oatmeal), cereal products and flours (wheat germ, wild rice, buckwheat, cornmeal, millet, rice bran, whole wheat), fruits (fresh fruits with skin, bananas and berries, dried fruits), vegetables (raw vegetables and those steamed in small amounts of water), legumes, nuts, seeds, popcorn.

in the American diet, although the recent favorable pattern of fat intake shows that more fat is being consumed from plants and less from animal sources. A major source of saturated fat in our diet is the food eaten in fast-food restaurants. Since saturated fat intake stimulates the production of cholesterol, it is important to reduce cholesterol intake to less than 300 milligrams daily and total saturated fat to less than 10 percent of daily calories.

Year 2000 National Health Objective

Because of the available evidence linking nutritional habits to cancer and heart and other diseases, the federal government is striving to reduce dietary fat intake to 30 percent or less of total calories consumed and saturated fat intake to less than 10 percent of total calories consumed among people age 2 and older. Current evidence shows a consumption of 36 percent total fat and 13 percent saturated fat among people age 20 to 74. The government is also striving to increase the intake of complex carbohydrates (fiber-containing foods) to five or more servings daily of vegetables (including legumes) and fruits, and to six or more servings daily of grain products, in order to prevent and eliminate obesity (see Chapter 8).

Protein

Protein, from the Greek word *proteios*, or "primary," is critical to all living things. In the human body, it is used to repair, rebuild, and replace cells. More specifically, protein aids in growth, fluid balance, salt balance, acid-base balance, and provides needed energy when carbohydrates and fats are insufficient or unavailable. Protein is produced in the body through protein building blocks called *amino acids.* Some amino acids are produced in the body; others are derived from food sources. **Nonessential amino acids** can be manufactured by the body if not obtained from the diet. These amino acids are alanine, aspartic acid, arginine, citrulline, cystine, glutamic acid, glycine, hydroxyglutamic acid, hydroxyproline, norleucine, proline, serine, and tyrosine. **Essential amino acids,** eight to ten of which must be present in the body in the proper amount and proportion to the nonessential amino

Fat Replacements: Having Your "Fat" and Eating It, Too

Artificial fats or fat substitutes have entered the marketplace. Although food chemists have been experimenting with artificial fats since the 1960s, manufacturers have only recently filed petitions with the FDA for approval of their products. Two such products that are certain to become as popular and common as NutraSweet® are Simplesse® and Olestra®. Each takes a different approach toward satisfying our appetite for products rich in fats and oils.[2] Each holds the promise of great taste without the calories or health consequences.

Simplesse® is a low-calorie, all-natural "fat substitute" with FDA approval that entered the market in early 1990 in Simple Pleasures Frozen Dairy Dessert ice cream (toffee crunch, chocolate, strawberry, coffee, peach, and rum raisin). Simplesse® is manufactured from egg white and milk protein through a "secret" cooking process, called microparticulation, which alters protein into tiny round particles that become creamy when placed on the tongue. The patented process inhibits the natural tendency of proteins to coagulate into a large mass when heated. This occurs by heating the protein under intense agitation, followed by rapid cooling to create uniform small, round protein particles. Due to the shape and size (0.1 to 3.0 microns; 50 billion per teaspoon of loosely packed complete protein molecules) of the protein in Simplesse®, the tongue perceives the particles as having the creamy rich texture of fat. Such a process counters the normal changes occurring when protein is heated. Unlike fat that contains nine calories per gram (1 teaspoon of fat = 5 grams and 45 calories), Simplesse® contains only $1\frac{1}{3}$ calories per gram.

Olestra® is a calorie-free fat replacement, formerly known as sucrose polyester, which was discovered over twenty years ago. Actually, it is a synthetic combination of sucrose and fatty acids (sugar and vegetable oil) that is not digestible. Olestra not only avoids absorption, it also interferes with the absorption of dietary cholesterol and the cholesterol recycled through the enterohepatic pathway. As a result, you can have the rich, creamy taste of fats and oils, zero calories, and a reduction in blood cholesterol. Olestra® will be used in oils, margarine, snacks, and desserts. It has the appearance, feel, and taste of dietary fat.

The good news is that wise use of Simplesse® and Olestra® could improve the health and nutrition of the American people by reducing saturated fat and cholesterol intake, by reducing total caloric intake, by making it easier to change eating habits, by improving nutrition density (the calorie to nutrient ratio) in foods such as baked potato, broccoli, and salads that traditionally involve high fat, butters, salad dressings, and sour creams, and by adding slightly more protein to the diet.

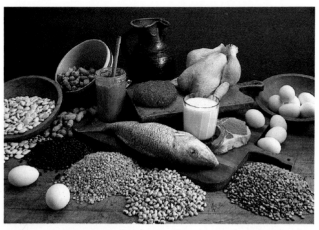

College students have little difficulty in consuming the recommended 12 percent of their daily calories from protein.

All twenty-two amino acids must be present simultaneously in order for the body to synthesize them into body proteins that will be used for optimal maintenance of body growth and function.

Humans obtain protein from both animal and plant foods. In general, animal protein is superior to plant protein because it contains all the essential amino acids and contains them in the proper proportions. If one essential amino acid is missing or in the incorrect proportion, protein construction may be blocked.

Eggs represent a complete protein source by which all other protein can be judged. Milk, cheese, other dairy products, meat, fish, and poultry compare favorably to eggs as excellent sources of protein. A recent one-year study by the U.S. Department of Agriculture revealed that eggs have less fat and 22 percent less cholesterol than previously believed—a relief to the egg industry, which has experienced steadily declining sales. The average large egg contains 213 milligrams of cholesterol instead of the 274 reported in the 1976 government guidelines, an extra large egg contains 230 milligrams, and a medium egg contains 180 milligrams. The average large egg unfortunately also contains 5 grams of fat, or 45 calories of the total 75 calories. An egg therefore contains 60 percent fat. On the positive side, however, eggs are a low-calorie source of protein (the best complete protein source in our diet), vitamin A, riboflavin, vitamin B_{12}, iron, zinc, phosphorus, calcium, potassium, and other nutrients. It is still advisable to consume no more than 2 or 3 eggs per week, never more than one in one day, to eliminate or substitute other food products in menus calling for eggs as an ingredient, and to purchase small eggs rather than medium, large, or extra large. The American Heart Association guideline of no more than 300 milligrams of cholesterol per day is difficult to follow if you start the day with eggs rather than with cold or hot cereal.

Protein containing all essential amino acids (ly-

acids for normal protein metabolism, cannot be manufactured by the body and must be acquired in our diet. The essential amino acids for adults are isoleucine, leucine, lysine, methionine, phenylalanine, threonine, tryptophan, and valine; children also need histidine.

water-soluble vitamins Those vitamins that are dissolved in water and are not stored in the body, such as vitamin C and the B complex vitamins.

fat-soluble vitamins Those vitamins that are dissolved in fatty acids and are stored in the body, such as vitamins A, D, E, and K.

megavitamin approach The practice, advocated by some, of taking large doses of vitamins to enhance health.

hypervitaminosis The name given to the serious toxic side effects that result from the overconsumption of vitamins.

sine, methionine, and tryptophan) is termed *high quality* or a *complete protein;* protein from most vegetable sources such as wheat and corn that are low in some amino acids and will not support growth and development when used as the only source of protein are termed *low quality* or an *incomplete protein.* Terms such as *low and high biological value* are also used to describe the quality of protein.

Approximately 54 grams of protein are recommended daily for males and 46–48 grams for females in the 15 to 65 age group. Larger individuals, pregnant and lactating women, adolescents, and those who are ill may need slightly more protein. Athletes generally do not need additional protein unless the weather is hot and profuse sweating occurs that produces additional nitrogen loss.[3] Individuals living in extremely hot climates may also need slightly more protein. Approximately 12 percent of calories in the American diet should come from protein.

It is not difficult for most college students to obtain their RDA in protein: approximately .8 grams/kilograms of body weight. A 130-pound person, for example, weighs 59 kilograms (130 divided by 2.2) and needs about 47 grams of protein per day (59 $\times$ .8). Meat contains approximately 7 grams of protein per ounce, milk has 8 grams per glass, and protein is plentiful in eggs and dairy products, and present in small quantities in vegetables and grains. Two glasses of milk, one ounce of cheese, and 3 ounces of beef, chicken, or fish provide all the protein the average person needs in one day.

There is some evidence that excess protein (more than 20 percent of one's daily calories) may contribute to a number of diseases, such as osteoporosis (see Chapter 17), heart disease, and certain types of cancer (see Chapter 16). When too much protein is ingested, the kidneys excrete more calcium—50 percent more when protein intake is doubled. Such losses over an extended period of time could lead to osteoporosis. The high saturated fat in meat protein elevates blood cholesterol and contributes to heart disease. High protein intake also increases the incidence of certain types of malignant tumors and accelerates tumor growth.[4] One way to regulate protein intake is to plan at least two meatless meals weekly, reduce egg consumption to two to three weekly, and cut down on dairy products.

Vegetarian Diets

Although the diets of many cultures contain more vegetables than meats, the American diet has traditionally prized meat as the centerpiece of well-balanced nutrition. However, this appears to be changing. Believing that vegetables are simply healthier than meats, or that it is morally wrong to consume meat, or that meat is "contaminated" with production-enhancing drugs, more and more Americans are shunning meats and becoming vegetarians.

There are three basic kinds of vegetarians. The *vegan vegetarian* eats vegetables only. The *lactovegetarian* eats vegetables and dairy products such as milk (the Latin word for milk is *lac*) and cheese. Finally, the *ovolactovegetarian* eats vegetables, dairy products, and eggs (the Latin word for egg is *ovum*). All vegetarians must plan their diets carefully because it is difficult to consume adequate protein and a balanced supply of amino acids from vegetable sources alone. However, because dairy products and eggs are excellent sources of protein, lacto- and ovolactovegetarians have much less difficulty than strict vegans in obtaining all the protein they need. Vegans must use *complementary protein* combinations of vegetables and grains to include proper amounts of protein in their diets. Traditional complementary protein diets include combinations of soybeans or tofu with rice (China and Indochina), peas with wheat (Fertile Crescent), beans with corn (Central and South America), and rice with beans, black-eyed peas, or tofu (United States and the Caribbean). Other complementary protein combinations readily available to American vegans include peanut butter and whole grain bread, brown bread and baked beans, and black bean and rice soup.

Because they have a low intake of saturated fat, cholesterol, and calories and a high intake of fiber, vegetarians tend to avoid heart disease for ten years longer than meat eaters. Vegetarians may also be able to avoid certain kinds of digestive system cancers. However, vegans are especially prone to dangerous deficiencies in iron, calcium, and vitamin B_{12} (which is usually only available in adequate amounts in animal products). In order to combat this serious disadvantage, the vegan vegetarian should meet these four special daily dietary requirements:

- Include 2 cups of legumes daily for proper levels of calcium and iron
- Include 1 cup of dark greens daily to meet iron requirements (for women)
- Include at least 1 gram of fat daily for proper absorption of vitamins
- Use a chemical supplement of fortified plant foods (like soy or nut "milks") to obtain vitamin B_{12}

Non-Energy Nutrients: Vitamins, Minerals, and Water

Vitamins

Vitamins are essential in helping chemical reactions take place in the body. They are required in very small amounts. Vitamins are divided into two major categories. **Water-soluble vitamins** are easily dissolved in water and are therefore easy for the body to get rid of in the urine, which is why these vitamins need to be consumed on a daily basis. Vitamin C and the B complex vitamins are the water-soluble vitamins. **Fat-soluble vitamins** are stored by the body in fatty tissues and the liver and are absorbed through the intestinal tract as needed.

Vitamin Supplements and Vitamin "Miracles" Some people take large doses of vitamin supplements in the belief that these are necessary to correct a dietary deficiency or to prevent or cure a variety of ills. However, consuming too many vitamins—especially fat-soluble vitamins A, D, E, and K, which the body stores for long periods—can be toxic. The U.S. Food and Drug Administration has restricted the addition of vitamin D to food products because studies have shown that excessive amounts of it can be toxic and produce body tissue damage. The **megavitamin approach,** followed by some health advocates and athletes who consume anywhere from 10 to 100 times the recommended daily vitamin allowance of fat- and water-soluble vitamins, may result in **hypervitaminosis,** the name given to the serious toxic side effects that result from the consumption of too many vitamins. Tables 7.4 and 7.5 list the functions of water-soluble and fat-soluble vitamins, respectively, and the problems and diseases associated with deficient or excess consumption of them.

Despite any concrete evidence, vitamin C holds a reputation for being a kind of miracle vitamin for the prevention or cure of practically any disease, ranging from high blood pressure, heart disease, and hepatitis to the common cold. Vitamin E has also generated considerable interest since claims were made that it could improve sexual potency and alleviate several other problems. There is no evidence to substantiate these claims.

Americans should realize two important things about vitamins and vitamin supplements: (1) the best

TABLE 7.4

Water-soluble Vitamins

Vitamin	Functions	Important Sources	Adult RDAs	Prolonged Deficiency Symptoms	Toxic Effects of Megadosages
Thiamin (B₁)	Helps convert carbohydrates, fats, and proteins to energy	Liver, pork, oysters; whole grain breads and cereals; enriched cereals and breads; peas; nuts	1.1–1.5mg	Moderate: depression, fatigue, constipation, muscle cramps Severe: beri-beri (nerve damage, paralysis, heart failure)	None presently known
Riboflavin (B₂)	Helps convert all fuel foods to energy; cell division; red blood cell formation	Liver, meat; dairy products; eggs; dark green vegetables; whole grain breads and cereals; nuts; produced in human intestine	1.3–1.7mg	Sore mouth, tongue, throat; dry, cracking skin; anemia; depression; personality shifts	None presently known
Niacin (nicotinic acid)	Release of energy from all fuel foods; protein and fat synthesis	Liver, poultry, meat; eggs; whole grain breads and cereals; nuts and legumes (peas, beans)	15–19mg	Pellegra (seen as rash, diarrhea, sleeplessness, confusion, and death)	Irritated stomach lining, diabetes, loss of liver function, jaundice; flushing of face, neck, and hands

TABLE 7.4 continued

Water-soluble Vitamins

Vitamin	Functions	Important Sources	Adult RDAs	Prolonged Deficiency Symptoms	Toxic Effects of Megadosages
Pyridoxine (B_6)	Release of energy from fuel foods; regulates nervous system activity; regenerates red blood cells; produces anti-bodies	High protein foods in general; bananas; some vegetables; whole grain cereals and breads; liver; green vegetables; fish; meat, poultry; nuts	1.6–2.0mg	Moderate: rash, mouth lesions Severe: nausea, vomiting, anemia, confusion, severe nervous disturbances	Nerve damage; depending on megadose, numbness, tingling in extremities, difficulty walking, poor coordination
Cobalamin (B_{12})	Helps produce red blood cells; growth and function of nervous system	Liver, kidney, meat, fish; eggs, dairy products; yeast	2.0mg	Moderate: fatigue, weakness, weight loss, tingling in extremities; sore tongue Severe: low immune response, paralysis; possibly fatal anemia	None presently known
Folacin (folic acid)	Helps produce nucleic acids; aids cell division; formation of red blood cells; fetal development	Liver; dark green vegetables; wheat germ; legumes; oranges, orange juice; fish; poultry, eggs	180–200mcg	Anemia; mouth and throat sores; rheumatoid arthritis; infections; toxemia in pregnancy; often deficient in alcoholics	Convulsions in some epileptics
Biotin	Helps release energy from fuel foods	Eggs; liver; dark green vegetables; widely found in foods	300–1000mcg	Rash; sore tongue; muscular pain; sleeplessness; nausea; loss of appetite; fatigue; depression	None presently known
Pantothenic acid	Release of energy; helps form cholesterol	Liver; whole grain cereals and breads; widely found in plant and animal foods	4–7mg	None known in humans on natural diet	Diarrhea and water retention
Ascorbic acid (C)	An antioxidant; promotes healing and fights infection; required for forming connective tissue; increases iron absorption	Citrus fruits; melons; tomatoes; strawberries; potatoes; dark green vegetables	60mg	Moderate: restlessness; swollen or bleeding gums; bruises; painful joints; energy loss; anemia Severe: scurvy (bleeding gums, poor wound healing, loose teeth, poor skin, irritability)	Diarrhea; bloating; abdominal pain; nausea; vomiting; kidney stones; loss of red blood cells; bone marrow changes

mcg = micrograms
mg = milligrams

Source: Adapted from the Food and Nutrition Board, National Academy of Sciences, National Research Council, *Recommended Dietary Allowances,* revised 1989.

✳ Fat-soluble Vitamins

Vitamin	Functions	Important Sources	Adult RDAs	Prolonged Deficiency Symptoms	Toxic Effects of Megadosages
A	Normal (especially night) vision; formation of cells, particularly skin; aids in resistance to infections	Fat-containing and fortified dairy products; liver; leafy dark green and yellow vegetables	800–1000 RE (2640–3300 IU)	Poor night vision, blindness; dry skin, dry eyes	Blurred vision; headaches; nausea; roughened skin; diarrhea; depression; spontaneous abortions and birth defects in pregnant women
D	Promotes absorption and use of calcium and phosphorus; bone growth; neuromuscular activity	Fortified milk, liver, cod liver; fish; egg yolk; formed in skin upon exposure to sunlight	5mcg	Children: deformed bones (rickets) Adults: softened bones (osteo-malacia); brittle bones (osteoporosis)	Children: poor appetite, retarded growth; deformed bones Adults: headaches; vomiting; diarrhea; weight loss; muscle weakness
E	Antioxidant to prevent cell membrane damage; helps form and protect red blood cells, muscles, and other tissue	Vegetables and fish oils; liver; whole grain breads and cereals; nuts and seeds	8–10 aTE (12–15 IU)	Rare in healthy children and adults; possible anemia; possible muscle loss	Reduced vitamin A storage; possible blood disorders in anemic children
K	Helps blood clot; promotes bone formation	Green leafy vegetables; other vegetables (peas, cabbage, cauli-flower); produced in human intestine	65–80mcg	Impaired blood clotting and bone formation; especially in some newborns; hemorrhaging, bruising	Rare, since not available in over-the-counter supplements; loss of red blood cells; jaundice; risk of brain damage

RE = retinal equivalents
IU = international units
mcg = micrograms
aTE = alpha tocopherol equivalents
Source: Adapted from the Food and Nutrition Board, National Academy of Sciences, National Research Council, *Recommended Dietary Allowances*, revised 1989.

way to obtain vitamins is from food, not from vitamin supplements, and (2) the vast majority of Americans get all the vitamins they need, in all the proper amounts, from their regular, balanced diets. Food has the added benefit over vitamin supplements of containing other nutrients, such as minerals, and non-nutrients, such as fiber and water. Studies have shown that most college students get more than 100 percent of their daily needs for all vitamins except Vitamin B_6 (pyridoxine), which is found in yeast, wheat germ, kidneys, eggs, and fish.

minerals Basic substances found in foods that are the key components of various hormones, enzymes, and other substances that aid in cell chemistry.

macrominerals Those minerals needed in large amounts by the body.

trace minerals Those minerals needed in small amounts by the body.

Minerals

Minerals are present in all living cells. They serve as key components of various hormones, enzymes, and other substances that aid in regulating chemical reactions within cells. Mineral elements play a part in the body's metabolic processes, and deficiencies can result in serious disorders. There are two major categories of minerals. **Macrominerals** are those needed by the body in large amounts (such as sodium, potassium, calcium, phosphorus, magnesium, sulfur, and chlorides). **Trace minerals** are those needed by the body in small amounts. A minimum of fourteen trace minerals must be ingested for optimum health; iron, iodine, copper, fluoride, and zinc appear to be the most important for proper body function. The body is composed of approximately thirty-one minerals, twenty-four of which are considered essential for sustaining life. A well-balanced diet will include the essential mineral elements (see Tables 7.6 and 7.7).

Iron is one of the body's most essential minerals. Approximately 85 percent of our daily iron intake is used to produce new *hemoglobin* (the pigment of the red blood cells that transports oxygen), with the remaining 15 percent used for the production of new tissue or held in storage. Iron needs also vary according to age and sex. Table 7.8 summarizes these variables.

TABLE 7.6

Macrominerals

Mineral	Functions	Important Sources	Adult RDAs	Prolonged Deficiency Symptoms	Toxic Effects of Megadosages
Calcium (Ca)	Bone and tooth formation; essential to blood clotting and membrane structure; fluid balance; nerve impulses; muscle contraction; enzyme activation	Dairy products; cheeses; liver; fish; egg yolk; green leafy vegetables; cereals; molasses; soybeans	800 mg	Muscle cramps, pain, spasms; tingling sensations and stiffness in hands and feet; deformed bones in children; osteoporosis in adults	Loss of appetite; nausea; vomiting; constipation; loss of weight; fever; weakness

Mineral	Functions	Important Sources	Adult RDAs	Prolonged Deficiency Symptoms	Toxic Effects of Megadosages
Phosphorus (P)	Bone and tooth formation; acid-base balance; energy release; fat transport; synthesis of enzymes, proteins, nucleic acids (DNA/RNA)	Liver; meats; dairy products; fish; egg yolk; legumes; dried fruit; nuts	800 mg	Loss of appetite; weakness; demineralization of bone and loss of calcium; bone pain	Reduced levels of calcium in blood; reduced bone-building capacity
Potassium (K)	Works with sodium to regulate blood pressure, transmit nerve impulses, regulate heart function; protein and carbohydrate metabolism	Meats; fish; poultry; potatoes; bananas; apricots; legumes; peanut butter; nuts; cocoa; molasses; cereals	1875–5625 mg	Vomiting and diarrhea; loss of appetite; irregular heartbeat; weakened pulse; lowered blood pressure	Weakened muscles; abnormal heart rhythm; kidney disorders
Sulfur (S)	Blood clotting; detoxification of body fluids; collagen synthesis	Protein foods (meat, dairy products, eggs, legumes)	Not established	Not clearly established	No toxic effects established
Sodium (Na)	Regulation of blood pressure; nerve impulse transmission; acid-base balance; formation of digestive secretions	Table salt, cured meats; cheese; sauerkraut; salted nuts	1100–3300 mg	Loss of appetite; thirst; vomiting; muscle cramps Extreme cases: convulsions; coma	Dehydration; higher body temperature; vomiting; depression
Chloride (Cl⁻)	With sodium and potassium, transmits nerve impulses; acid-based balance; helps blood cells transport carbon dioxide	Table salts, cured meats; cheese	1700–5100 mg	Vomiting; diarrhea; sweating; alkalinity of body fluids	No toxic effects established
Magnesium (Mg)	Energy production; regulates heart function; activates enzyme system; release of energy	Leafy green vegetables; whole grains; soybeans; nuts; molasses; animal proteins; milk	280–350mg	Muscle pain, tremors, spasms; vertigo; convulsions; altered heart rhythm; apathy; depression	Depressed respiration and central nervous system function

Source: Adapted from the Food and Nutrition Board, National Academy of Sciences, National Research Council, *Recommended Dietary Allowances*, revised 1989.

TABLE 7.7

Trace Minerals

Mineral	Functions	Important Sources	Adult RDAs	Prolonged Deficiency Symptoms	Toxic Effects of Megadosages
Iron (Fe)	Oxygen and carbon dioxide transport; red blood cell formation	Liver, heart, shellfish; beans and peas; vegetables	10–15 mg	Iron-deficiency anemia	Liver damage
Manganese (Mn)	Nerve action, muscle action; bone and connective tissue formation	Meat; fruits; vegetables; whole grains and cereals	2.0–5.0 mg	No specific description	No specific description
Copper (Cu)	Hemoglobin synthesis; energy release of fats and carbohydrates; bone formation	Meat, liver; shellfish; whole grain cereals	1–3 mg	Occurs along with kwashiorkor and cystic fibrosis	Ingestion of large amounts toxic to humans
Iodine (I)	Thyroid regulation of metabolism; synthesis of vitamin A	Iodized table salt; shellfish; green vegetables	150 mcg	Cretinism (stunted growth) Goiter (thyroid gland enlargement)	Hypothyroidism (toxic goiter)
Cobalt (Co)	Part of vitamin B_{12} molecule	Shellfish; nuts	Not established	No specific description	No specific description
Zinc (Zn)	Promotes healing and growth; immune functions	Meat; shellfish; whole grain cereals; nuts	12–15 mg	Impaired wound healing; decreased sense of taste and smell	Ingestion of large amounts is toxic to humans
Fluorine (F)	Tooth and bone formation	Drinking water	1.5–4.0 mg	Tooth decay	Mottled stains on teeth

Source: Adapted from the Food and Nutrition Board, National Academy of Sciences, National Research Council, *Recommended Dietary Allowances,* revised 1989.

TABLE 7.8

Summary of Iron Needs

Group	Daily Needs	Daily Loss	Comments
Nongrowing adult men	10 mg	1 mg	Little need for iron; body absorbs 10 percent of iron ingested
Women during childbearing years	18 mg	5–45 mg*	Great need for iron
Adolescent boys and girls	18 mg		Slightly greater need than categories above
Growing children	16–18 mg		Additional iron needed during periods of growth (infancy and childhood)

*Loss during menstrual period.

Issues in Health

Is NutraSweet Safe or Does It Cause Health Problems?

NutraSweet (trade name for aspartame) experienced immediate success when it was approved and declared safe by the Food and Drug Administration and the American Medical Association in 1981. Since that time, it has appeared in thousands of products, including sodas, candy, and ice cream. The consumer also adds aspartame to coffee, tea, cereal, cocoa, grapefruit, and hundreds of other products on a daily basis. In fact, aspartame is so popular that experts are quite concerned about the effects of widespread use and overuse among the American people.

Over one-half of scientists surveyed by the General Accounting Office as part of a two-year investigation expressed concerns over the safety of the widely used artificial sweetener NutraSweet (aspartame). NutraSweet is suspected of causing behavioral problems, headaches, and seizures in some users.[5] Aspartame was originally approved by the FDA in 1974; however, because of concern

over the possible link to mental retardation and brain tumors, approval was put on hold. In addition, complaints of dizziness, blurred vision, menstrual changes, and depression have been received. Although these symptoms could be attributed to other ailments, aspartame has not yet been ruled out. Until more conclusive evidence is found, it is argued, aspartame should be taken off the market to protect the American people.

Supporters of aspartame point out that safety issues were addressed by the FDA and that, regardless of initial concerns and mixed opinions among FDA members, it was approved for use in dry foods in 1981 and in soft drinks in 1983. Approval was based on the assumption that no one will consume more than 34 milligrams per kilogram of body weight in a day. Even in studies revealing questionable findings, a 150-pound individual would have to consume about seventeen cans of soda sweet-

ened with aspartame daily (four to five cans for a 40-pound child) to reach that level. Research shows that people of all ages are consuming much less than these amounts.[6] Leading experts also indicate that three to four servings of aspartame-containing products daily are safe for pregnant women. Aspartame is also a substitute sweetener for individuals who are forced to avoid sugar for medical reasons such as diabetes and obesity. In addition, people who avoid sugar reduce their number of dental caries. The fact that aspartame was approved by health regulatory agencies in thirty-three countries and the World Health Organization and that the FDA stands by its original judgment declaring aspartame safe is strong support for its place on the market.

What do you think? Should aspartame be taken off the market? With moderate use, is aspartame safe?

iron deficiency anemia A major health problem in the United States among certain population groups, iron deficiency anemia is caused by a lack of iron in the diet, resulting in a low hemoglobin level in the blood.

iron overload The ingestion of too much iron in the diet resulting in constipation and possible liver damage.

Iron deficiency results in loss of strength and endurance, rapid fatigue during exercise, shortening of attention span, loss of visual perception, impaired learning, and numerous other physical disorders. Despite its importance, many people do not get enough iron in their diet. Iron intake in the United States has been reduced due to the removal of iron-containing soils from the food supply and the diminished use of iron cooking utensils. Whereas animals can ingest iron from muddy water and soil, we humans are concerned with cleanliness, so our intake is restricted to selected foods.

Iron deficiency anemia, a major health problem in the United States, is common in older infants, children, women of childbearing age, pregnant women, and people of low income and minority groups. Nevertheless, people should be aware that too much iron can be dangerous to the body. Iron toxicity is rare, but a condition called **iron overload** occurs when the body is overwhelmed by too much iron given by vein (blood transfusions) or when too much iron is absorbed due to hereditary defects, heavy supplementation, and alcohol abuse (which increases absorption). Iron overload can cause tissue and liver damage as well as infections. And rapid ingestion of large amounts of iron can even cause sudden death: iron overdose is the second most common cause of accidental poisoning in small children. The body absorbs iron from food more easily than from iron supplements, which need to be in doses as high as 50 milligrams per day. Always consult a physician or registered dietician when considering an iron supplement.

Water

The most critical food component is water. Though it has no nutritional value, water is necessary for energy production, temperature control, and elimination. Inadequate water intake will decrease endurance, cause early fatigue, and restrict the function of all body systems. Although water is present in all foods, experts recommend a minimum of four to six glasses daily, exclusive of other fluids.

Even with proper nutrition from the basic four food groups, there is a danger of vitamin and mineral deficiency for some individuals. These people and their special dietary needs are shown in Figure 7.1.

Regulating Your Diet for Good Health

The U.S. Department of Agriculture and the U.S. Department of Health and Human Services have listed seven dietary guidelines for Americans that have implications for good health:[7]

1. Eat a variety of foods.
2. Maintain ideal weight.
3. Avoid too much fat, saturated fat, and cholesterol.
4. Eat foods with adequate starch and fiber.
5. Avoid too much sugar.
6. Avoid too much sodium.
7. If you drink alcohol, do so in moderation.

Table 7.9 compares the current American dietary intake (food and drink) and the proposed dietary goals or recommendations of numerous expert groups and nutrition specialists. In most areas, our current dietary intake in terms of percent of daily calories fails to meet the proposed dietary goals. There is too much total fat in our total daily calories (42 percent instead of 30 percent), too much saturated fat (16 percent instead of 10 percent), too much concentrated sugar (24 percent instead of 10 percent—more than 125 pounds annually

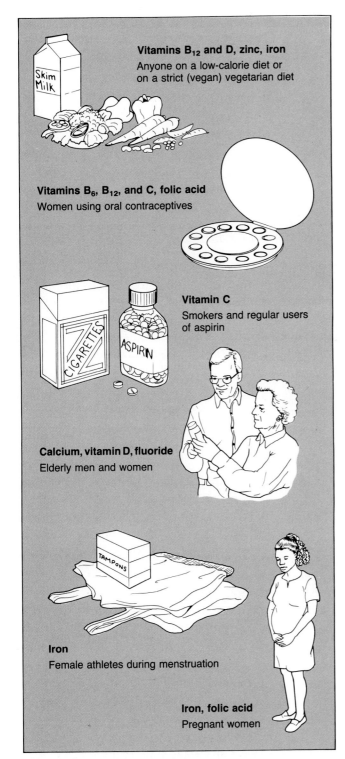

Vitamins B₁₂ and D, zinc, iron
Anyone on a low-calorie diet or on a strict (vegan) vegetarian diet

Vitamins B₆, B₁₂, and C, folic acid
Women using oral contraceptives

Vitamin C
Smokers and regular users of aspirin

Calcium, vitamin D, fluoride
Elderly men and women

Iron
Female athletes during menstruation

Iron, folic acid
Pregnant women

FIGURE 7.1 • People Who Should Consider Dietary Supplements

per person), and too little total carbohydrate (46 percent instead of 58 percent) and complex carbohydrates (22 percent instead of 48 percent). In addition, we consume too much cholesterol (500–1,000 milligrams instead of less than 300 milligrams), salt (6–18 grams daily instead of 4 grams), too much alcohol, too many

carbonated drinks, too much coffee and tea, too many calories, and not enough water. It is obvious that our eating habits are much more influenced by taste than by health.

Study Table 7.9 carefully. Later in this chapter, you will be asked to compare your nutritional practices to these standards.

Food Density

You can easily determine whether a food item or meal is nutritionally dense by examining calorie and nutrient content. A high-density food or meal is one that provides more nutrients than calories, or, in other words, is low in calories and high in vitamins and minerals. A good cold cereal with skim milk, for example, provides about 190 calories and 20–30 percent of practically all vitamins, minerals, carbohydrates, and protein for the day. The RDA for the average adult woman is 2,000 calories. Since the cold cereal breakfast contains only 190 calories or about 8 percent of her RDA in calories and 20–30 percent of her RDA in nutrients, the meal is said to be nutritionally dense. Fruits, vegetables, and grains are other examples of foods that are dense for a given nutrient or a group of nutrients. Potato or corn chips and cake are examples of low-density foods that supply mainly calories and little nutrition.

Regulating Sugar Intake

Sugar is consumed in four forms: sucrose, glucose, fructose, and lactose. Annual cane and beet sugar (sucrose) intake in the United States exceeds 100 pounds per person; 20 to 25 pounds of sugar syrups (glucose and fructose) are also consumed, bringing the total to 125 to 150 pounds of yearly sugar intake per person. Consumed in these large quantities, sugar contributes to dental cavities, excessive weight, and indirectly to such degenerative diseases as heart disease and diabetes.

As you can see from Table 7.10 it is not unusual for a person to consume the equivalent of fifty teaspoons of sugar per day. Sugar intake should be man-

Year 2000 National Health Objective

To help prevent early tooth decay, the federal government is striving to increase to at least 75 percent the proportion of parents and caregivers who use feeding practices that prevent baby bottle tooth decay.

TABLE 7.9		

Summary of Dietary Recommendations to the American Public

	Current Dietary Intake	Proposed Dietary Goals
Calories	Excess calories are consumed by the average person	Per lb. weight: Active: 17; moderately active: 12–13; sedentary: 10–11
Carbohydrate	46% of daily calories	58% of daily calories
Simple Concentrated sugar, sugar in fruits, vegetables and grains	24%	10% 5% 5%
Complex (fruits, vegetables and grains)	22%	48%
Protein	12% of daily calories	12%
Total Fat	42%	30%
Saturated	16%	10%
Monounsaturated	13%	10%
Polyunsaturated	13%	10%
Cholesterol	500–1,000 milligrams	less than 300 milligrams
Salt*	6–18 grams	less than 4 grams (1100–3300 milligrams)
Dietary Fiber	11 grams	25–35 grams
Fluid		
Water	2–3 glasses**	6–8 glasses, 10–12 if on any type of diet
Alcohol	——	Less than 10% of daily calories, 1–2 drinks
Carbonated Drinks	——	No more than 1–2 daily
Coffee or Tea	——	No more than 1–2 daily

* Salt substitutes that contain potassium chloride may not be wise choices. Some evidence indicates that it is the chloride in salt (sodium chloride), not the sodium, that is associated with high blood pressure in some individuals. Salt substitutes containing potassium also contain chloride.

** Results of four-year survey of students at Virginia Commonwealth University, 1986–1990.

TABLE 7.10

Sugar Content of Common Foods and Drinks

Food	Size	Approximate Content in Teaspoons	Food	Size	Approximate Content in Teaspoons
Beverages	12 oz.		**Breads**		
Sodas		5–9	White	1 slice	$\frac{1}{4}$
Sweet cider		$4\frac{1}{4}$	Hamburger/hot dog bun	1	3
Jams and jellies, candies	1 tbsp	4–6	**Dairy products**		
Milk chocolate	$1\frac{1}{2}$ oz.	$2\frac{1}{2}$	Ice cream cone	Single dip	3
Fudge	1 oz.	$4\frac{1}{2}$	Sherbert	One scoop	9
Hard Candy	4 oz.	20	**Desserts**		
Marshmallow	1	$1\frac{1}{2}$	Pie (fruit, custard cream)	1 slice	4–13
Fruits and canned juices			Pudding	$\frac{1}{2}$ cup	3–5
Dried raisins, prunes, apricots, dates	3–5	4			
Fruit juice	8 oz.	$2\frac{1}{2}$–$3\frac{1}{2}$			

Year 2000 National Health Objective

In an attempt to improve the healthy nature of foods available to Americans in supermarkets, restaurants and fast-food chains, schools, homes, and worksites, the federal government has established several health objectives: (1) to increase the availability of processed food products that are reduced in fat and saturated fat to at least 5,000 brand items (2,500 items were available in 1986); (2) to increase to at least 90 percent the proportion of restaurants and institutional food service operations that offer identifiable low-fat, low-calorie food choices, consistent with the *Dietary Guidelines for Americans* (about 70 percent of fast-food and family restaurant chains with 350 or more units had at least one low-fat, low-calorie item on their menu in 1989); (3) to increase to at least 90 percent the proportion of school lunch and breakfast services and child care food services with menus that are consistent with the nutrition principles in the *Dietary Guidelines for Americans;* and (4) to increase to at least 80 percent the receipt of home food services by people age 65 and older who have difficulty preparing their own meals or are otherwise in need of home-delivered meals.

aged beginning in infancy. Infants begin to show a preference for sweet foods by 12 to 18 months of age, and it is not until early adulthood (around age 19 or 20) that the desire for sugar slowly decreases. To control a child's intake and desire for sugar, parents can serve desserts high in sugar as an occasional treat rather than as part of every meal.

It is not necessary to eliminate all foods high in sugar from the diet, only to limit their use. You can reduce your own daily sugar intake by reading the labels for sweeteners and sugars in products you are considering buying (the terms sucrose, glucose, dextrose, fructose, corn syrups, corn sweeteners, natural sweeteners, and invert sugar all mean that the product contains sugar), substituting water and unsweetened fruit juices for sodas and punches, buying fruit canned in its own unsweetened juice, cutting back on desserts, purchasing cereals low in sugar, reducing the amount of sugar called for in recipes, and avoiding sweet snacks.

Regulating Salt Intake

Approximately one-third of our salt intake occurs naturally in food, another third comes from processed food, and the remaining third comes from the salt shaker. Recent analysis of dietary intake has shown that the average salt ingestion for adults, excluding salt added at the table, was within the Established Safe and Adequate Daily Dietary Intake range of 1100 to 3300 milligrams devised by the National Academy of Sciences in 1980. Salt intake for children appears to be above these guidelines. Although a decrease in salt in-

carcinogen Any substance that acts as a cancer-causing agent.

take has occurred in the United States in the past few years, some experts still feel that the typical diet contains three to six times more salt than is necessary.

If you wish to reduce your salt intake, consider using less salt in cooking and substitute other spices and flavorings such as garlic, pepper, onion, or lemon; taste food before adding table salt; remove salt from the table; learn to count the milligrams of sodium consumed daily and stay within the recommended ranges,

and reduce consumption of cured meats (bacon, ham), luncheon meats, sausages, canned fish (crab, salmon, tuna), American cheese, instant potatoes, and table salt. Salt may be mildly habit-forming, and some people develop a craving for it. Because eating habits established in the early years tend to carry over into adult life, extra salt in children's diets may become a difficult habit to shed later in life. "Lite" or diabetic salt may be indicated for some individuals. To discourage the salt habit, parents can serve their children unsalted foods beginning in infancy. The only time salt may be needed is when a child's salt and other mineral loss (potassium, chloride) is high due to heavy work or athletics.

Managing Fat and Cholesterol Consumption

High blood cholesterol levels have been strongly linked to early heart disease; therefore, it is important to regulate your dietary intake of foods high in animal fats (saturated fats). To reduce cholesterol intake significantly and manage fat consumption, three measures are recommended: (1) Cut total fat consumption, (2) reduce saturated fat intake, and (3) increase the ratio of polyunsaturated to saturated fat.

Some examples of high-fat foods that you should

A hamburger, fries, and soda is still the most popular fast food meal. It is also too high in calories, fat, and salt.

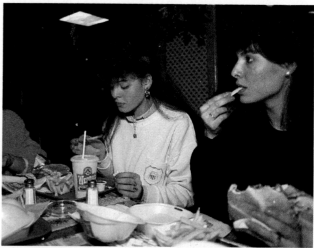

consume only in limited quantities are whole milk, butter, and meats such as bacon, ham, beef, hot dogs, pork, lamb, and lunch meat. In place of these meats, eat more fish and poultry.

Although milk is a vital source of calcium and an excellent source of potassium, whole milk is a high-fat food. Each quart of whole milk contains approximately 34.14 grams of fat, or 47 percent of the total calories. More than half of whole milk is saturated fat. The Commission for Heart Disease Resources recommends that we consume no more than 10 percent of our total calories in the form of saturated fat and no more than 300 milligrams of cholesterol. One quart of whole milk contains 110 milligrams.

One solution is to switch to fortified skim (nonfat) milk, which provides the following benefits: (1) 25 percent fewer calories; (2) additional calcium, protein, and vitamins (with the exception of vitamin A); and (3) less saturated fat (30 percent of total calories rather than 47 percent). Skim milk is also slightly less expensive than whole milk. Another solution is to eat uncreamed cottage cheese. It contains little fat (3 percent of calories) and cholesterol (15 milligrams in 3.5 ounces). All other cheeses are high in cholesterol and fat content. Butter is all fat, with over half the contents in saturated fat. Margarine has a similar number of calories but contains no cholesterol, and some brands contain limited saturated fat. Thus, using margarine for eating and cooking is preferable to using butter, if you are concerned with reducing your fat intake.

Some other foods that are particularly high in cholesterol are eggs, organ meats (like liver), and shellfish. To manage your cholesterol intake, eat them in moderate amounts. For example, eat only three eggs per week, and eat shellfish and organ meats, such as liver, only occasionally.

Many cooking oils are high in saturated fats. Avoid those that are labeled hydrogenated or partially hydrogenated, and substitute polyunsaturated and monounsaturated oils.

Now that you have learned about the six different kinds of nutrients and how to regulate your intake of certain foods, you can use Exploring your Health 7.2 to identify your current eating habits and develop a healthier diet plan.

Government Regulation of Foods

Food Additives

Two basic kinds of additives appear in foods: *intentional additives* (used to improve nutrient content, shelf life, or quality) and *incidental additives* (such as pollutants). Food additives are used to protect against the spread of infection and food poisoning, lengthen the storage time of food, change the taste of food to improve sales, change its color to make it more appealing, and change its texture. Hundreds of additives fall into such categories as multipurpose additives, anticaking agents, chemical preservatives, emulsifying agents, nutrients and dietary supplements, sequestrants, stabilizers, flavoring agents, coatings and films.

Manufacturers may legally use any additive that has been approved by the FDA, including those designated GRAS (Generally Recognized as Safe). In 1975, food additives were rated sixth and last among the main hazards identified by the FDA, behind food-borne infection, malnutrition, environmental contaminants, naturally occurring toxicants in foods, and pesticide residues. The fear that additives are an increasing hazard may not be unwarranted. The FDA 1958 Food Additives Amendment to the Food, Drug, and Cosmetic Act requires extensive testing on the chemistry, use, function, and safety of an additive before it is approved for use in food. If an additive is found to be a **carcinogen** (cancer-causing agent) in any test on animals or humans, it is discarded (Delaney Clause). Additives that involve risk are permitted only at levels one hundred times lower than the risk level. This margin of safety of $\frac{1}{100}$ appears quite adequate, because it is known that potentially harmful, naturally occurring substances appear at levels with a margin of safety of only $\frac{1}{10}$. Moreover, toxicity has been found not to be additive; a $\frac{1}{100}$ dose of one hundred different compounds still results in a $\frac{1}{100}$ toxic dose. The distinction between toxicity and hazard is very important. *Toxicity* refers to the potential capacity of a chemical to harm living organisms, and *hazard* is the potential of a chemical to produce injury under conditions of use. Most substances are potentially toxic but only hazardous if consumed in very large quantities. For an even greater margin of safety, individuals should avoid consumption of any one additive (such as drinking six to eight diet drinks with saccharin or NutraSweet daily) by selecting a variety of foods and drinks from the basic four food groups. A quick look at the label will also reveal how much of the product is food and how much is artificial color, preservative, and other additives.

Several food additives remain controversial. Saccharin is one example. In 1977 the FDA proposed a ban on the use of saccharin as an artificial sweetener. Critics of this proposal argued that saccharin is a very weak cancer-producing agent and is useful to certain individuals, such as diabetics, who need to reduce their sugar intake. Consequently, saccharin is back on the market.

Nitrites and nitrates, used in bacon, sausages, and luncheon meats to prevent *botulism* (food poisoning that can affect the central nervous system) and improve flavor, are potentially dangerous. Cooking at high heat and the digestive process convert nitrites to nitrosamines, a potential carcinogen. Nitrates and nitrites also occur naturally in vegetables in amounts higher than those added to bacon, sausages, and luncheon meats.

Exploring Your Health 7.2

Do You Meet the Dietary Recommendations for Americans as Shown in Table 7.9?

The first step toward developing healthy eating habits is to identify your current behavior. This requires careful recording of everything you eat and drink for a 7-day period. Estimate the portion size and secure the calories, fiber, salt, cholesterol, and fat content from the tables in this chapter and Appendix C. Reproduce copies to complete your 7-day log.

FOOD AND DRINK DIARY OF _____ **DATE** _____

Time	Food and Drink/ Quantity	Estimated				
		Calories	Fiber	Salt	Chol.	Fat
Breakfast						
Between Meal						
Lunch						
Between Meal						
Dinner						
Evening						

Record the percentage of your daily calories that come from the following:

Simple carbohydrates: Complex Carbohydrates: Protein
Saturated fat: Polyunsaturated fat: Monounsaturated fat:

Are you consuming too much salt?   Cholesterol?

Are you consuming enough fiber?   Water?

Summarize the strengths and weaknesses of your diet in terms of food and fluid intake. What steps can you take toward a healthier diet?

The controversy over saccharin, nitrites, and nitrates hinges on the issue of risk versus benefit and whether the decision should be left up to the FDA or the individual. If a benefit of an additive is purely esthetic, the FDA imposes much more stringent restrictions. An example is FDA removal of all food-color additives that are not thoroughly investigated. For additives serving valuable functions, however, the decision is not quite so clear, and some potentially hazardous additives remain on the market because of their benefit in preventing food poisoning and in helping certain individuals with specific medical problems.

Food Labeling

You now have enough knowledge about RDAs for carbohydrate, fat, protein, vitamins and minerals, salt, sugar, cholesterol, and calories to evaluate the contents of a food item from the label. In 1973, a law was passed establishing a set of standards to enable Americans to choose food products based upon sound nutritional information. This set of standards resulted in nutritional labeling or the listing of major nutrients found in a food product on the label. The law requires every food label to state:

- The common name of the product.
- The name and address of the manufacturer, packer, or distributor.
- The net contents in terms of weight, measure, or count.
- The ingredients in descending order of predominance by weight, to be prominently displayed in ordinary words. A product that lists sugar as its first ingredient and whole wheat as its last, for example, has a much greater amount of sugar than whole wheat.

The nutrition labeling section of the law states that, if a nutrient is added to a food or any claim is made on the label, an informational panel must be provided that complies fully with the nutrition labeling requirements. The panel must conform to the following format under the heading "Nutrition Information":

- Serving or portion size.
- Servings or portions per container.
- Food energy in kilocalories per serving.
- Carbohydrate and fat, in grams, per serving.
- Protein, vitamins, and minerals as percentages of the U.S. RDA. A claim may not be made that a food is a significant source of a nutrient unless it provides a minimum of 10 percent of the U.S. RDA in a single serving.
- Eight nutrients, known as *indicator nutrients,* must be listed:

Indicator nutrients:

Protein	Niacin
Vitamin A	Vitamin C
Thiamin (B_1)	Calcium
Riboflavin (B_2)	Iron

Optional listings:

Vitamin D	Phosphorus
Vitamin E	Iodine
Vitamin B_6	Magnesium
Folacin	Zinc
Vitamin B_{12}	

If you secure these eight indicator nutrients in sufficient quantities from the basic four food groups, you are likely to be obtaining 100 percent of the other nutrients also.

Reading a Food Label   By applying what you have learned from this chapter, it will only require a little practice before you can quickly determine whether a product is a healthy or unhealthy food choice. Refer to the two labels shown in Figure 7.2 (cream cheese and fortified milk) and master these steps. Practice on other products until you can make a wise decision in less than 15 seconds.

1. Notice the weight or measure, sodium, and calories on the front of the package. Although not shown on this panel, this information will help focus your thoughts.
2. Read the ingredients on the front or side of the package. Whatever appears first on the list is present in the largest quantity. Milk and cream, both high in fat, are listed first and second on the cream cheese label. Be alert also for multiple ingredient names for similar items. A product with sugar, salt, and beef fat listed first, second, and third is not likely to be purchased. Tricky labeling, however, may not make the problem so ob-

Your first step to wise food purchasing and nutritious, healthy eating begins with a thorough understanding and regular use of label reading.

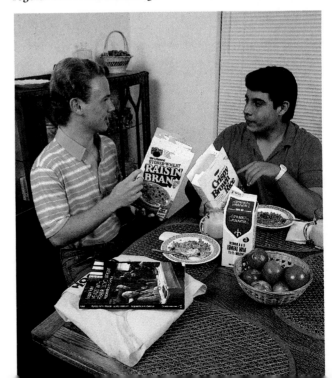

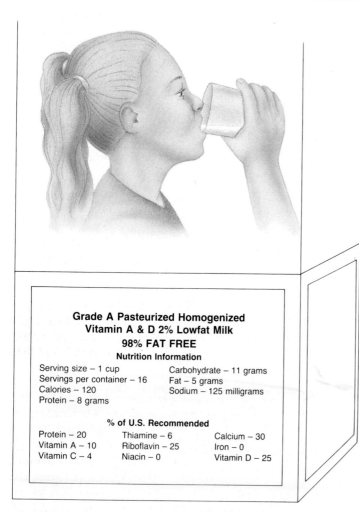

Grade A Pasteurized Homogenized
Vitamin A & D 2% Lowfat Milk
98% FAT FREE
Nutrition Information

Serving size – 1 cup	Carbohydrate – 11 grams
Servings per container – 16	Fat – 5 grams
Calories – 120	Sodium – 125 milligrams
Protein – 8 grams	

% of U.S. Recommended

Protein – 20	Thiamine – 6	Calcium – 30
Vitamin A – 10	Riboflavin – 25	Iron – 0
Vitamin C – 4	Niacin – 0	Vitamin D – 25

Cream Cheese
NUTRITION INFORMATION PER PORTION

PORTION SIZE .... 2 TBSP.(28 g)
PORTIONS PER CONTAINER 8
CALORIES 100
PROTEIN .... 2 GRAMS
CARBOHYDRATE .... 2 GRAMS
FAT .... 10 GRAMS
SODIUM .... 100 mg

PERCENTAGE OF U.S. RECOMMENDED
DAILY ALLOWANCES (U.S. RDA)

PROTEIN	4	RIBOFLAVIN	2
VITAMIN A	4	NIACIN	*
VITAMIN C	*	CALCIUM	2
THIAMINE	*	IRON	*

CONTAINS LESS THAN 2% OF THE
U.S. RDA OF THESE NUTRIENTS.

INGREDIENTS: MILK, CREAM, CHEESE CULTURE,
SALT AND VEGETABLE GUM.   KEEP REFRIGERATED

FIGURE 7.2   ◆   Food labels for cream cheese and fortified milk

vious: sugar may be listed in several places lower on the ingredients label as sugar, corn syrup, maple syrup, or dextrose, when combining all these would require sugar to be listed first. Salt, sodium potassium, monosodium glutamate, and other names for salt provide the same opportunity to hide the true total salt content. Check for salt, fat, cholesterol, and sugar under a variety of different names.

3. Compare the servings per container and the serving size to be sure it is the same amount you normally eat. Some manufacturers reduce the portion size from the standard cup or 8 ounce drink to a 6 ounce drink, or from a 3 ounce to a

2 ounce serving to make their products look like low calorie food. Such a change for an unsuspecting consumer can make a product appear quite low in calories when it is actually higher in calories than other brands. Still other products marketed for weight gain may increase portion sizes to give the impression of higher calories per serving. A portion size of 2 tablespoons for cream cheese and 8 ounces of milk is appropriate for one serving for most people.

4. Check the total calories per serving and compare with the U.S. RDA to determine whether this is a high-density or low-density food. Protein, vitamins, and minerals are listed in percentages of

U.S. RDA. A serving of a product that uses one-fourth of your daily allotted calories and provides less than 10 to 15 percent of your RDA in key nutrients is a low-density food choice. Cream cheese contains 200 calories per serving or approximately 4 to 5 percent of the total calories needed daily. This is a rather low-density food and should be consumed in moderation. By comparison, one glass of skim milk meets 20 percent of the U.S. RDA for protein, 30 percent for calcium and 4 to 25 percent for thiamine, vitamin C, vitamin D, and riboflavin—all for 5 to 6 percent of your total daily calories.

5. Notice that sodium is listed in milligrams; protein, carbohydrate, and fat is listed in grams. A breakdown of simple and complex carbohydrates may be listed to tell you how much simple sugar and how much starch is in the product. A fat breakdown may also show the amount of each of the three types of fat (saturated, polyunsaturated, and monounsaturated). Fiber and cholesterol content may also be listed here. In general, fiber will be listed if the product has 2 to 3 grams or more; the cholesterol content will be specified if the product is low in cholesterol. If no information is provided, the product probably has little or no fiber and too much cholesterol.

6. Study the percentage of U.S. Recommended Daily Allowances (U.S. RDAs). Use the U.S. RDAs to determine what percent of the product is fat. Go over the calculations below for cream cheese and fortified milk and learn to quickly identify what percentage of the total calories in one serving are made up of fat. You can do the same for sugar in cereal and in other products. Cream cheese has 10 grams of fat (9 calories per gram × 10 = 90 calories) per serving and is actually 90 percent fat (90 of 100 calories). Fortified milk contains 5 grams of fat (9 calories per gram × 5 = 45 calories) per serving and contains 37.5 percent fat (45 divided by 120 calories = 37.5 percent). Skim milk, with 0 grams of fat, would be a much better choice. McDonalds

7. Master the Dietary Recommendations in Table 7.9 to help you decide whether a product is a wise or unwise food choice. One easy method is to avoid any food item that either exceeds these standards or will make it difficult for you to stay within the standards after your daily food intake. A product that has more than 30 percent fat or more than 10 percent saturated fat is an unwise choice. Processed food that has one-fourth or more of your recommended daily salt or cholesterol intake should also be avoided. A cold or hot cereal or a loaf of bread with less than 2 to 3 grams of fiber per serving is also an unwise choice. Depending upon your nutritional concerns, you can monitor intake of various vitamins, minerals, carbohydrates, protein, and fat at a glance through use of this information.

8. Be aware of products labeled ''Cholesterol Free,'' 90 percent fat free, or 2 percent fat. These products often contain saturated fat, which stimulates the body's production of cholesterol. Such products are unwise choices for individuals with high cholesterol. As we determined previously, the 2 percent fat milk shown in Figure 7.2 contains 37.5 percent fat, not 2 percent. By comparison, whole milk contain 150 calories and 48 percent fat. Only skim milk meets our standard of no more than 30 percent fat or 10 percent saturated fat.

9. Be alert to the use of dark food dye in breads to give the impression that they contain wheat and fiber. Unless products list whole wheat and whole grain as major ingredients, fiber content is probably low.

A number of terms have been standardized and manufacturers must conform if the terminology is used: *sodium free* (must be less than 5 milligrams/serving), *very low sodium* (35 milligrams or less per serving), *reduced sodium* (processed to reduce the regular amount by 75 percent or more), *unsalted* (processed with the normally used salt), *low in calories* (no more than 40 calories per serving or 0.9 calories per gram), *reduced-calorie food* (at least a third lower in calories than the food it most closely resembles), *enriched* (returning the mineral iron and the B vitamins thiamin, riboflavin, and niacin to refined products), *fortified* (nutrients have been added to the food that may or may not have been in the original product).[8]

Saturated and polyunsaturated fats and cholesterol information may also be provided. Protein is listed twice, once in grams and second as a percentage of the U.S. RDA. The percentage is the most important listing since not all protein quality is identical. Eight grams of protein in milk, a complete protein, yields 20 percent of the U.S. RDA for protein, while an identical amount of protein in spaghetti, an incomplete protein, yields only 10 percent of the U.S. RDA.

Because wise food purchasing is critical to nutritious eating, the federal government has established a national health objective to increase to at least 85 percent the proportion of people age 18 and older who use food labels to make nutritious food selections. In 1988, approximately 74 percent of these people used labels to make food selections.

The federal government has also established a national health objective to achieve useful and informative nutrition labeling for virtually all processed foods and for at least 40 percent of fresh meats, poultry, fish, fruits, vegetables, baked goods, and ready-to-eat carry-away foods. Only 60 percent of processed foods that were regulated by FDA had nutrition labeling in 1988.

Nutrition Myths

Americans spend more than half a billion dollars each year on special health foods. Some people believe that such foods will prevent and cure practically any illness. Some eat fish eggs, raw oysters, organic foods, or flavored insects as brain foods or foods that will nourish a specific body part. The truth is that eating a balanced diet of foods from the basic four food groups will supply you with the proper vitamins and minerals and make special foods unnecessary.

There are hundreds of food fallacies and misconceptions that you may encounter. List your nutrition biases in Exploring Your Health 7.3. Here are some common misbeliefs:

- **The best food plan is a vegetarian diet.** It is difficult to get enough cell-building protein without eating some meat, fish, or poultry. For vegetarians who avoid dairy products and eggs, which are good protein sources, the difficulty is even greater. Certainly, too much meat, particularly beef, can increase the risk of heart disease. A good compromise is to eat fish, poultry, and cheese as sources of protein.

- **Special "energy" foods, such as honey, improve your strength and vitality.** Honey, candy, and other highly sugared products are a form of quick energy, but they will not improve your overall vitality. Only a balanced diet and exercise can do that. In fact, if you eat an excess amount of sugar (an entire candy bar, for example), an insulin reaction occurs that removes sugar from the blood and may leave you with less quick energy than you would have had without the sugar.

- **Natural foods are always more nutritious.** *Organic,* or so-called natural foods are those that are grown in soil enriched with natural rather than chemical fertilizers. These foods are never sprayed with pesticides, and no artificial substances are added to the soil in which the foods are grown. Nevertheless, even organically grown products have traces of artificial chemicals. Food plants break all fertilizers (chemical or natural) into the same organic components. Consequently, organic foods are no more nutritious than foods grown

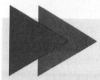

Exploring Your Health 7.3

Your Nutrition Biases

Do you purchase any special foods with the hope of receiving particular health benefits from them? If so, list them here. Then ask your instructor to discuss whether these foods really do have special benefits.

Food or Drink	Reason for Purchase
1.	
2.	
3.	
4.	
5.	

with chemical fertilizers; in fact, chemical fertilizers can sometimes help produce more nutritious food by improving the nutrients in the soil. There is no evidence that taste or nutritional quality is affected by the nature of the fertilizer. In addition, locally grown and marketed organic foods are not subject to the safety regulations applied to commercially grown foods.

- **Pasteurized milk is not very nourishing.** Pasteurization makes milk safe from harmful bacteria. In this process the only nutrient lost is vitamin C, and raw milk before pasteurization has very little vitamin C anyway.

- **Yogurt is a health food providing special nutrition.** Yogurt is made from cultured whole milk evaporated to two-thirds its original volume, forming a solid that can be eaten with a spoon. It is neither more nor less nourishing than milk.

- **White eggs are more nourishing than brown eggs.** Eggshell color depends on the breed of the hen and has nothing to do with nutritive value.

- **The modern practice of food processing robs foods of their nutritional value.** Food is processed for our protection, and processed food is the most nutritious food possible.

- **Food manufacturers destroy all the nutrients and include dangerous additives in their processing.** Some nutrients are lost during food processing but the key nutrients in most products are added back and often contain more than the product had prior to processing. Additives often improve a food's nutritional value, freshness, texture, appearance, and preparation. Before a new additive can be used, the U.S. government requires the manufacturer to prove its safety.

- **Certain foods prevent or even reverse the effects of aging.** No one in our society wants to grow old. Americans spend large sums of money on special foods and treatments that claim to delay the aging process. There is no evidence that any of these products is the slightest bit effective. The best protection against premature aging is proper nutrition, adequate exercise and rest, meaningful work, and the maintenance of good mental and emotional health.

Special Nutritional Needs of Athletes and Active Individuals

Athletes and active individuals have a few special nutritional needs to meet the demands of vigorous activity, to prevent heat exhaustion and heat stroke and to maximize and store energy from food.[9]

More Calories

If you are neither losing nor gaining weight and have sufficient energy, you are probably taking in the correct number of calories daily. Weigh yourself at the same time and under the same conditions daily, preferably upon rising. If no weight gain or loss is occurring, there is no need to keep complicated records in caloric intake and expenditure. In general, very active male college-age athletes need approximately 25 to 27 calories per pound compared to 20 to 21 per pound for female athletes. Moderately active individuals need approximately 20 to 23 (males) and 16 to 18 (females) calories per pound. Sedentary individuals, on the other hand, need approximately 15 to18 (males) and 11 to 12 (females) calories per pound.

More Water

To avoid dehydration, electrolyte imbalance, and heat-related disorders, as well as early fatigue, it is necessary to hydrate approximately fifteen minutes before exercising by drinking 12–48 ounces of cold water (one to four glasses), then drinking water freely during and after exercise. Since thirst will underestimate your needs, you must form the habit of drinking when no thirst sensations exist.

Proper Nutrition

Electrolytes—water, sodium, potassium, and chloride—lost through sweat and water vapor from the lungs should be replaced as rapidly as possible. It is the proper balance of each electrolyte that prevents dehydration, cramping, heat exhaustion, and heat stroke. Too much salt without adequate water, for example, actually draws fluid from the cells, precipitates nausea, and increases potassium loss. Although water alone will not restore electrolyte balance, it is the single most important element in preventing heat-related disorders. Eating extra portions of potassium-rich foods several days before a contest and using extra table salt is all most individuals need. If commercial electrolyte drinks are used, they should be diluted with twice the normal amount of water to reduce the sugar content. Lower sugar content will speed absorption time and prevent the body's release of insulin and possible reduction of quick energy.

Iron Supplements

Iron deficiency can lead to a loss of strength and endurance, early fatigue during exercise, loss of visual perception, and impaired learning. Needs vary according to age, activity level, and sex. Iron is the only nutrient that adolescent female and male athletes need in greater quantity. Adolescent female athletes in particular are more apt to be iron deficient because of their

carbohydrate loading A special diet used by athletes in the seven days before competition to help improve their performance.

concern for their appearance and their avoidance of iron-rich foods. In addition, female athletes of all ages may benefit from an iron supplement during their menstrual periods.

The Pre-event Meal

Research shows that you cannot significantly improve your athletic performance by eating a special meal before the event. At the same time, eating light meals at various times (varying from three hours to half an hour) before the event is not detrimental to your performance in sprinting, middle-distance running, running a mile, or swimming. Nevertheless, many athletes seem to derive a sense of psychological well-being from eating a special meal before an important event. The real object of the pre-event meal, however, should be to fill energy reserves completely before exercise and to be comfortable during the workout or contest. Bear in mind that fats and proteins are absorbed so slowly that they will not supply fuel for competition even when eaten up to four hours beforehand. Because the body absorbs sugar in about two hours, small amounts of sugar could have some temporary, positive effect on performance. But if food is to alter your energy quotient, you should change your pattern of eating for three to four days before a contest for maximum nutritional benefit.

Carbohydrate Loading

For normal activity, the body has an adequate supply of energy available in the form of glucose and glycogen:[10]

Blood glucose
20 grams $\times$ 4 calories per = 80 calories
Muscle glycogen
300 grams $\times$ 4 calories per = 1,200 calories
Liver glycogen
75 grams $\times$ 4 calories per = 300 calories
Total energy in calories = 1,580 calories

Individuals who compete in marathons, triathlons, and other endurance contests lasting several hours need additional energy and can benefit from a technique referred to as **carbohydrate loading,** consisting of three to four days of vigorous exercise and a high-protein and high-fat/low-carbohydrate diet (the depletion stage), followed by three days of little or no exercise and a high-carbohydrate diet (the loading stage). New evidence indicates that the depletion stage is unnecessary. By merely increasing carbohydrate intake three to four days before the contest, liver glycogen stores double and muscle glycogen stores have been shown to more than double. Such an increase provides approximately 3,040–3,640 calories of energy—enough for practically any endurance event. Two large high-carbohydrate meals (300 grams, 1,200 calories per meal) daily for three to four days are recommended.

The value of carbohydrate loading for events other than those mentioned above is questionable. Carbohydrate loading may also be an inadvisable technique for growing children. A safer approach for everyone is to concentrate on glycogen loading of the liver by merely increasing carbohydrate consumption drastically for two days before the big event. Plan a big family meal with lots of tasty pasta dishes!

High Protein

Excess protein in the diet adds extra cholesterol and calories, is expensive, is a poor source of fuel for muscular work, and does not guarantee increased muscle mass or body weight. Athletes have been shown to perform equally well on 50, 75, 100, or 150 grams of protein daily (approximately 75–85 grams are needed daily). There is little evidence to suggest that increasing protein intake will improve strength, muscular or heart-lung endurance, muscle mass, or performance in any sport. Only when there are drastic changes in an exercise program (greatly increased intensity) is there evidence to suggest a possible need to increase protein intake for one to two weeks to avoid nitrogen imbalance.[11]

Get Involved!

Working for Better Nutrition

There can be no doubt that health, wellness, and nutrition are very closely related. Nevertheless, surveys of American eating habits reveal some alarming trends. Fast food restaurants and fast cooking in high-fat, high-salt, and high-calorie foods dominate our lives. Childhood and adult obesity are on the rise. Osteoporosis, cardiovascular disease, and cancer remain major health problems whose development, control, and even prevention have been linked to dietary habits. Generally, we continue to consume too much saturated fat, cholesterol, salt, sugar, alcohol, coffee, tea, soft drinks, and calories, and too little water, fruits, vegetables, and grains. What things can you start doing now to help yourself and others adopt healthier nutritional habits?

1. First—and perhaps toughest—of all, adopt healthier eating habits for yourself and set an example for friends, family, and acquaintances. As a college student, it's easy for you to eat "on the run" and not really think about what you're eating. Make a conscious effort every day to cut out all fast foods and high-calorie, high-fat, and high-salt snacks by brown-bagging healthy breakfasts, lunches, and snacks that feature healthy breads, no-sugar-added fruit juices, and fresh fruit and vegetables.

2. Do your student union and dormitory buildings have row after row of snack food vending machines? Start or get involved with student groups that work for the availability of healthier food choices for students and a reduction in the number of high-calorie, high-fat, and high-salt snack food vending machines. Ask about such groups at your student council or fraternity or sorority council offices. (While you're at it, try to get rid of those cigarette vending machines, too!)

3. Are good, tasty, and varied food choices available in your school's cafeterias to vegetarians or people considering a vegetarian diet plan? If not, why not? Make up brief survey forms for distribution to students in dormitories and cafeterias. (You may want to clear this with university administrators first.) See the box at right for one possible format for your survey form.

You may be able to use the results of your survey to convince food service managers and university administrators of the need for certain changes in nutritional offerings in the cafeteria.

4. Create a series of "Nutrition Tips" you can write or have printed out on single sheets of 8½ × 11 paper or on larger sheets of colored construction paper. Designate

This is a survey to find out how many of the students who use this cafeteria would like to see more vegetarian food choices.

Are you a vegetarian? _____ Yes _____ No
If so, what kind of vegetarian are you?:

_____ Vegan (I eat vegetables only; no milk or other dairy products or eggs)

_____ Lactovegetarian (I eat vegetables and all dairy products; no eggs)

_____ Ovolactovegetarian (I eat vegetables, all dairy products, and eggs)

If you're NOT a vegetarian, would you nevertheless like to see more vegetarian food choices in your cafeteria? _____ Yes _____ No

General Question I: If more vegetarian food choices were made available in this cafeteria, do you believe you would include them more often in your own diet? _____ Yes _____ No

General Question II: Do you have any suggestions for changing or improving the nutritional choices available to you in this cafeteria?

Thank you for your answers!

a day of each week as "Nutrition Awareness Day" and post your "Nutrition Tips" on bulletin boards or walls in your house, dormitory, or cafeteria.

5. Working with classmates or other interested friends, develop a brief (15 to 30 minute) presentation on sound basic nutrition. Be sure to make use of pictures, charts, slides, overhead transparencies (sheets of acetate and special felt pens are available at many office supply stores), and even recorded music. Plan on testing your program in your dormitory or to a group of friends or family members. Then take the program out into the community, perhaps to local elementary, middle, and secondary schools. Call local PTAs and school administrators to discuss appropriate formats and dates for your presentation.

Conclusion

Adequate nutrition is essential to proper body function and freedom from numerous diseases associated with excesses and deficiencies in vitamins, minerals, protein, carbohydrates, and fats. Nutritional needs vary, depending on age, sex, weight, metabolism, and lifestyle. The typical American diet is currently too high in calories, fats, protein, salts, and sugar, and too low in fruits, vegetables, and water. The real secret to good nutrition is not multiple vitamins, organic foods, special diets, or miracle foods; it is a balanced diet coupled with wise food purchasing and adequate rest, sleep, and exercise.

Summary

1. Six nutrients are needed daily to satisfy the body's basic needs: carbohydrates, fats, and proteins (the energy nutrients); and vitamins, minerals, and water (the non-energy nutrients).

2. The Food and Nutritional Board of the National Academy of Sciences' National Research Council reviews the recommended dietary allowances (RDAs) every five years for possible changes. RDAs are recommendations, not minimum requirements.

3. The Four Food Group Plan offers an alternative to the complex RDA tables for determining whether you are obtaining an adequate diet.

4. Carbohydrates and fats provide the body with its two main sources of energy. Energy is measured in calories.

5. Protein is used in the body to repair, rebuild, and replace cells.

6. Although the number of vegetarians in the United States is on the rise, non-meat eaters must plan their diets carefully because it is difficult to consume adequate protein from vegetable sources alone.

7. Vitamins are required in very small amounts and are essential in helping chemical reactions take place in the body.

8. There is no evidence that consuming large quantities of vitamin supplements improves health or prevents disease. Hypervitaminosis can occur in people who resort to the megavitamin approach.

9. Present in all living cells, minerals serve as key components of various hormones, enzymes, and other substances that aid in regulating chemical reactions within cells.

10. Iron is one of the most essential minerals, and iron intake should be increased at certain times in our lives (early childhood, adolescence, during pregnancy, and while lactating). The body only absorbs about 10 percent of the total iron consumed daily.

11. Water is the most critical food component. Though it has no nutritional value, water is necessary for energy production, temperature control, and elimination.

12. For optimum health, Americans should increase the amount of carbohydrates, fiber, and water, and decrease the amount of sugar and salt in their diets.

13. Nutritionally dense foods contain a high amount of nutrients and a low amount of calories and are excellent food choices.

14. It may be inadvisable to use salt tablets on hot, humid days. Excess salt may actually increase salt and potassium loss.

15. High blood cholesterol levels and heart disease are good reasons to reduce the intake of high-fat foods.

16. Food additives are designed to protect us against the spread of infection and food poisoning. Although many substances are potentially toxic or carcinogenic (cancer-causing), they are hazardous only if consumed in very large quantities, which are rarely ingested by human beings.

17. The federal government requires food products to carry proper nutritional labeling. With a little practice, anyone can learn to read a food label quickly and accurately.

18. There are many nutritional myths. Keep in mind that no special foods prevent or cure disease, nor do any special diets improve health or cause rapid weight loss.

19. Athletes and active individuals may need extra calories if energy levels are low or if weight loss occurs. Additional water is needed before, during, and after exercise to maintain proper electrolyte balance. Extra servings of potassium-rich foods may be called for several days before a contest.

20. Adolescent male and female athletes, and female athletes during menstruation, may need an iron supplement.

21. A pre-event or pre-exercise meal is an individual meal and provides only limited energy and value for improved performance.

22. Carbohydrate loading improves energy levels and performance in endurance-type events, such as marathon running.

23. Little evidence exists to suggest the need for additional protein in athletes' diets.

Questions for Personal Growth

1. What nutritional areas do you and your friends need to change the most? Discuss at least four things you can do now to initiate these changes.

2. If you are drinking any milk other than skim milk, begin using skim milk now and continue to do so for one month. (Remember: skim milk contains only 90 calories and 0 grams of fat in every serving.) Store and use the milk quite cold. Record your thoughts about the taste and consistency of the milk at the beginning of your trial month and once again at the end of the month. Have you adjusted to skim milk? Do you feel you are making a "sacrifice" by drinking skim rather than whole, 1 percent fat, or 2 percent fat milk? Do you think the health benefits are worth it?

3. Choose three of your favorite processed snack foods (for example, potato chips, candy, ice cream bars) and carefully analyze their labels. For each item determine: (1) Is this a high-density or a low-density food? (2) Does it have too much fat, cholesterol, salt, sugar, or calories? (3) Is there a healthy food substitute for this item?

4. Ask five of your friends about their water consumption habits. Write down five ways you could tactfully encourage them (1) to stop at water fountains instead of soda machines and (2) to drink one glass of water immediately upon rising every morning, one glass with each meal, and one glass before going to bed every night. Now put your plan into action!

5. Briefly describe how the things you learned in this chapter will affect your choice of restaurants and restaurant menu choices.

6. List all of the foods you enjoy eating that contain 2 to 3 grams of fiber per serving. How often do you eat these foods? Could you add several fiber-rich foods to you daily diet? What would they be?

7. Develop a one-week menu plan for yourself. Use the Four Food Group Plan and make sure you are meeting your RDAs in the key areas.

8. Make a chart to list the advantages and disadvantages of three different kinds of diets: (1) standard diet (all foods, including meat), (2) ovolacto-vegetarian diet (vegetables plus dairy and egg products), and (3) vegan vegetarian diet (vegetable foods only). You might use a simple "T" chart design like the following:

	Standard Diet	Ovolactovegetarian Diet	Vegan Diet
Advantages			
Disadvantages			

References

1. Food and Nutrition Board, *Recommended Dietary Allowances*, 10e (Washington, D.C.: National Academy of Sciences, 1989).

2. David C. Nieman, Diane E. Butterworth, and Catherine N. Nieman, *Nutrition* (Dubuque, Iowa: Wm. C. Brown, 1990).

3. George B. Dintiman and Robert Ward, *Train America! Achieving Peak Performance and Fitness for Sports Competition* (Dubuque, Iowa: Kendal-Hunt, 1988), p. 124.

4. Corrine B. Cataldo, Jacquelyn R. Nyenhuis, and Eleanor N. Whitney, *Nutrition and Diet Therapy: Principles and Practice*, 2e (Minneapolis: West, 1989), pp. 220–226.

5. "America's Diet Wars," *U.S. News and World Report* (January 20, 1986): 62–66

6. Tufts University, *Diet and Nutrition Letter* 3, 7 (September 1985): 31

7. Science and Education Administration/Human Nutrition, *Nutrition and Your Health: Dietary Guidelines for Americans* (Washington, D.C.: U.S. Government Printing Office, 1981).

8. Melvin H. Williams, *Nutrition for Fitness and Sport* (Dubuque, Iowa: Wm. C. Brown, 1988).

9. George B. Dintiman, Robert G. Davis, Stephen Stone, and June C. Pennington, *Discovering Lifetime Fitness: Concepts of Exercise and Weight Control* (St. Paul, Minn.: West, 1989).

10. Eleanor Ness Whitney, Eva May Nunnelly Hamilton, and Sharon Rady Rolfes, *Understanding Nutrition*, 5e (St. Paul, Minn.: West, 1990), p. 419.

11. Ibid., p. 420.

CHAPTER

8

Weight Control

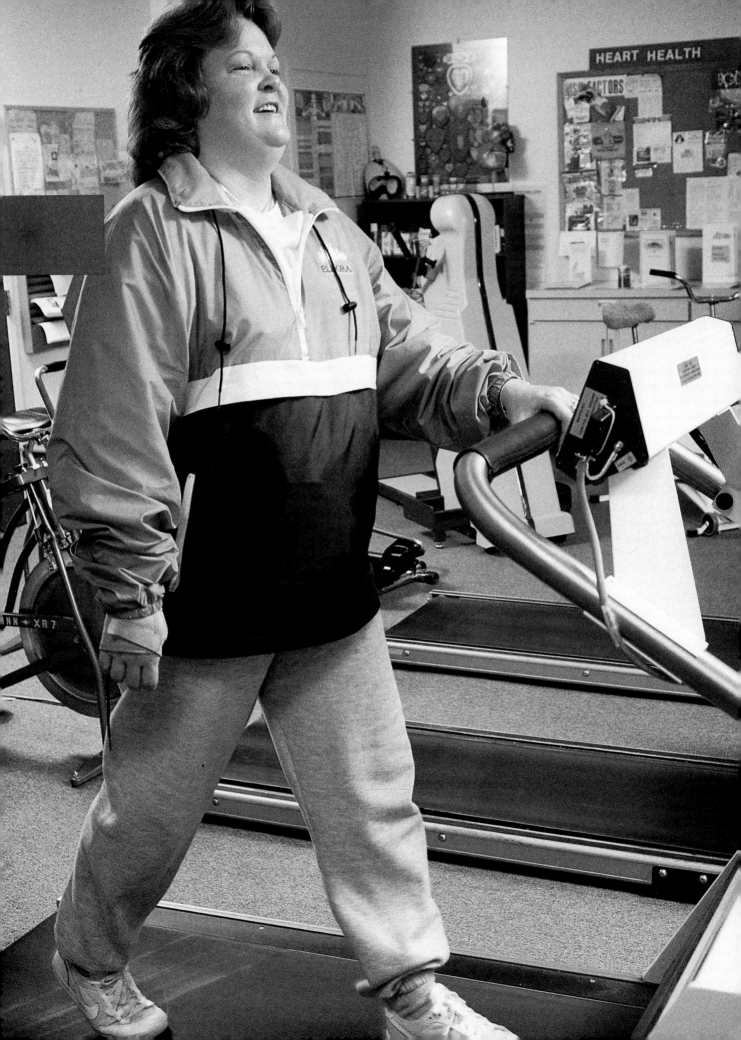

obesity An overweight condition in which there is an abnormally high proportion of body fat, usually 25 to 30 percent or more of total body weight.

skinfold measurement An accurate method of determining body fat (adipose tissue) and ideal body weight.

Judging from television, magazines, and books, no topic is more important to Americans than weight control. Dieting has become a national obsession, as people of all ages strive to be thinner and thus more "attractive." Many Americans are indeed overweight, but some of the techniques they use to reduce are unsound or potentially harmful. In this chapter, we present the problems of being overweight, obese, and underweight, and suggest how a healthy diet, combined with regular exercise, can set you on the right course.

Evaluating Body Weight, Body Fat, and Caloric Intake

Estimating Overweight, Underweight, and Obesity

There are two basic methods of determining whether you are overweight, underweight, or obese. A person who is *overweight* merely has an increase in body weight above some arbitrary standard defined in relation to height, usually 10 percent to 19 percent above desirable weight. **Obesity** refers to an abnormally high proportion of body fat (adipose tissue), usually 25 to 30 percent or more of total body weight or a single tricep skinfold measure falling at the 95 percentile or higher (see Table 8.3). The most common procedure to determine whether you are overweight or underweight is to use a standard chart (see Table 8.1) to compare your body weight to the suggested ranges. As we will discover later in this chapter, however, this method is crude and often inaccurate. The second method to identify obesity is to determine your percent of body fat (see Figure 8.1). This method can also be used to judge more accurately whether you are overweight or thin. If you possess more than 15 to 20 percent (men) or 20 to 25 percent (women) body fat, you are considered to be overweight; more than 25 percent (men) or 30 percent (women) classifies you as obese, and less than 5 percent (men) or 10 percent (women) as *underweight* or thin.

Estimating Body Fat

Weight charts, such as Table 8.1, provide only a rough guide to the determination of desirable weight and entail several pitfalls:

- It is possible to be within the range of suggested weight and still possess excessive fat. The key to obesity is not total body weight but total fat. Weight charts fail to reveal the presence of fat.

- It is possible to be classified as overweight or obese when you are at a desirable weight and possess little fatty tissue. Among thick-muscled athletes with low body fat, this is common.

- Some charts allow you to gain weight with age, suggesting that it is fine to be fat at age 30, 40, or 50, but not at age 20. Actually, weight should decrease slightly with age. If you weigh the same now as you did twenty years ago, you may be overweight. Loss of muscle mass from earlier active years is now made up by an increased proportion of fatty tissue. Ideally, you should be five to ten pounds lighter at age 50 than your ideal weight at age 25.

- The three categories of small, medium, and large frame encourage cheating. Very few individuals take their recommended weight from the small or medium frame range, yet not everyone has a large frame.

To use the new weight chart in Table 8.1 correctly, it is important to determine your frame size and height accurately. Frame size can be estimated by wrapping the thumb and index finger around the opposite wrist. If the thumb and finger do not meet, you have a large frame. If they just meet or barely overlap, you have a medium frame, and if they overlap, you have a small frame. A more accurate method involves measuring your elbow with a tape measure. Follow the directions provided in Table 8.2. Since clothed subjects were used to secure height and weight in Tables 8.1 and 8.2, add an inch to your barefoot height.

Several methods of determining body fat are more accurate than weight charts. Underwater weighing, or *hydrostatic weighing,* is one accurate method for assess-

TABLE 8.1

Metropolitan Life Insurance Height-Weight Tables

Men[a]					Women[b]				
Height					Height				
Feet	Inches	Small Frame	Medium Frame	Large Frame	Feet	Inches	Small Frame	Medium Frame	Large Frame
5	2	128–134	131–141	138–150	4	10	102–111	109–121	118–131
5	3	130–136	133–143	140–153	4	11	103–113	111–123	120–134
5	4	132–138	135–145	142–156	5	0	104–115	113–126	122–137
5	5	134–140	137–148	144–160	5	1	106–118	115–129	125–140
5	6	136–142	139–151	146–164	5	2	108–121	118–132	128–143
5	7	138–145	142–154	149–168	5	3	111–124	121–135	131–147
5	8	140–148	145–157	152–172	5	4	114–127	124–138	134–151
5	9	142–151	148–160	155–176	5	5	117–130	127–141	137–155
5	10	144–154	151–163	158–180	5	6	120–133	130–144	140–159
5	11	146–157	154–166	161–184	5	7	123–136	133–147	143–163
6	0	149–160	157–170	164–188	5	8	126–139	136–150	146–167
6	1	152–164	160–174	168–192	5	9	129–142	139–153	149–170
6	2	155–168	164–178	172–197	5	10	132–145	142–156	152–173
6	3	158–172	167–182	176–202	5	11	135–148	145–159	155–176
6	4	162–176	171–187	181–207	6	0	138–151	148–162	158–179

[a] Weights at ages 25–59 based on lowest mortality. Weight in pounds according to frame (in indoor clothing weighing 5 pounds, shoes with 1-inch heels).
[b] Weights at ages 25–59 based on lowest mortality. Weight in pounds according to frame (in indoor clothing weighing 3 pounds, shoes with 1-inch heels).
Source: Basic data from *1979 Build Study*, Society of Actuaries and Association of Life Insurance Medical Directors of America, 1980. Courtesy *Statistical Bulletin*, Metropolitan Life Insurance Company.

ing body fatness. The density of fat is different from that of lean body tissue. By dunking the entire body in a pool of water, the amount of body fat can be estimated by either (1) comparing the difference between underwater and dry weighings or (2) measuring the amount of water displaced.

A newly popular method for determining fatness is *electrical impedance analysis*. A mild electric current is passed through several electrodes attached to the body at various points. Since the electricity more easily passes through lean than through fatty tissues, a computer can calculate fat percentage based on measurements of the electric currents.

Unfortunately, hydrostatic weighing and electrical impedance analysis are both rather inconvenient and not widely available methods for determining body fat.

Skinfold measures are the most practical for home and school use. Since most body fat (adipose tissue) lies just under the skin, it is possible to pinch certain body parts, measure the thickness of two layers of skin and the connected fat, and refer to charts to estimate the percent of body fat (see Figure 8.1). You can evaluate your body weight and fat by using Exploring Your Health 8.1.

Estimating Your Caloric Needs

An individual's weight, age, sex, and activity patterns determine how many calories he or she needs daily. Certainly, if you experience no weight gain or loss, you are consuming an appropriate number of calories.

caloric balance When caloric intake per day equals caloric expenditures per day, at which point no weight loss or gain occurs.

TABLE 8.2

Determining Frame Size

Extend your arm and bend the forearm upward at a 90 degree angle. Keep fingers straight and turn the inside of your wrist toward your body. If you have a caliper, use it to measure the space between the two prominent bones on *either* side of your elbow. Without a caliper, place thumb and index finger of your other hand on these two bones. Measure the space between your fingers against a ruler or tape measure. Compare it with these tables that list elbow measurements for *medium-framed* men and women. Measurements lower than those listed indicate you have a small frame. Higher measurements indicate a large frame.

Height in 1-inch Heels	Elbow Breadth	Height in 1-inch Heels	Elbow Breadth
Men		Women	
5′2″–5′3″	$2\frac{1}{2}''-2\frac{7}{8}''$	4′10″–4′11″	$2\frac{1}{4}''-2\frac{1}{2}''$
5′4″–5′7″	$2\frac{5}{8}''-2\frac{7}{8}''$	5′0″–5′3″	$2\frac{1}{4}''-2\frac{1}{2}''$
5′8″–5′11″	$2\frac{3}{4}''-3''$	5′4″–5′7″	$2\frac{3}{8}''-2\frac{5}{8}''$
6′0″–6′3″	$2\frac{3}{4}''-3\frac{1}{8}''$	5′8″–5′11″	$2\frac{3}{8}''-2\frac{5}{8}''$
6′4″	$2\frac{7}{8}''-3\frac{1}{4}''$	6′0″	$2\frac{1}{2}''-2\frac{3}{4}''$

Source: Courtesy *Statistical Bulletin,* Metropolitan Life Insurance Company.

Exploring Your Health 8.1

Evaluating Your Body Weight and Body Fat

1. Locate your ideal weight on the weight charts (Table 8.1). Measure the space between the two prominent bones on either side of your elbow to determine the size of your frame (Table 8.2). With your shoes on, determine your correct height. Now locate your weight range in the table.

2. Using a skinfold caliper, have a partner obtain your triceps skinfold measurement. With your arm resting comfortably at your side, have your partner take a vertical fold midway between the tip of the shoulder and the tip of the elbow using the index finger and the thumb. The skinfold calipers are now placed approximately one-sixteenth of an inch under your finger and thumb. Preset tension determines how hard the skin is pinched by the caliper. Caliper readings are in millimeters. This one site test provides an estimate of your total body fat.

3. Find the triceps fatfold percentile for your age from Table 8.3. This reveals the estimated percent of males and females who have triceps fatfold scores higher and lower than yours. Another way to evaluate your score is to categorize percentiles: 5th or below—very low fat, 25th—low fat, 50th—average fat, 75th—above average fat, and 95th—high fat.

4. Compare the two methods. Did both methods obtain similar results? Were you normal weight on the charts and overly fat in the skinfold test? Were you overweight on the charts and found to possess only average fat on the skinfold test? Discuss how this can happen.

TABLE 8.3

Triceps Fatfold Percentiles (Millimeters) for Males and Females

Age	Male					Female				
	5th	25th	50th	75th	95th	5th	25th	50th	75th	95th
1–1.9	6	8	10	12	16	6	8	10	12	16
2–2.9	6	8	10	12	15	6	9	10	12	16
3–3.9	6	8	10	11	15	7	9	11	12	15
4–4.9	6	8	9	11	14	7	8	10	12	16
5–5.9	6	8	9	11	15	6	8	10	12	18
6–6.9	5	7	8	10	16	6	8	10	12	16
7–7.9	5	7	9	12	17	6	9	11	13	18
8–8.9	5	7	8	10	16	6	9	12	15	24
9–9.9	6	7	10	13	18	8	10	13	16	22
10–10.9	6	8	10	14	21	7	10	12	17	27
11–11.9	6	8	11	16	24	7	10	13	18	28
12–12.9	6	8	11	14	28	8	11	14	18	27
13–13.9	5	7	10	14	26	8	12	15	21	30
14–14.9	4	7	9	14	24	9	13	16	21	28
15–15.9	4	6	8	11	24	8	12	17	21	32
16–16.9	4	6	8	12	22	10	15	18	22	31
17–17.9	5	6	8	12	19	10	13	19	24	37
18–18.9	4	6	9	13	24	10	15	18	22	30
19–24.9	4	7	10	15	22	10	14	18	24	34
25–34.9	5	8	12	16	24	10	16	21	27	37
35–44.9	5	8	12	16	23	12	18	23	29	38
45–54.9	6	8	12	15	25	12	20	25	30	40
55–64.9	5	8	11	14	22	12	20	25	31	38
65–74.9	4	8	11	15	22	12	18	24	29	36

Source: Adapted from A. R. Frisancho, "New norms of upper limb fat and muscle areas for assessment of nutritional status," *American Journal of Clinical Nutrition* 34 (1981): 2540–2545.

Table 8.4 shows the recommended number of calories per pound per day for males and females of various age groups and activity patterns. To estimate your caloric needs, complete Exploring Your Health 8.2.

Caloric Balance You can determine whether you are in a state of caloric balance (food intake not excessive) by weighing yourself once a week. Weigh yourself at exactly the same time of day and under the same conditions (preferably upon rising). When the total daily caloric intake is equal to energy costs or expenditure and calories lost in excreta, a **caloric balance** has been attained and no weight loss or gain will occur. When you eat more calories than you use, these excess calories are stored as fat. With the accumulation of ap-proximately 3,500 excess calories, one pound of fat is stored. Remember, the body is extremely thrifty. Every unused calorie is stored as fat. Often a change to an alternative food or drink will cause weight loss. An individual who drinks three glasses of whole milk daily (165 calories per 8-ounce glass), for example, takes in nearly one pound of fat per week (3,485 calories). A change to skim milk (85 calories per glass) results in a weight reduction of one-half pound weekly or two pounds monthly.

Once unused calories are placed in your fat bank, they cannot be withdrawn at a moment's notice. It takes weeks of deprivation and suffering to remove them. To top it off, you have to carry the bank around with you until a withdrawal is made.

morbid obesity Usually refers to extreme cases of obesity that are obviously life-threatening; however, all obesity is potentially life-threatening.

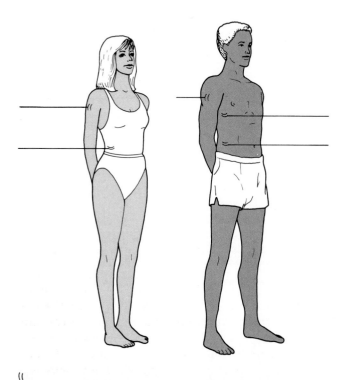

((

This merely shows the direction of the skinfold after being grasped between the tester's thumb and index finger at the proper location.

FIGURE 8.1 • Location of skinfold measures for men and women. This symbol merely shows the direction of the skinfold after being grasped between the tester's thumb and index finger at the proper location.

The incidence of childhood obesity continues to rise—it has increased 15 percent in the last fifteen years alone. Unfortunately, an overweight child eventually becomes an overweight adult.

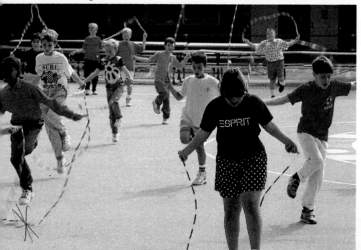

Overweight and Obesity

Overweight and obesity are serious problems in our society. Childhood obesity is reaching epidemic proportions. Between 1963 and 1980, there was a 54 percent increase in the prevalence of obesity among children age 6 to 11 and a 39 percent increase among adolescents age 12 to 17. This trend appears to have continued through 1990 and is responsible for the rise in the prevalence of adult obesity and its consequences.

- There is a direct relationship between percent of body fat and age. The percent of body fat increases with each passing decade.

- The younger you are when you are overweight, the more likely you will grow out of the problem. The later in life you are overweight, the less likely you are to ever return to normal body weight and fat. The fatter you are, at any age, the less likely you are to return to normal body weight and fat.

- It is estimated that over 15 percent of children in grades one to six are overweight or obese. These percentages have been rising steadily over the past two decades.

- Fifty percent of males between 30 and 39 years of age are at least 10 percent overweight.

- Sixty percent of males between 50 and 59 years of age are at least 10 percent overweight, and 33 percent are at least 20 percent overweight.

- The percentage of overweight women under age forty is lower than that of men; it is identical for ages 40 to 49; and more women are obese than men in the over-49 category.

- Approximately 10 percent of the school population is obese (in some high schools, this figure reaches approximately 20 percent).

The average woman in the United States is 5'4'' and weighs 142 pounds, slightly heavier than a decade ago; the average man is 5'9½'' and weighs 173 pounds, slightly less than a decade ago.

The term **morbid obesity** is usually reserved for cases of obesity that are obviously life-threatening. However, all obesity is associated with a number of disorders, including atherosclerosis, high blood pressure, stroke and heart disease, diabetes, gallstones, ar-

TABLE 8.4

Approximate Number of Calories Needed Daily Per Pound of Body Weight

Age Ranges	7–10	11–14	15–22	23–35	36–50	51–75
Males						
Very active[a]	21–22	23–24	25–27	23–24	21–22	19–20
Moderately active[b]	16–17	18–19	20–23	18–19	16–17	11–15
Sedentary[c]	11–12	13–14	15–18	13–14	11–12	10–11
Females						
Very active[a]	21–22	22–23	20–21	20–21	18–19	17–18
Moderately active[b]	16–17	18–19	16–18	16–17	14–15	12–13
Sedentary[c]	11–12	13–14	11–12	11–12	9–10	8–9

[a]Very active—Involved in a regular aerobic exercise program four to six times weekly, expending more than 2,500 calories per week during physical activity.

[b]Moderately active—Involved in a regular exercise program at least three times weekly.

[c]Sedentary—No physical activity beyond attending classes and desk work.

Source: Reprinted by permission from *Discovering Lifetime Fitness: Concepts of Exercise and Weight Control,* by George B. Dintiman, Stephen E. Stone, June C. Pennington, and Robert G. Davis, p. 176. Copyright © 1989 by West Publishing Co. All rights reserved.

thritis, orthopedic problems, varicose veins, snoring, kidney stones and kidney failure, and cancer of the breasts, uterus, cervix, and gall bladder.[1]

Causes of Obesity

A number of factors contribute to overweight and obesity in the United States population. Inactivity and overeating, in that order, are the two leading causes among both children and adults. Early eating patterns, the number of fat cells acquired early in life, metabolism, age, and environmental and genetic factors also play a significant role.

Early Eating Patterns   Most experts agree that environmental forces influence eating patterns more than physiological forces such as hunger. Negative eating behavior may begin in infancy. Some researchers feel that bottle feeding predisposes infants to obesity. Approximately three times more bottle-fed than breast-fed babies are overweight. The researchers suggest that bottle feeding fails to provide the solace of breast feeding, and an unsatisfying bottle produces anxiety, which provokes overeating. Breast-fed babies also learn to stop feeding after removing the richest portion of the milk (the highest fat content). The bottle does not provide such a natural mechanism, so that bottle-fed babies require more calories to satisfy hunger.

Exploring Your Health 8.2

Estimating Your Caloric Needs

Estimate your daily caloric needs by using this formula:

$$\frac{\text{Desirable weight}}{\times}$$

$$\overline{\text{Calories per pound}}$$

$$= \text{Calories per day}$$

To find your desirable weight, refer to Tables 8.1 and 8.2. The recommended number of calories per pound is shown in Table 8.4. Use these tables as guides only. You may know

from experience that you'll gain or lose weight by consuming a certain number of calories. What's right for you will also depend upon your metabolism and exercise habits.

set point theory A theory that postulates that each individual has an ideal weight (the set point), and that the body will attempt to maintain this weight against pressures to change it.

Year 2000 National Health Objective

Because of the association between obesity and disease, the federal government is striving to reduce overweight to a prevalence of no more than 20 percent among people age 20 and older and no more than 15 percent among adolescents age 12 through 19. This national health objective is designed to reduce the upward trend in the United States toward higher body weight and higher body fat content at all ages. An additional national health objective has been established to increase to at least 50 percent the proportion of overweight people age 12 and older who have adopted sound dietary practices combined with regular physical activity to attain an appropriate body weight.

Perhaps a more important problem is feeding babies solid foods too early. Researchers believe that starting solid foods early in infancy contributes to the production of excess fat cells. They recommend that parents not start their infants on solid foods before the age of six months (a month or two earlier for very large or fast-developing babies). Another behavior that may continue long after infancy is the general parental tendency to foster overeating. Many children are forced to clean their plate after they are full.

Fat Cells and Overweight Our fat cells are formed early in life and increase in both size and number until puberty. Weight loss decreases only the size of the fat cells, not the number (see Figure 8.2). With a large number of fat cells formed, return to an overweight condition is much easier. This explains why adults who were heavy babies have difficulty keeping their weight down. These extra cells also may affect metabolism and result in the need for fewer calories to maintain normal weight than are needed by someone who has always maintained normal weight.[2]

The number of fat cells in the human body grows rapidly during three stages of development: (1) the last trimester of pregnancy, (2) the first year of life, and (3) the adolescent growth spurt. Fat is acquired by storing

FIGURE 8.2 • Fat cell quantity is constant. Dieting decreases only the size of fat cells, not the quantity. Fat cell size can only be reduced by modifying diet and exercising regularly.

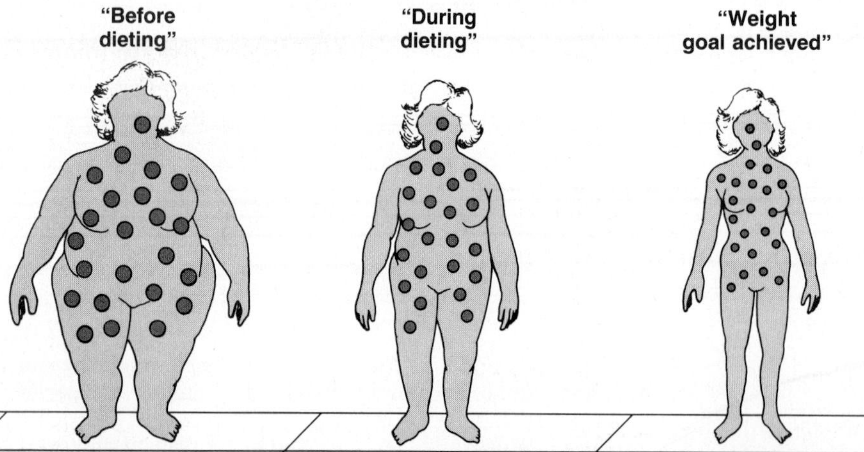

	"Before dieting"	"During dieting"	"Weight goal achieved"
Body weight	190 lb	160 lb	130 lb
Fat cell size	0.9 µg/cell*	0.6 µg/cell	0.2 µg/cell
Fat cell number	75 billion	75 billion	75 billion

*µg = "micrograms"

larger quantities of fat in existing fat cells *(hypertrophy)* and by new fat cell formation *(hyperplasia)*. It is unlikely that new fat cells are formed in humans after age twenty-one or so.

There is a large difference in the number of fat cells in different individuals. A nonobese person has approximately 25 to 30 million fat cells, and an extremely obese person has as many as 260 billion cells. A formerly obese person is never "cured," because weight loss does not change the number of fat cells. Research indicates that fat cell size (anytime in life) and number (before adulthood) can only be reduced by modifying nutrition and exercising regularly. Prevention of excessive fat cells centers around developing healthy eating and exercise habits early in life and during the growth spurt. Children who exercise have been found to develop fewer and smaller fat cells. In the adult, the same approach will successfully reduce the size of existing fat cells and cause weight and fat loss.

Set Point Theory and Overweight The human body regulates many functions with tremendous precision. It may also regulate body weight. **Set point theory** postulates that each individual has an ideal biological weight (the set point), and the organism will defend its body weight against pressure to change. Individuals who do succeed in losing or gaining weight generally come back to their set point weight over time. The body defends its weight in several ways. Within a very short time after initiating a low-calorie diet (less than twenty-four hours), metabolic rate (number of calories burned at rest) slows by 15 to 30 percent as a means of conserving calories and making it more difficult to lose weight. In addition, once excessive fat cells become depleted, they signal the central nervous system to alter feeding behavior through an increase in caloric intake so that the set point can be maintained. In other words, an internal "thermostat" regulates body fat and weight and triggers an increase in food intake when fat and weight are lowered too much. Unfortunately, this "one-way" thermostat does not key the body to reduce its caloric intake when excess weight and fat accumulate. Overcoming the set point is difficult. Willpower and other factors that aid in tolerating physical discomfort are poor matches for a computerlike system that never quits.[3]

Research suggests that one way to "take it off and keep it off" may be to lower the thermostat. "Seesaw" approaches to weight loss may have the opposite effect and actually result in a higher set point. The thermostat now keys the body to defend a higher weight. Regular aerobic exercise and weight training appear to lower the thermostat over time and allow you to lose weight and maintain a lower weight.

Issues in Health

Weight and Longevity

The Metropolitan Life Insurance Company developed charts of so-called ideal weight (later referred to as desirable weight) for men and women based on data associating average weights by height and age with longevity. Early data indicated that those who weighed less than average lived up to 20 percent longer. These charts, which became the national guide for determining overweight and obesity for the general public, advocated the theory that "the greater the weight, the greater the risk of death." Recent research, such as the Framingham Project, has questioned the validity of such data. Findings revealed that less-than-average weight involved health risks greater than those associated with overweight and that the American preoccupation with "thin" may not be healthy. Even more dramatic results were found by a team of researchers from Northwestern University Medical School. Overweight (not obesity) was found to be associated with longevity. In fact, subjects with the greatest longevity were as much as 20 to 25 percent above the old Metropolitan chart's ideal weight. As Alfred Harper, chairman of the National Academy of Sciences Food and Nutrition Board, states, "The man in the street certainly deserves to know that desirable weights have been underestimated by ten to fifteen pounds." Not everyone agrees. Some medical authorities feel that the new weight charts shown in Table 8.1 give people the impression that it is all right to be heavier when this is not the case; excess weight is still associated with greater health risks.

Authorities do not dispute that people who are much heavier than average (more than 20 percent above ideal weight) obtain health benefits from weight reduction. For those in normal health who are at average or near average weight, there is no health benefit in losing weight. In fact, one should beware the lean and hungry look.

anorexia nervosa *An eating disorder, found most often in women, that involves lack of appetite to the point of self-starvation and dangerous weight loss.*

bulimia *An eating disorder, found most often in women, that involves eating binges followed by self-induced vomiting or the use of laxatives to expel the unwanted food.*

Genetic Factors and Overweight   Research has demonstrated that the genes we inherit do influence our weight. Thus, children of overweight parents are more likely to be overweight. One study indicates that only 9 percent of children of normal-weight parents are overweight, whereas 40 percent of those with one overweight parent were also overweight, and with both parents overweight, the proportion of overweight children rose to 80 percent.

Genetics also affects what the body does with unneeded calories. Some people tend to store excess calories more as fat, others lay them on as muscle. In other words, for a given amount of calories that results in overfeeding, there are differences in body composition and the topography of fat deposition. Controlled studies that overfed twins by 1,000 calories per day for 84 days (84,000 extra calories) produced much less weight gain for some than for others (an average weight gain of 17 pounds with a range of 9.5 to 29 pounds). Almost 40 percent of the weight gain was explained by the propensity to store calories in the form of lean or fat tissue. When one individual gained considerable weight, his twin did the same. There was three times more variation in weight gain between pairs than within pairs. Researchers concluded that genetic factors played a major role in determining how much weight was gained, the distribution of fat, and the tendency to store energy as either fat or lean tissue.[4] Other studies have supported the influence of heredity on obesity. Environment had little effect on twins raised by different parents. Pairs tend to have the body builds of their biological parents rather than those who raised them. Where fat tends to accumulate is also determined by genetics. Android (upper body) obesity is characterized by excess fat in the trunk and abdominal areas and is associated with medical complications such as an increased risk of heart disease. Unlike men, who typically develop android obesity, most women develop gynoid obesity carrying excess fat in the hip and thigh areas. While carrying excess fat anywhere on the body is unhealthy, it is far better to possess fat away from the heart.

Environmental Factors   Although genes play an important role, environment is still critical; our exercise and eating and drinking habits can overcome the genetic tendency to be either thin or fat. One of the clearer causes of obesity, overweight, and overfatness is the act of watching television. People on TV programs eat approximately eight times per hour. Those who watch TV pick up on these cues and tend to eat more often and eat more high fat, high calorie foods. In addition, TV is a passive activity that could be replaced by activities that burn more calories. While it is a good idea to restrict the number of TV-watching hours for children and teenagers, it is an absolutely critical change for the overweight child. Other environmental influences, such as the eating and exercise habits of parents, food availability, and nutrition knowledge, may not be as important as previously indicated. Studies show that genetic influences account for about 70 percent of the differences in body-mass index that are found later in life and that childhood environment has little or no influence. These studies are designed to measure hereditability and their conclusions should not leave the impression that environment has absolutely no influence on the incidence of obesity. Nongenetic factors are important determinants of body fat. These factors are also reversible and capable of overcoming some of the problems associated with genes that make us fat.

Metabolic Factors and Overweight   It is estimated that a 10-percent error in metabolism would result in an annual weight gain of approximately twenty-six pounds. The role of metabolism in weight control is receiving considerable attention, since it is obvious that minute changes in either direction can result in significant weight/fat loss or gain. Aerobic exercise, for example, will increase metabolic rates by thirty to fifty calories per hour for as long as six hours after exercise ceases. The longer and more vigorous the exercise bout, the longer this "after-burn" tends to continue. Walking, for example, burns almost as many calories as running the same distance; the after-burn, however, may last less than an hour. Caffeine (coffee, colas), amphetamines, and other drugs increase metabolic rate. In midafternoon, the metabolism of most people is quite low; this may be a good time for exercise to boost metabolic rates.

Age In middle and late adulthood, people experience a number of progressive alterations in body compositions as lean body mass shrinks and the mass of adipose tissue expands. The reduction in lean body mass is a result of atrophy of the skeletal muscles, liver, kidney, spleen, skin, and bone. There is also a clear relationship between age and body weight and body fat—with each decade people become fatter. Although once considered an unavoidable part of aging, it is now evident that regular aerobic exercise, strength training, and proper nutrition that avoids weight gain can reduce the loss of lean body mass and limit the increase in adipose or fatty tissue. One of the genetic causes of lean body mass loss is the declining activity of the growth hormone—insulin-like growth factor I—with advancing age. When healthy men from 61 to 81 years of age received biosynthetic human growth hormone (0.3 milligram per kilogram of body weight), an 8.8 percent increase in body mass and a 14.4 percent decrease in adipose tissue mass occurred. In addition, skin thickness increased 7.1 percent.[5] In combination with diet and exercise, growth hormone therapy shows great promise in helping men and women retain body mass and skin thickness, and in avoiding the addition of fatty tissue with age.

As we age, metabolism slows until, at age 50, metabolic rate may have decreased significantly, particularly in those individuals who do not exercise regularly. As we approach the sixth and seventh decades of life, metabolism slows significantly in almost everyone.

Underweight and Eating Disorders

The problems of gaining weight can be just as complex as those associated with weight loss. Hunger, appetite, and satiety irregularities, psychological factors, or metabolic problems can cause an underweight condition. Underfeeding during infancy may limit fat cell number; early eating habits such as food aversions and physical activity may add to the problem. For some athletes who need additional weight and muscle for sports and others who merely want to be and appear stronger, gaining a pound is just as difficult as it is for others to lose one.

Gaining Weight

A drug-free muscle-weight gain program requires considerable dedication to both diet and exercise. Sound approaches to muscle-weight gain strive to add no more than one-half pound of muscle per week, two pounds per month. This is about as quick as the body can add lean muscle tissue. Faster approaches involv-

ing too many calories are almost certain to add adipose or fatty tissue to the bodies of most individuals.

A sound strength training program, such as weight training, is an absolute must for muscle-weight gain. Athletes who want to add considerable muscle weight will train for several hours daily, alternating muscle groups each day, in a rather complicated low repetition, heavy weight, multiple set free weight lifting program that involves bimonthly or less frequent changes in the choice of exercises, repetitions, weights, and rest intervals (periodization).

The nutritional support for a sound weight gain program involves an increase in food (approximately 400–500 additional calories daily) that provides high calories in as small a volume as possible to keep the individual from getting uncomfortably full, slight increases in protein intake (14–15 percent of daily calories), and a slight reduction in total fat intake (18–20 percent of daily calories). Where should these extra calories come from if they don't come from protein and fat? Complex carbohydrates, in the form of fruits, vegetables, and grains, should make up 65–68 percent of total daily calories. Complex carbohydrates are a major source of long-term fuel that will provide the energy for the increased exercise and produce a protein sparing effect to keep the body from utilizing lean body tissue for energy. Most individuals who have difficulty gaining weight simply do not eat enough calories to support their vigorous exercise schedule. Muscle weight can also be acquired without the use of amino acid or protein tablets and the dangerous use of anabolic steroids. Amino acid supplements will not significantly increase production of the muscle growth hormone beyond that caused by strength training. It is also important to keep in mind that although a thin person expends fewer calories to exercise than a heavy person does, the only real solution for the person who wants to gain weight is an increase in daily food intake to counter the increase in activity. If there is no existing medical condition affecting metabolism, the result will be a weight gain.[6]

Eating Disorders

The current overemphasis on flat stomachs, lean thighs, firm buttocks, and slimness in the United States is at least partially responsible for aggravating two serious eating disorders that can lead to death: **anorexia nervosa** and **bulimia.** Both disorders are known only in developed nations and are more common in higher economic groups.

Anorexia The number of cases of *anorexia* (loss of appetite) *nervosa* (nervous or psychogenic) is increasing and now occurs in almost one of every one-hundred females;[7] nineteen out of twenty of these patients are

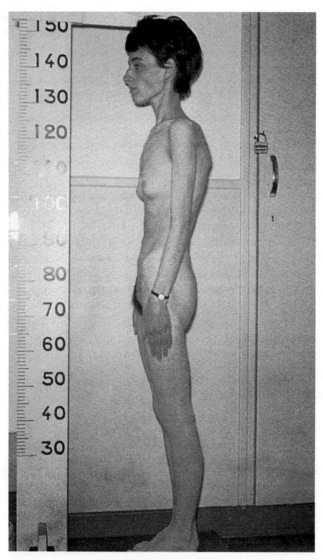

Despite obvious malnutrition and lack of body fat, anorexics nevertheless continue to view themselves as "fat" and continue to try to lose weight.

young women. The disease is four to five times more common in identical than in nonidentical twins, suggesting an inherited predisposition to the disease.[8] Unfortunately, our culture encourages its development. A typical case involves a young woman from a middle-class family who values appearance more than self-worth and self-actualization. Typically, family ties are

strong and the patient is efficient, eager to please her parents, and somewhat of a perfectionist. An absentee or distant father is also common in families of anorexic children. The characteristic behavior of anorexia is obsessive and compulsive, resembling an addiction. Patients may become obsessed with the idea that they are or will become fat. They may fear the transition from girlhood to womanhood resulting in a more curvaceous figure, and become determined to stave it off by controlling their weight. This starvation approach is then carried to the extreme point of undernourishment until total adolescent/adult body weight may reach seventy pounds or less. Even at that extreme, patients may still feel fat and continue to starve themselves.

Young female anorexics generally have amenorrhea. Females must acquire 17 to 22 percent body fat before the menstrual cycle resumes. Young male anorexics lose their sex drive and become impotent. Thyroid hormone secretions, adrenal secretions, growth hormones, and blood pressure-regulating hormones reach abnormal levels. The heart pumps less efficiently as cardiac muscle weakens; the chambers diminish in size, and blood pressure falls. Heart rhythm disturbances (see Chapter 14) and sudden stopping of the heart may occur due to lean tissue loss and mineral deficiencies, producing sudden death in some patients. Other health problems include anemia, gastrointestinal problems, atrophy of the digestive tract, abnormal function of the pancreas, blood lipid changes, dry skin, decreased core temperature, and disturbed sleep.

Early treatment by an experienced physician or clinic is essential if permanent damage is to be avoided. Without treatment, approximately 10 percent of anorexics die of starvation. Forced feeding may temporarily improve health, but the condition can reappear unless proper psychological and medical therapy is successful.[9] Treatment is aimed at restoring adequate nutrition, avoiding medical complications, and altering psychological and environmental patterns that have supported or permitted the emergence of anorexia.[10] Teams of medical, psychiatric, psychological and nutrition personnel working together are most successful. According to Whitney, Hamilton, and Rolfes,[11] 5 percent of those in treatment reach a point within 25 percent of their desired weight, and 50 to 75 percent resume normal menstrual cycles. However, follow-up studies reveal that 66 percent fail to eat normally after treatment ends. Six percent die, 1 percent by suicide.

Bulimia Bulimia is more common than anorexia nervosa and occurs in males as well as females. Ten to twenty percent of college students are estimated to be bulimic. Only 5 percent of these individuals meet the criteria for anorexia nervosa, and less than 1 percent are actively anorexic. The disclosure by exercise and weight-control enthusiast Jane Fonda that she was bulimic from age 12 to age 35 has helped to focus attention on the problem of bulimia.

The typical profile of victims is similar to those suffering from anorexia nervosa, although they tend to be slightly older and healthier. Though they tend to be malnourished, they are close to their normal weight. Bulimics tend to eat a tremendous volume of food secretly and follow the binge with vomiting or the use of large quantities of laxatives to eliminate the food. The binge is generally not a response to hunger, and the food is not consumed for nutritional value. As the binge/vomiting cycle is repeated, medical problems grow. Fluid and electrolyte imbalance can lead to abnormal heart rhythm and kidney damage. Infections of the bladder and kidneys may cause kidney failure. Vomiting results in the irritation and infection of the pharynx, esophagus, and salivary glands, erosion of the teeth, dental caries. In some cases, the esophagus or stomach may rupture. The use of emetics to induce vomiting, a bulimic behavior, caused the death of singer Karen Carpenter in 1983. Bulimia patients are more cooperative and somewhat easier to treat than anorexia nervosa patients since they seem to recognize that the behavior is abnormal. Although the number of treatment clinics and qualified physicians is growing, the disease is still poorly understood. Most programs attempt to help people gain control over their binge-eating and encourage a minimum of 1,500 calories per day for proper nutrition. Lithium and other drugs have been shown to reduce the incidence of bulimic episodes by 75 to 100 percent. Most patients are also clinically depressed and may be helped by antidepressant medication.

Weight Control and Nutrition

Hunger and Appetite

Hunger is said to be physiological, an inborn instinct, whereas *appetite* is psychological or a learned response to food. Therefore, it is not uncommon to experience appetite and eat when one is not hungry; conversely, some very thin people or those with eating disorders may experience hunger without appetite. Hunger is said to be a negative experience, whereas appetite is positive.

The feeling of fullness or satisfaction that prompts us to stop eating is referred to as *satiety,* perhaps the main regulator of eating behavior. Some experts feel that eating behavior is always in operation except when the satiety signal turns it off. Just how that happens is unknown, although a number of theories have been forwarded. The *glucostatic theory* of hunger regulation suggests that the exhaustion of liver glycogen may account for the starting and stopping of eating. The liver stores approximately 75 grams of glycogen or 300 energy units (calories). When liver glycogen levels fall significantly, feelings of hunger may occur. The *lipostatic theory* suggests that hunger is regulated in some way by the number of fat-storing enzymes on the surfaces of fat cells. The messenger that the cells send to the brain has still not been identified. The *purinegic theory* is relatively new and untested and proposes that the circulating levels of purines, molecules found in DNA and RNA, govern hunger. Exactly where and how the brain receives these messages is also unknown. The hypothalamus appears to be important in regulating eating. Damage to this area can produce eating disorders and severe weight loss or gain. Eating behavior appears to be a response to numerous signals. The possibility also exists that an inherited, internal regulatory defect is at least partially responsible for obesity, rather than its being a purely learned behavior. A summary of research efforts currently in progress to discover the answers to these and other questions appears in Figure 8.3. An understanding of the difference between hunger and appetite and the factors suspected of controlling food intake will help you control your body weight and fat.

Controlling Appetite

From the limited information available, it is known that two basic approaches to controlling appetite are somewhat effective: keeping the stomach full of low-calorie food and drink and raising the body's blood sugar level. Increasing your fluid intake (particularly water) and consuming complex carbohydrates such as raw fruits and vegetables between meals and at mealtime will keep the stomach relatively full and help you control your appetite. Small amounts of candy, such as one chocolate square, twenty to thirty minutes before a meal is another technique you can use. This approach will raise blood-sugar level and help curb your appetite. Slow eaters (twenty minutes or more) at mealtime also experience this elevated blood sugar level and are less likely to overeat.

A Sensible Approach to Dieting

Weight loss should occur gradually (no more than two to four pounds per week for a fairly heavy person) over a period of months and in combination with exercise.

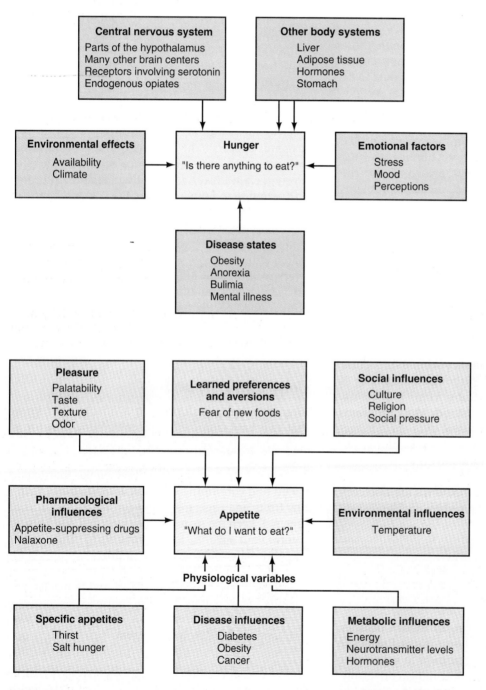

FIGURE 8.3 • Hunger and appetite: some of the factors suspected of controlling food intake.

Source: Adapted from T. W. Castonguay et al., ''Hunger and Appetite: Old Concepts/New Distinctions,'' *Nutrition Reviews* 41(April 1983): 101–110. © ILSI-Nutrition Foundation. Used with permission.

TABLE • 8.5

Daily Caloric Deficits and Weekly Weight Loss

Caloric Deficits Daily (Minus Calories from Reduced Food Intakes and Exercise Expenditure − 3,500 = 1 lb fat)	Approximate Weekly Weight Loss (in lbs)
250	$\frac{1}{2}$
500	1
750	$1\frac{1}{2}$
1,000	2
1,250	$2\frac{1}{2}$
1,500	3

Such an approach is more likely to produce a permanent change in eating habits and result in a high proportion of fat loss and little loss of lean muscle tissue. A nutritious low-calorie diet is well rounded and consists of foods chosen from each of the basic four food groups. It is a diet scaled down in calories but not in nutrition. You can tailor your diet to your own needs. Healthy dieting involves learning how to gauge portion sizes, estimate calories closely, and create a daily caloric deficit. When a deficit of approximately 3,500 calories exists, you will lose one pound. Most low-calorie diets recommend approximately 1,000 or 1,200 calories per day for women and 1,200 to 1,500 for men. This represents a daily deficit of approximately 800 to 1,700 calories, depending on your weight, metabolism, and activity patterns. It also represents a potential weight loss of two to four pounds per week, as shown in Table 8.5.

Follow the suggestions below for a healthy approach to a low-calorie diet:

- Determine how much you should weigh for your height, frame, and age. If your desired weight loss exceeds 5 percent of your body weight or if you have any health problems, consult your physician before beginning a diet. Determine the number of calories you must cut out daily to reach this desired weight gradually. Count calories carefully and eat only this number daily. Weight loss will occur with reduced calories regardless of the diet's percentage of carbohydrates, fats, and proteins.

- Make sure you need to go on a diet. If you are 5 percent or less above your desirable weight, merely increase your aerobic exercise activity to achieve your desired weight. If you are trying to change your body type such as trying to eliminate inherited large hips, avoid dieting and increase your activity.

- Eat three meals a day from the four basic food groups. Do not skip a meal. Choose the foods from each group that you enjoy and can continue to eat over a period of several months.

- Consume a minimum of 1,200 calories daily.

- Drink a minimum of ten glasses of water daily.

- Consume sufficient vitamins and minerals from the four basic food groups. If your doctor recommends it, take one multiple vitamin tablet per day.

- Consume the RDA in protein daily.

- Consume enough fat for satiety (10–15 percent of daily calories).

- Consume a minimum of 100 grams of carbohydrates daily (400 calories; no more than 80 from concentrated sugar) to spare protein and prevent ketosis.

- Gear your program to a weight loss of between two and three pounds weekly, and stay with it until you reach your goal.

- Make your evening meal light, consuming less than 30 percent of your daily calories at this time. Research suggests that those who eat a big traditional evening meal gain more weight and do not lose as much weight as those who eat a light dinner. In fact, four or five light meals (total calories must conform to your desired weight) will produce the greatest weight loss.

- Premeasure each portion.

- Keep records of your food and drink intake, identify problem areas, and take steps to change.

- If you snack, eat low-calorie snacks, such as carrots or celery.

- Combine dieting with exercise in an activity or aerobic program you enjoy. Exercise three or four times weekly, at least thirty minutes each time.

Fats and Carbohydrates: Reduce, Don't Eliminate

There is no doubt that too much fat in the diet contributes to obesity. However, people try so hard to minimize the amount of fat in their diets that it is easy to overlook the fact that fat does serve a valid function. Up to 65 percent of caloric intake should come from carbohydrates, 10 to 15 percent from protein, and the remainder from fats. Fat plays a vital part in digestion and the transportation of vitamins, and it is the main fuel for some muscle fibers in most muscle groups. Fat intake should therefore be reduced but not eliminated.

Similarly, starches and naturally occurring sugars have an important place in the diet. They should be restricted, not eliminated. Exercise, for example, draws from available carbohydrate supply for energy. If the supply is limited, the body must resort to fat for fuel, resulting in loss of fatty tissue. In women, too little fat may lead to amenorrhea (temporary loss of menstruation). A constant supply of glucose is also needed by the brain. This need is so essential that the body has a built-in mechanism to convert protein to carbohydrates when the supply is absent.

Snacking: It Can Have a Place

Between-meal and late-evening snacking is a leading cause of obesity and overweight. Yet it is unrealistic to expect people to avoid snacking altogether. In fact, planned snacking on the right foods can help you control hunger and eat less.

Snacks likely to be low in calories are those that are:

- Thin and watery, such as tomato juice.
- Crisp but not greasy (celery, carrots, radishes, cucumbers, broccoli, cauliflower, apples, berries, and other fresh fruits and vegetables).
- Bulky, such as salad greens.

No Place for Sugar

As an important source of energy, as fuel for cell building, or as an aid to the functioning of body systems, sugar is nearly worthless. And as a by-product, it can

It is unrealistic to try to eliminate snacking altogether. Make an effort to have nutritious snacks handy. Fresh fruit and vegetables are ideal.

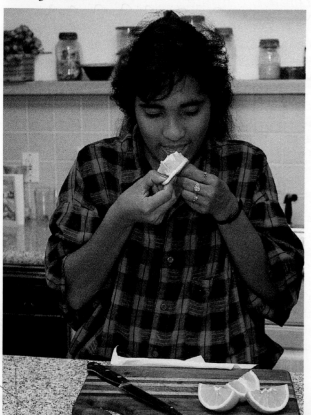

Exploring Your Health 8.3
Food as Rewards

All of us have been rewarded with food, and we often reward ourselves with food. Describe three occasions on which you rewarded yourself with food and try to explain why you did so.

1. _____

2. _____

3. _____

Now list three nonfood rewards you could substitute:

1. _____

2. _____

3. _____

lead to a pattern of eating that will encourage future obesity.

Most of the body's need for sugar can be supplied by eating foods that are naturally high in sugar, such as fruit. A common mistake people make is to reward children (or themselves!) with candy or other sweets. This reinforces the belief that sweets are better than other foods. In addition, it associates warmth and love with food—a link that remains throughout life.

The Need for Water

As we stated in Chapter 7, water is essential to the proper functioning of every body system. In addition, it is helpful to weight loss because it helps keep the stomach full and, when consumed in large quantities, can actually serve as a diuretic. About 80 percent of excessive weight is fat, not water. Thus, a person on a diet should not expect to lose weight by reducing water intake.

During the past ten years, we have moved toward

a "waterless" society, drinking more sodas, beer, and other high-calorie drinks. Consuming four glasses of orange juice or beer daily provides 120 to 150 calories per 12-ounce glass. This can add approximately 8,400 calories to the diet each week, or two pounds of fat. Water, on the other hand, can help to reduce hunger without adding a single calorie.

Fluid Retention

People in the early stages of dieting (during the first four weeks) frequently experience a temporary retention of water, which obscures their actual weight loss. This temporary water retention can be discouraging and cause the scales to record only moderate weight loss even when strict dieting has been observed. Nevertheless, actual weight loss has occurred and will be more apparent in terms of reduced pounds following this period. The problem is that vacated fat cells retain fluids. Many disappointed dieters discontinue the diet before this phase runs its course.

Some sound diets require the consumption of large quantities of water in order to prevent water retention; as we've already noted, increasing water consumption actually results in the elimination of water. A more accurate measure of weight loss during the ini-

tial stages of diet is the reduction of adipose tissue in fatty body areas. Both observation and pinching fatty tissue or the skinfold measures described previously will reveal benefits even in the early stages.

The Best Times to Diet

There are particular times when dieting is likely to be more successful. For example, controlled eating after splurges (such as eating out or parties) can prevent the need for a diet. Dieting is easier if you don't allow too much excess weight to accumulate. Other times to consider starting a diet are:

- At the beginning of your vacation. Although this often is difficult to do, you will save money and avoid additional weight gain during a time when everybody has a tendency to overeat.
- After the November–December holiday season, when temptation is reduced. Or if you are well disciplined, begin during the holiday season.
- After the cold and virus season. The winter months are particularly troublesome due to flu epidemics and colds; avoid lowering resistance due to dieting.
- When finances are particularly low in your house-

A Question of Ethics

Diet Books: Should Laypeople Be Permitted to Write Them?

By the end of 1984, it was possible to buy a book about how to write a best-selling diet book. Hardly a year passes without a new diet book reaching the top-ten list. Often, the diet book is written by a layperson, the diet has not been tested on humans, the book contains inaccurate information (some use the term "quackery"), and the total program may be slightly harmful to everyone and fatal to some. One point of view is that such books should not be permitted on the market unless dieticians, physicians, or other equally qualified reviewers give their stamp of approval. Literary freedom has its limits, and no one has the right to harm another's health. The FDA, for example, has indicated that a number of deaths have been attributed to the liquid protein diet and to some of the popular very low-calorie formula diets. When the motives of lay writers, unqualified in the area of nutrition and health, are purely

financial, the theme and contents of the book move toward sensationalism: fast loss of pounds and fat, and quick, easy methods of shaping up and taking weight off and keeping it off. The book may be based on one unfounded gimmick or claim that is new to the public, and such claims may be too much to resist for people who have tried and failed at hundreds of diets, have limited knowledge of nutrition, and must rely on so-called experts for guidance. Or the book may be a part of a business scheme in which groups of "counselors" join to promote the program, recruit other counselors who work under them, and give testimony on what the product and the approach did for them. Such vested-interest writing and promotion is unethical and unsafe, it is argued.

Another point of view is that individuals have full responsibility for making their own health decisions. They must learn to read and

sort out fact from fiction and use what is safe and sound. If they are unsure, they should consult their family physician or research the problem more carefully. In addition, people have been trying various types of diets for centuries and will continue to do so in the future. It is far safer for them to try one that has been researched and at least looks sound on paper. In actual practice, it is argued, few people suffer permanent bodily harm from diets of this type. If they follow the instructions carefully, no harm of any kind is likely to occur. It is when readers carry the approach to extremes that harmful effects occur. In addition, a democratic society requires freedom of the press.

An ethical dilemma exists. Do we control who writes what in the area of nutrition in order to protect the consumer? Or do we continue to allow people to interpret and sort things out for themselves?

cellulite The name commonly given to fat that accumulates on the legs and buttocks in overweight individuals; medically speaking, it is no different from fat in other parts of the body.

hold. Your chances of eating in a restaurant or stocking empty high-calorie treats are minimized.

- After finishing an organized sport or exercise program. Since the decrease in activity will not be followed by a decrease in appetite, this is a dangerous time when you can't afford to overeat.

Keeping It Off Permanently

A return to an obese or overweight state tends to occur within a perior proportional to that spent losing a specific amount of weight. Reducing over an extended period (minimum of three months) is preferred and generally results in the acquisition of sensible new eating habits, which are more likely to be continued. Rapid weight loss, through fasting and other crash programs, can be dangerous and often results in a rapid return to old eating habits and weight gain. Losing weight over an extended period also involves a pleasant personal adjustment to clothes and a new positive self-image so vital to weight control. Controlled weight loss, then, has the advantages of safety and permanence.

Fad Diets and Weight Loss Gimmicks

There are several reasons why the average diet lasts only five to seven days: boredom, monotony, lack of energy, fatigue, depression, complicated meal planning and purchasing, and failure to lose weight and body fat. These problems are much less likely to occur for individuals on a sound diet. Unfortunately, diet choices are often a direct result of magazine, book, or television publicity that reveals some "secret," easy method of shedding pounds and fat.

Very Low-Calorie Formula Diets   Some of the most common and potentially dangerous types of commercial diets involve very-low calorie formula intakes that provide only 400 to 800 calories and produce large weight loss while preserving vital lean body mass. These diets come in powdered form and contain relatively large amounts of protein, limited fats and carbohydrates, and supplemented vitamins, minerals, and

electrolytes to meet the RDAs. Water is added to the powder and the liquid is consumed three to five times daily. The Liquid Protein Diet, introduced in 1976, and the Cambridge Diet of the early 1980s marked the start of very low-calorie formula diets. Unfortunately these diets were poorly supervised and fifty-eight deaths were reported among users of the Liquid Protein Diet and six in individuals who used the Cambridge Diet Plan. When Oprah Winfrey disclosed to 18 million viewers in November 1988 that she had lost 67 pounds in four months by consuming a medically supervised diet, interest again surfaced in very low-calorie formula diets. According to the American Medical Association, very low-calorie formula diets are relatively safe when administered to carefully selected patients by physicians trained in their use. Selection is limited to patients who are at least 30 percent (and 18 kilograms/ 28 pounds) overweight who have received a recent medical examination and electrocardiogram with satisfactory results, are free of contraindicating conditions (including a recent myocardial infarction; a cardiac conduction disorder; a history of cerebrovascular, renal, and hepatic disease, cancer, type I diabetes, or significant physiatric disturbance). Unfortunately, no physician screening or care occurs for the several hundred thousands of people who use the Oprah Winfrey plan, the Ultra Slim Fast plan, or other very low-calorie formula diets. For these individuals, health risks are common and such diets are not safe.

> "It is the position of the American Dietetic Association that while very low-calorie diets promote rapid weight loss and may be beneficial for certain individuals, such diets have health risks and should be undertaken only with the supervision of a multidisciplinary health team with monitoring by a physician and nutrition counseling by a registered dietitian."[12]

The two most common problems with unsupervised patients is the use of the diets as the sole source of nutrition without the recommended consumption of conventional foods (at least one meal per day), and the use of the diet by those who are not severely overweight. Short-term misuse of very low-calorie formula diets can result in dehydration, electrolyte imbalance, hypotension, increased uric acid concentrations, and the common complaints of cold intolerance, fatigue, light-

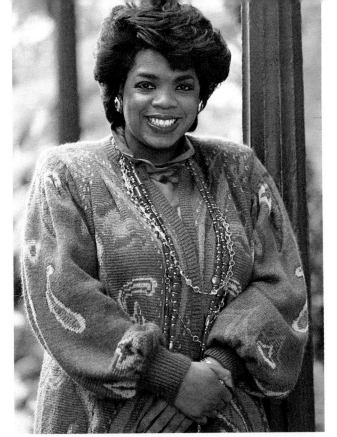
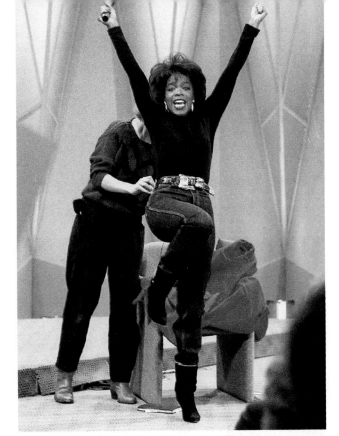

Talk show host Oprah Winfrey's stunning weight loss in 1988 caused a widespread resurgence of interest in very low-calorie formula diets.

headedness, nervousness, euphoria, constipation or diarrhea, dry skin, thinning and reddened hair, anemia, and menstrual irregularities. Long-term misuse includes the risk of severe ventricular arrhythmias and death. There is also no guarantee of long-term, permanent weight loss. High dropout rates and poor long-term maintenance are common. Most people regain the weight lost after returning to their conventional diet.

Weight Control and Exercise

For most people, maintaining ideal weight without exercise means remaining mildly or acutely hungry most of their lives. In reality, if you expect to either maintain or lower body weight and fat, you will have to manage both food intake and exercise. If you remain physically active, you will be able to eat a greater number of calories daily. In addition, your muscle tone and conditioning level will improve. There are a number of other important ways exercise helps to control body weight and body fat.

How Exercise Helps

The human body regulates many functions with tremendous precision. It also regulates body weight and fat. Each individual seems to have an ideal biological weight, or set point (see our previous discussion of set point theory and overweight). Regular exercise (minimum of four aerobic workouts weekly for thirty minutes or more) appears to permanently lower the set point over time and allow you to lose weight and maintain a lower weight.

Fatty Tissue Loss, Fat Cell Reduction, and Cellulite There is a difference between weight loss in terms of pounds and fatty tissue loss in terms of inches (weight loss versus fat loss). A diet without exercise can result in about 70 percent fatty tissue loss and 30 percent lean muscle loss. With the combination of exercise and diet, fatty tissue loss can be increased to 95 percent. A greater percentage of fatty acids is used for energy during exercise: 50 percent of the fuel for exercise bouts of from thirty to sixty minutes and as high as 70 to 85 percent for longer sessions.

Research indicates that regular exercise reduces the size of fat cells at any age and can reduce the number of fat cells that would be developed if regular activity and proper nutrition occur during the first year of life and up to adulthood.

One type of fat that women in particular are concerned about getting rid of is cellulite. **Cellulite** is really nothing but plain old fat, but its special label has helped many cosmetic and health care companies reap

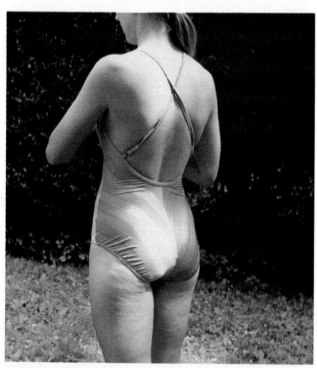

Cellulite is a label given to fatty deposits that commonly appear on the back and front of the legs and the buttocks, primarily in women. It does not necessarily appear in overweight people only, though it is usually more obvious in overweight people.

Exercise, Appetite, and Nutrition Studies of both humans and animals indicate that physical activity decreases appetite. This was first reported in 1954, in rat experiments showing that females rats decreased food intake and body weight with exercise. These findings have been confirmed with other studies on humans.

If the body has no energy-producing foods (carbohydrates) to draw upon for fuel during exercise, it must resort to its fat supply. The result is a reduction in adipose tissue in the areas of greatest concentration. Obviously, if you exercise in the morning before breakfast and have not eaten since the previous evening, the only available fuel will be fatty tissue. On the other hand, when the body can utilize energy-producing foods for energy, no loss of fatty tissue occurs. If your carbohydrate intake is high, you will burn a greater proportion of carbohydrates with exercise. If your intake is low, you will metabolize a greater amount of fat through exercise.

One disadvantage of performing on an empty stomach is that the blood-sugar level is rather low, and headache and dizziness may occur. A more sound approach, when loss of fatty tissue is desired, is to cut down on carbohydrate intake and increase protein consumption. This will produce similar results without negative side effects.

Your Exercise Choices for Weight Control

Many kinds of exercise can help in weight reduction. If you are already overweight, keep in mind that excess pounds do put extra strain on the knees, hips, back, and ankles. Low impact aerobics or walking, for example, are better exercise choices than high impact aerobics, jogging, or sports such as tennis and racquetball, at least until some reduction has taken place. Your exercise choice should allow for a gradual increase in intensity to strengthen muscle and bone slowly and to lessen the risk of injuring the orthopedic system. If you also replace the majority of dietary fat with complex carbohydrates, you will immediately improve your health during your weight loss program.

enormous profits by selling all sorts of potions, lotions, and devices that supposedly reduce the occurrence of this fatty dimpling that resembles the peel of a navel orange. Cellulite commonly appears on the back and front of the legs and on the buttocks of overweight women, though it may also appear on the legs and around the armpits of overweight men, too. However, it does not necessarily appear in overweight people only; many a young (even teenaged!), thin, otherwise healthy body may show some evidence of this fatty buildup if it is not properly fed and exercised. The best way to treat cellulite is to prevent it by maintaining normal body weight and starting a regular schedule of exercise—preferably before age 35, when the skin still has enough elasticity to shrink back to a smooth surface.

TABLE 8.6

Activity Rating Chart

Sport/Activity	Caloric Expenditure	Potential for Heart-Lung Development	Sport/Activity	Caloric Expenditure	Potential for Heart-Lung Development
Apparatus/Tumbling	L	L	Horseshoes	L	L
Archery	L	L	Judo/Karate/Kung Fu	M–H	M
Badminton	M–H	L–M	Running programs	H	H
Baseball	L	L	Rugby	H	H
Basketball (full court)	H	M–H	Skating	M	M
Bicycling	M–H	M–H	Skiing (cross country)	H	H
Bowling	L	L	Soccer	H	H
Calisthenics	M	M	Softball	L	L
Canadian Air Force Program exercises	M	M–H	Swimming (competitive)	M–H	M–H
Field hockey	H	M	Table tennis	L–M	L–M
Football	H	M	Tennis (singles)	M–H	M–H
Golf	L–M	L	Volleyball	L	L
Hiking	M	L–M	Wrestling	H	M

Note: L = low, M = medium, H = high.

Some sports and activities provide little more than relaxed movement and good fun, but others develop heart and lungs and aid weight loss. Consult Table 8.6 for a rating of various activities according to their potential for caloric expenditure and heart-lung development.

The best type of exercise program for you is one that is enjoyable, expends a high number of calories, develops the heart and lungs, can be continued throughout life, requires no special equipment or facilities, provides the chance for progressive improvement of conditioning, and allows you to start and progress at your present level of fitness.

The importance of exercise as a means of controlling weight and fat can't be overemphasized. The secret is to exercise daily, emphasizing volume or time, rather than occasional efforts for short durations. A three-mile walk, for example, burns almost as many calories as a three-mile run. To lose weight by burning calories, it is far better to exercise for a longer time at a less strenuous pace. The more vigorous or intense the pace, the less likely you are to exercise for the recommended 45 minutes to one hour. The longer you exercise in one session, the more fat is utilized as an energy source. A long one and one-half hour session not only burns more calories than a short, intense session, it also utilizes more of your fat supply as energy.

Behavior Modification and You

Behaviors Linked to Obesity

Eating behaviors identified as important to weight control with high potential for behavioral change were: drinking high-calorie drinks instead of water, consuming too much sugar, consuming too many foods high in saturated fats, binge eating, between-meal snacking at school and college on high-calorie foods, overeating at lunch and dinner, skipping breakfast, eating a high-calorie breakfast, and failing to plan snacks.

Exercise behaviors rated important and having the potential to be changed were: no weekend leisure activity, long hours spent watching television in the afternoons, evenings, and on weekends, and no regular exercise program.

Use Exploring Your Health 8.4 to reveal your own negative eating behaviors and to develop strategies for putting a permanent end to these behaviors.

Behavior Modification Techniques

It is important to recognize that you are in complete control of your own eating behavior. You have the

TABLE 8.7

Behavioral Principles of Weight Loss Cited in Books on the Subject

Principles	Principles

1. STIMULUS CONTROL
  A. Shopping
    1. Shop for food after eating
    2. Shop from a list
    3. Avoid ready-to-eat foods
    4. Don't carry more cash than needed for shopping list

  B. Plans
    1. Plan to limit food intake
    2. Substitute exercise for snacking
    3. Eat meals and snacks at scheduled times
    4. Don't accept food offered by others

  C. Activities
    1. Store food out of sight
    2. Eat all food in the same place
    3. Remove food from inappropriate storage areas in the house
    4. Keep serving dishes off the table
    5. Use smaller dishes and utensils
    6. Avoid being the food server
    7. Leave the table immediately after eating
    8. Don't save leftovers

  D. Holidays and Parties
    1. Drink fewer alcoholic beverages
    2. Plan eating habits before parties
    3. Eat a low-calorie snack before parties
    4. Practice polite ways to decline food
    5. Don't get discouraged by an occasional setback

2. EATING BEHAVIOR
    1. Put fork down between mouthfuls
    2. Chew thoroughly before swallowing
    3. Prepare foods one portion at a time
    4. Leave some food on the plate
    5. Pause in the middle of the meal
    6. Do nothing else while eating (read, watch television)

3. REWARD
    1. Solicit help from family and friends
    2. Help family and friends provide this help in the form of praise and material rewards
    3. Utilize self-monitoring records as basis for rewards
    4. Plan specific rewards for specific behaviors (behavioral contracts)

4. SELF-MONITORING
  Keep diet diary that includes:
    1. Time and place of eating
    2. Type and amount of food
    3. Who is present/How you feel

5. NUTRITION EDUCATION
    1. Use diet diary to identify problem areas
    2. Make small changes that you can continue
    3. Learn nutritional values of foods
    4. Decrease fat intake; increase complex carbohydrates

6. PHYSICAL ACTIVITY
  A. Routine Activity
    1. Increase routine activity
    2. Increase use of stairs
    3. Keep a record of distance walked each day

  B. Exercise
    1. Begin a very mild exercise program
    2. Keep a record of daily exercise
    3. Increase the exercise very gradually

7. COGNITIVE RESTRUCTURING
    1. Avoid setting unreasonable goals
    2. Think about progress, not shortcomings
    3. Avoid imperatives like "always" and "never"
    4. Counter negative thoughts with rational restatments
    5. Set weight goals

Exploring Your Health 8.4

Negative Eating Behaviors

Circle those behaviors in Table 8.7 that you feel contribute to your weight problem or to a potential weight problem. Now list each circled behavior on a separate sheet of paper, along with some things you might try in order to increase the barriers to the behavior, decrease the motivation for the behavior, and eventually avoid or alter the behavior.

power to alter behavior that is contributing to obesity or overweight. In the early part of this chapter, you had the opportunity to calculate exactly how many calories you need to consume to reach your desired weight. The next step is to discover what your eating patterns are and what circumstances prompt you to overeat. With this information, you can discover the "cues" that cause you to overeat or to eat inappropriate foods and devise ways to substitute or ignore those cues.

Get Involved!

Helping "Fat America" Slim Down

Overweight and obesity represent a major health problem in the United States. The number of obese adults and children has now reached epidemic proportions, translating into tremendous health costs to manage the numerous disorders and diseases associated with being overweight. Medical experts are alarmed not only at the physical, but also at the emotional impact of "Fat America." Society continues to discriminate heavily against the obese of all ages in the workplace, in the home, and in leisure pursuits. To date, little has been done on national or local levels to reverse these powerful trends in our affluent society. Their causes are complicated and confusing, and a simple solution is unlikely. However, there are steps we can take right now to help increase our own and other people's awareness of this serious problem and, perhaps, begin to defeat its effects.

1. First, inventory your own health status in terms of body weight and fat. Are you overweight? If so, identify and implement immediately five changes you can make in your diet to reduce your caloric intake. Also identify and implement five exercise activities you can do every day (such as situps, riding a bike or walking to school, or swimming). Record your progress over a period of three to six months. If you are not overweight, help an overweight friend inventory her or his body weight and fat and implement a similar weight-loss program.

2. Prepare a six-month program to help yourself or a friend gain ten to twelve pounds of muscle weight. As in the program described above, be sure to include both nutritional and exercise aspects in your muscle-weight gain program.

3. Snacking is a part of most college students' lives. Nutritious snacking on high-density foods need not contribute to overeating. In fact, the right snack choices can actually help to control appetite and reduce the occurrence of snacking on high-calorie, low-density foods. What snack food choices do your college or university food service and vending machines offer? Develop a simple program to increase other students' awareness that it's OK to snack but that there are healthy snack food choices.

4. Although they are always potentially unhealthy and dangerous, fad diets that promise rapid weight loss will probably always appeal to the impatient American public. Identify and analyze several diet fads in your college or local community. Focus on these questions: (1) Can the weight-loss claims be substantiated by the total calories in the diet? (2) Does the diet contain sufficient calories to maintain basal metabolism? (3) Are there sufficient carbohydrates? (4) Is there sufficient fat for satiety? (5) Does the diet encourage adequate fluid intake? (6) What are the three main factors that lead you to believe that the diet is unhealthy? Submit your findings for publication in a student or community newsletter.

5. Working by yourself or with several of your classmates, develop a survey of elementary school children in your community to determine how many of these children are or may be in danger of becoming overweight. Start by collecting data on height and weight and collect any information you can about dietary and exercise habits. Your surveys could be directed to the children's teachers or to the children themselves, but be sure to work in conjunction with school administrators and teachers. Include as many children in the survey as you can. Use the results to make specific suggestions for weight control among these children to teachers, administrators, and PTA members.

Conclusion

In the final analysis, you are responsible for your own eating and exercise behavior. If you are gaining weight and body fat, you are probably overeating and under-exercising. Once you decide to do something about it, you can apply the information in this chapter to your personal life by evaluating your body weight and fat, discovering the factors that contribute to your weight problem, and altering your eating and exercise behavior to eliminate these factors. Weight gain and weight loss are calorie counts. You gain weight by consuming more calories than you expend and lose weight by burning up more calories than you consume. Although it is not easy, you can alter your behavior in several specific areas and slowly reach your weight and fat loss or weight gain objective.

Summary

1. There is little evidence to support the contention that being overweight, not obese, is a health hazard.

2. Weight charts serve only as a guide to determine whether you are overweight, obese, under-weight, or of normal weight. Skinfold measures (pinching various body parts), on the other hand, provide an accurate evaluation of both weight and body fat.

3. The main cause of obesity is inactivity, combined with overeating.

4. Bottle feeding, overeating by the pregnant mother, and overeating and inactivity the first year of life and during the adolescent growth period result in the production of a high number of permanent fat cells, making it easier for the individual to gain weight throughout life.

5. The body defends a certain biological weight against pressure to change (set point theory); taking weight off and keeping it off may require a lowering of your set point through proper nutrition and regular exercise.

6. Minute changes in body metabolism can translate into large changes in body weight and fat over a period of years.

7. Gaining weight may be just as difficult for some as losing weight is for others.

8. Anorexia nervosa and bulimia are underweight conditions that can lead to serious health problems if qualified medical treatment is not secured.

9. Hunger and appetite are not the same; hunger is physiological and inborn, whereas appetite is psychological and a learned response to food.

10. Calories do count. To lose weight and body fat and to keep firm, you must burn, through exercise and daily activity, more calories than you eat. This is best achieved through a combination of diet and exercise.

11. Nutritious snacking on low-calorie, bulky foods is an important part of a weight control program.

12. Six to eight glasses of water should be consumed daily, whether or not you are on a diet.

13. Weight loss should occur slowly, at the rate of no more than two to four pounds per week. This slow approach is safe and more apt to produce permanent weight loss, as eating habits change and remain changed when the diet is discontinued.

14. Fad diets are potentially dangerous and offer little chance for permanent weight loss.

15. Extra calories are burned both during exercise and for six to eight hours following the exercise session. These calories are very important to weight and fat loss.

16. Exercise assists in the control of appetite. Regular aerobic exercise helps to maintain normal body weight and fat by depressing appetite, burning fat as fuel, shrinking existing fat cells, inhibiting the production of new fat cells in the young, and firming the body.

17. Behavior modification programs help the individual to control his or her eating habits by discovering the cues that cause overeating and by devising ways to substitute or ignore those cues.

18. There are no exercise or diet shortcuts to permanent, safe weight loss.

Questions for Personal Growth

1. How common is "binge" eating in your life? Review and total the number of calories you consume in a one-week period while binging.

2. What simple changes in your lifestyle could you make starting right now that would help you to maintain or lose body weight? Try to identify as many of these changes as you can. For example, how about parking your car several blocks away from and walking to your destination, using the stairs instead of elevators and escalators, and taking a walk at lunchtime?

3. How much water do you consume daily? By keeping your stomach full of zero-calorie fluids such as water, you are less likely to allow hunger to lure you into patterns of overeating.

4. One general way to avoid eating too many high-calorie foods is to apply the principle of "nutrition density." At the end of the day today, take a moment to analyze each meal for nutrition density. Did you receive a large number of nutrients relative to a lower number of calories in each meal? What foods could you have substituted for greater nutrition density?

5. Weight loss quackery is big business in the United States. Identify the current exercise and weight-loss plan that is receiving the most media attention. What claims are being made about the plan that cannot be substantiated?

6. If you are not overweight, when was the last time you had to deal with a person who was overweight? Do you think that the way you dealt with that person was influenced by her or his overweight condition? How?

7. If you are overweight, describe one or more experiences you have had in which you believe your overweight condition contributed negatively to the way you were treated by another person. How did you respond to this treatment? Did these experiences make you feel pressured to lose weight?

8. Why do you think that, in a country as wealthy as the United States, there is such a serious obesity problem? Identify and discuss at least five things that you believe contribute to this problem and suggest remedies for each of these things.

References

1. Patricia A. Kreutler and Dorice M. Czajka-Narins, *Nutrition in Perspective,* 2e (Englewood Cliffs, N.J.: Prentice-Hall, 1987).

2. "Dieting: The Losing Game," *Time* (January 20, 1986): 54–60.

3. George B. Dintiman, Robert G. Davis, Jude C. Pennington, and Stephen S. Stone, *Discovering Lifetime Fitness: Concepts of Fitness and Weight Control* (St. Paul, Minn.: West, 1989).

4. Claude Bouchard et al., "The Response to Long-Term Overfeeding in Identical Twins," *New England Journal of Medicine* 322, 21 (May 24, 1990): 1477–1482.

5. Daniel Rudman, "Effects of Human Growth Hormone in Men over 60 Years Old," *New England Journal of Medicine* 323, 1 (July 5, 1990): 321–323.

6. George B. Dintiman and Robert Ward, *Train America! Achieving Peak Performance and Fitness for Sports Competition* (Dubuque, Iowa: Kendal-Hunt, 1988).

7. Ibid.

8. Eleanor Noss Whitney, Eva May Nunnelley Hamilton, and Sharon Rady Rolfes, *Understanding Nutrition,* 5e (St. Paul, Minn.: West, 1990) pp. 366, 383–384, 389–394.

9. Ibid., p. 391.

10. Ibid., pp. 390–391.

11. Ibid., pp. 391–392.

12. American Dietetic Association position on very low-calorie formula diets approved by the House of Delegates on October 21, 1989, to be in effect until December 31, 1994, unless it is reaffirmed or withdrawn as directed in the position development procedures of the House of Delegates.

Fitness

CHAPTER OBJECTIVES

After reading this chapter, you should understand:

- That although more and more Americans are engaging in regular exercise, few people can actually be classified as active.

- How regular aerobic exercise can foster health-related fitness.

- That by applying a few basic conditioning principles, you will be able to achieve and maintain a good level of basic fitness.

- How you can use training to achieve specific fitness objectives, such as muscular and heart-lung endurance, strength, flexibility, girth control, and an improved general level of conditioning.

- What exercise program might work best for you, how to begin that program, and how to measure your progress.

- Why weather conditions, what you eat, and how much water you consume are important factors to consider in your exercise habits.

CHAPTER OUTLINE

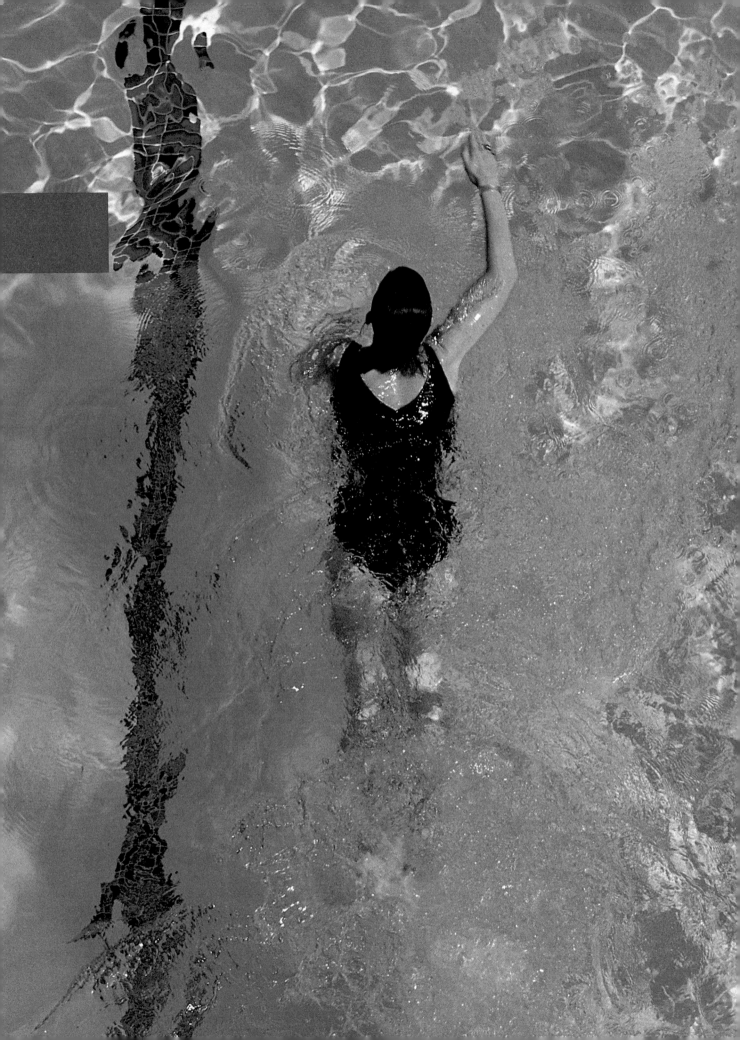

plaque The fatty deposits that may build up on the walls of arteries, causing coronary heart disease.

resting metabolic rate Calories used while an individual is at rest, but not while sleeping.

maximum oxygen uptake The maximum amount of oxygen breathed in and then used at the tissue level.

Fit for Life

Each year more and more Americans engage in regular exercise, as it is defined by the surgeon general of the United States. Unfortunately, best estimates from survey results indicate that only 10 to 20 percent of the adult population, ages 18 to 64, can be classified as active, including college students. Fitness data on our nation's youth, ages 6 to 17 is even more discouraging. A survey of 18,857 public school pupils at 187 schools, the largest study of its kind ever conducted in the United States, revealed a low level of performance in running, jumping, flexibility, and strength:

- Forty percent of boys 6 to 12 and 70 percent of all girls could not do more than one pull-up.

- Fifty percent of girls and 30 percent of boys, ages 6 to 12, could not run one mile in less than 10 minutes.

- Forty-five percent of boys 6 to 14 and 55 percent of all girls could not hold their chin over a raised bar for more than 10 seconds.

- Forty percent of boys ages 6 to 15 could not reach beyond their toes when seated on the floor with the legs outstretched.

Overall, the performance of children did not change from surveys taken in 1965 and 1975. A more recent survey completed in 1987, *The Shape of the Nation: A Survey of State Physical Education Requirements,* revealed that only one state, Illinois, met the minimum physical education requirement recommended by the American Alliance of Health, Physical Education, Recreation and Dance—30 minutes daily in grades K through 6 and 50 minutes daily in grades 7 through 12. Only four states (Illinois, New Jersey, New York, and Rhode Island) required all students to take physical education for a specific amount of time in grades K through 12. It is obvious that fitness is not a priority in our nation's schools.

On the positive side, it must be said that millions of people participate in a number of sports on a regular basis: swimming (74.4 million), bicycle riding (51.0 million), running and jogging (29.5 million), aerobic exercise (24.4 million), basketball (21.2 million), tennis (19.5 million), racquetball (9.9 million), soccer (9.0 million), and cross-country skiing (4.5 million).

Year 2000 National Health Objective

In recognition of the value of physical education in our nation's schools, the government is striving to increase to at least 50 percent the proportion of children and adolescents in grades 1 through 12 who participate in school physical education, and to increase to 50 percent the proportion of school physical education class time that the students spend being physically active, preferably in lifetime activities.

The government is also interested in promoting physical activity in the workplace and community by striving to increase the proportion of worksites offering employer-sponsored physical activity and fitness programs, and by increasing availability and accessibility of physical activity and fitness facilities to the community.

Each of these sports meet the surgeon general's definition of proper physical activity (frequency—three or more times weekly, intensity—at or above target heart rates, duration—20 to 30 minutes) and each has the potential to improve health-related fitness. This chapter presents an overview of exercise and health so that you can evaluate your current fitness and make wise exercise choices that will meet your interests and needs. Regular exercise is the best and least expensive approach to health insurance.

Benefits of Exercise

Regular aerobic exercise has long been recognized as a healthy behavior. Unfortunately, researchers have been unable to identify the exact contribution of exercise in preventing, and helping people recover from, various physical and mental disorders. The issue has been clouded by extremists whose opinions vary from wild, unsupported claims of benefits to vigorous condemnation of regular exercise as dangerous and of no health value.

A number of sound research studies have revealed some interesting new information on the value of regular exercise. A summary of the findings that can be substantiated by research follows. Regular aerobic exercise (three or more times per week for thirty continuous minutes at or above one's target heart rate) has been shown to have the health-related fitness benefits described in the next section.

Health-Related Fitness

Exercise has been shown to:

- Help prevent cardiovascular disease and lessen the severity of and speed recovery from a heart attack. Regular exercise also lowers triglycerides, lowers LDL or the so-called bad cholesterol, increases HDL or good cholesterol, and, in combination with altered nutrition, actually begins to reverse **plaque** buildup in the coronary arteries (see Chapter 15). This latter evidence, coupled with previous evidence that exercise increases the diameter of the coronary arteries and allows more blood to pass through, is one of the most critical findings in recent years concerning the importance of regular exercise in preventing early heart disease.

- Reduce the risk of developing hypertension and help control mild hypertension.

- Help prevent and control obesity and reduce excess body weight and fat. Keep in mind that you are burning calories both while you exercise and for the next 20 minutes to four hours after exercise through an elevated resting metabolic rate *(afterburn)*. The longer and more intensely you exercise, the longer your resting metabolic rate remains elevated. Expending 20 to 50 extra calories per hour for several hours after your workout ends, in addition to those burned during exercise, makes a significant contribution to weight and fat loss.

- Assist in the prevention of *osteoporosis* (porous bone mineral loss and bone weakening with age). Weight-bearing exercise such as walking, jogging or running, aerobic dance, aerobic exercise, tennis, racquetball, team sports, and so forth, help bring dietary calcium to the bones.

- Delay some of the physiological changes that occur with aging. With each passing decade in the sedentary individual, **resting metabolic rate** (calories used while in a resting state) slows, **maximum oxygen uptake** declines (amount of oxygen one can take in and utilize at the tissue level—the higher the oxygen uptake, the higher one's aerobic fitness level), muscular strength declines, and physical appearance changes as a protruding stomach, hip handles, and fat become evident on various body parts.

- Help in the treatment of adult-onset diabetes mellitus by contributing to weight loss, helping to normalize glucose tolerance, and increasing insulin sensitivity.

- Increase life expectancy. Large numbers of subjects who have been exercising on a regular basis throughout their lives are still not available for

Year 2000 National Health Objective

Regular aerobic exercise 3 to 4 times weekly has been shown to produce a number of health benefits at all ages. In recognition of the health values of exercise, the federal government is striving to increase to at least 30 percent the proportion of people age 6 and older who engage regularly, preferably daily, in light to moderate physical activity for at least 30 minutes per day. In 1965, data indicated that 22 percent of people age 16 and older were active for at least 30 minutes five or more times per week and 12 percent were active seven or more times per week.

Exercise-related National Health Objectives have also been determined for other age groups: to increase to 20 percent the proportion of people age 18 and older, and to 75 percent of children and adolescents age 6 to 17, who engage in vigorous activity promoting the development and maintenance of cardiorespiratory fitness three or more days weekly for 20 minutes or more; and to reduce to no more than 15 percent the proportion of people age 6 and older who engage in no leisure-time physical activity.

study, and it is for this reason, experts say, that some studies indicate that exercise will add only one year to your life. It has been predicted that regular exercise could add as many as ten to twenty years to the lives of many individuals.[1]

- Strengthen the orthopedic system, making the body less susceptible to muscle and joint injury.

- Assist in reducing mental tension, anxiety, and depression.

Feeling and Looking Good

Regular exercise has been shown to:

- Aid in weight reduction, improve energy levels, and impart a feeling of vitality.
- Improve sleeping habits.
- Assist in reducing, withstanding, and adapting to psychological stress; reduce mental tension, anxiety, and depression.
- Increase muscle strength and endurance and improve muscle tone.
- Improve the efficiency of the lungs and circulatory system: *stroke volume* (amount of blood ejected per contraction of the heart), *cardiac output* (amount of blood ejected into the circulatory system minute by minute), and physical work capacity are increased.

Principles of Conditioning

Mere participation in an exercise program or sport is no guarantee that you will become more physically fit. By keeping some simple records and applying a few

work hypertrophy A physiological process whereby there is a temporary decline in conditioning level following a strenuous workout, followed by the development of a higher level of conditioning after recovery.

Exploring Your Health 9.1

How Fit Are You?

You can roughly evaluate your fitness level in just a few minutes. Test yourself in each of the areas described below to estimate your body fat, flexibility, muscular strength and muscular endurance, and cardiovascular fitness.

What did you discover? How fit are you? Regular exercise can bring about tremendous improvement in each of the test areas and in your health.

Test	Purpose	Procedure	Scoring
Pinch Test	Measure body fat	Using the thumb and index finger, take a deep pinch of skin and fat on the back of the upper arm, thigh, back of upper leg, and the abdomen (to the right of the umbilicus).	A pinch of more than an inch at any site indicates excess fat.
Sixty-second Sit Up	Determine abdominal strength and endurance	Lie on your back with the knees bent and feet drawn up to the buttocks. On the signal, "go," raise your upper body until your chest touches both knees; return to the starting position. Continue as rapidly as possible for sixty seconds.	Adequate (men) Ages 19–29; 42 or more Ages 30–39: 33–41 Ages 40–49: 28–32 Adequate (women) Ages 19–29; 33 or more Ages 30–39: 29–32 Ages 40–49: 8–32
Toe Touch	Determine lower body flexibility	With the feet together and knees straight, bend forward at the hips and touch the thumbs to the floor. Bend slowly without bouncing.	Adequate: floor contact with any part of the hand
1.5-mile Run	Cardiovascular/ aerobic fitness	After a proper warm-up of light jogging and stretching, complete six laps around a one-quarter mile track. If you have been inactive, avoid the test for 6–7 weeks; instead, begin a walking program at Level I (see Table 9.1). The test can be dangerous for older individuals and those who have been inactive, or overweight or obese, or have high blood pressure.	See Table 9.1. College students should strive for a Fitness Category of *Good* (less than 12:00 minutes for men and 15:54 for women)

basic conditioning principles, however, you can make tremendous gains in fitness with little risk of injury or illness. Fitness involves five basic elements: heart-lung endurance (cardiovascular and cardiorespiratory efficiency), muscular endurance, muscular strength, body fat reduction (see Chapter 8), and flexibility. You can show improvement in each of these components of fitness by following the conditioning principles discussed in this section.

TABLE 9.1

1.5-Mile Run Test Time (Minutes)

Fitness Category		13–19	20–29	Age (Years) 30–39	40–49	50–59	60+
I Very Poor	(Men)	>15:31*	>16:01	>16:31	>17:31	>19:01	>20:01
	(Women)	>18:31	>19:01	>19:31	>20:01	>20:31	>21:01
II Poor	(Men)	12:11–15:30	14:01–16:00	14:44–16:30	15:36–17:30	17:01–19:00	19:01–20:00
	(Women)	16:55–18:30	18:31–19:00	19:01–19:30	19:31–20:00	20:01–20:30	21:00–21:31
III Fair	(Men)	10:49–12:10	12:01–14:00	12:31–14:45	13:01–15:35	14:31–17:00	16:16–19:00
	(Women)	14:31–16:54	15:55–18:30	16:31–19:00	17:31–19:30	19:01–20:00	19:31–20:30
IV Good	(Men)	9:41–10:48	10:46–12:00	11:01–12:30	11:31–13:00	12:31–14:30	14:00–16:15
	(Women)	12:30–14:30	13:31–15:54	14:31–16:30	15:56–17:30	16:31–19:00	17:31–19:30
V Excellent	(Men)	8:37–9:40	9:45–10:45	10:00–11:00	10:30–11:30	11:00–12:30	11:15–13:59
	(Women)	11:50–12:29	12:30–13:30	13:00–14:30	13:45–15:55	14:30–16:30	16:30–17:30
VI Superior	(Men)	<8:37	<9:45	<10:00	<10:30	<11:00	<11:15
	(Women)	<11:50	<12:30	<13:00	<13:45	<14:30	<16:30

* < Means "less than"; > means "more than."

Source: From *The Aerobics Program of Total Well-Being*, by Kenneth H. Cooper, M.D. Copyright © 1982 by Kenneth H. Cooper, M.D. Reprinted by permission of the publisher, M. Evans & Co., Inc., New York, N.Y. 10017.

Atrophy — get when you dont use muscles

Work Hypertrophy get when set up program

Any improvement in physical work capacity is based on **work hypertrophy**—a process in which one's conditioning level temporarily declines after exercise but improves beyond the original level after recovery. Let's examine what happens to your body when you first begin an exercise program. You start that program with a certain functioning or conditioning level (level A in Figure 9.1). During and immediately after your first workout, this conditioning level temporarily declines (to point B). You are now actually in worse shape (physically) than you were before you exercised. During the recovery phase, however, tissue will rebuild

beyond the original level of conditioning to point C. You are now able to perform more work than before with no more strain or effort. You are in better condition twenty-four hours later than before you completed your first workout.

Repetition of this simple process will lead to continued improvement of conditioning levels, as indicated by A-2, A-3 and A-4 in Figure 9.1, providing that certain basic principles are followed:

- Exercise must be sufficiently strenuous to cause an initial decrease in the conditioning level; the depth of the valley is in proportion to the intensity and duration of the workout.

- Sufficient time must be allowed for the recovery; improvement will not occur and conditioning will suffer if your second workout is performed before the recovery phase is complete (forty-eight hours for weight training and eighteen to twenty-four hours for other workouts).

- The next workout must occur within twenty-four to forty-eight hours; a greater time lapse will cause your fitness level to decline.

- Each workout must be progressively more strenuous than the previous one to ensure a deep valley, continued progression, and increased capacity to perform exercise.

FIGURE 9.1 • Concept of Work Hypertrophy. (A) preexercise functioning level; (B) functioning level following exercise; (C) elevated functioning level following recovery; (A-2) elevated functioning level at the proper point to reconvene exercise.

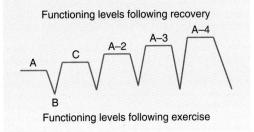

Functioning levels following recovery

Preexercise functioning level

A-2   A-3   A-4

A   C

B

Functioning levels following exercise

target heart rate The heart rate, measured as pulse per minute, needed to be attained and maintained during exercise to produce a training or conditioning effect.

Issues in Health

Is Exercise Dangerous?

Exercise is advocated not only for normal, healthy individuals but also for patients with known underlying ailments such as heart disease. Most people who exercise feel good, have better endurance than those who do not exercise, weigh less, have lower blood pressure and lower blood lipids, and may even live longer. According to some experts, however, exercise may be dangerous and even fatal to some individuals, including the highly conditioned young person under the age of 25.

Con Opponents of exercise point out that sudden death during exertion seems to occur with unusually high frequency, as was found by University of North Carolina researchers who studied a group of exercising adults with known risks of heart disease. Although men who exercised were sixty times less likely to die from a sudden heart attack at rest, they were at four to five times higher risk during exercise. In addition, sedentary adults who haphazardly engage in occasional exercise are at a much higher risk of sudden death during this unaccustomed exercise than at rest. Orthopedic surgeons have also voiced concern about the dangers of jogging, aerobic exercise, calisthenics, handball, tennis, and other forms of exercise as causes of back injuries, knee deterioration, foot, ankle, elbow, and shoulder problems, and so forth. Too much exercise eventually results in "over-

use injuries." In addition, it is argued, exercise is dangerous for everyone during the early stages of a newly started program.

Pro Exercise proponents argue that the dangers of injury or death are grossly exaggerated and often represent isolated, well-publicized cases such as the death of running guru Jim Fixx. Newspapers often fail to reveal significant facts such as previous heart and other health conditions (as was the case with Fixx), drugs found in the body, congenital disorders, or heat conditions. Exercise gets the blame and reinforces the sedentary living habits of millions of Americans. The incidence of sudden death in healthy males aged 45 to 54, for example, is one per 1,000 per year. The incidence is less than half that expected for this age group among runners. Even in people with known heart disease, sudden death during exercise occurs in only one in every 150,000 to 305,000 patient exercise hours. Sudden death in young athletes and exercising individuals in normal health during physical activity is even more rare. The causes of instantaneous death are usually cardiac, particularly in the 25-and-under age group. In the 25-to-50 age group, coronary artery disease due to undiagnosed *atherosclerosis* is usually the cause. The third major cause is heart illness. Although a heart attack is generally

cited in the sudden death of exercising individuals, it can be documented only 20 percent of the time. Most victims show atherosclerosis without *coronary thrombosis* (blockage). Death appears to be caused by lack of oxygen to the heart muscle, producing irregular heartbeats. Information gathered from surviving relatives shows that the majority of the individuals experienced and ignored heart attack symptoms. Proponents of exercise do admit that the potential does exist for injury, illness, or death unless sound exercise principles are applied. Learning to "read" the body's signals, such as fatigue, chest distress, sudden changes in resting pulse, pain; resorting to rest instead of a workout; securing an exercise EKG and risk analysis; and consulting an exercise specialist who will make certain you progress slowly and safely (avoiding too much, too soon) go a long way toward assuring that you will avoid injury and illness. Although minor muscle and joint injuries may occur, a careful approach can greatly reduce the risk. Rarely does a properly conceived program result in serious illness or injury, it is argued.

Exercise can be misused, and incorrect practices may lead to serious injury or illness. Whether this is also the case with properly conceived programs is another matter.

What do you think?

Source: George B. Dintiman, Stephen E. Stone, June C. Pennington, and Robert G. Davis, *Discovering Lifetime Fitness: Concepts of Exercise and Weight Control* (St. Paul, Minn.: West, 1989).

Exploring Your Health 9.2

Determining Your Target Heart Rate

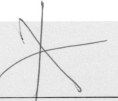

For exercise to produce a cardiovascular "training effect," you must reach and maintain your target heart rate for approximately twenty to thirty minutes during each workout, three to four times weekly. The following procedure, based upon your resting heart rate, accurately identifies your personal target heart rate range.

Steps and example for a 20-year-old:

1. Find your predicted maximum heart rate (PMHR):

   220 minus your age = PMHR, or 220 − 20 = 200

2. Find your resting heart rate for 60 seconds. After sitting quietly for 15 minutes, take your pulse at the carotid artery (either side of the neck) or use the radial pulse (thumb side of the wrist).

Because your thumb has its own pulse and will cause inaccurate readings, use only the fingers to find and count the pulse. Count for an entire minute. Let's assume, for our example, that a resting heart rate of 70 was found for our 20-year-old.

   Resting heart rate (RHR) = 70

3. Subtract your resting heart rate (RHR) from your predicted maximum heart rate.

   200 (PMHR) minus 70 (RHR) = 130

4. Multiply this figure by 60%.

   130 × 60% = 78

5. Add your resting heart rate to this amount.

   70 (RHR) + 78 = 148 (Lower end of your target heart rate)

6. Find the upper end of your target heart rate by repeating steps 4 and 5, but using 80 instead of 60 percent.

   130 × 80% = 104

   70 (RHR) + 104 = 174 (Upper end of your target heart rate)

Your target heart range is 148–174. An exercise program that keeps your heart rate within this range will produce a training effect in as safe a manner as possible. If your heart rate does not reach the lower limit, increase the intensity (exercise more vigorously, walk or ride faster) on your next workout. If your heart rate exceeds the upper limit, reduce your intensity, particularly in the early months of a newly started exercise program.[2]

Intensity, Duration, and Frequency

Although results can be attained without lengthy training periods, there are no shortcuts to improving conditioning levels. Ten-second contractions, massage, mechanical devices, steam baths, three-minute slimnastic programs, and other such approaches vary from slightly effective to worthless.

Exercise intensity (work per unit of time) should be such that sweating is evident in the early stages of the workout. More important, exercise must be intense enough to cause you to reach and maintain your **target heart rate** (the exercise heart rate needed to produce a training effect) for twenty to thirty minutes each workout. Complete Exploring Your Health 9.2 to find your target rate.

Exercise duration is affected by intensity. Obviously, you cannot sprint at near-maximum effort for fifteen minutes. If aerobic conditioning is your goal, the exercise session should maintain your target heart rate for twenty to thirty minutes. If the purpose of your program is cosmetic—to lose body weight and fat and to trim down—duration is the key. Long, slow runs are preferable to short, fast runs.

Exercise regularity is the key to the success of your program. Exercising three to five days a week rather than doing one hard workout per week will greatly increase your chances of meeting your training objectives. It is important to start slowly (low intensity) and gradually work up to your target heart rate and twenty to thirty minutes of continuous exercise.

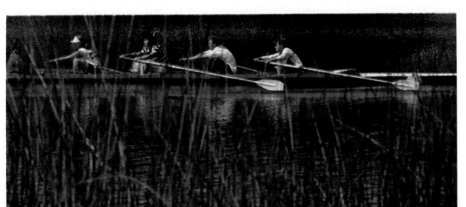

Regularity is the real key to the success of your fitness program. You will meet your training objectives much more easily by exercising three to five days a week at similar levels of intensity for relatively short periods of time rather than by exercising one day a week at a high level of intensity for a longer period of time.

postexercise peril The physiological factors that occur immediately after strenuous exercise that can lead to illness or sudden death.

Alternate Light and Heavy Days

The body responds best to a conditioning program that alternates light and heavy workouts. This approach reduces the risk of injury, provides several relaxing exercise sessions each week, and allows the body to repair fully between workouts. Consider the following suggestions:

- Do stretching exercises at the beginning of every workout immediately following five to ten minutes of light jogging or walking.
- Alternate hard and easy days; never train hard on consecutive days.
- Exercise hard no more than four times weekly.
- Schedule one extra hard workout each week.
- Know your body and allow it to direct you; if pain continues or worsens or your legs feel heavy, stop, regardless of whether it is a light or heavy day.

Warm-up

Warm-up is the preparation of the body for vigorous activity through stretching, calisthenics, and running movements designed to raise core temperature. The purpose of warm-up is to improve performance and prevent muscle injury. The theory behind warm-up is that muscle contractions depend on temperature, and increased muscle temperature improves work capacity. Warm-up increases muscle temperature and the amount of fluid in the knee. It also improves oxygen intake, so that the amount of oxygen needed for exercise is reduced.

Research findings suggest the following facts about warm-up:

- A general warm-up routine involving the large muscle groups, such as light jogging and walking, should be performed for five to ten minutes, or at least until you are perspiring, to raise core body temperature.
- Stretching or flexibility exercises, such as those described in this chapter, should immediately follow the general warm-up routine.
- Only a few minutes should elapse from completion of the stretching exercises and the start of the activity.
- A longer warm-up period is required in a cold environment to allow the body to reach the desired temperature.
- Warm-up will not cause early fatigue or hinder performance.

Cool-down

A cool-down, or the use of five to ten minutes of very light exercise movements at the end of a vigorous workout to slowly cool the body to near-normal temperature, is recommended following any type of strenuous activity. Walking, light jogging, swimming, and any activity at an easy pace are good ways to cool down.

Blood returns to the heart through the veins and is pushed along by the contraction of the heart and the "milking" action of the muscles. The veins are contracted or squeezed through muscular action, which moves the blood forward against the force of gravity, while valves prevent the blood from backing up. If you stop exercising suddenly, the milking action of the muscles, which occurs only through muscle contraction, will stop; the blood return will drop quickly and may cause blood pooling in the extremities (blood remaining in the same area), leading to deep breathing. The deep breathing in turn lowers the level of carbon dioxide, and muscle cramps can develop. It is at this point also that blood pressure can drop precipitously and cause trouble. The body compensates for the unexpected drop in blood pressure by increasing norepinephrine tenfold and epinephrine threefold over baseline levels during the first three minutes after exercise. These high levels can cause cardiac problems for some individuals during the recovery phase of vigorous exercise, such as a marathon or triathlon.

A number of studies have been conducted in the area of **postexercise peril** (sudden death or illness immediately after exercise) to determine the most effective approach to reducing the danger during this period. The behavior producing the most deaths and illness was standing. Lying down flat or walking or jogging (light exercise) reduced the risk of illness immediately following exercise.[3]

Exploring Your Health 9.3

Developing a New Mind Set About Exercise

When students develop a new habit, they are often plagued with self-doubts and thoughts of failure. During the early stages of your newly started exercise program, you can become your own worst enemy. Examine the following list of excuses. Do any of these look familiar to you? Take a minute to prepare your own list of self-defeating thoughts about exercise. Prepare a list of positive thoughts, too.

Learn to use the lists wisely. When self-defeating thoughts enter your mind, counteract them immediately with your positive ones. Write your positive thoughts on a card that you carry in your wallet or purse and refer to the list when you are about to avoid your scheduled exercise session. List both long-term benefits of your program, such as more energy, weight loss, improved appearance, disease prevention, emotional release, and other benefits.

Negative Thoughts About Exercise	**Positive Thoughts About Exercise**
1. I'm too busy to exercise today. I'm working too hard anyway and need a break.	1. I can find time to exercise today. I just have to think about my routine and plan carefully.
2. I'm too tired to exercise today, and if I do work out, I won't have enough energy to do the other things I must do.	2. I may feel tired today, but I'll do a light exercise routine instead of the heavy one I usually do. If I keep working out on a regular basis, I'll build my stamina so I won't feel so tired during the day.
3. I missed my workout today. I might as well forget all this fitness stuff. I don't have the self-control to keep at it.	3. Just because I missed one exercise session doesn't mean I should give up. I'm not going to let this small setback ruin everything I've accomplished all week.
4. None of my friends are fit or trim and they don't worry about it. I'm not going to either.	4. What my friends do about exercising has nothing to do with my exercise habits. I'll make additional friends who do exercise.
5. I'm already "over the hill." I should let myself go and enjoy life more.	5. I can get in shape and stay there. All I have to do is stick to my schedule. Knowing I can control my behavior is something I can enjoy every day.

Negative Exercise Thought

1. _____

   _____

   _____

2. _____

   _____

   _____

3. _____

   _____

   _____

4. _____

   _____

   _____

Positive Exercise Thought

1. _____

   _____

   _____

2. _____

   _____

   _____

3. _____

   _____

   _____

4. _____

   _____

   _____

strength Physiologically speaking, strength is the total amount of force a person can apply with a particular muscle or group of muscles at one time.

muscular endurance The maximum number of times (repetitions) a particular amount of weight can be moved through a complete range of motion by a muscle or a muscle group.

Specific Objectives of Training

Training for Strength

Strength is the total amount of force you can apply with a particular muscle group at one time, such as the amount of weight you can lift over your head once. **Muscular endurance** is the maximum number of times (repetitions) you can move a particular amount of weight through the complete range of motion, such as lifting weight over your head as many times as possible. Among Americans of all ages, upper body (arms and shoulders) and abdominal strength and muscular endurance are generally poor.

Weight training is the most popular and effective activity to develop muscular strength. Numerous types of exercise equipment are available to provide you with a sound weight training workout. *Isotonic exercise* involves muscle shortening during the positive (contraction) phase and lengthening during the negative (relaxation) or lowering phase of each repetition. Free weights, universal gym, Nautilus, Cam II, and Polaris equipment are examples of isotonic equipment. *Isokinetic exercise* requires special equipment designed to provide maximum resistance for a muscle throughout the full range of movement. The Mini-Gym uses the accommodating resistance principle to provide an isokinetic movement—the harder you pull or exert, the harder the Mini-Gym resists your pull. You therefore apply force at a constant speed. Combinations of isotonic and isokinetic movements can be performed using the Hydra-Fitness and Eagle Performance Systems. *Isometric* exercise involves the application of force

As you age, your body's ratio of fat to lean muscle mass increases. This in turn slows metabolism and contributes to weight and fat gain. Strength training contributes to weight loss and maintenance by reversing this trend.

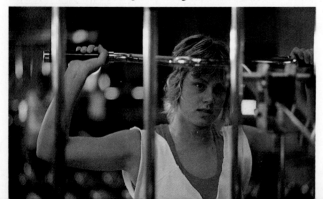

against an immovable object causing the muscle to contract without any change in its overall length. Isotonic and isokinetic strength training or combinations of the two are the best way to develop strength. The effects of isometric exercise on overall strength, fitness, and sports performance is limited.

Although some equipment is more effective than others in meeting specific training objectives, both free weights and special isotonic and isokinetic equipment will produce rapid results. *Free weights* (dumbbells, bar, colars, and iron or plastic weights of various sizes) allow you to simulate specific muscular movements in practically any sport or activity and tend to produce rapid strength and muscular endurance gains. One serious limitation is the danger of injury and need for a spotter, an assistant, on most exercises. Special machines are much safer and do not require an assistant. In addition, the neck station and other machines often allow movements to strengthen key body areas that cannot be done with free weights.

To gain strength, muscles must be exercised against gradually increasing resistance. Loads that are increased beyond the demands regularly made on the organism determine the ultimate effectiveness of a strength training program, such as weight training. The *overload principle* is applied in exercise programs by increasing the resistance (amount of weight to be lifted or moved), the number of repetitions (number of times you lift the weight), and the speed of contraction (speed at which you perform one repetition), or by decreasing the rest interval (amount of rest between exercises). The closer to maximum capacity a muscle is worked, the greater the increase in strength.

Table 9.2 lists some popular training objectives and the variable control recommended to meet that objective. To develop strength, for example, a heavy weight such as the 3 RM (maximum amount of weight you can lift only three times) is chosen for each exercise selected. On the first workout, three sets of three repetitions are performed with one minute of rest allowed between each set and exercise. The object is to reach complete muscle failure on the final repetition of each set. In other words, the third and final repetition should be the last you are physically capable of completing. If you can perform more than three repetitions, increase the weight. On the next workout, four

TABLE 9.2

Weight Training Objectives and Variable Control

Desired Physical Outcomes	Variable Control
Cardiovascular endurance	Moderate to heavy weight, rapid contractions, the use of repeated power exercises, 6 to 10 repetitions for 3 sets, 5 to 15 seconds rest between each set and exercise.
Muscular endurance	Light weight, 10 to 15 repetitions, 3 sets, moderate contractions, and minimum rest interval.
Explosive power/speed	Moderate weight, 1 to 5 repetitions, rapid contractions, decreasing rest interval, 1 to 5 sets, and use of power exercises.
Flexibility	Moderate weight, slow contractions, 6 to 10 repetitions, 1 to 3 sets, carrying each exercise to the extreme range of motion and applying static pressure for several seconds before returning to the starting position. Avoid ballistic movements that force the joints quickly beyond the normal range of movement.
Muscle mass or bulk	Heavy weight, maximum number of repetitions, 5 to 8 sets, slow contractions, repeated heavy or maximum lifts, use of "flushing," or activation of the same muscle groups repeatedly to provide a prolonged flow of blood to a specific area.
Rehabilitation of injured muscles and joints	Light weights, slow contractions, 6 to 10 repetitions after initial training sessions involving no weight and 3 to 5 contractions, 3 sets, utilizing exercises that activate the supporting muscles of a joint such as those of the ankle, knee, and shoulder. Also helpful for prevention of injury to these areas.
Strength	Heavy weights (2 to 5 RM), low repetitions, slow contractions, minimum rest between sets and exercises, maximum lifts, and 3–5 sets.
Strength and endurance (general body development)	Moderate weight (8 RM), 6 to 10 repetitions, moderate contractions, decreasing rest interval, 3 sets, varied exercises to activate all major muscle groups.

repetitions are completed, five on the following workout. On the fourth workout, return to three repetitions and increase the weight five pounds for each upper body exercise and ten pounds for each lower body exercise. This is one of the many methods of applying the progressive resistance principle to weight training. Weight training workouts should occur every other day to allow full recovery and to benefit from the previous session. *Body building,* not included on Table 9.2,

Year 2000 National Health Objective

Recognizing the value of fitness components other than cardiorespiratory development and maintenance, the federal government has established a national health objective to increase to at least 40 percent the proportion of people age 6 and older who regularly perform physical activities that enhance and maintain muscular strength, muscular endurance, and flexibility.

requires well-defined musculature and bulk in practically every muscle in the body, long hours of daily weight training, and the use of hundreds of different exercises to bring out muscle definition. Dumbbells, barbells, and resistance-designed machines are used to carve out and define individual muscles. Beauty of physique is much more important than feats of strength in body building.

Training for Heart-Lung Endurance

Respiration (oxygen absorption and elimination of carbon dioxide) and *heart efficiency* (ability to deliver oxygenated blood to tissues) form the foundation of any sound exercise program. Programs that improve efficiency of the heart and lungs also bring about improvements in general health. If heart-lung endurance is your training objective, your exercise program must result in your reaching a target heart rate, in terms of heartbeats per minute, during exercise and maintaining this rate for twenty to thirty minutes. Only sustained, nonstop programs are strenuous enough to do this—activities such as vigorous walking (four miles per hour or faster), jogging and running, lap swimming, bicycling, rope jumping, aerobic dance, and sports such as soccer, cross-country skiing, field hockey, lacrosse, and rugby. Immediately after your workout, before cool-down, take your heart rate. If your heart rate has not reached the target rate, you need to increase the intensity of the workout. Remember, this target heart rate is the minimum level at which cardiovascular improvement begins to occur. Your task is to work up slowly to continuous exercise that elevates your heart rate to this minimum level for twenty minutes or more.

Training for Flexibility

Stretching exercises to improve flexibility have received considerable attention in recent years, inspired by the yoga and aerobic exercise boom. Considerable controversy exists over the importance of extreme flexibility and even the importance of stretching before and after exercise. Although the evidence is conflicting, it does appear that a sound stretching program reduces the incidence of injury and improves performance.[4]

Orthopedic surgeons have developed what is now termed the "hit list" of exercises that have been shown to cause muscle or joint damage to some individuals. Specific stretching movements such as straight-leg toe touching, straight-leg sit-ups and straight-leg lifts are suspect and may cause lower back problems. Full squats, squat jumps, the duck walk, hurdler's stretch, and sitting on the ankles and bending backwards may cause damage to the knee. Exercises that hyperextend the back are also being condemned as dangerous. The yoga plow (lying on back, feet lifted and brought overhead), for example, places pressure on spinal disks and ligaments and may cause permanent damage. Some experts feel that the extreme flexibility sought in yoga is unnecessary and unnatural and can result in soft tissue injuries.[5] It is therefore important to select flexibility exercises that are both safe and effective.

The range of motion that is possible at any joint is determined by bone structure, the state of the connective tissue maintaining a particular joint, the soft tissues, and the state of the muscle itself. The last two qualities can be altered significantly by stretching procedures that increase the total range of movement in a specific joint. Flexibility in the major joints can be improved in a relatively short period of time (two to three weeks).[6]

A number of sound approaches to improving flexibility have been used in the past:

- **Ballistic exercises.** Vigorous bouncing forces the joint beyond the normal range of motion. This technique, which is effective, has been virtually abandoned by nearly all experts because of the danger of injury. Force generated by the jerks may be greater than the extensibility of the tissues.

- **Static exercises.** Steady pressure is applied at the extreme range of motion in a particular joint for fifteen to thirty seconds, and the exercise is repeated two or three times. No bouncing is permitted to force the joints beyond the normal range of motion. This procedure improves flexibility and reduces the probability of injury and the likelihood of muscle soreness.

- **Slow-reversal-hold.** With this technique, a partner will apply pressure to a body area at the extreme range of motion until you feel slight discomfort (while you are lying on your back with leg extended and ankle flexed to ninety degrees, a partner lifts the leg and applies steady pressure to raise it overhead). At this point, you begin to push against your partner's resistance by contracting the muscle being stretched. After a ten-second push, relax again while your partner applies pressure for ten seconds. Repeat two to three times. This procedure alternately relaxes and contracts both the *agonistic* (contracting) and *antagonistic* (relaxing) muscles and increases flexibility.

- **Contract-relax and hold-relax.** In the contract-relax method, the hamstring muscle, as described in the above example, will actually contract and move the leg toward the floor during the push phase. The hold-relax method involves an isometric hamstring contraction (no leg movement occurs) during the push phase. During the relaxation phase, both techniques result in relaxing the hamstrings and quadriceps while the hamstrings are passively stretched by a partner.

Experts suggest that you take your time and enjoy the stretching phase of your exercise session, spending five to ten minutes before the workout and five to ten minutes after your workout. The period following your workout may be even more important. Although there are many other exercises, the ten shown in Figure 9.2 are both safe and effective and stretch the major body joints. Each extreme exercise position should be held statically for approximately fifteen to thirty seconds before relaxing for fifteen seconds and repeating the exercise two to three times. See also Exploring Your Health 9.4.

FIGURE 9.2 • Stretching exercises for flexibility.

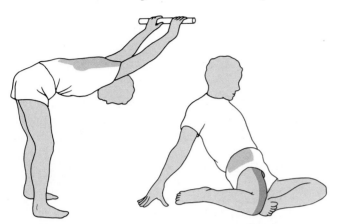

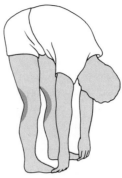

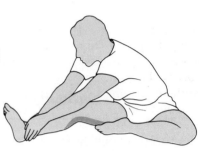

Shoulder stretch
Hold onto an object about shoulder height. With hands on the support, relax and keep arms straight and chest moving downward, feet under hips, and knees slightly bent.

Hip and upper thigh
Tighten left side of the buttocks as the hip is turned in that direction for five to ten seconds. Relax the buttocks, and repeat the exercise on the right side.

Hamstrings (a)
With knees slightly bent, slowly bend forward from the hips until you feel a stretch in the back of your legs.

Hamstrings (b)
Keep only a slight bend in the front leg, with the other foot next to the inside of the leg. Bend forward at the hips until you feel slight pressure.

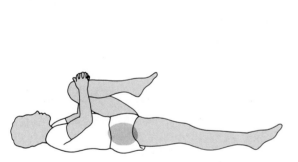

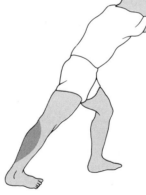

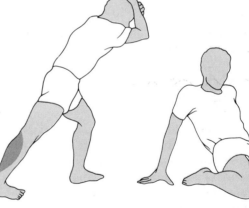

Hip
Lying on your back, relax and straighten both legs. Pull the left foot toward the chest. Repeat using the right foot.

Calf
Stand slightly away from a wall and lean forward with the lead leg bent and the rear leg extended. Move the hips forward with the heel of the straight leg on the ground until you feel a stretch in the calf.

Quadriceps
Sit with right leg bent and the heel just to the outside of the right hip. Bend the left leg, with the sole next to the inside of the upper right leg. Lean back until you feel an easy stretch.

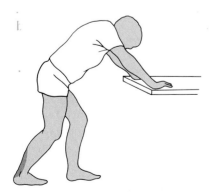

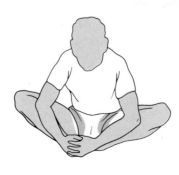

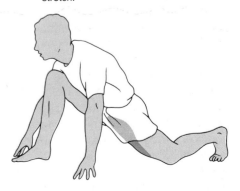

Achilles tendon and soleus
Bend the back knee slightly with the heel flat. Lean forward as in the calf stretch.

Groin (a)
With soles of the feet together, place hands around the feet and pull yourself forward.

Groin (b)
Move one leg forward until the knee is directly over the ankle. The back knee rests on the floor. Lean forward and hold.

aerobic Aerobic means "with oxygen" and describes extended vigorous exercise that stimulates heart-lung activity and conditioning.

Exploring Your Health 9.4

Flexibility Training

Sit on the floor with your legs almost fully extended. Without warm-up or practice, bend forward at the waist and reach for your toes. Pay close attention to how close you got to your toes or how far past your toes you were able to reach without bending your knees. Now assume a position on your knees with your feet tucked under the body. Lean backward slowly and carefully while sitting on your ankles and hold your maximum position of comfort for fifteen seconds. Quickly return to the sit-up position and repeat step number one. What did you discover? Why were you so much more flexible on your second attempt to touch your toes in the sit-up position?

During the first sit-up you were stretching the hamstring muscle group. You quickly followed with an exercise that stretched your quadricep muscle group and completely relaxed the hamstring muscles. This complete relaxation before restretching resulted in greater extensibility of the muscles and enabled you to reach much farther on the second sit-up. This method can be used with practically all muscle groups by first stretching and then completely relaxing a particular muscle group to be stretched.

Girth Control Training

Every college student seems to want a flat "tummy." In fact, a flat stomach has become strongly associated with fitness and wellness although some fat around the midsection is not necessarily unhealthy. As time passes, almost everyone acquires both a small "spare tire," in the form of fat on both sides of the hips, and some abdominal fat. Becoming obsessed with this somewhat natural change is a mistake. Depending upon your body type, it may be next to impossible to maintain the flat stomach you had in high school after the third or fourth decade of life.

Many people try to solve the girth control problem by using unnatural and worthless devices, such as girdles, corsets, weighted belts, rubberized workout suits, and special exercise equipment that promises flat stomachs in only minutes a day. It is important to keep in mind that fatty or adipose tissue cannot be converted into muscle tissue. One thousand sit-ups per day, for example, will not eliminate stomach fat unless your sit-up program is combined with caloric reduction that causes abdominal fat cells to shrink. Without diet control, you will merely develop very strong abdominal muscles underneath layers of fatty tissue. Your outward appearance will also change very little. The truth is that it is very difficult to develop the perfect tummy. You will need several months of both diet control and exercise before you notice a difference in the way your stomach muscles look and feel.

Before beginning your program, measure your waist with a tape measure, and take skinfold measures on both hips and next to the navel. You must also follow the suggestions in Chapter 8 to reduce your caloric intake if fat cells are to decrease in size. In addition, a high number of repetitions must be used for each exercise described below, working toward 100 for each exercise daily. Begin with the maximum number you can perform in one set. Add two to five repetitions daily until you reach 100.

1. **Sit-ups.** Lie flat on your back with knees slightly bent and both hands resting on your chest. Pull your chin to the chest and sit up slowly to an angle of approximately 60 degrees.
2. **Crunches.** Lie flat on your back with arms against the sides of your body and knees bent and pulled toward your chest. Raise your head and shoulders off the floor as you thrust your upper body towards the knees and then return to the starting position.
3. **Twisting crunches.** Lie flat on your back, hands behind your head, and touch your elbow to the opposite knee while the other leg straightens. Keep your feet flexed.
4. **Alternate knee kicks.** Lie flat on your back

with your hands under the buttocks. Bend one knee, and with the other leg straight, raise the other leg 6 inches off the floor. Straighten your bent knee and bend the other leg as in walking or marching, and repeat the exercise with the other leg.

5. **Back scissors.** Lie on your stomach with hands at your sides, palms down for support. Start with your legs apart and feet off the floor, and bring the feet together, then apart.

Training for the Lower Back

Lower back pain is common among college students. In fact, over 50 percent of middle school, high school, and college students who participated in the NASE Speed Camps throughout the United States from 1979 to 1990 complained of lower back problems severe enough to cause them to miss school or athletic practice. If you exhibit poor hip flexibility and poor abdominal strength, you are more likely to develop lower back problems in the future.

The exercises described below, in combination with adequate abdominal strength, hip flexibility, and the avoidance of the orthopedic exercise "hit list" described previously, improve lumbar (lower back) and gluteal (buttocks) musculature and are designed to help prevent lower back problems. They are also recommended for those who already suffer from lower back pain. For each exercise, the starting position is the same: The knees and hips are bent, with the back flat and the neck comfortably supported; arms are to the side, feet flat on the floor.

1. Take in a deep breath and exhale slowly. Tighten your stomach and buttock muscles and hold the back flat against the floor for 5 seconds. Relax. Repeat very slowly five times.

2. With both hands on one knee, bring your knee up as near to the chest as possible. Return it slowly to the starting position. Relax, Repeat ten times, alternating each leg.

3. Tighten your abdominal muscles and hold your back flat, then bring both knees up to the chest, grasp the knees with both hands, and hold them against your chest for thirty seconds. Return slowly to the starting position. Relax. Repeat five times.

Year 2000 National Health Objective

The federal government is striving to increase to at least 50 percent the proportion of worksites with 50 or more employees that offer back injury prevention and rehabilitation programs. Only 28.6 percent offered back care activities in 1983.

4. Bring one knee to the chest; straighten that knee, extending the leg as far as possible; bend knee and return to the original position. Relax. Alternate with the opposite leg and repeat five times. This exercise is not recommended for patients with sciatic nerve pain.

5. Lie on your back with the knees bent; feet flat on the floor. Pull up to a sitting position and hold for five seconds before returning to the starting position. Relax. Repeat five times.

Training for Maintenance

It is possible to alter your training program to maintain the level of conditioning you have acquired. Strength, for example, can be maintained by doing one hard weight training workout weekly. Maintaining heart-lung endurance requires two to three workouts weekly.

Selecting an Exercise Program

Any basic exercise program for people of all ages should emphasize development of the heart and lungs. An exercise program is judged by the demand it places on the heart and lungs and its caloric expenditure. You should select an exercise program according to your physical objectives, the amount of time you can devote to exercising, and your particular interests. Table 9.3 compares characteristics of various exercise programs.

Aerobic Programs

The term **aerobic** means "with oxygen" and describes extended vigorous exercise that stimulates heart and lung activity enough to produce a training effect. The primary objective is to increase the amount of oxygen processed by the body within a given period (*maximum oxygen uptake*). Any of the following types of sustained, vigorous exercises can be selected for achieving aerobic fitness: cycling, aerobic dance, jogging/running, calisthenics, rope jumping, swimming, walking, tennis (singles), handball, racquetball, basketball, and the like. A few of these activities are discussed below.

Cycling   Cycling has several advantages over jogging and running as an aerobic exercise: joint trauma (ankles, knees, and hips) is only mild and rarely results in injury; associated back problems are uncommon; and mild cycling can be used while recovering from certain types of injuries to the back, feet, or arms. A road bike is expensive and requires special protective head gear. Target heart rates can be reached and held for twenty to thirty minutes with either a road or stationary bike. Your task is to locate the speed that ele-

Selecting an Exercise Program   •   231

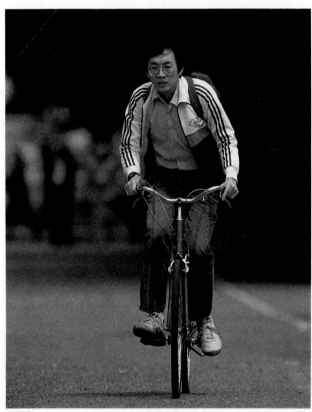

Walking or bicycling to campus from a distant dormitory or off-campus housing is an excellent way to incorporate some exercise into your daily routine. However, be aware that casual cycling may not give your body the regular workout it needs to be fit—unless, of course, you have a lot of hills to climb on your way to school!

Low impact aerobic exercise develops the cardiovascular system and aids in fat loss and weight management without overstressing the orthopedic system.

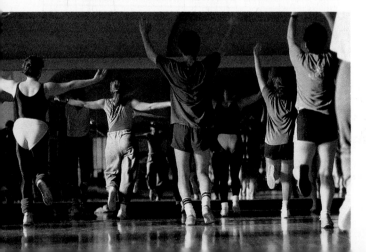

vates your heart rate to the target level; in most cases, this requires rather vigorous pedaling as opposed to slow, recreational cycling. When performed correctly, cycling can be one of the best aerobic fitness choices for all age groups.

Aerobic Dance *Aerobic dance* (movement to music aimed at increasing aerobic fitness) can be an excellent form of aerobic exercise for attaining your target heart rate. Formal classes by certified instructors provide continuous activity and careful monitoring of the exercise heart rate. However, many classes that are called aerobic dance do not monitor heart rate carefully or record progress. You need to be certain your instructor is well qualified before signing up for classes in aerobic dance.

Jogging/Running Although *jogging* (running at a steady slow trot at a 9-minute-per-mile pace or slower) and *running* (8:59-minute-per-mile pace or faster) are excellent forms of aerobic exercise, they may not be ideal choices for everyone. Current popularity is based on low cost, safety, minimum hassle (no special equipment or partner is required), and high fitness value (physical and mental). Negative aspects include foot, ankle, knee, and back problems from pounding on hard surfaces and a difficult adaptation to a strenuous form of activity for those unaccustomed to running. After years of activity, most runners eventually discover they need an alternate form of aerobic exercise that is less stressful to the body while they recover from minor injuries and illnesses.

Calisthenics *Calisthenic* exercises are designed to develop and maintain muscular strength and endurance and flexibility. A specific movement that uses the body as resistance is one of the oldest forms of conditioning in existence. Exercises such as sit-ups, toe touching, trunk rotation, jumping jacks, and push-ups must be performed with many repetitions because the resistance (body weight) is relatively low. Moreover, resistance remains constant, so the number of repetitions must be gradually increased, the rest interval between exercises decreased, the speed or rate of exe-

TABLE 9.3

Evaluation of Exercise Programs

Characteristics of the Ideal Program	Aerobic Exercise and Dance	Anaerobics	Calisthenics	Cycling	Rope Jumping	Running Programs	Sports[b]	Walking	Swimming (Lap)	Weight Training
Easily adaptable to individual's exercise tolerance	P	Y	Y	Y	Y	Y	P	Y	Y	Y
Applies the progressive resistance principle	Y	Y	Y	Y	Y	Y	P	Y	Y	Y
Provides for self-evaluation	Y	Y	P	Y	Y	Y	P	Y	Y	Y
Practical for use throughout life	Y	N	N	N	Y	Y	P	Y	Y	Y
Scientifically developed	Y	Y	P	Y	Y	Y	U	Y	Y	Y
Involves minimum time	Y	P	N	Y	Y	Y	N	Y	Y	Y
Involves little or no equipment	P	Y	Y	N	Y	Y	N	Y	Y	N
Performed easily at home	N	N	Y	Y	Y	Y	N	Y	Y	N
Widely publicized	Y	N	N	Y	Y	Y	Y	Y	Y	Y
Accepted and valued	Y	P	N	Y	Y	Y	P	Y	Y	Y
Challenging	Y	Y	N	Y	Y	Y	Y	Y	Y	Y
Firms body	Y	Y	Y	Y	Y	P	P	Y	Y	Y
Develops flexibility[a]	Y	N	Y	N	Y	Y	Y	N	P	N
Develops muscular endurance	Y	Y	Y	Y		Y	Y	Y	Y	Y
Develops cardiovascular endurance: prevents heart disease	Y	N	Y	Y	Y	Y	Y	P	Y	P
Develops strength	P	P	Y	P	P	Y	Y	P	P	Y
High caloric expenditure: weight loss	Y	P	P	Y	Y	P	Y	Y	Y	N

Note: Y = yes, P = partially, N = no provision, U = unknown (referring to meeting ideal characteristics).

[a]Flexibility can be improved only if the complete range of movement is performed in each exercise, applying static pressure at the extreme range of motion before returning to starting position.

[b]The value of the sports approach depends on the activity and the level of competition.

Source: Adapted from John Unitas and George B. Dintiman, *Improving Health and Fitness in the Athlete* (Englewood Cliffs, N.J.: Prentice-Hall, 1979), p. 180.

radial pulse The pulse, that is, heart beats per minute, as taken at the inside of the wrist on the same side as the thumb.

anaerobic Anaerobic means "without oxygen" and describes short, all-out exercise efforts.

---

cution increased, and the duration of the workout increased. In other words, you must perform more work each day through a longer, faster workout with less rest between each exercise. A sound practice is to add two to four repetitions every workout to each calisthenic exercise. With little or no rest between exercises, aerobic conditioning will also improve.

Rope Jumping Jumping rope is an inexpensive, effective way to develop aerobic fitness by elevating and maintaining the heart rate at the target level. You can easily stop jumping during your workout, take a **radial pulse** (at the wrist), compare this exercise pulse rate to your target rate, and adjust the intensity of the rope jumping accordingly. For variety, the type of jump and rope manipulation can be altered. By counting the number of jumps per minute, regulating the rest period between different jumps, and using some difficult high-energy jumps, a program can be designed that will improve both agility and aerobic endurance. During the first week or two it may be helpful to warm up by jogging in place fifty to 100 steps. The following program includes three warm-up jumps (to be completed slowly) and five basic jumps (to be completed at the rate of seventy to seventy-five jumps per minute). The boxer's shuffle and single-foot jumps are performed at a rate of seventy to seventy-five per minute; the double jump is restarted when missed and continued for the specified number of repetitions.

Warm-up Jumps

- **Two-foot jump with an intermediate jump (double beat).** After the rope passes under the feet, a small hop is taken before jumping again to clear the rope.
- **Two-foot jump (single beat).** No intermediate jump is taken.
- **Single-foot hop (single beat).** The left foot is used for a specified number of jumps, followed by the right foot.

Basic Program

- **Boxer's shuffle (single beat).** Use alternate right and left foot jumping as the rope passes under.
- **Running forward (single beat).** Jump while

running forward; repeat running backward to starting position.
- **Cross-overs (double beat).** Jump with the rope turning forward; cross the rope by fully crossing the arms as the rope clears your head; repeat with rope turning backwards.
- **Single-foot hops (single beat).** Same as warm-up jump; progress from slow to fast or pepper jumping.
- **Double jumps (double beat).** The rope must pass under the feet twice while you are in the air. Perform one double jump, one single jump, one double jump, alternating until completing the specified number.

Swimming Swimming is one of the best overall aerobic exercise programs. The combination of cardiovascular development, muscular strength and endurance, and freedom from injury makes it superior in many ways to other forms of exercise. Initially you may find any stroke difficult to sustain for twenty to thirty minutes. The side, breast, and elementary back strokes can be used as resting strokes so movement can be continuous as you swim laps using either the front or back crawl stroke. Again, your task is to swim for twenty to thirty minutes at a pace that maintains your target heart rate. Slowly add one to two laps each workout over a period of several months, depending on your conditioning level, until you are capable of thirty minutes of continuous swimming.

Walking Walking can be an excellent form of aerobic exercise for people of all ages. To elicit your target heart rate, you will have to walk at a pace of three and a half to four miles per hour (15-minute mile). Slowly, over a period of several months, add one-fourth to one-half mile to each workout until you are capable of walking for three to five miles at this brisk pace. With this approach, you will expend a high number of calories and improve heart-lung endurance.

Anaerobics

The term **anaerobic** means "without oxygen" and describes short, all-out exercise efforts, such as a 100-,

200-, or 400-meter dash. Anaerobic metabolism comes into action at the beginning of any type of exercise as the immediate energy source for all muscle work. The energy source, called *ATP (adenosine triphosphate)* is formed in the muscles through the metabolizing of carbohydrates and fats. Every muscle needs ATP to perform its work. The process is termed anaerobic because ATP is metabolized without the need for oxygen. For short sprints, the heart and lungs cannot deliver oxygen to the muscles fast enough; anaerobic energy sources therefore must provide the fuel. The very second that the amount of oxygen breathed in is not enough to supply active muscles, oxygen debt occurs. In the absence of oxygen to fire working muscles, anaerobic metabolism comes into play. After exercise stops, this oxygen debt is repaid.[7]

Getting Started

You now have enough basic information to begin your fitness program. By following the step-by-step approach described below you can safely and efficiently progress from your present conditioning level to a higher level. When necessary, return to the appropriate section in this chapter for more detailed information.

Analyze Your Medical History   If you are over 40 years of age, have been inactive for more than two to three years, regardless of age, or are in the high-risk group (obese, high blood pressure, diabetic, high blood lipids), a thorough physical examination is recommended. Although the chances of a serious problem for college students are slight, it's better to be safe than sorry.

Begin Gradually and Progress Slowly   It takes three to four months to get into fair physical conditioning. Attempting to progress any faster is dangerous. "Too much, too soon" is a common cause of muscle and joint injuries.

Use Your Target Heart Rate to Elevate Each Workout   Immediately after completing your aerobic exercise session, take your radial (wrist) pulse to determine whether your workout elevates heart rate to the target level. If it does not, increase the intensity of the workout (run or walk faster, swim faster, cycle faster). If your heart rate is too high, reduce the intensity of your workout. Remember, you are not expected to be able to exercise at your target heart rate for twenty to thirty minutes in the early stages of your program. It may take several weeks or months before your conditioning level is sufficient to perform this task.

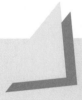

A Question of Ethics

The Dangers of Steroids and Muscle Weight Gain: A Personal Decision for the Individual or the Responsibility of Society?

The use of steroids by athletes and nonathletes of all ages who want to add muscle weight is becoming more common in the United States. A high school or college student can easily purchase black market anabolic steroids in practically any part of the country. This synthetic version of testosterone, the male hormone, stimulates increased water retention and adds muscle mass. Because individuals also find that strength gains occur at a more rapid rate, anabolic steroids remain extremely popular despite the extreme dangers of their use. Regular use has been shown to produce hostility, aggression and violent rages, high blood pressure and clogged arteries (which can lead to a heart attack and clogging of the vessels supplying the extremities), acne, liver and prostate cancer, sterility and atrophied testicals in men, and growth interference in adolescents. Women who use steroids may experience body hair growth, facial hair growth, scalp hair loss, and voice changes.

Neither making steroids illegal nor mandatory testing in the United States has had much effect on the incidence of steroid use. Certainly, it is the ethical responsibility of coaches and trainers to place the health of their athletes above winning and money. In addition, athletic role models need to demonstrate healthy rather than dangerous behaviors to our nation's youth. Opponents of steroid use also point out that drug-free muscle weight gain programs will produce the same results. Adequate, not excessive, protein and carbohydrate intake, a sound diet with sufficient calories, and a vigorous weight-training program that involves a six-day workout, alternating muscle groups every other day, has been shown to add muscle weight safely at the rate of one-half pound per week. Certainly, twenty-six pounds of muscle weight gain in a twelve-month period makes this approach effective and safe.

Proponents of steroid use argue that numerous drugs are utilized in the United States to relax, energize, or alter mood and that it is absurd to ban the use of a drug that will improve performance. In addition, some college and professional-level athletes complain that they cannot compete against the additional strength and muscle weight that an opponent has acquired through the use of anabolic steroids.

Exploring Your Health 9.5

Your Exercise Contract

Make a written agreement with yourself about exercise. Set specific goals in Section 1 for increasing your energy and specific goals in Section 2 for increasing activity. Start slowly. Even a 100 calorie expenditure per day produces a weight loss of ten to twelve pounds in one year.

Remember to motivate yourself through a reward system in Section 3. List specific daily and weekly rewards for meeting your exercise goals. Self-payments may range from eating special foods to treating yourself to a night out. Choose rewards that are not destructive to your overall fitness program.

During this week _____ 19 ____, I hereby agree to work as hard as possible at achieving the following:

1. Physical activity goals for increasing my energy use during occupational time:
   A. I will park my car or leave public transportation and walk _____ additional minutes per day.
   B. I will spend _____ minutes daily standing instead of sitting while I work.
   C. I will walk up _____ flights of stairs each working day.
   D. I will walk around my work area _____ minutes every day.
   E. I will spend _____ minutes during each coffee break standing instead of sitting.
   F. I will spend _____ minutes during each lunch break walking outside in the open air.

2. Physical activity goals for increasing my energy use during recreational time:
   A. I will spend _____ minutes daily doing stretching activities to increase my flexibility.
   B. I will spend _____ minutes at least three times per week doing aerobic activities to improve my endurance.
   C. I will spend _____ minutes at least three times per week doing strength activities.
   D. I will spend _____ minutes Saturday and Sunday in active recreational activities.

3. My rewards and consequences:
   A. I will reward myself daily with one of the following pleasures when I achieve my daily goals in increased activity:

      1) _____   4) _____
      2) _____   5) _____
      3) _____   6) _____

   B. When I do *not* make my daily goals I agree to do the following:

      1) _____   2) _____

   C. I will reward myself every week with one of the following pleasures when I achieve my weekly exercise goals:

      1) _____   4) _____
      2) _____   5) _____
      3) _____   6) _____

   D. When I do *not* make my weekly goals I agree to do the following:

      1) _____   2) _____

I now agree to the above contract and with the goals and consequences. I also agree to follow this contract until my goals are reached.

Signed _____ Date _____ Witnessed _____

Get Involved!

Getting Others to Get the Message About Regular Exercise

In the last decade a number of alarming trends have emerged that have serious implications for our nation's health. These trends include a reduction in the number of required hours of physical education in public schools, chronic low-level fitness among children, adolescents, and young adults, and increased incidence of childhood obesity. Furthermore, the number of all Americans who exercise according to the Surgeon General's definition (three times weekly at the individual's target heart rate for a minimum of twenty minutes) are well below the Year 2000 National Health Objectives.

You can begin to alter some of these trends right now. The health behaviors of college students are well known to the American public. A nation of physically active college students can positively influence other people to include regular exercise in their own lifestyles as well as to support exercise programs and opportunities in their schools and communities. One of the most important messages you need to get across to other people, however, is that exercise is not only for "the young and the beautiful." Exercise—like good nutrition and weight control—is for people of all ages. Here are some specific things you can do to convey this message:

1. Encourage family and friends to eliminate unhealthy behaviors such as sedentary living, dangerous weekend exercise sessions, and, of course, tobacco, alcohol, and drug use. Help these people in your immediate circle to develop exercise regimens that are appropriate for them.

2. Become involved as a counselor or coach in a college or local community-affiliated sports and recreation program for children. Such programs might involve day camps for elementary or junior high school students or even extended week- or month-long sports and recreation programs. Some of these programs qualify as internships, many of them involve some sort of stipend or other form of payment, and all of them can be extremely valuable experiences in your own life!

3. Locate one or more faculty members or community health officers (such as doctors or physical therapists) who specialize in the care of older people. Discuss with these people how you could contribute your time and energy to the improvement of exercise opportunities for older people, especially for those currently confined to their homes or in nursing homes. There are many simple, healthful exercises that older people—even those who cannot leave a wheelchair—can perform that will help them to develop better muscle tone, feel better, and have higher energy levels.

4. Get politically involved in supporting physical education and exercise programs and opportunities in public schools, colleges, and universities. Inform yourself about the physical education elements in local school budgets and in your own college's budget, and lobby and rally voters and other students for support when necessary.

5. Encourage exercise and recreation programs in your own college community by participating in and otherwise supporting intramural sports, fitness, and recreation activities. Actively encourage other students to participate in these activities, too.

Warm Up and Cool Down Properly at Each Workout Use an appropriate warm-up and cool-down period as described earlier in this chapter.

Apply the Progressive Overload Principle Plan your program so that your workout is slightly more strenuous each session. You can increase the length of the total workout or the intensity of the workout (work per unit of time). For example, you can swim thirty minutes today and add two to three minutes each workout or swim slightly farther in the thirty-minute period each workout.

Exercise a Minimum of Four Times Weekly for Thirty Minutes or More Daily or alternate-day programs are necessary to improve aerobic capacity, change the way your body handles fats, improve strength and endurance, and so forth.

Avoid the Weekend-Athlete Approach to Fitness One sure way to guarantee numerous injuries and illnesses is to exercise vigorously only on weekends. The older weekend athlete is particularly susceptible to heart attack, while individuals of all ages increase their chances of muscle, tendon, and ligament injuries.

Pay Close Attention to Your Body Signals Pain and other distress signals should not be ignored. It is sound advice to stop exercising immediately if you notice any abnormal heart action such as pulse irregularity; fluttering; palpitations in the chest or throat; rapid heartbeats; pain or pressure in the middle of the chest, teeth, jaw, neck, or arm; dizziness; lightheadedness; cold sweat; or confusion. After each session let your body analyze the severity of the workout. It was too light if sweating did not occur. It was too heavy if breathlessness persisted ten minutes after, if your pulse

FIGURE 9.3 • The RICE technique is an excellent way to deal with many muscle, ligament, and tendon problems in an emergency. There are four simple steps:

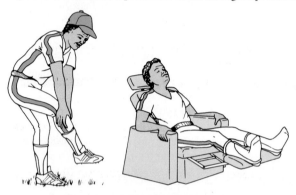

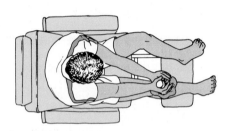

1. *Rest.* To prevent additional damage to injured tissue, stop exercising immediately; if the lower extremities are affected, use crutches to get around.

2. *Ice.* To decrease blood flow to the injured body part and prevent swelling, apply ice immediately for fifteen to nineteen minutes. Place the ice in a pack or create a makeshift ice pack with a towel to avoid direct contact of the ice with skin.

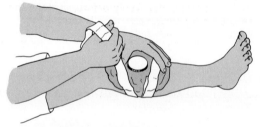

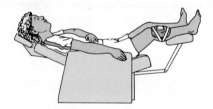

3. *Compression.* To limit swelling, wrap the ice pack firmly to the affected area with a bandage or another towel.

4. *Elevation.* Gravity will help drain fluid buildups that lead to swelling and pain. Raise the injured limb above the level of your heart.

Based on information presented in George B. Dintiman and Robert Ward, *Train America! Achieving Peak Performance and Fitness for Sports Competition* (Dubuque, Iowa: Kendal/Hunt, 1988).

rate was above 120 beats per minute two hours after stopping, if prolonged fatigue remained for more than twenty-four hours, if nausea or vomiting occurred, or if sleep was interrupted. To remedy these symptoms, you should exercise less vigorously and lengthen your cool-down period. When you are ill or not "up to par," rest a few days and return to a lower level or easier workout.

In spite of all precautions, problems may still occur. Fortunately, the majority of exercise injuries can be managed through emergency home treatment methods.

Emergency treatment and initial home treatment for most muscle, ligament and tendon strains, sprains,

suspected fractures, bruises, and joint inflammation involve four simple actions known as the RICE (*Rest, Ice, Compression, Elevation*) approach. See Figure 9.3 for an explanation of how RICE works.

Exercise, the Weather, and Your Body

Coping with the Weather

Very warm or cold weather affect you as you exercise. Some factors are discussed in Table 9.4.

TABLE 9.4

Weather and Exercise

	Hot, Humid Weather	Cold Weather
Intensity of Exercise	Avoid vigorous exercise if the temperature is above 90 degrees and the humidity is above 70 percent. Make hot days your light workout.	Avoid vigorous exercise if the temperature and wind-chill factor approach zero.
Food	Avoid salt tablets; increase consumption of fruits and vegetables.	Eat well during cold months; the body needs more calories.
Warm-ups	Avoid lengthy warm-up periods.	Warm up carefully.
Clothing	Wear light-colored, porous cloth to promote evaporation.	Use two to three layers of clothing rather than one heavy warm-up suit.
	Avoid using a hat (unless it is an open visor with brim) since considerable heat loss occurs through the head.	Protect the head (warm hat), ears, fingers, toes, nose, and genitals.
	Avoid rubberized suits that hold sweat in and increase fluid and salt/potassium loss.	Avoid rubberized, airtight suits that keep the sweat in. When the body cools, sweat begins to freeze.
	Wet clothing increases salt and sweat loss. Replace.	Keep clothing dry, changing wet items as soon as possible.
Duration of Exercise	Slowly increase the length of your workout five to ten minutes daily for nine days to acclimate yourself to the heat.	Slowly increase the length of your workout five to ten minutes daily for nine days to acclimate to the cold.
Water	Drink cold water (24 to 48 ounces) fifteen minutes before, during, and after exercise.	Drink cold water freely before, during, and after exercise.

Exercise After Eating

Most of us were taught as children to avoid exercise after eating because it was supposed to hinder digestion and bring on stomach cramps. It is true that vigorous exercise slows acid secretion and peristaltic movements of the stomach during exercise and for a short time afterward (about one hour). Following this period, there is increased activity in these areas beyond the normal state. With mild exercise, however, gastric motility and acid secretion actually increase. In the final analysis, exercise has little effect on the entire digestive process. Performance could be hindered, however, by discomfort due to overeating, a psychological feeling of lethargy or sickness, or a full stomach that does not allow the diaphragm to descend completely during inhalation.

For over a hundred years, parents have warned against swimming immediately after eating. The fear of stomach cramps and drowning, supposedly caused by eating, continues to keep many swimmers out of the water for one to two hours after eating. The truth is that stomach cramps are not common. One researcher who studied 30,000 swimmers did not observe even one case of stomach cramps.

Need for Water During Exercise

The average person needs about six 12-ounce glasses of pure, soft water daily for sound nutrition. This is in addition to the water obtained from food materials—vegetables (90 to 95 percent water), fruits (80 to 85 percent water), and meat (up to 70 percent water).[8] An athlete or exercising individual needs much more. In hot, humid weather, additional water is needed to keep up with loss from perspiration. A rapid water loss of 2 percent will decrease performance slightly, a 5 percent loss can reduce muscle performance by as much as 20 to 30 percent, and 6 to 8 percent can result in heat exhaustion, heat stroke, and even death.

Water should be consumed freely before, during, and after exercise. Regardless of its availability, most athletes do not consume enough to prevent a water deficit during exercise. Keep in mind that thirst will

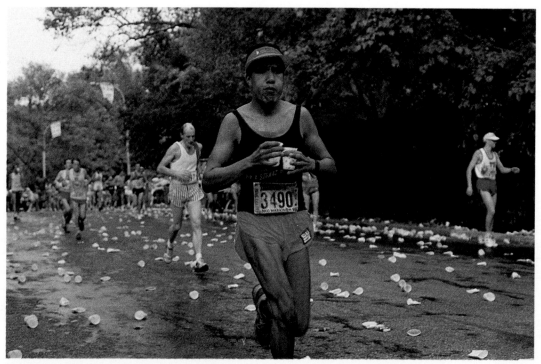

Everybody needs at least six 12-ounce glasses of water a day to maintain good health. People who are working out or participating in competitive sports, however, need to consume water freely before, during, and after exercise.

underestimate your needs. It is therefore necessary to drink an extra twenty-four to forty-eight ounces of cold (40 degree) water approximately fifteen minutes before you begin your exercise even though thirst sensations do not exist. Drinking water earlier than 15 minutes before exercise may fill the bladder and make you uncomfortable during activity. Cold water is ab-

Year 2000 National Health Objective

To protect participants in organized competitive and recreational activities, the federal government has established a national health objective to extend requirement of the use of effective head, face, eye, and mouth protection to all organizations, agencies, and institutions sponsoring sporting and recreational events that pose risks of injury.

TABLE 9.5	
Exercise, Weight Loss, and Water Replacement	
Weight Loss	**Water Needed to Replace Loss**
1 pound	Two 8-ounce glasses
4 pounds	Eight 8-ounce glasses
8 pounds	Sixteen 8-ounce glasses

sorbed faster than warm or room-temperature water. In addition, forced drinking (hydrating) has been shown to significantly delay fatigue and improve performance. In fact, one study demonstrated that consuming thirty-six to forty-eight ounces of water before activity not only delayed fatigue by 50 percent but also kept body temperature under 101 degrees even after six hours.[9] This hydrating turned out to be nearly the exact amount of water the subjects lost through perspiration.

Weight loss following exercise provides an indication of how much water is needed to replace the loss[10] (see Table 9.5). Weighing yourself just before and immediately after exercise will provide you with this valuable information.

Drinking too much water is not a problem; water is not toxic and the kidneys will excrete it efficiently. The kidneys are also capable of conserving water when the body is deprived of it by excreting more highly concentrated urine. On hot, humid days, however, the kidneys can be helped by drinking extra water.[11]

Conclusion

It is evident that the choice of an exercise program depends on the outcomes desired, as well as on time pressures, available equipment, and personality. The degree to which a program contributes to the development of physical fitness depends on both the activity selected and the extent to which the principles of conditioning are applied. In terms of overall fitness, aerobic programs are the most desirable choice for adult men and women. They offer the advantages of high caloric expenditures for weight control, heart-lung development, and possible protection from early heart disease. In addition, the time required to follow aerobic programs of exercise is relatively limited.

Summary

1. The majority of Americans are still unfit, and fewer than 20 percent engage in regular aerobic exercise.

2. Overall fitness is associated with limited body fat, heart-lung endurance, muscular strength and endurance, and body flexibility. Each of these components can be improved with regular exercise.

3. Regular aerobic exercise has been shown to contribute to both physical and mental health.

4. To continue to improve your conditioning level, you must perform more work in each exercise session.

5. Aerobic fitness is attained by following an exercise program that maintains your target heart rate for twenty to thirty minutes, three to four times weekly.

6. The key to weight loss through exercise is volume (length of workout); long, easy workouts expend more calories than short, intense sessions.

7. Sufficient warm-up and cool-down periods are needed to prevent muscle injuries and illness.

8. Once you have attained your desired fitness objective, two to three workouts weekly will maintain this level.

9. Flexibility is best improved through the use of static exercises that apply steady pressure at the extreme range of motion without undue bouncing.

10. Flexibility and calisthenic exercises must be selected carefully. A number of movements have been shown to cause injuries to the lower back and knees.

11. Cycling, calisthenics, rope jumping, aerobic dance, jogging/running, swimming, and fast walking are excellent forms of aerobic exercise.

12. Anaerobic training is important for individuals who participate in sports requiring repeated short sprints (tennis, racquetball, squash, handball, football, baseball, basketball).

13. Exercise can be dangerous. It is important to know your limitations, begin gradually and progress slowly, exercise regularly, take weather conditions into account, warm up and cool down properly, and pay close attention to your body signals.

14. Additional water is needed before, during, and after exercise on hot humid days.

15. Attaining a high level of aerobic fitness through participation in recreational sports is difficult but possible if you select the right activity.

16. Weight training with free weights is one of the most effective programs to develop muscular strength and endurance. Weight training does more than just make you stronger; it adds muscle weight, increases resting metabolic rate, tones muscles, and improves body appearance. Variables, such as the number of repetitions and sets, the weight to be lifted, the speed of con-

traction, and the rest interval, can be altered to meet your training objective.

17. To flatten your stomach it is necessary to combine girth control exercises and diet. Unless a calorie deficit is achieved, stomach fat cells will not shrink and you will strengthen your abdominal muscles with little or no change in the appearance of your stomach.

18. You can help prevent lower back pain in the future by avoiding the orthopedic "hit" list of dangerous stretching exercises, strengthening your abdominal muscles, improving your hip flexibility, and performing the basic lower back flexion exercise routine.

19. The use of anabolic steroids is extremely dangerous to your health and can and has caused death from heart attack, liver failure, and other problems. You can add muscle weight with a combination of weight training and nutritional support without the use of drugs.

Questions for Personal Growth

1. Design an ideal exercise program that you can continue throughout life. In the program, include the three major components of fitness: exercise for cardiovascular fitness, flexibility, and strength. Schedule a typical week, fitting workouts into your present schedule.

2. How is RICE used to treat common soft tissue injuries, such as an ankle sprain or muscle contusion? How does each of the four steps help prevent further swelling and injury, and aid the healing process?

3. After several weeks of regular flexibility exercises, repeat the toe touch test in Exploring Your Health 9.1. Did your flexibility improve?

4. Anaerobic and aerobic exercises produce entirely different results. Which of the two programs are more important to you? Which of the two are likely to produce more health-related benefits? Why?

5. An adequate cool-down period will protect you from a dramatic drop in blood pressure and the potential harmful health consequences. Design a five to ten minute cool-down routine you can use at the end of your aerobic workout. Try it out, burn the extra calories, enjoy the feeling of accomplishment for completing your exercise routine, and see how it makes you feel.

6. Memorize your target heart rate range. Try several of the following activities and take your pulse immediately after you finish exercising: A 1-mile walk in 15 minutes, or 20 minutes of each of the following: rope jumping, lap swimming, aerobic dance, aerobic exercise, racquetball, tennis, basketball, or other sports activity. Was your activity intense enough to reach your target heart rate? How could you change the activity to elevate your heart rate to within your target heart rate range? Did you exceed your range? If so, what change could you make to reduce the intensity of the exercise session?

7. Although it is difficult, you can reduce your waistline and even obtain a flat stomach with a combination of diet, aerobic exercise, and abdominal exercises. Record your waist measurements and start an abdominal fitness program. Be sure to reduce your caloric intake (see Chapter 7). Try the program for one month. What changes do you observe?

References

1. "Exercising Options," *Review Magazine* (September 1986).

2. Kenneth H. Cooper, *The Aerobic Program for Total Well-Being* (New York: Evans, 1982).

3. Joel E. Dimsdale, Howard Hartley, Timothy Guiney, Jeremy Ruskin, and David Greenblatt, "Post-exercise Peril: Plasma Catecholamines and Exercise," *JAMA* 251, 5 (February 3, 1984): 630–632.

4. Pat Croce, *Stretching for Athletics* (Champaign, Ill.: Leisure Press, 1982).

5. R. Dominguez, *Total Body Training* (New York: Scribners, 1982).

6. George B. Dintiman and Robert Ward, *Sportspeed* (Champaign, Ill.: Human Kinetics Publishers, 1988), p. 68.

7. Ibid, p. 112.

8. Eva May Nunnelley Hamilton, Eleanor Noss Whitney, and Frances Sienkiewicz Sizer, *Nutrition: Concepts and Controversies*, 4e (St. Paul, Minn.: West, 1988), pp. 226–231.

9. M. G. Hardinge, *Water-Water-Water* (film) (Loma Linda, Calif.: Loma Linda University School of Health, 1972).

10. J. W. McFarland, "The Real Fountain of Youth," *Life and Health,* July 1981.

11. George B. Dintiman, Robert G. Davis, Stephen S. Stone, and Jude C. Pennington, *Discovering Lifetime Fitness: Concepts of Exercise and Weight Control,* 2e (St. Paul, Minn.: West, 1989), p. 244.

CHAPTER 10

Using and Abusing Drugs

CHAPTER OBJECTIVES

After reading this chapter, you should understand:

- Why Americans are becoming overly reliant on medication and mood-altering substances and how you can work toward responsible drug use for yourself and for your community.

- The difference between "drug misuse" and "drug abuse."

- How various factors such as dosage, potency, and individual response influence the effects that drugs have on the body.

- What we know about the effectiveness of several common over-the-counter (OTC) drugs.

- How psychoactive drugs—stimulants, depressants, psychedelics and hallucinogens —affect the central nervous system.

- Why people use drugs, why "use" is sometimes actually misuse, and some of the reasons for drug abuse.

- Several different approaches to the treatment of drug addiction.

- That it is not enough to know about how drugs affect your body in order to avoid drug abuse. You must also *know yourself.*

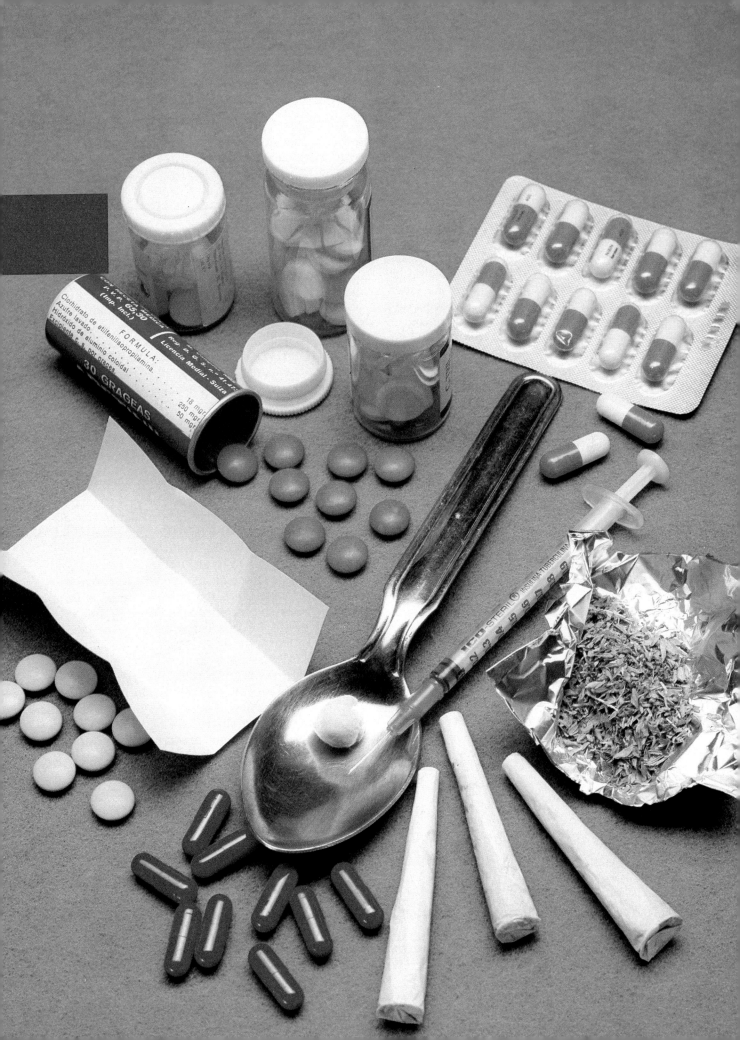

FORMULA:
Clorhidrato de etilfenilisopropilamina.
Azufre lavado.
Hidróxido de aluminio coloidal.
Excipiente c.s. por grageas

R.C.P. 65.30
(Imp. Incl.)
Licencia Modial - Suiza

30 GRAGEAS

18 mgr.
250 mgr.
50 mgr.

drug Any substance that by its chemical nature alters the structure or function in a living organism.

responsible drug use The wise and prudent use of pharmaceuticals and over-the-counter medications with a conscientious regard for the physiological, psychological, social, and legal factors and effects of their use.

A **drug** is any substance that by its chemical nature alters the structure or function in a living organism. This definition includes such substances as aspirin or antibiotics, as well as psychoactive drugs that alter mood, thought, and perception. Thus tranquilizers, antidepressants, and marijuana are drugs, as are coffee, tea, alcohol, and the nicotine in tobacco. You will find detailed discussions of alcohol and tobacco in Chapters 11 and 12 respectively. Here our focus will be on the other kinds of drugs mentioned above.

Whether drugs have a beneficial or harmful effect is largely determined by how they are used. Just as nuclear power can be used to create energy or wreak destruction, drugs can be used either to enhance or to destroy life. In this chapter we will explore a variety of drugs and look at how some of them affect the body and the mind. In addition, we will examine some of the reasons people abuse drugs and propose some alternative ways in which people can meet the needs they feel are met by drugs. In light of the information presented and your own values and needs, your task is to decide how you will use drugs responsibly.

America: A Drug-Taking Society

Perhaps the most important drug discoveries have been vaccines (providing protection from many diseases that used to wipe out whole populations), antibiotics (which control many previously fatal bacterial diseases), tranquilizers (a major breakthrough in the treatment of mental illness), and oral contraceptives (an extremely reliable means of birth control, with important social consequences). These discoveries show clearly that drugs have had a significant beneficial impact on our lives.

But for all the good that has come from drugs, many people believe that Americans have become too reliant on medication and mood-altering substances. For many of us, the remedy for anxiety is taking a tranquilizer or smoking a cigarette rather than managing the anxiety. The remedy for a headache is aspirin. Problems are forgotten with alcohol, and social occasions are made more stimulating with cocaine. We Americans have access to vast quantities of prescription and nonprescription drugs, as well as psychoactive drugs, and there is no doubt that we use them freely.

Several factors have contributed to this situation. For one thing, we've come to believe that technology is the answer to our problems. Rather than prevent disease from occurring in the first place, for example, we try to find a technological solution to eliminate it once it exists. Consider the vast amounts of money the government and private foundations pour into research to *cure* illness compared to the relatively small amount spent on research concerned with *preventing* illness.

Another factor contributing to the prevalence of drugs in society is the attitude that life should be entirely free of stress and anxiety. As evidence for this view, consider the fact that some physicians prescribe tranquilizers to patients who, in many instances, might be better off managing in other ways; or consider the barrage of television advertisements for medications that will alleviate "tension" headaches. Advertising by drug manufacturers exerts a powerful influence. Much

---

▶▶ *Exploring Your Health* 10.1

Revolutionary Drugs

Before reading on, can you think of four discoveries of drugs that have revolutionized society? Which four drugs would you list? Why?

1. _____   3. _____

2. _____   4. _____

of the enormous expenditure on drug advertising is aimed at a society that takes drugs too readily.

Political and economic factors play a role in drug use as well. One need only consider the government's continued subsidies to tobacco farmers, despite the known hazards of smoking, to realize that this is so. Social factors also contribute to the abuse of drugs in our society. We'll look at some of these factors later in the chapter.

Responsible Drug Use

The information in this chapter will allow you to use drugs in a manner that best meets your needs. We will refer to such use of drugs as responsible. **Responsible drug use** means looking at such factors as dosage, potency, interaction effects, solubility, location of action on the body, individual response, dependence, tolerance, and reverse tolerance. It means considering the psychological, physiological, societal, and legal implications of administering a particular drug. It means judging the effectiveness of the drug and its safety. And it means understanding your motivation for and the influences on your drug-related behavior. If this sounds like a tall order, read on. All these subjects are discussed in this chapter, with the intention of helping you become a responsible user of drugs.

In addition to effects on the individual, we will also consider the implications of drug use and abuse on the nation. We know that drugs are pervasive and that their effects can be devastating. For example, in 1978 alone, there were 2.7 drug-related deaths (excluding alcohol) for every 100,000 Americans. That prompted the federal government to develop a national health objective to decrease this rate to 2 per 100,000 by 1990. These deaths were attributed, in particular, to the use of heroin and cocaine, and to the use of drugs in combination with alcohol. Data from 1987 indicated drug-related mortality to be 3.8 per 100,000.

The government is concerned not only about drug deaths, but also with the overall abuse of drugs. A decrease in drug abuse should decrease a range of health-related problems, including physical, social, mental, emotional, and spiritual components. In this regard, another national health objective seeks to check the

Year 2000 National Health Objective

Because data from 1987 indicated that drug mortality was 3.8 per 100,000 people, the original Year 1990 National Health Objective of 2 per 100,000 was unattainable. The Year 2000 National Health Objective is a more realistic goal of reducing drug-related deaths to 3 per 100,000 people.

Year 2000 National Health Objective

In 1988, 6.4 percent of those age 12 to 17 and 15.5 percent of those age 18 to 25 had used marijuana within the month prior to being polled. The Year 2000 National Health Objectives seek to cut those rates in half. Further, in 1988 1.1 percent of those age 12 to 17 and 4.5 percent of those age 18 to 25 used cocaine within a month of the survey. The year 2000 objectives seek to cut those rates in half as well.

increase of drug abuse. To achieve this objective, the government is encouraging the private sector, as well as various federal, state, and local governmental agencies, to educate and inform Americans—young Americans in particular—regarding drugs so that drug abuse levels will not exceed the 1988 rates.

What Is Drug Abuse?

On a sheet of paper, list the last ten times you can remember taking a drug. Your list probably includes an occasion when you were ill and took either a drug prescribed by a physician or one available "over-the-counter." Such remarks as "I took an aspirin when I had a headache last Tuesday," or "I took some antibiotics that were prescribed by my physician for a urinary tract infection" would fit into this category of drug taking. If used properly (for example, as recommended by a physician), drugs can be helpful. In fact, in some cases, physical harm might result if drugs were not used. If you contract pneumonia, for instance, and do not take the drugs prescribed for you, you may die. Drug use of this type is approved in our society.

The federal government is so concerned about the use of marijuana by college-age Americans that one of the Year 2000 National Health Objectives is directed at decreasing the use of that drug in this population.

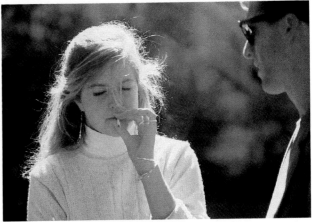

drug misuse The inappropriate and excessive use of pharmaceuticals and over-the-counter drugs in ways or in dosages not originally intended.

drug abuse When the use of drugs for either medical or recreational purposes results in physiological or psychological harm to the users or to others.

dosage The specific amount of a specific drug needed to produce a pharmacological effect.

potency A measure of a drug's pharmacological strength. The greater the potency, the smaller the dosage needed to produce an effect.

solubility A measure of the amount of a substance that can be dissolved in a given solvent under certain conditions.

Drug Misuse versus Drug Abuse

Some drugs, however, have useful purposes but are frequently used in ways they were not intended to be used. Aspirin is one of these. Some people swallow aspirin for every headache, muscle tension, pain, or other small discomfort. Prescription drugs are also frequently misused. For example, many people take a larger dosage than is indicated on the principle that, if two pills will help, three will really do the trick. We call this practice **drug misuse.**

Drug abuse is a more difficult concept than drug misuse. Whether the use of a drug constitutes abuse depends largely on how a society regards the drug at a particular time. In our culture, for example, people who use heroin to achieve a state of euphoria are considered abusers. But in some cultures, use of opium (the naturally occurring drug from which heroin is derived) is regarded as acceptable.

Drug abuse is often defined as use of drugs that are forbidden by law. According to this definition, in most states, people who use marijuana or minors who smoke cigarettes would be considered abusers. The important point is that what constitutes drug abuse depends on societal norms and attitudes at a particular time.

Nevertheless, to discuss the problems that can occur with drugs, we must at least try to define drug abuse. For the purposes of this discussion, we will use the following definition:

Drug abuse occurs when the use of drugs for either medical or recreational purposes results in physiological or psychological harm to the user or to others. Would you define drug abuse differently? If so, how? In what ways do your own values enter into your definition?

Now look again at your list of the last ten times you took drugs. Next to each item on your list write the word that best describes that episode: drug use, drug misuse, or drug abuse.

The symptoms of drug abuse may differ for different drugs. Table 10.1 indicates the most common symptoms that occur with the abuse of drugs.

FIGURE 10.1 • Trends in reported drug use in last 30 days for young adults age 18 to 25.

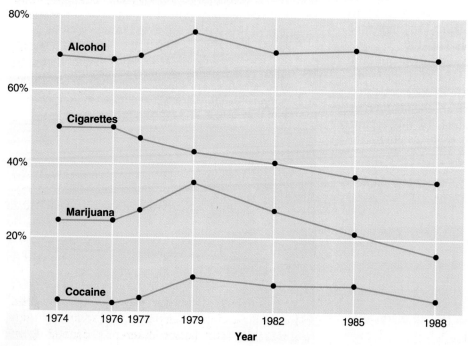

Factors Related to Drug Effects

Many factors influence the effects of drugs. It is useful to discuss some of these factors, so that you will be aware of them if you consider using particular drugs.

Interaction with Other Drugs

Two drugs that, when used together, have opposite effects on the body are said to be *antagonistic*. An amphetamine abuser taking barbiturates to come down from a high is employing antagonistic drugs.

When two drugs used together have a similar effect on the body, the physiological effects cannot be easily predicted because of a process called *synergism*. Synergism refers to the effect on the body of the two drugs taken together, which is greater than the sum of the effects of the two drugs ingested on separate occasions. For example, barbiturates ingested with alcohol have resulted in coma and death, whereas separate dosage of either would not have been lethal.

Dosage

A drug needs to be taken in certain amounts—or a **dosage**—in order to have an effect. Too small a dosage may have no effect; too high a dosage may be harmful. At a particular dosage, some drugs may be toxic or poisonous to the body. The dosage required depends on such factors as the user's size, metabolism, sensitivity to the drug, and the way it is administered.

Potency

A drug's **potency,** or "strength," also influences its effect. Potent drugs require small dosages for the effect

sought. Also, two drugs that are initially equal in potency may differ with subsequent use because one may have chemicals that are maintained within the body, whereas the other's chemicals are excreted from the body. A drug whose chemicals are stored within the body—for example, THC in marijuana—may result in the same effect as another drug but will require a lower dosage.

Solubility

The effects of some drugs may be diluted by the manner in which they are taken. **Solubility** refers to the amount of a substance that can be dissolved in a given solvent under certain conditions. For example, most water-soluble drugs—those that dissolve in water—cannot reach the brain, because their molecules are blocked by what is termed the blood-brain barrier. (Alcohol, however, is an exception.) Fat-soluble drugs, in contrast, can reach the brain, because they can penetrate cell walls, which are composed largely of fat. Most psychoactive drugs are fat-soluble.

Location of Action in the Body

Certain drugs act upon certain sites within the body. For example, some antibiotics are termed broad-spectrum—that is, they act throughout the body, whereas other antibiotics act on only one site.

Individual Response

As noted before, the same dosage of a drug can affect different people in different ways, according to weight, height, body fat, and metabolism. In addition, drugs may affect the same person differently, depending on

TABLE 10.1

Terms and Symptoms of Drug Abuse

This chart indicates the most common symptoms of drug abuse. However, all of the signs are not always evident, nor are they the only ones that may occur. Any drug's reaction will usually depend on the person, his mood, his environment, the dosage of the drug, and how the drug interacts with other drugs the abuser has taken or contaminants within the drug.	Slang Terms	Symptoms of Abuse										
		Drowsiness	Excitation and Hyperactivity	Irritability and Restlessness	Belligerence	Anxiety	Euphoria	Depression	Hallucination	Panic	Irrational Behavior	Confusion
Morphine	M, dreamer, white stuff, hard stuff, morpho, Miss Emma, monkey	■				■	■		■			
Heroin	H, snow, junk, horse, dope, smack, skag	■				■	■					
Codeine	Schoolboy	■					■					
Hydromorphone	Dilaudid, Lords	■					■					
Meperidine	Demerol, Isonipecaine, Dolantol, Pethidine	■					■		■			
Methadone	Dolophine, Dollies, dolls, amidone	■					■					
Exempt preparations	P.G., P.O., blue velvet (paregoric with antihistamine), red water, bitter, licorice	■					■					
Cocaine/Crack	The leaf, dynamite, gold dust, coke, flake, speedball (when mixed with heroin), rock		■	■		■	■		■		■	
Marijuana	Smoke, weed, grass, pot, Mary Jane, joint, reefer, tea, hash, roach	■	■				■		■	■	■	■
Amphetamines	A's, pep pills, bennies, uppers, whites		■	■		■	■					
Methamphetamine	Speed, meth, splash, crystal, methedrine, crank, ice		■	■		■	■					
Other stimulants	Pep pills, uppers		■	■		■	■					
Barbiturates	Yellow jackets, reds, seccy, pink ladies, blues, red and blues, barbs, phennies	■			■			■			■	■
Other depressants	Candy, goofballs, sleeping pills	■			■			■			■	■
Lysergic acid diethylamide (LSD)	Acid, cubes, sugar, instant Zen			■		■	■		■	■	■	■
STP	Serenity, tranquility, peace, DOM, syndicate acid			■		■	■		■	■	■	■
Phencyclidine (PCP)	PCP, peace pills, synthetic marijuana	■		■		■			■	■	■	■
Peyote	P, Mescal button, cactus, Mesc.		■			■	■		■		■	■
Psilocybin	Sacred mushrooms, mushroom		■			■	■		■		■	■
Dimethyltryptamine (DMT)	DMT, 45-minute psychosis, businessman's special		■			■	■		■		■	■

Source: Bureau of Narcotics and Dangerous Drugs.

TABLE 10.1

	Symptoms of Withdrawal	Dangers of Abuse*	How Taken

Column headers (left to right):

Talkativeness · Rambling Speech · Slurred Speech · Laughter · Tremor · Staggering · Impairment of Coordination · Dizziness · Hyperactive Reflexes · Depressed Reflexes · Increased Sweating · Constricted Pupils · Dilated Pupils · Unusually Bright Shiny Eyes · Inflamed Eyes · Runny Eyes and Nose · Loss of Appetite · Increased Appetite · Insomnia · Distortion of Space or Time · Nausea and Vomiting · Abdominal Cramps · Diarrhea · Constipation · Physical Dependence · Psychological Dependence · Tolerance · Convulsions · Unconsciousness · Hepatitis · Psychosis · Death from Withdrawal · Death from Overdose · Possible Chromosome Damage · Orally · Injection · Sniffed · Smoked

* One of the most significant dangers facing drug abusers today is AIDS. Not only is the AIDS-causing HIV virus passed between drug users who share intravenous needles or who are sexual partners, it is also passed between people who sell and buy drugs in exchange for sexual acts. The AIDS danger applies potentially to all the drugs listed in this table.

physical dependence Physiological changes in an individual that result in a physical need for a particular drug.

withdrawal syndrome Physiological changes that occur when the physical need (physical dependence) for a particular drug is denied.

psychological dependence The habit, or keenly felt need, for a particular drug, without necessarily the physical dependence on it.

tolerance A measure of the tendency of an individual to need more and more of a drug, that is, a higher dose, to achieve a given effect.

Therapeutic Index A measure of a drug's safety as based on testing to determine its lethal dosage and its effective dosage.

over-the-counter (OTC) drugs Drugs that can be purchased at a pharmacy without a prescription.

---

the setting in which the drug is taken. For example, drinking with friends at a baseball game may produce a different effect than drinking alone. Further, your mood can affect how you'll react to a drug. A depressed person may become more depressed on a drug, a happy person happier. Finally, the expectations you have about a drug, based on prior experience, can affect your response.

Drug Dependence and Tolerance

Some drugs cause physical dependence. Sometimes termed addiction, **physical dependence** refers to physiological changes that result in a physical need for the drug. Should this need not be satisfied, the body may experience what we call the **withdrawal syndrome,** a complex of symptoms, including severe discomfort, pain, nausea, vomiting, and convulsions. These symptoms sometimes even result in death. Withdrawal from barbiturates, for instance, is very dangerous, and the abuser who goes "cold turkey" without being under a physician's care is taking a serious risk.

Other drugs create a **psychological dependence.** Sometimes referred to as a habit, psychological dependence means that, in the absence of the drug, the person misses it deeply, though no physical symptoms are present. LSD, for example, does not result in physical dependence or withdrawal symptoms when it is not available. It does, however, provide a feeling that is so desired by abusers that they rely on it to feel good or to be stimulated. The inability to obtain this drug is a real loss for such persons.

Related to physical and psychological dependence upon drugs is the need to take increasingly larger doses. The body builds up a **tolerance** to many kinds of drugs. A heroin addict, for example, might not get the same high feeling ("rush") on the amount of heroin that once provided it; a larger dose is needed. Some drugs seem to work in the opposite manner and are said to develop *reverse tolerance* in the user. Marijuana was thought to be one such drug. It was believed that, as an individual smoked more and more marijuana, that person would need less of it to get "high." We know now that marijuana does not result in a reverse tolerance and that the early high by experienced mari-

juana users has been related to their learning how to get high rather than to the drug's effect on the body. Alcohol, however, does create a reverse tolerance in the latter stages of addiction. In other words, it takes less alcohol for an alcoholic to get drunk in the latter stages of alcoholism than in the early stages.

The Therapeutic Index

The safety of a drug is calculated by determining its **Therapeutic Index.** To employ the index, pharmacologists spend a good deal of time, money, and effort testing drugs to determine their lethal and effective dosages. The Lethal Dose for 50 percent of test animals (termed the LD-50 dose) and the Effective Dose for 50 percent of the population (termed the ED-50 dose) are used in the calculation of the Therapeutic Index. The Therapeutic Index, then, consists of the following formula: LD-50 Dose/ED-50 Dose. Any drug's safety can be evaluated once you know this index and the components appropriate for that particular drug.

The practical implications of the Therapeutic Index is that some drugs are much more powerful than other drugs and, therefore, need to be prescribed in smaller dosages to be safe.

Another implication of the Therapeutic Index relates to the safety of drugs of abuse. It is impossible to evaluate the safety of a drug whose lethal and effective dosages have not been determined (for example, illegal drugs of abuse purchased on the streets or in other uncontrolled settings). It stands to reason then that the safety of drugs of abuse cannot be assured because not enough information regarding their lethal and effective dosages is available to the user.

The Effectiveness of Common Over-the-Counter (OTC) Drugs

We all use drugs that we purchase at pharmacies without prescriptions. These are called **over-the-counter (OTC) drugs.** We will discuss some of the more common of these and what we know about their effectiveness.

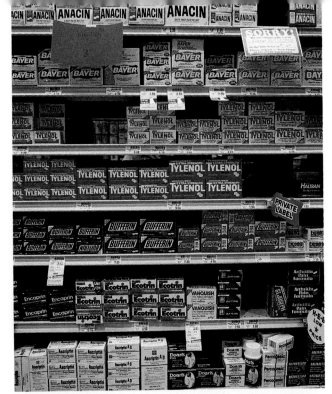

When you have pain or fever, there are several products from which you can choose. Some of these products alleviate inflammation and others do not. Some decrease fever and others do not. Make sure you choose the right product for your condition.

Aspirin Is Aspirin

Any brand of aspirin is effective in providing some relief from fever, aches, grippe, flu, and tension headaches. *Aspirin* is a white, crystalline powder which is chemically called acetylsalicylic acid. In 1899, H. Dreser, a German chemist, found that this acid could be compounded without *spirea*, the plant in which the acid naturally occurs. Dreser therefore named this manufactured acetylsalicylic acid "aspirin" (literally: "without spirea"). Although all aspirin is essentially the same substance, some name brand aspirins contain additional substances ("buffers") that may help make the aspirin easier on your stomach by neutralizing some of the acid. To save money, ask your druggist for the least expensive generic aspirin. Using any of the highly advertised products will only divest you of a little more money.

Aspirin works by reducing the level of a substance called prostaglandin E, a natural hormonelike substance in the body. This substance increases the sensitivity of the body's pain receptors. With less prostaglandin E, pain receptors become less sensitive and pain is relieved. In addition, aspirin reduces fever by both increasing perspiration and increasing the blood flow to the skin. Both of these changes result in heat loss from the body and, thereby, a reduction in body temperature. Finally, aspirin also thins out the blood, thereby helping to reduce the accumulation of harmful substances that can clog the blood vessels and lead to coronary heart disease.

Using Aspirin

Aspirin is the most commonly used medicine in the American household. Follow these suggestions for proper use:

- Avoid aspirin if you react with hives, swelling of mucous membranes, or asthma.

- If you suffer stomach upset from taking aspirin, take it immediately after eating, and always drink a full glass of water with each dose.

- Discard aspirin that has been in your medicine cabinet longer than two or three months. High humidity and moisture cause a chemical decomposition of the tablets. If aspirin have a vinegary odor or crumble when held between the fingers, discard them immediately. In this condition, they are less effective and much more likely to irritate the stomach.

- Avoid purchasing special-flavored children's aspirin. Any medicine that tastes like candy increases the risk of aspirin poisoning.

- Avoid using aspirin for extended periods without medical supervision. See a physician if symptoms continue for more than ten days (five days in children under twelve) or if new symptoms develop.

- Read the label carefully and follow directions.

- Avoid aspirin if you are allergic to it or if you have ulcers or a bleeding problem.

- Seek medical assistance immediately if you experience any bleeding or vomiting of blood after taking aspirin.

- Avoid administering aspirin-containing products to a child who has cold or flu symptoms or chicken pox. Give the child acetaminophen instead (see the next section). Some children who are given aspirin appear to be more likely to develop *Reye's syndrome*. This is an acute illness in children up to twelve years of age that often follows the flu or other viral infection and affects the upper respiratory tract. Vomiting, progressive damage to the central nervous system, and fatty liver symptoms may occur, with 30 percent of the victims dying from cerebral damage.

In addition to its ability to decrease fever and inflammation, aspirin taken daily has been found effective when used with people who have experienced a heart attack to prevent a second heart attack. The thinning of the blood that results from aspirin use is believed to be the reason for this effect. The preventive nature of aspirin has also been verified. An article in the January 28, 1988, issue of the *New England Journal of Medicine* reported a study that found an aspirin tablet every other day reduced the risk of heart attack by nearly 50 percent.[1] Research is presently being conducted to further validate the preventive benefits of aspirin.

expectorant A medication that causes an increase in the flow of respiratory tract secretions and facilitates the removal of irritating substances that cause coughing.

laxatives Substances that loosen feces in the bowels and relieve constipation.

Acetaminophen

Acetaminophen, the active ingredient in such brand name drugs as Tylenol, Allerest, Tempra, Anacin–3, and Datril, can substitute for aspirin in many instances. Acetaminophen and aspirin are similar in their abilities to lower a fever and reduce pain. Acetaminophen, however, has not been associated with Reyes syndrome and is therefore the drug of choice for children. The disadvantage of acetaminophen is that it is not effective in reducing inflammation, whereas aspirin is. In using acetaminophen, follow the dosage recommendations. This is very important, because acetaminophen has the potential to cause severe liver damage if too large an amount is ingested.

Ibuprofen

Ibuprofen—marketed under brand names such as Advil, Nuprin, and Mediprin—works like aspirin and acetaminophen by inhibiting production of prostaglandins. In particular, ibuprofen inhibits prostaglandins in the uterus, recommending its use to alleviate menstrual cramps. Unlike acetaminophen, ibuprofen reduces inflammation as well as fever and is less toxic than aspirin.

Although ibuprofen causes fewer side effects than does aspirin, recent concern for its misuse has developed. If used repeatedly, in too high a dosage, ibuprofen can cause itching, skin rash, stomach upset, and dizziness. It can also wear out the stomach lining and cause ulcers (cuts in the lining of the stomach and just outside the stomach). If an ulcer happens to appear where a major blood vessel is located, bleeding ulcers can result and, if severe enough, the loss of blood can even cause death. Obviously, as with all medications, if you are using ibuprofen make sure to follow the directions on the package that instruct how many tablets should be ingested at one time, how much time should elapse before taking another dose, and how many days you should take ibuprofen before consulting with your physician.

Ibuprofen should not be used by people with gout or ulcers, who are allergic to aspirin, who are younger than 14 years of age, or by women who are in the last trimester of a pregnancy.

Antacids

An *antacid* is any substance that neutralizes stomach acid. There are hundreds of antacids on the market to treat indigestion. Nothing is more effective than precipitated chalk (precipitated calcium carbonate U.S.P.), which can be purchased cheaply at any drugstore. If constipation occurs, use magnesium carbonate U.S.P. instead, or combined precipitated chalk with magnesium oxide U.S.P. Sodium bicarbonate (baking soda), a common home remedy, is proven safe and effective for indigestion if used sparingly. The closer a product is to a simple antacid, the more effective it is. If you purchase antacid tablets, make sure you suck or chew them thoroughly so that they are dissolved in the stomach before moving into the small intestine.

Sleep Aids

All people have difficulty sleeping at times. Sleeplessness is often caused by tension or stress; only rarely is it caused by some physical disorder. There is no evidence that lack of sleep by itself is detrimental to health. Even people who have been deprived of sleep for long periods suffer no long-term ill effects once they are permitted to sleep again. Nevertheless, many people believe that if they lose sleep, their functioning will be impaired. Thus, they respond to occasional sleeplessness by using over-the-counter sleep remedies.

These nonprescription sleep aids contain small amounts of antihistamine and a painkiller (aspirin). Used infrequently, they offer little danger, providing the user follows directions and does not take stronger doses than are recommended. Overuse of sleep preparations containing antihistamines can produce side effects such as dizziness, lack of coordination, blurred vision, skin rashes, and possibly blood changes. If loss of sleep is only occasional, medication is not recommended. If it becomes chronic, a physician should be consulted because the condition may indicate other problems, such as stress or depression.

Cough Medicine

Coughing is a reflex action controlled by a cough center in the brain. It is nature's response to irritation

Checklist for Correct Drug Use

Drugs can kill! Even safe drugs, when taken incorrectly, can be dangerous. However, following the directions below should result in your using OTC drugs or prescribed drugs effectively and safely. Remember, altering the state of your body or mind with drugs is serious business. Read these directions carefully.

✓ Never mix two or more medications without consulting a physician or a pharmacist. Only an expert can evaluate the effects of synergistic and antagonistic drugs.

✓ Never take prescription drugs unless they are specifically prescribed by a physician for a particular ailment. Drugs prescribed for one illness should not be taken for another without consulting a physician.

✓ Make sure you know which medications you are allergic to and keep away from them.

✓ Never drink alcoholic beverages while on medication.

✓ Keep all your medication out of reach of children and preferably in a locked cabinet.

✓ Remember that too much of a good thing might be a bad thing. Know the proper dosage and adhere to it. This will tend to limit any negative side effects.

✓ Don't take any medication continually unless it's recommended by a physician.

✓ Remember to stop all medication until you consult a physician if you become pregnant. Most drugs will pass through the placenta to the fetus. This can sometimes affect the normal growth and development of the fetus.

✓ Ask the pharmacist for the generic rather than the brand name of a drug. The generic drug is the same but is often less expensive.

✓ When taking prescription drugs, don't discontinue use when you start feeling better. For example, if you stop using an antibiotic before you've taken the whole dosage, the infection may reappear.

✓ Don't use someone else's prescription medication.

✓ Ask your doctor or pharmacist about the side effects associated with any drug you are thinking of using.

in the respiratory tract or pleural lining of the lungs. Coughing is often caused by the common cold and can also be associated with a bacterial infection, pneumonia, and tuberculosis.

More than a hundred over-the-counter remedies are available to the consumer. Medication for coughs come in several different forms. Some medications actually depress the cough center in the brain. These are called *suppressants* or *antitussives.* Codeine, which is only available with a prescription, and dextromethorphan, which is contained in some over-the-counter cough medications, are examples of cough suppressants.

Other cough medications increase the flow of respiratory tract secretions that facilitate the removal of the irritating substances causing the cough. These medications are called **expectorants.** Expectorants also soothe tissues irritated by coughing. Physicians recommend expectorants when the cough is accompanied by large amounts of fluid and when phlegm is produced. Examples of commonly available expectorants are quaifenesin, ammonium chloride, and terpin hydrate. These substances are contained in many over-the-counter products that are advertised to provide relief from the symptoms of a cough.

You can take other actions to make a cough less bothersome. These actions do not involve drugs but can help soothe irritated tissue. For example, sucking on hard candies or cough drops, swallowing hot drinks, or using a vaporizer to moisten the air breathed into the air passages can lessen the discomfort of a cough (cool-mist vaporizers and hot-steam ones are equally effective in relieving irritation).

If a cough persists longer than seven to ten days, a physician should be consulted.

Nasal Decongestants

Many people use nasal decongestants for stuffiness related to colds and allergy. Nasal *decongestants* shrink small swollen blood vessels inside the nose. As the decongestant effect wears off, these capillaries begin to swell once again. A rebound nasal congestion may occur that is actually worse than the original stuffiness, and a vicious cycle is in effect, with the decongestant bringing on the very symptoms it was supposed to eliminate.

Labels on all decongestants warn against use for more than three days, yet the typical container has 0.5 fluid ounces, enough for three or four weeks. Unfortunately, many people ignore this warning. Many severe sufferers greatly exceed the recommended maximum use of twice per day. Breaking the habit requires withdrawal over a period of several weeks. If this procedure doesn't work, an ear, nose, and throat specialist can provide special medication and advice.

Laxatives

Makers of **laxatives**—substances that loosen feces in the bowels and relieve constipation—try to convince us that we all need a laxative from time to time. This is certainly not true. In fact, bowel habits vary greatly from one person to another. A movement once or twice a day may be common for one individual, whereas once every three days may be perfectly normal for another. Constipation is generally not accompanied by stomach pain. If you skip a day, this is not necessarily an indication that constipation is developing. For occasional, temporary constipation, a laxative is not needed. If an uncomfortable feeling persists, a very mild laxative, such as milk of magnesia, may be used. For chronic constipation, add roughage to your diet (fruits, vegetables, whole grain cereals), drink plenty of fluids, and see your physician.

caffeine A common stimulant drug found in many foods, drinks, and medications, including coffee, tea, soft drinks, and over-the-counter drugs.

amphetamines A powerful stimulant drug with dangerous side effects and addictive qualities; found in pharmaceuticals and in illegal drug compounds.

crank The street name for the pill form of a common methamphetamine.

ice A highly addictive methamphetamine that is even more potent than crank.

cocaine A highly dangerous and illegal stimulant-type drug with serious side effects and addictive properties. It has been a very commonly used drug in the past decade and is found in various forms with various street names.

Psychoactive Drugs

Drugs that affect the central nervous system (the brain and the spinal cord) are called *psychoactive drugs*. Generally speaking, these drugs can be categorized as stimulants, depressants, psychedelics, or hallucinogens. These categories will be discussed briefly, in order to give you a general familiarity with them. Consult Table 10.1 for more information about these drugs.

Stimulants

Stimulants are psychoactive drugs that stimulate the central nervous system and cause blood vessels to dilate, thereby speeding up body processes. Three of them are caffeine, amphetamines, and cocaine.

Caffeine
The drug **caffeine** is present in coffee, tea, and cola drinks, as well as in some other soft drinks. For example, a toddler who drinks a six-ounce glass of Sunkist orange soda is consuming the equivalent, by body weight, of one cup of coffee for an adult. In response to society's new emphasis on health, soft drink companies have successfully marketed caffeine-free sodas. However, caffeine is also present in some medications; one dose of Excedrin contains as much caffeine as two cups of instant coffee.

Depending on the amount consumed, caffeine can increase heartbeat, stomach acid, and production of urine. Excessive caffeine consumption (six cups of coffee or a six-pack of cola a day) can lead to disturbed sleep, irritability, nervousness, irritation of the stomach, diarrhea, and headache. The chronic use of caffeine is now usually referred to as caffeine intoxication or *caffeinism*. However, some evidence suggests that even moderate amounts of caffeine are harmful.

Amphetamines
The use of **amphetamines** speeds up the body processes so the user feels more energetic, alert and active. These drugs can also cause irritability, restlessness, anxiety, depression, and high blood pressure. Amphetamines are sometimes precribed for hyperactive (hyperkinetic) children, but this treatment of hyperkinesis is controversial. Although they curb appetite, amphetamines are no longer used as diet pills because of their potentially harmful side effects.

Crank and Ice
When the government began cracking down on amphetamine usage in the 1970s, people who used amphetamines for dieting, staying awake on long drives or long job shifts, as well as for getting "high" found a new and cooperative—though illegal—source in laboratories that manufacture *methamphetamines*, more powerful variations on amphetamines. Two such illicit stimulants are called crank and ice.

Crank is the street name for the pill form of a common methamphetamine. Although the most common forms of methamphetamine are injected, crank seems to have gained a wide popularity among truck drivers and other workers who must stay awake for long periods of time. In the late 1980s, many people feared that crank would become a new, widespread drug "fad." Although it is popular in some parts of the country, this fear seems unwarranted at the moment.

An even newer and scarier stimulant that appeared in the United States only a few years ago is **ice**. A highly addictive drug that is even purer than crank, ice can be manufactured in a simple laboratory using chemicals that are easily obtainable. Ice is also inexpensive and, when smoked, a small amount is enough to keep a person in highs for as long as a week. Addicts call the euphoric feeling they get from smoking ice "amping."

However, there is nothing euphoric about the long-term effects of methamphetamines. Drugs like crank and ice can cause fatal kidney and lung damage as well as major psychological difficulties, including highly aggressive behavior, that have been shown to last up to two and a half years after use has stopped.

Cocaine
The drug **cocaine,** which is also called "coke," "blow," "nose candy," or "snow," is derived from the coca plant found in Central and South America. Cocaine was once an ingredient in Coca Cola but is no longer legal in the United States, except as a topical anesthetic. Cocaine is usually sniffed through the nose but is sometimes injected intravenously or smoked;

| TABLE 10.2 | | | |

Use of Cocaine by American Youths: 1974–1988

Age and Year	Percent Who Used Cocaine:		
	Ever	Last Year	Last Month
18 to 25 years:			
1989	19.7	12.1	4.5
1985	25.2	16.3	7.6
1982	28.3	18.8	6.8
1979	27.6	19.6	9.3
1974	12.7	8.1	3.1
12 to 17 years:			
1989	3.4	2.9	1.1
1985	4.9	4.0	1.5
1982	6.5	4.1	1.6
1979	5.4	4.2	1.4
1974	3.6	2.7	1.0

Source: National Institute on Drug Abuse, *Highlights: 1988 National Household Survey on Drug Abuse,* (Washington, D.C.: NIDA, 1989).

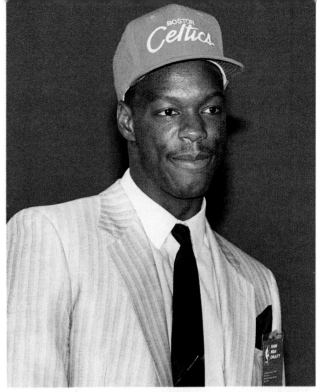

Even the most healthy of bodies can be placed in serious danger when confronted with cocaine use. Len Bias was a well-conditioned, All-American college basketball player who died right after being selected as the first player chosen in the NBA draft. His dream to be a Boston Celtic player was tragically short-circuited by his death from cocaine use.

and it is even eaten mixed into food on occasion. The high from cocaine is almost immediate, peaks within thirty to sixty minutes, and usually disappears within a few hours.

The use of cocaine has decreased in recent years after it had dramatically increased from the 1970s to the 1980s. In 1985, 5.8 million Americans reported using cocaine within the previous month. In 1988, that number was down to 2.9 million. In 1985, 12.2 million Americans reported using cocaine during that year. In 1988, that number had decreased to 8.2 million. Although these decreases are encouraging, there are still large numbers of Americans using a very dangerous drug. As noted in Table 10.2, about 25 percent of college-age people have used cocaine at some time in their lives, 16 percent used it last year, and almost 8 percent used cocaine in the last month. These figures for college-age people have remained fairly constant since 1979 when they increased dramatically.

Cocaine has both psychological and physiological consequences. Sniffing regularly can result in a constant running nose, burns and sores on the nasal membranes, sore throat, and hoarseness. Tremors may also occur. Use of cocaine speeds up the heart rate (tachycardia) and can be dangerous for even a fit person. This fact was dramatically evidenced by basketball player

Len Bias who, after being drafted by the Boston Celtics, celebrated by sniffing cocaine with some friends. Bias convulsed and soon died of heart failure. New studies also indicate that cocaine can bring on acute high blood pressure, causing strokes. In addition, cocaine diminishes one's appetite with the potential to lead to malnutrition and lowered immune system defenses. Psychologically, cocaine can result in confusion, anxiety, or depression. Cocaine users are sometimes referred to as "coked out" when they exhibit these symptoms. They can become short-tempered and grow suspicious of friends, loved ones, and co-workers. In a few cases, a "cocaine psychosis" has developed in heavy users, in which the person experiences delusions, may become paranoid, and often reacts violently.

Freebasing When cocaine is smoked, it is called *freebasing*. Freebase cocaine is the purified base form of cocaine processed from the hydrochloride salt using volatile chemicals, usually ether. Freebase is increasingly popular in spite of its being very dangerous. In 1982, almost 7 percent of clients admitted to drug treatment facilities were freebasing cocaine, up from 1 percent in 1979. Of the almost 200,000 drugs related to hospital emergency room visits reported to the National Institute on Drug Abuse's Warning Network in 1988, 26 percent involved cocaine; and about 25 percent of these were related to smoking cocaine. Freebase cocaine is smoked in a water pipe and reaches the

barbiturate A common depressant-type drug, found in pharmaceuticals and in illegal forms.

opiates Those drugs derived from opium, which comes from the opium poppy.

narcotics A term originally used to indicate several of the opiate or opiate-like drugs, including morphine, heroin, and codeine. The term "narcotic" is now used to indicate a wide variety of illegal drugs.

heroin A common, illegal, dangerous, and addictive opiate. Often injected by syringe, its use has contributed to the spread of AIDS and hepatitis.

marijuana The crushed leaves of the *cannabis sativa* or hemp plant, which contain the chemical tetrahydrocannabinol (THC), a depressant drug.

---

brain in seconds, resulting in a sudden and intense high. However, the high dissipates in a few minutes, resulting in the need to take more and more of the drug. Dependence on freebase quickly develops, and the dosage needed increases. Freebase can result in weight loss, increased heart rate and blood pressure, depression, paranoia, and hallucinations.

Crack Another form of cocaine is called "crack." "Crack" is the street name given to freebase cocaine that has been processed from hydrochloride to a base, using ammonia and baking soda and water (rather than the volatile ether) and heating it to remove the hydrochloride. It is called "crack" after the crackling sound that is heard when the mixture is smoked (heated). The use of crack also seems to be increasing in the United States. It is sold in small vials, in folding papers, or in heavy tinfoil. Crack results in such an intense high that its user can't stand when the "fireworks" stop. Consequently, they use more and more crack to obtain that high. It is the intense high that makes the crack habit so difficult to break.

Although "crack" is sometimes referred to as "rock," it should not be confused with "rock cocaine." "Rock cocaine" is a cocaine hydrochloride product that is designed for snorting, not smoking. It is white, and a dosage is about the size of a pencil eraser.

Because of its intense high, easy availability, and relatively low cost, crack use has become one of the most serious drug problems in the United States. Particularly threatened are inner-city communities of major cities, where crack babies (babies of crack-addicted mothers), crack houses (houses—often abandoned—where crack is exchanged for money or sexual acts), and crack-related crime have drawn intense media attention since crack first came on the scene in 1986. Those in trouble with cocaine can get help by telephoning the cocaine hotline at Fair Oaks Hospital in New Jersey at 1-800-COCAINE. The hotline operates twenty-four hours a day, and the call is free of charge.

Depressants

Depressants are drugs that lower the rate of activity in the central nervous system. Some common psychoactive depressant drugs are barbiturates, tranquilizers, and opiates.

Barbiturates Taken orally, **barbiturates** are used medically to induce sleep, relieve tension, and control epileptic seizures. These drugs are fat soluble and are consequently absorbed into the fatty tissue of the brain. Used on a short-term basis, barbiturates can reduce anxiety and produce euphoria. They do this by generally slowing down bodily functions. Consequently, they are referred to as "downers." Over the long term, however, they are physically addictive. Severe withdrawal symptoms, including convulsion, psychosis, and even death, can occur when the drugs are no longer taken. Consequently, barbiturates can only be legally obtained with a prescription, and those withdrawing from barbiturate dependence are advised to seek medical assistance.

Major and Minor Tranquilizers Before tranquilizing drugs were made available in the 1950s, severe forms of mental illness were much more difficult to treat. There was no effective way to calm patients so they could profit from psychotherapeutic counseling. With the availability of *major tranquilizers,* such as chlorpromazine (Thorazine), the management of mental illnesses, such as schizophrenia, became somewhat easier. The *minor tranquilizers,* which include such drugs as diazepam (Valium) and chlordiazepoxide (Librium), are used to treat anxiety and muscle tension. Long-term use of these tranquilizers may produce psychological and physiological dependence and withdrawal symptoms whenever their use is discontinued. Some experts believe the minor tranquilizers are overprescribed, whereas others believe these drugs are an important precursor to other forms of anxiety treatment.

Opiates The **opiates,** drugs that are synthesized from opium (a derivative of the opium poppy), include morphine, heroin, black tar heroin, and codeine. Generally known as **narcotics,** these drugs create both psychological and physiological dependence. Some drug experts call all natural and synthetic derivatives of opium *opioids,* while others reserve opioid for references to synthetic opiates such as methadone. The medical use of narcotic drugs has been debated every since morphine was first synthesized in the early 1800s. *Morphine* was administered to relieve pain but was often abused. As a result, the Harrison Narcotic Act of 1914 was passed to prohibit the nonmedical use of narcotics.

Heroin has no medically and legally approved use, although it too was once used to relieve pain. Heroin—either in the form of a white powder or as a black, sticky, and smelly substance called black tar heroin—is derived from morphine and was originally believed to be a nonaddictive pain reliever. However, it soon became known that heroin *is* addictive, that tolerance built up, and that discontinuance of heroin use could lead to severe withdrawal symptoms. Heroin can be injected just under the skin ("skin-popping") or intravenously ("mainlining"), smoked, eaten, or sniffed. Use of an unclean hypodermic needle can result in hepatitis or AIDS (Acquired Immune Deficiency Syndrome). Other effects of heroin are loss of appetite (and the accompanying illnesses and diseases associated with malnutrition), loss of sexual interest, and lethargy.

Codeine is a weaker painkiller than either morphine or heroin but can also be psychologically and physiologically addictive. It is medically prescribed on a short-term basis to relieve coughs and sometimes is injected to relieve pain. Most codeine is produced from morphine.

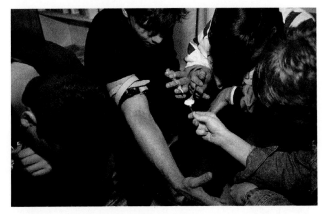

Not only is heroin dangerous and addicting, its use can also transmit AIDS and other diseases (for example, hepatitis) if contaminated needles are shared.

Marijuana

Marijuana is made from the crushed leaves and flowers of the *cannabis sativa* plant, which grows best in warm, moist climates. The common name for the marijuana plant found in India is hemp. The ingredient in marijuana that causes the psychoactive effect is *tetrahydrocannibinol (THC)*. THC can be taken into the body by smoking marijuana or by eating it. Although 66 million Americans have tried marijuana at least once, its use has decreased in recent years. As noted in Table 10.3, in 1979, 68.2 percent of college-aged Americans had tried marijuana at least once and 35.4 percent used

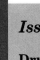

Issues in Health

Drug Abuse and AIDS

AIDS is discussed in detail in Chapter 14. However, since this is a fatal disease for which there is no known immunization or cure and since drug abusers are one of the high-risk groups for contracting AIDS, a brief mention of it appears in this chapter as well. AIDS is caused by a virus which is passed from person to person by the exchange of bodily fluids such as blood and semen. It results in the inability of the immunological system to combat threats to the body. Consequently, no one dies of AIDS *per se;* instead, they die from some other condition (such as pneumonia) that develops out of control because the immunological system can't protect the body. Drug abusers are at risk because of the habit of sharing hypo-dermic needles ("works"). When needles are shared, the AIDS virus may be passed from one addict's bloodstream to another's. Recognizing the threat that AIDS poses to our society—not only to drug abusers and homosexuals, but to all of us—governmental agencies have proposed various methods to prevent its spread. These proposals vary from traditional methods such as educating drug abusers about the dangers of sharing needles through media campaigns and the distribution of pamphlets to the more unusual. For example, Maryland appointed an AIDS advisory council to recommend actions to the governor; in 1987, that council recommended distributing free sterile syringes to intravenous drug abusers. This sort of response, which creates moral dilemmas while solving health problems, is not without controversy. In Maryland, the State Department of Health objected to the council's recommendation, arguing that it would be condoning drug abuse and would not be effective. The Health Commissioner of the District of Columbia was also opposed to the free distribution of sterile syringes, believing that it would send a "dangerous double message" to the drug community, and Washington, D.C. has a large drug-abusing community. How would you decide this issue if you were the Health Commissioner?

psychedelics A broad group of drugs that produce extreme changes in mood, behavior, and perception, sometimes causing hallucinations and other symptoms associated with mental illness.

hallucinogens A term used interchangeably with the term "psychedelics" to describe drugs that alter mood, behavior, and perception, and which sometimes cause hallucinations.

flashback A hallucination that occurs sometime *after* the use of a psychedelic or hallucinogenic drug, indicating that the drug has some sort of retroactive effect on the user.

phencyclidine (PCP) An illegal depressant drug that can act as a psychedelic with highly unpredictable and dangerous effects. It is sometimes falsely sold as THC, the active ingredient in marijuana, to unsuspecting users.

TABLE 10.3

Use of Marijuana by American Youths: 1974–1988

Age and Year	Percent that Used Marijuana:		
	Ever	Last Year	Last Month
18 to 25 years:			
1988	56.4	27.9	15.5
1985	60.3	36.9	21.8
1979	68.2	46.9	35.4
1974	52.7	34.2	25.2
12 to 17 years:			
1988	17.4	12.6	6.4
1985	23.6	19.7	12.0
1979	30.9	24.1	16.7
1974	23.0	18.5	12.0

Source: National Institute on Drug Abuse, *Highlights: 1988 National Survey on Drug Abuse*, (Washington, D.C.: NIDA, 1989).

---

it regularly. In 1980, 7.2 percent of college students used marijuana *daily*. If you were in high school during 1979, almost 31 percent of your classmates had tried marijuana at least once and almost 17 percent were using it regularly. In fact, in 1978, 11 percent of high school seniors reported *daily* use of marijuana. By 1988, experience with marijuana by college-aged Americans was down to 56.4 percent, with almost 16 percent using it on a regular basis; 17.4 percent of youth age 12 to 17 had at some time used marijuana, with 6.4 percent using it regularly. By 1989, only 3 percent of high school seniors reported *daily* marijuana use.

At doses commonly used, marijuana impairs memory, perception, judgment, and fine motor skills which increases the risk of accidents while performing such complex tasks as driving an automobile or operating machinery. In fact, marijuana use impairs driving ability a full four to six hours after smoking a single marijuana cigarette. If marijuana is used with alcohol, as is often the case, driving behavior will be even more erratic. Lung abnormalities suggestive of precancerous lesions have been found in marijuana users, although no instance of lung cancer has been solely attributed to marijuana use. As a matter of fact, there are more known carcinogens (cancer-causing chemicals) in marijuana smoke than in regular cigarettes. In addition, marijuana speeds up the heart rate and can raise blood pressure, may result in birth defects in babies whose mothers used marijuana during their pregnancy, and may lead to decreased effectiveness of the immunological system. Some of these effects are still under investigation to determine their prevalence and severity.

Marijuana also has beneficial outcomes. For people with high intraocular pressure in the eye, a condition known as glaucoma, marijuana use seems to decrease that pressure. It has even been prescribed on a regular basis to glaucoma patients. In addition, marijuana can alleviate nausea and vomiting caused by chemotherapy treatments that some cancer patients must endure; it has been studied as an adjunct to chemotherapy for these patients.

There are also psychological effects of marijuana use. Some researchers speak of marijuana users developing an "amotivational syndrome." This syndrome is characterized by apathy, loss of ambition, loss of effectiveness, diminished ability to carry out long-term plans, difficulty in concentrating, and a decline in school or work performance.[2] However, there is no widespread agreement as to the actual existence or extent of this syndrome; it may have more to do with preexisting personal and psychological factors.

Marijuana has also been referred to as the "gateway" to other drugs. That is, those who use marijuana heavily tend to move on to other more serious drugs. For example, 74 percent of those who have used marijuana one hundred or more times have tried cocaine.[3] However, the great majority of those who are not heavy users of marijuana never go on to other more serious drugs.

During the 1960s and into the 1970s, there

seemed to be sympathy for the legalization of marijuana use. Groups formed to lobby this cause, and many legislators were supportive. Several states passed laws decriminalizing marijuana; that is, it is now treated as a violation similar to a traffic ticket rather than as a crime. However, with more research validating the negative physiological effects of marijuana, the movement to legalize it has lost its momentum.

Psychedelics and Hallucinogens

Psychedelics and **hallucinogens** are a broad category that includes LSD and PCP, among others. All psychoactive drugs alter mood and behavior, but psychedelics are more likely than others to produce extreme alterations, such as hallucinations and feelings of paranoia.

LSD The drug *lysergic acid diethylamide (LSD)* was first synthesized in 1938 by Swiss chemist Albert Hoffman. Use of the drug peaked in the 1960s and 1970s after it was advocated as a means of enlightenment by such gurus as Timothy Leary, who was at the time a professor at Harvard University. As the "flower children" grew into adulthood and as the potential harmful effects of LSD became known, its use tapered off.

Taken in capsule or liquid form (sometimes poured on sugar cubes), LSD results in excitation, anxiety, euphoria, distortion of perception, and hallucinations involving exotic colors, shapes, and images. The hallucinations have been reported to sometimes be very frightening, and some people experiencing "bad trips" act in a bizarre manner, even jumping out of a window to escape an image. In addition, some users report recurring hallucinations when the drug is no longer being used. This experience is called a **flashback.** Researchers have found that long-term use of LSD is related to chromosomal damage and birth defects, although the evidence is not conclusive. Other dangers include paranoid reactions, psychosis, and serious depression.

PCP Another psychedelic drug is **phencyclidine (PCP),** a white crystalline powder, soluble in water, which is used orally, smoked, injected, or sniffed. It is sold on the streets in tablets, capsules, or powders, or sprinkled on marijuana. PCP is actually a depressant, although in large doses it acts as a psychedelic. It is the active chemical in many street drugs sold as THC (the active chemical in marijuana) and is easily manufactured illicitly. Thus dosage levels and effects vary and are difficult to control.

Originally developed for medical use as an anesthetic (Sernyl), PCP was found to cause agitation, visual disturbances, delirium, increased heart rate, elevated blood pressure, poor speech, lack of muscular coordination, and dizziness. With large doses, convulsion and coma can occur. As a result, it is no longer used for human beings but is instead used as an anesthetic for animals.

Other effects of PCP include disturbances of memory, perception, concentration, and judgment, and, when used in large doses over a period of time, brain and nervous system damage. The drug can result in the development of long-lasting anxiety and depression, as well as psychosis and, in some cases, even death.

In 1989, 2.4 percent of high school seniors used PCP, with 1.4 percent reporting use during the previous month. Almost 4 percent of high school seniors in 1989 had used PCP at some time during their lives.

PCP users are often unaware that they have used the drug because, when it is sold on the street, it is almost always misrepresented, usually as THC. This problem, along with the harmful effects noted previously, make PCP an extremely dangerous drug.

Designer Drugs

Designer drugs are structural analogs (chemically identical except for one minor, insignificant difference) of substances already identified as illegal under the Controlled Substances Act. That is, because they are not structurally identical to drugs which are specified, their manufacture and distribution are not illegal.

Examples of types of designer drugs are the PCP analogs, the fentanyl analogs, the meperidine analogs, and the amphetamine and methamphetamine analogs.

PCP analogs are not widespread, although they do exist, and they result in similar reactions to PCP itself.

Fentanyl analogs have pharmacological properties similar to heroin or morphine. They also create addiction, as do heroin and morphine. Fentanyl analogs are known as "synthetic heroin," "China White," and "new heroin." These drugs have been known to cause many deaths, and, as a result, several of them have now been placed under the Controlled Substances Act, for example, alphamethylfentanyl and 3-methylfentanyl.

Meperidine, commonly known by its trade name, Demerol, is a narcotic drug. Two designer drugs that are structurally similar to meperidine—MPPP and PEPAP—can be even more dangerous than meperidine itself. It seems that an impurity formed during the manufacture of MPPP—called MPTP—has toxic effects on nerve cells and can result in irreversible brain damage.

Amphetamine and methamphetamine analogs are hallucinogenic and result in euphoric feelings. One of these designer drugs has received a great deal of publicity: 3,4-methylenedioxymetham-phetamine (MDMA). Commonly referred to as Ecstasy or Adam, MDMA is reported to be widely used on college campuses by students wishing to achieve a state of euphoria. However,

MDMA can result in confusion, depression, anxiety, and paranoia. It can also lead to muscle tension, nausea, blurred vision, faintness, chills, and sweating. In addition, MDMA increases heart rate and blood pressure. For these reasons, MDMA has been placed on the list of controlled substances as of July 1985. MDA is another amphetamine and methamphetamine analog. It has been found to be harmful to nerve cells.

Tables 10.4 and 10.5 depict the prevalence of drug experience among high school seniors and others. It should be noted that alcohol and cigarettes are more prevalent than any of the other drugs. We discuss these drugs—alcohol and cigarettes—in the chapters that follow.

TABLE 10.4

Percentage of High School Senior Drug Use (Class of 1988)

Drug	Ever used	Used in last 30 days	Used daily in last 30 days
Marijuana/hashish	47	18	2.7
Inhalants	17	3	0.2
Hallucinogens	9	2	0.0
Cocaine	12	3	0.2
Heroin	1	0	0.0
Other opiates	9	2	0.1
Stimulants	20	5	0.3
Sedatives	8	1	0.1
Tranquilizers	9	2	0.0
Alcohol	92	64	4.2
Cigarettes	66	29	18.1

Source: Lloyd D. Johnston et al., *Drug Use, Drinking, and Smoking: National Survey Results From High School, College, and Young Adult Populations* (Rockville, Md.: Alcohol, Drug Abuse, and Mental Health Administration, 1989).

TABLE 10.5

Percent of Drug Usage

Drug	Age 12–17 ever/last month	Age 18–25 ever/last month	Age 26+ ever/last month
Marijuana/hashish	24/12	60/22	27/6
Hallucinogens	3/1	11/2	6/0
Cocaine	5/2	25/8	10/2
Heroin	0/0	1/0	1/0
Stimulants	6/2	17/4	8/1
Sedatives	4/1	11/2	5/1
Tranquilizers	5/1	12/2	7/1
Alcohol	56/31	93/71	89/61
Cigarettes	45/15	76/37	80/33

Source: National Institute on Drug Abuse, *National Household Survey on Drug Abuse* (Washington, D.C.: U.S. Government Printing Office, 1988).

Anabolic Steroids

So you want to be strong and appear "tight?" So you want to run faster than you ever thought you could? Well, forget about all that work involved with weight training or exercise that makes you perspire. Try steroids. In today's quick-weight loss, quick-fitness, quick-everything society why not engage in quick-bulking up? Right? *Wrong!* The use of anabolic steroids subjects you to liver cancer, high blood pressure, heart disease, sterility, and increased hostility. In men it can lead to atrophied testicles, prostate cancer, and breast growth. In women it can lead to menstrual irregularities, a deepening of the voice, decreased breast size, baldness, and facial hair growth. In both men and women, it can lead to clogging of the arteries, eating compulsions, and increased aggressiveness. All of these side effects are possible even when the muscle enhancing effects have not been truly verified. In fact, the 1989 *Physician's Desk Reference*, the source doctors use for drug information, states that "anabolic steroids have not been shown to enhance athletic ability."

Anabolic steroids, as we saw in the last chapter's *A Question of Ethics* box, are derivatives of the male sex hormone testosterone. Steroids are prescribed as treatment for such conditions as anemia, growth problems, and as an aid in recovery from surgery. However, a black market has developed and steroids are illegally used to increase body weight and muscle mass, gain power, and increase speed. One of the most publicized users of steroids was Ben Johnson, the Canadian sprinter. Johnson had his Olympic gold medal stripped from him in the 1988 Olympic Games after testing positive for steroids. It is estimated that over a million Americans use steroids for nonmedical purposes. Steroid use is particularly prevalent on college campuses where the desire to look "strong" is pervasive.

Steroids can be taken in pill form or injected. It is not unusual for steroid abusers to take more than one steroid at a time, believing its effects will be hastened. This practice is called "stacking." Although the effects sought by muscle builders, athletes, and others may never be able to be verified—asking people to take a dangerous substance for research purposes is unethical —the harmful effects of steroids as described previously are clear. They have been documented in numerous case studies of people who have taken steroids illegally.

Causes of Drug Use, Misuse, and Abuse

Reasons for Use and Misuse

Drugs are often used socially and have sometimes become a part of the culture itself. Wine, for example, is used in certain religious ceremonies. Distilled beverages are consumed at cocktail parties, and beer is consumed at ballparks. These uses are generally accepted in our society.

The *misuse* of drugs is mainly a matter of ignorance. People misuse drugs either because they lack information concerning the drugs or their side effects, or because they do not carefully follow instructions concerning their use or dosage. An example of this would be mixing alcohol and a prescription drug because you don't realize this is dangerous.

Reasons for Abuse

The *abuse* of drugs is a different story. Although some drug abusers are ignorant of a drug's side effects, long-term hazards, and the legal consequences of using it, many are quite knowledgeable. There is clear evidence that knowledge alone has little effect on drug abuse. People abuse drugs for many and varied reasons. Still, researchers have been able to identify some of the reasons for some people's drug-related behavior.

Alienation As described in Chapter 2, alienation is composed of three subfactors: social isolation, powerlessness, and normlessness. People who have no "significant others," who feel unable to control their own destinies, and who have not accepted a set of standards for their behavior have been found to abuse drugs to a greater extent than those not so alienated.

Self-esteem Many drug education programs emphasize the development of a healthy sense of self-esteem rather than knowledge about drugs. The reason for this focus is that those who have a low regard for themselves have been found to abuse drugs to a greater degree than those with positive self-esteem.

Lack of Confidence Related to low self-esteem, lack of confidence is one reason for abuse of drugs. People who lack confidence can't relate well to others unless they are high. They get high at every party they attend and then, and only then, become the life of the party. Using drugs for confidence is only a temporary solution.

Peer Pressure It is reasonable to assume that people who have low self-esteem will not have a great deal of confidence in their own opinions and, consequently, will be unduly influenced by their peers. Many researchers have cited peer pressure as a factor in drug abuse, and it is the objective of some drug education programs to lessen the influence of this pressure in the decision-making process. The consequence of being excessively influenced by one's peers is that one is less able to be oneself.

Adult Modeling We learn adult behavior by observing adults and copying them. Some symbols of adulthood have special meaning to young people who want to feel adult. One of these symbols is having a job and earning money. Another is owning a car and being free to travel. A third is moving out of one's parents' house. Unfortunately, some "adult" behavior is unhealthy, but it too is copied. If children see parents using alcohol, they may imitate this behavior in order to feel adult. If parents misuse or overuse medication, children may also misuse it. Studies have indicated, for instance, that children whose parents smoke cigarettes have a greater tendency to be cigarette smokers than do children whose parents do not smoke.[4]

Coping Coping may take positive forms, such as making friends, getting a job, or acquiring a hobby, or it may take the form of drug abuse. Positive coping focuses on changing the *external* situation. But when drugs are used to cope, the goal is to change the *internal*

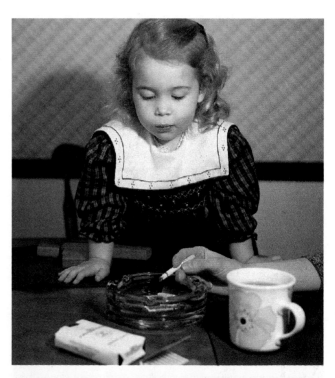

Children model their behavior on the adults in their lives. If these adults use drugs, it is likely that children who look up to them will also use drugs.

environment so the situation doesn't seem as bad. However, when the effects of the drug wear off, the situation remains unchanged and the problem unsolved. There are situations in which changing the internal environment may be the only solution. For example, terminally ill people have been given LSD or marijuana to relive pain or psychological suffering. In most instances, however, the temporary nature of the drug's effect does not argue for its use. Either more drugs would be needed or the problem would reappear.

Mood Alteration Some people abuse drugs for the psychological high they provide. The mellow feeling obtained from some drugs, the excitation from others, and the feeling of invincibility from still others lead some people to seek this experience over and over again. For them, the high is everything.

Exploring Your Health 10.3

Addictive Personalities

Place a check mark alongside each of the following statements with which you agree:

_____ 1. I am easily bored.

_____ 2. I vomit often.

_____ 3. I often got into trouble with the principal in grade school.

_____ 4. I sweat easily.

_____ 5. I believe in the second coming of Christ.

_____ 6. I enjoy reading crime news.

_____ 7. I have had periods when I couldn't remember what I'd done.

_____ 8. I enjoy a game more when I can bet on it.

_____ 9. I enjoy big noisy parties.

_____ 10. I stole things as a child.

Addicts and potential addicts tend to agree with these statements more often than others.* In addition, addicts tend to:

• Be impulsive.

• Be risk takers.
• Be outgoing and sociable (but superficial in interpersonal relationships).
• Have high-energy and high-activity levels.
• Often feel empty and meaningless.
• Usually make a good first impression.
• See themselves as leading unsuccessful lives.
• Often look for excitement and stimulation.
• Have problems with authority.

*Don Oldenburg, "The Addictive Personality," *The Washington Post* (June 30, 1982): B5.

Treating Drug Addiction

It is very difficult to determine the most effective method of treatment for drug abuse. The circumstances differ widely from one addict to another. Each addict brings to whatever treatment is being considered his or her own level of motivation to get off drugs. Also, addicts differ in background and in situation. Some are fortunate, in that they will receive a great deal of family support; others receive none. The financial resources available to treatment programs also vary, and community support services range from generous to nonexistent.

Several approaches to the rehabilitation of drug addicts follow.

Therapeutic Communities

These communities are designed to house drug addicts trying to kick the habit. They try to meet the addicts' needs (except, of course, drugs) and provide counseling, medical care, and gainful work. They try to instill in community members a sense of personal and social responsibility. Ex-addicts reside within these communities until they are ready to be eased back into society. Some examples of therapeutic communities are the Delancey Street Family in San Francisco, Phoenix House in New York City and elsewhere, and Daytop Village in New York City.

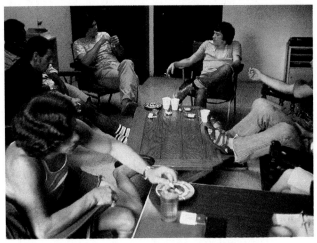

Drug rehabilitation communities bring drug abusers and health care professionals together so that they can work intensively toward the goal of a drug-free life for the drug abuser.

Therapy Combined with Medical Help

For those fortunate enough to be able to afford it or whose health insurance will cover its cost, psychological counseling, accompanied by medical care, is available. Former First Lady Betty Ford received this sort of help for her dependence on alcohol and other unspecified drugs as an in-patient in a hospital. Out-patient counseling services are also available at many hospitals and have the advantage of allowing the patient to re-

methadone A synthetic drug developed during World War II that is used to treat heroin addiction.

main with family and friends. Of course, for addicts who are negatively influenced by family and friends, counseling as an in-patient or joining a therapeutic community is recommended.

One setting in which counseling for drug-related problems can be effective is the workplace. Recognizing this potential, the federal government is seeking, through the national health objectives, to encourage at least 70 percent of major U.S. firms to provide substance abuse prevention and referral programs. A 1976 survey found that 50 percent of Fortune 500 firms offered some type of employee assistance program for substance abuse. By 1979, that number had increased to 57 percent. It appears that the government is making significant progress toward the achievement of this objective.

Pharmacological Support

Another method of treating addicts is to provide them either with the drug to which they are addicted (for example, heroin maintenance in England) or with a drug that will block the pleasurable effects of the drug to which they are addicted (for example, methadone maintenance or methadone withdrawal). The rationale behind providing drugs to drug addicts is that they will then not have to resort to crime to get the money to support their addiction. Methadone withdrawal programs are designed to wean the addict from a heroin addiction to a methadone addiction. **Methadone,** a synthetic drug developed during World War II, can then be withdrawn with less difficulty than heroin—at

least, that was the original thought. Recently, however, drug researchers have begun to question the value of methadone and to look for other drugs that will act in a similar way but with longer-lasting effects.

Get Involved!

The War on Drugs and You

At the time of this writing there is a declared "war on drugs." Considering yourself a soldier in that war, you can contribute to a successful outcome. Here are a few ideas to consider:

1.   You are influenced by your physician, but you also influence your doctor. For example, if you expect your doctor to prescribe medications every time something is wrong—the "miracle drug syndrome"—your doctor may feel pressured to recommend drug use more than is desirable. He or she may do so because of a concern for satisfying patients so that they will return to that practice when needing medical services. Your doctor also wants you to be satisfied so you will recommend friends and relatives to that medical practice when they need medical services. You can do your part by expressing to your doctor the attitude that medications should only be prescribed for you when they are clearly needed.

2.   Companies do not remain in business if their products do not sell. When someone buys drugs, that sale contributes to the demand side of the drug equation. You are either part of the problem because you buy drugs, or part of the solution because you do not! Which will you choose?

3.   Your campus health center or health education department may have peer drug education or peer drug counseling programs. Consider volunteering for one of those programs or suggest the idea for the development of such programs if they do not now exist. Usually you can acquire academic credit for participating, and you will be contributing to the elimination of the drug problem on your campus.

4.   Consider volunteering to coach a community team or working in a community center to assist your neighborhood in offering alternatives to drugs.

5.   Support politicians willing to fund the "war on drugs."

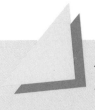

One such promising drug is cyclazocine; another is naltrexone.

Another method that has been tried is requiring addicts convicted of crimes to join rehabilitation programs. Community drop-in centers and telephone hotlines also have been developed. It is evident that no one method is a panacea. Rather, what is needed is a multimethod approach, with addicts somehow being directed to the treatment most appropriate for them.

Alternatives to Drugs

There are alternatives to drug abuse that will meet the needs of drug users. In order to choose one or more of these alternatives, however, you must know yourself.

Recalling how psychological and social factors influence our health behaviors (Chapter 2), can you now see why we sometimes adopt self-destructive behaviors to alleviate boredom or loneliness, impress friends, appear adult, and attain more self-worth? If we cannot assert our own needs, feel alienated from society, and perceive events affecting our lives as beyond our control, we may take drugs in spite of the physical harm we know we are risking. As with other health-related behavior, it is not enough for us to *know* about drugs

for us to adopt appropriate drug behavior. Certainly this knowledge is necessary and important. However, the psychosocial influences upon us are so pervasive and so strong that, in addition to the knowledge about drugs, we must have knowledge about ourselves—about our needs and motivations, our perceptions and philosophies, and our goals and desires. Only self-knowledge will allow us to make decisions that are right for us.

Such activities as meditation, exercise, yoga, sky diving, hang gliding, kiting, participation in religion, and social service are alternative ways to feel the "high" or "rush" that drugs provide—only in a health-enhancing manner. Some people get so involved in the Special Olympics, for example, that when they see the thrill on the faces of the young competitors, they feel high. Others find their work so absorbing that they feel a rush when they've accomplished a job-related goal. Still others report that the experience of learning a new skill or acquiring new knowledge is akin to a drug-induced state.

There are many alternatives to drugs that will hold appeal for you. The trick is to match one of these alternatives to your personality and needs. Only you can do that for yourself.

Conclusion

This chapter has presented information about types of drug-related behavior (use, misuse, and abuse), classification of drugs and their physiological effects, and reasons for the abuse of drugs. Whether to use drugs is not the question. Each of us probably ingests drugs, applies drugs to our skin, or has drugs injected into our bodies at one time or another. The question we must answer for ourselves is: Considering the presentation made in this chapter and all that we have learned elsewhere, and considering the validity of these sources, how and when will we use drugs? This question is of profound importance, should be given most serious consideration, and should be reconsidered periodically as health scientists learn more about drugs and their effects upon human beings.

Why not take some time *now* to contemplate your

drug-related behavior? Your instructor or staff at your campus health center might be good sources of help and information. If you wait until you're confronted with a situation necessitating a decision related to drugs, you may have to make a hasty decision, and a decision made hastily is more likely to be wrong for you than one well thought out.

Summary

1. A drug is any substance whose chemical nature alters structure or function in the living organism.

2. Americans tend to rely on drugs to relieve their anxious feelings, make them happier, and help them to relax.

3. Drug use involves a legal drug taken as recommended by a physician or approved by society. Drug misuse involves the improper use of prescribed or over-the-counter drugs. And drug abuse is the use of a chemical substance so as to cause the user serious physiological or psychological harm.

4. The effect of a drug depends on such factors as its interaction with other drugs, the dosage taken, its solubility, and its location of action within the body, and on such individual user characteristics as weight, height, body fat, and personality. In addition, the user's frame of mind and the setting in which the drug is taken affect its action.

5. People can learn to take care of minor health problems at home with a few basic medications used wisely. The conditions for which self-care are appropriate include colds, coughs, diarrhea, constipation, hemorrhoids, pain, fever, and stomach upset. Follow-up care is recommended for some of these conditions, but initially self-care is appropriate.

6. People can become dependent on drugs—psychologically, physiologically, or both. Physical dependence occurs as the user builds up a tolerance to the drug and needs increasingly larger doses to obtain a drug effect. When the drug is discontinued, withdrawal from physiological dependence may be marked by shaking, sweating, and convulsion, and may even lead to coma or death.

7. Psychoactive drugs can be classified as stimulants, depressants, psychedelics, or hallucinogens. Caffeine, amphetamines, and cocaine are examples of stimulant drugs. Barbiturates, tranquilizers, and the opiates are examples of depressant drugs. Marijuana, LSD, and PCP are examples of psychedelic or hallucinogenic drugs.

8. Drug abuse can be caused by alienation, poor self-esteem, lack of confidence, peer pressure, adult modeling, an attempt at coping, or a desire to seek mood alteration.

9. Drug abuse is treated in residential therapeutic communities, in nonresidential therapy programs combined with medical help, by providing pharmacological support (for example, methadone maintenance), or through a combination of these treatments.

10. Alternatives to getting high on drugs are involvement in family, religion, community service, hang gliding, sky diving, meditation, or some other means appropriate to the individual's personality and needs.

Questions for Personal Growth

1. When did you last take medication? Did you really need it? What would have happened if you did not take that medication?

2. When is the last time you used a drug (for example, alcohol) for recreational purposes? Who were you with? Where did that occur? Why did

you choose to use that drug; in other words, what were your motivations?

3. How similar is your drug-related behavior to your parents' and siblings' behavior? To your friends'? Do you want your children or your younger brother or sister to adopt similar drug-related attitudes and behavior? If so, why? If not, why not?

4. Which drugs have you decided not to use? Which of the following reasons for not using those drugs is most important to you: It's against the law? My family would not approve? It would affect my schooling or my job? It might harm my health? I would lose control? Any other reasons?

5. What would you say to a close friend—someone whose friendship you desperately want to maintain—who offered you drugs? What if he or she refuses to just allow you to say no? What would you do?

6. If you were asked to speak with a group of 10-year-olds about preventing drug abuse, what would you tell them? What do you wish someone told you when you were 10?

7. If you were the president of your college's student government, what would you recommend to limit the abuse of alcohol? Which groups and individuals would you involve in this campaign? Can you do that now even though you are not the president? Could you organize others on your campus to begin an alcohol education effort?

8. Numerous athletes and celebrities have recently admitted to alcohol abuse or abuse of other drugs. How many of those people can you name? Do you think they serve as good role models because they overcame drug abuse? Or do you think they are bad role models because they used drugs in the first place?

References

1. "Aspirin and the Heart," *Harvard Medical School Health Newsletter* 13 (1988): 7–8.

2. Ray Oakley and Charles Ksir, *Drugs, Society, and Human Behavior* (St. Louis: Times Mirror/Mosby, 1990), p. 339.

3. National Institute on Drug Abuse, "Marijuana," *NIDA Capsules* (August 1986): 2.

4. Ellen W. Bonaguro and John A. Bonaguro, "Tobacco Use Among Adolescents: Directions for Research," *American Journal of Health Promotion* 4 (1989): 37–41, 71.

CHAPTER 11

Using and Abusing Alcohol

CHAPTER OBJECTIVES

After reading this chapter, you should understand:

- Some of the research findings about the use and abuse of alcohol by various groups of people in the United States and why alcohol abuse remains a serious problem in this country.

- How alcohol travels through the body and why all forms of alcohol are really the same, whether it is in the form of beer, wine, or hard liquor.

- The immediate and long-term psychological and physiological effects of alcohol, including the consequences of combining alcohol with other drugs and the effects of alcohol on unborn children (fetal alcohol syndrome).

- What constitutes the responsible use of alcohol, some specific guidelines for serving and using alcohol, and the consequences of drinking and driving.

- The basic psychological and physiological factors and sociocultural correlates that contribute to alcoholism, the stages in the development of alcoholism, and the effects and treatment of alcoholism.

CHAPTER OUTLINE

Alcohol in American Society

Alcohol's Trip Through the Body

Psychological and Physiological Effects of Alcohol

Using Alcohol Responsibly

The Tragedy of Alcoholism

This chapter was written by Dr. Lawrence A. Cappiello, State University of New York at Buffalo, and John G. Rousselle, D'Youville College.

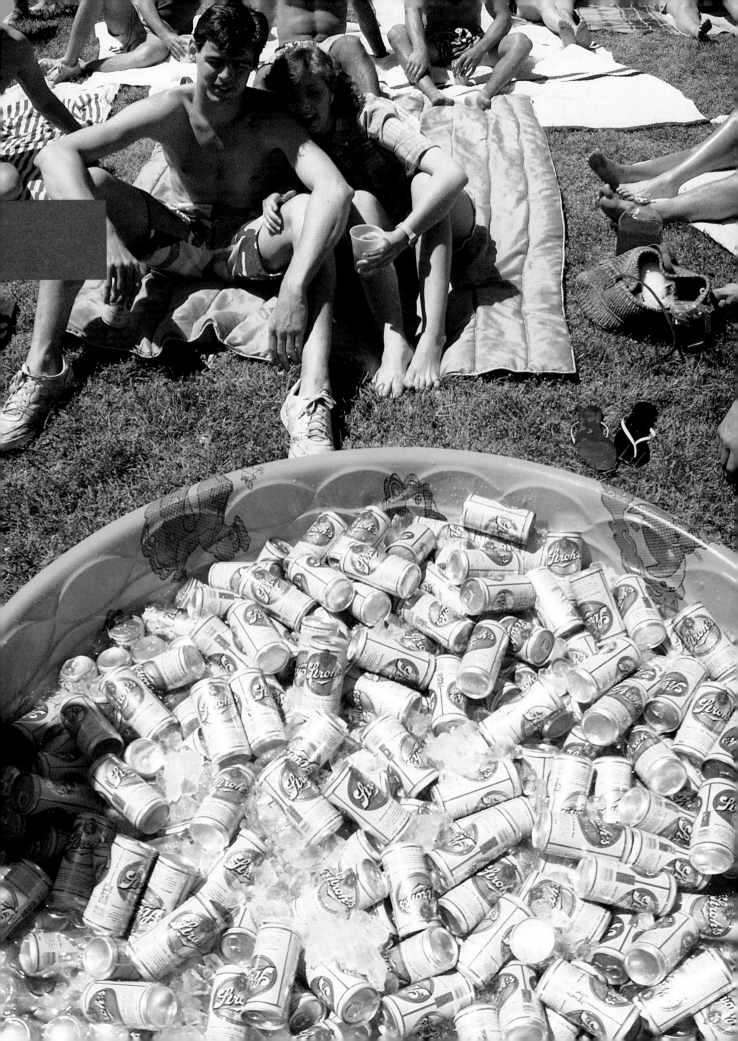

Was there ever a time in your teenage years when you couldn't wait to drink "legally"; when you and your friends thought that sneaking bottles of beer, wine cooler, or even bourbon out of your parents' liquor cabinets was one of the greatest accomplishments for a Saturday night? Why did drinking alcoholic beverages seem so appealing then? Was it the "buzz," the feeling of being grown up, the fun of being "illegal"? Do any of these reasons still account for why you would drink alcoholic beverages now?

The consumption of alcoholic beverages for social and religious purposes has long been a part of the traditions of many cultures. Unfortunately, the abuse of alcohol has been another tradition in many of these same cultures. In the United States, alcohol abuse and alcoholism were long seen as signs of immaturity or weakness. Later, people began to realize that the abuse of alcohol, like the abuse of any other drug, is a disease that must be dealt with firmly yet compassionately. Although alcohol consumption in the United States has declined in recent years, health problems that are linked with alcohol consumption and abuse still constitute one of the most dangerous health problems in this country.

In this chapter we will try to answer several questions concerning alcohol use, alcohol abuse, and the compulsive use of alcohol, alcoholism. Why is alcohol such a widespread problem? What do you need to know about alcohol abuse so that you can avoid it and help friends and relatives avoid it as well? What is the responsible use of alcohol? We will also consider specific problems associated with alcohol use and abuse, such as drinking and driving and the effects of drinking during pregnancy.

Alcohol in American Society

Research Findings

The National Institute on Alcohol Abuse and Alcoholism (NIAAA) provides a regular special report to Congress on the latest research developments in the entire field of alcohol consumption, abuse, etiology, and treatment. Among the findings of the 1990 report are the following:

- As Figure 11.1 depicts, the consumption of alco-

holic beverages has declined steadily since 1977 to an equivalent of 2.54 gallons of pure alcohol per capita for people age 14 years and older in the United States. Even though this is the lowest level since 1970, alcohol continues to be used by more Americans than any other drug. Among persons 12 and older, 36.2 percent report smoking cigarettes during the past year, while 73.4 percent report drinking alcohol over the same year period.

- Over 46,000 people died in motor vehicle crashes in 1987 and *half* of these accidents were alcohol-related.

- The risk of being involved in a fatal motor vehicle accident is eight times greater for a drunk driver than for a sober one.

- Intoxication is not only highly related to accidental deaths, suicides, homicides, drownings, boating accidents, and associated trauma but it may also exacerbate the effects of the trauma and thus cause more damage or longer rehabilitation than would have been the case without alcohol.

- It was estimated that the cost of alcohol abuse and dependence was $116.9 billion in 1983, with over 60 percent attributed to lost employment and productivity reductions.

- The population group most at risk for having high rates of heavy drinking, along with the largest number of alcohol-related problems, are young (under 35), single males.

- The highest rates of alcohol-related problems among women (single or married) are found in young, unemployed women who have a heavy drinker partner. Women living with children seem to be less at risk.

- Even though the consumption pattern is continuing to decline, still more than 91 percent of all high school seniors report some consumption of alcohol within the past year, making it by far the most widely used drug. (This is far above the rate for tobacco or marijuana use.) More alarming still is that 64 percent of high school seniors report being current drinkers, with 34 percent reporting consuming five or more drinks in one sitting during the previous two weeks. Four percent of high school seniors report daily consumption of alcohol.

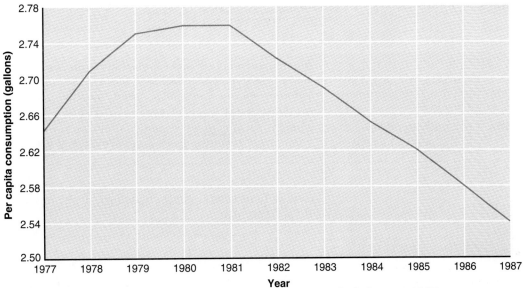

FIGURE 11.1 • Apparent U.S. per capita consumption of pure alcohol, 1977–1987.
Source: NIAAA 1989.

- One of the most at risk groups in the U.S. population for alcoholism is the homeless. The proportion of those who abuse alcohol or are dependent on it among this growing population has been reported to be as high as 45 percent. This is most likely due to the fact that alcohol abusers are much more at risk of becoming homeless, but also it is due to the fact that many homeless report that their use of alcohol is a means of coping with the physical and emotional stresses of being homeless.

- Black men seem to have slightly lower overall consumption rates than white men but they report more alcohol-related problems. Both black men and black women are at much higher risk for developing alcohol-related diseases such as cirrhosis, hepatitis, heart disease, and cancers of the mouth when compared with their white counterparts.

- Young male Hispanics are at even higher risk for developing alcohol-related problems than young black males.

- Drinking patterns vary widely among the Native American population, thus it is impossible to generalize about all native groups. However, among those tribal populations that drink, the rates of alcohol-related problems, diseases, and alcohol-related mortality are extremely high.

- Asian Americans show the lowest rates of alcohol consumption and thus the lowest rates of alcohol-related problems for any ethnic group in the United States.

- Estimated costs for the alcohol abuse problem in the United States during 1983 were almost $117 billion. Of this amount, $71 billion were attributed to lost employment and reduced productivity, while $15 billion were associated with direct health care costs.

Children, Young People, and Alcohol

A recent *Statistical Bulletin*[1] study surveyed the beliefs and perceptions about alcohol held by elementary school children. Some of the alarming results of this investigation include:

- Less than half (42 percent) of fourth through sixth graders consider alcohol to be a drug, and only 21 percent realize that wine coolers are drug-containing beverages.

- Only 17 percent of sixth graders sampled believed "great harm" would come about by daily consumption of wine coolers.

- 46 percent of sixth graders felt strong peer pressure to try wine coolers.

- 42 percent of sixth graders, 31 percent of fifth graders, and 26 percent of fourth graders report having tried wine coolers.

Children's perceptions about the use of alcoholic beverages seem to show ever-increasing acceptance. More alarming than this may be the increasing perception of alcohol being socially "important" by a wide majority of children. The U.S. Secretary of Health and Human Services has outlined several important "protective factors" that can help reduce alcohol and drug use by American youth. Among these factors are:[2]

- We need to have clear "nonuser" messages given by families, communities, peers, and the media.

- We need to start prevention programs at early ages.

- We need to establish community-based teams to implement comprehensive and well-coordinated prevention programs.

alcohol abuser A person who frequently drinks alcoholic beverages to excess, who suffers from psychological and physical problems from drinking alcohol, but who is not yet dependent on alcohol.

alcohol dependent person A person who drinks alcoholic beverages excessively to the point of dependence upon alcohol, and who suffers from chronic alcohol-related psychological and physical problems. These people are commonly called "alcoholics."

morning drinking A technique used by alcohol dependent persons to alleviate the after-effects or "hangover" resulting from excessive alcohol use.

Year 2000 National Health Objectives

The Year 2000 National Health Objectives recognize the continuing problem of alcohol in younger populations. Consequently, several objectives relate to high school and college students. These objectives include:

1. Increase by at least one year the average age of first use of alcohol by adolescents age 12 through 17. In 1988, 13.1 was the average age of first use of alcohol in this age group.
2. Reduce the proportion of young people who have used alcohol in the past month. In 1988, 25.2 percent of young people age 12 to 17 and 57.9 percent of 18 to 20-year-olds reported using alcohol in the past month. The objective is to reduce these numbers to 12.6 and 29 percent, respectively.
3. Reduce the proportion of high school seniors and college students engaging in recent occasions of heavy drinking of alcoholic beverages to no more than 28 percent of high school seniors and 32 percent of college students. In 1989, 33 percent of high school seniors and 41.7 percent of college students reported recently engaging in heavy drinking.
4. Increase the proportion of high school seniors who perceive social disapproval as being associated with the heavy use of alcohol from the 1989 baseline of 56.4 percent to 70 percent.
5. Increase the proportion of high school seniors who associate risk of physical or psychological harm with the heavy use of alcohol from the 1989 baseline of 44 percent to 70 percent.

- We need to foster the development of parent groups and to educate parents and other adults about the warning signs of substance abuse by youth, the effects of their own alcohol use on children's behavior, and available resources for help.
- We should build social skills among youths and promote relationships with nonusing peers.
- We should continue to work in every community to reduce the availability of alcohol to youth.
- And finally, we must empower young people to ask for help when confronted with peer or societal pressures to drink, dating or social problems, seemingly insurmountable challenges, or the onset of substance use.

Drinking Patterns

History has taught us that people differ greatly in their alcohol drinking patterns and that these differences seem to affect dramatically all aspects of prevention and treatment. After many years of struggling over the best way to describe these patterns, the NIAAA (1990) has attempted to clarify the definitions to be used in the description of different drinking patterns.

Social Drinkers The majority of drinkers fall into this social drinking category. These individuals do not report any long-term health consequences. In addition, the discontinuation of the use of the alcohol seems to pose no problem. The "social drinker" label does not come without caution, however. Clearly, there is evidence that even a single bout of moderate alcohol ingestion may contribute to some serious health consequences, as in alcohol-related motor vehicle accidents or in the case of the ingestion of alcohol during early pregnancy.

Alcohol Abusers Individuals who experience one or several serious social, physical, and medical problems as a result of their drinking but who are not yet dependent on alcohol are called **alcohol abusers** or "nondependent problem drinkers." Frequent bouts of moderate to heavy drinking often render these individuals with severely impaired judgment or physical problems that begin to adversely affect their lives. These drinkers may begin to have marital or family troubles or may even have encounters with the law.

Alcohol Dependent Persons The distinguishing characteristic of **Alcohol Dependent Persons** is their lack of control of their drinking behavior. These persons, sometimes called "alcoholics," may suffer many of the same acute or chronic alcohol-related problems as the alcohol abuser, but this individual is powerless over the drug. Once drinking has commenced, it typically does not stop until stupor results. These indi-

Exploring Your Health 11.1

Your First Drink

Can you remember your first alcoholic drink? _____

What was the setting? _____

How old were you? _____

Were you frightened? _____

Were you with your family? _____

Were you sneaky about it?* _____
Were you afraid your folks would find

out?* _____

Were you pressured into it?* _____

Were you alone? _____

Most of you have already decided whether or not to drink alcoholic beverages. If you have decided not to: Have you been embarrassed by that

decision? _____

Do you have trouble defending it? ___

Has it restricted your social life? ___

If you classify yourself as a social drinker:
Do you very often not order an alcoholic beverage when others you are

with do? _____
Do you have trouble refusing a

drink? _____

If you do have trouble, can you analyze why? _____
Do you ever feel that you really *need*

a drink? _____
Do you ever become aware that you change your behavior patterns after

a drink or two? _____

As you can see, our alcohol-related behavior (drinking or abstinence) is a function of various influences, and the consequences of that behavior can necessitate coping skills. For example, you must manage the peer pressure either to join others who are drinking or to abstain from drinking.

* Note that peer pressure and experimentation are implied here.

viduals often attempt to alleviate the unpleasant aftereffects of a bout of heavy drinking with continued alcohol consumption. This is sometimes called **morning drinking.** We will discuss other symptoms and effects of alcohol dependency later in this chapter.

Societal Factors in Alcohol Use

It might sometimes appear as though some of the decisions that we are called on to make have already been made for us, at least in part. In this country, when we drive to a fast food restaurant for lunch, we are programmed to expect a flat portion of ground meat placed between two circles of soft bread. We are further programmed to lift one of those pieces of bread and place a bright red or yellow sauce on top of the

meat. Our programming goes on, and we find ourselves ordering a flavored, bubbling fluid to drink. We have been programmed by our society to make a meal of the hamburger and soft drink. What this means is that a nutritional decision has been made for us by the tastes and customs of our peers.

In a similar way, society influences our individual decisions concerning the use of alcoholic beverages. Your own first encounter with alcohol probably did not even take the form of an active decision. For many of us, our first drink containing alcohol was handed to us at a social gathering, or we were confronted with a situation where, if we wanted to quench our thirst, the only beverages available were alcoholic drinks. Others were introduced to alcoholic beverages in an even more deeply cultural manner: through rituals asso-

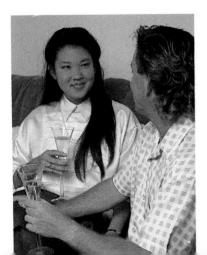

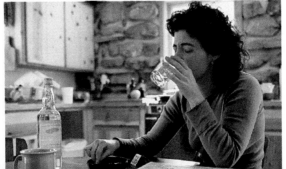

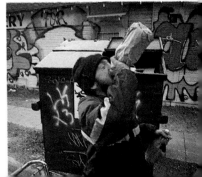

Consumption of alcohol can take several forms: from the least problematic (social drinking), to more serious problems with alcohol (alcohol abusers), to being dependent on alcohol (alcoholism).

ciated with ethnic eating habits or religious ceremonies, such as communion rite or a bar mitzvah. Still other people learned on their own by a friend's or relative's example that a bottle or shot glass represented a convenient place to hide from feelings, problems, and other people.

Much has been said about the possible influences of mass advertising on our individual decisions as consumers. Certainly that cannot be downplayed in the case of alcohol. We are constantly exposed to advertising portraying people who drink as young, "with it," popular, and attractive. Many people find this image hard to resist.

We recognize that many people do not drink alcoholic beverages and were just as programmed to that decision as were those who do drink. In both cases, one's parents, church or synagogue, experiences, and peers have influenced the decision.

Alcohol's Trip Through the Body

How often have you heard people say something like, "How can you drink vodka? That stuff really hits me hard." We have probably all known people who claim that one type of drink is, for them, more or less potent than another.

What Is Alcohol?

However, all alcoholic beverages contain the same kind of alcohol, *ethyl alcohol,* also called ethanol or "grain" alcohol. Because ethyl alcohol consists of very small molecules that are highly soluble in both fat and water, organs of the human body—including the brain—can rapidly absorb it.

There are two basic processes for producing alcohol: *fermentation* and *distillation.* Beer (fermented barley), wine (fermented grape juice), and rum (fermented molasses) are all examples of alcoholic beverages produced by fermentation. Fermentation naturally ceases when alcohol content has reached 14 percent. Distillation is actually an extension of fermentation and produces stronger alcoholic beverages, such as whiskey and vodka, which are often referred to as "spirits" or

"hard liquor." Because alcohol has a lower boiling temperature than water, fermented liquids or "mashes" derived from grains, fruits, sugar cane, and other materials can be gently heated and their alcohol vapors condensed and mixed with water in a still to produce a beverage. The alcohol content of distilled beverages is expressed in "proof," which is simply double the alcohol percentage. For example, 80 proof Scotch whiskey is 40 percent alcohol.

In recent years, beer and wine products have become the undisputed favorite alcoholic beverages among teenagers and adults. Part of the reason for this is the increasing cost of distilled products. Distilled products have traditionally been priced higher than beer and wine, but in recent years many states have introduced frequent increases in "sin taxes" in order to raise state tax revenues and discourage alcohol use simultaneously. Another reason is undoubtedly beer and wine company advertising, which promotes beer and wine products as the best beverages for parties and other good times. Figure 11.2 depicts recent data that show that between 1977 and 1987 Americans have increasingly shown a preference for beer and wine over spirits. Perhaps it is no coincidence that beer and wine companies spent a great deal of money during those years—and continue to spend a great deal of money today—to promote their products on television and radio.

Determining Alcohol Content in the Body

Now that we know a little about where alcohol comes from, let's examine why all forms of alcoholic beverages present us with important and potentially dangerous choices. What follows are some simple mathematics for determining alcohol content in the body for a variety of alcohol-containing beverages.

The most common-size bottle or can of beer is 12 fluid ounces. Most beer brewed in the United States is roughly 5 percent alcohol. If we multiply the 12 fluid ounces by the 5 percent alcohol, we find that the amount of alcohol in beer is 0.60 fluid ounces.

The standard wine glass for most restaurants and drinking establishments holds 5 fluid ounces of wine.

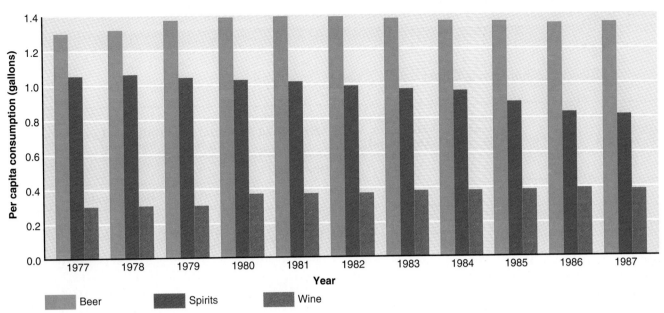

FIGURE 11.2 • Apparent U.S. per capita consumption of beer, wine, and spirits, 1977–1987.
Source: NIAAA 1989.

The alcohol content of wine is determined by the sugar in the grapes and by the fermentation process, with the natural limit at about 12 percent. If we multiply 5 fluid ounces by 12 percent, we find that the amount of alcohol in a glass of wine is 0.60 fluid ounces.

Repeating the procedure for hard liquors (gin, vodka, scotch, bourbon, rye, and so forth), we multiply the contents of a standard "shot" (1.5 fluid ounces) by the percentage of alcohol in the drink (one-half its proof, as stated on the label). Thus, one shot of an 80-proof bourbon whiskey translates to 1.5 times 0.40, or 0.60 fluid ounces of alcohol.

These calculations show that we are only fooling ourselves if we think that one type of drink is less potent than the others; each contains roughly the same amount of alcohol. Obviously, if you drink an 8-ounce rather than a 12-ounce beer, or a small glass of wine, or a whiskey of lower proof, you will reduce the amount of alcohol ingested. However, the fact is that anyone who drinks beer or wine as a protection against intoxication is making a decision based on misconception. It is the alcohol that intoxicates, and we ingest just about the same amount, whichever of the three drinks we choose.

"Light" Beers and Wine Coolers Some information concerning the so-called light beers is needed here. These beers are characterized by reduced *calorie* content: some have half or fewer than half the calories of the regular product of that brewer. The advertising strongly implies that, because it has fewer calories, light beer can be consumed in greater quantity than regular beer. You should keep in mind that, although the calories have been reduced significantly, the alcohol content may not have been. People who drink a greater quantity of light beer may not get as fat but they get just as drunk.

In the 1960s, wine coolers were the "in" drink with the young beach crowd, in California in particular. Recently, interest in wine coolers has reemerged. These drinks are marketed for the young who have not yet learned to like the taste of alcohol. Wine coolers mask the alcoholic taste in a fruit-juice flavor. However, most wine coolers contain as much alcoholic content as do ales (5 percent); and some contain as much as other beers (6 percent). Since they are sold in 12-ounce bottles, as are beers, the effect of drinking wine coolers is similar to that of drinking beers. However, given its fruity taste, people don't often equate drinking a wine cooler with drinking a beer and erroneously think they can drink as much as their thirst dictates.

Brewers and vintners have now recognized that a portion of the public is concerned about its alcohol intake. The new "low-alcohol" beers and wines, advertised as having the same taste qualities as their more potent cousins, were developed in response to that market. Even with beverages of low alcohol content you will have to figure your "safe" capacity, by using Table 11.1.

Absorption and Metabolism

Alcohol is absorbed directly into the bloodstream through the walls of the stomach and the small intestine. Once into the bloodstream, it is carried to all water-bearing parts of the body, and to the liver, where

Blood Alcohol Levels Chart

Alcoholic Beverages	Alcohol Content (%)	Normal Measures Dispensed	Estimated Potential Blood-Alcohol Level Achieved with Normal Measure*				
			One Drink				
					Body Weight		
			Alcohol Content (Oz.)	100 (% w/v)	140	180	220
Beer							
Ale	5	12-oz. bottle	0.60	0.05	0.04	0.03	0.02
Malt beverage	7	12-oz. bottle	0.72	0.06	0.05	0.04	0.03
Regular beer	4	12-oz. bottle	0.48	0.04	0.03	0.02	0.02
Wines							
Fortified: Port, Muscatel, etc.	18	3-oz. glass	0.54	0.04	0.03	0.02	0.02
Natural: Red/ white champagne	12	3-oz. glass	0.36	0.03	0.03	0.02	0.02
Wine coolers	5	12-oz. bottle	0.60	0.05	0.04	0.03	0.02
Cider (Hard)	10	6-oz. glass	0.60	0.05	0.04	0.03	0.02
Liqueurs							
Strong: B & B, Cointreau, Drambuie	40	1-oz. glass	0.40	0.03	0.03	0.02	0.02
Medium: Fruit brandies	25	2-oz. glass	0.50	0.04	0.03	0.02	0.02
Distilled Spirits	45	1-oz. glass	0.45	0.04	0.03	0.02	0.02
Brandy, cognac, rum, scotch, vodka, whiskey							
Mixed Drinks and Cocktails							
Strong: Martini, manhattan	30	3½-oz. glass	1.05	0.08	0.06	0.04	0.04
Medium: Old fashioned, daiquiri, alexander	15	4-oz. glass	0.60	0.05	0.04	0.03	0.02
Light: Highball, sweet and sour mixers, tonics	7	8-oz. glass	0.56	0.05	0.04	0.03	0.02

* This constitutes one, two, or three drinks consumed in a normal period, or within one hour. For each additional hour, subtract 0.015% w/v from the number shown.

Source: Data from the U.S. Department of Transportation, National Highway Traffic Safety Administration.

Two Drinks					Three Drinks				
	Body Weight					**Body Weight**			
Alcohol Content (Oz.)	100 (% w/v)	140	180	220	Alcohol Content (Oz.)	100 (% w/v)	140	180	220
1.20	0.08	0.06	0.05	0.05	1.80	0.11	0.09	0.08	0.07
1.44	0.09	0.07	0.06	0.05	2.16	0.15	0.12	0.09	0.08
0.96	0.07	0.05	0.04	0.03	1.44	0.10	0.08	0.06	0.05
1.08	0.07	0.05	0.04	0.03	1.62	0.10	0.08	0.06	0.05
0.72	0.06	0.05	0.04	0.03	1.08	0.08	0.06	0.04	0.04
1.20	0.08	0.06	0.05	0.05	1.80	0.11	0.09	0.08	0.07
1.20	0.08	0.06	0.05	0.05	1.80	0.11	0.09	0.08	0.07
0.80	0.07	0.05	0.04	0.03	1.20	0.08	0.06	0.05	0.05
1.00	0.08	0.06	0.04	0.04	1.50	0.10	0.08	0.06	0.06
0.90	0.07	0.05	0.04	0.03	1.35	0.09	0.07	0.06	0.05
2.10	0.15	0.12	0.09	0.08	3.15	0.22	0.16	0.12	0.10
1.20	0.08	0.06	0.05	0.05	1.80	0.11	0.09	0.08	0.07
1.12	0.08	0.06	0.05	0.04	1.68	0.12	0.09	0.07	0.06

blood alcohol level (BAL) A measure of the amount of alcohol present in the total blood of an individual, presented as a percentage of the total blood volume.

cirrhosis The final stage of a liver disease directly related to alcohol abuse. At this stage, liver cells are dying and damage to the liver is permanent.

fetal alcohol syndrome (FAS) A condition found in babies born to women who are heavy users of alcohol. The condition is characterized by low birth weight and serious developmental problems.

fetal alcohol effect (FAE) A term used to describe less serious cases of fetal alcohol syndrome.

---

it is metabolized (broken down chemically). When the amount ingested is greater than the capacity of the liver to metabolize (or remove) it, the **blood alcohol level (BAL)**—the amount of alcohol present as a percentage of total blood—increases and the signs of intoxication begin to appear.

It is true that you can slow the absorption of alcohol into the bloodstream by eating immediately before or while you are drinking. However, only a very small percentage of the alcohol is absorbed through the stomach wall. Eventually it reaches the small intestine where the major absorption takes place. Your protective action was really no protection at all, since the alcohol does not disappear; you merely postponed the beginning of a closed process over which you have no control once alcohol is ingested.

The key organ in this closed process is the liver. By understanding the role of the liver in alcohol metabolism, one can guard against intoxication and understand the sobering-up process. Most important to the whole discussion is the fact that the liver metabolizes alcohol at a constant rate per hour, no matter how much you drink or what you might do to speed it up, such as attempting to speed up the sobering process. Interestingly enough, that hourly rate is just about equal to the amount of alcohol previously shown to be present in a can of beer, a shot of liquor, or a glass of wine.

Thus, simple logic gives you the formula for remaining sober: simply restrict your intake to no more than one drink, containing no more than 0.60 fluid ounces of alcohol, per hour. That same logic tells you that the only way to achieve a sober state is to wait for the liver to metabolize the alcohol you have ingested, thus reducing the BAL to an acceptable level.

Because the liver does not begin the metabolizing process until the alcohol reaches an equilibrium state in all water-bearing parts of the body, your body weight becomes an important part of the intoxication and sobering-up time factors. By studying Table 11.1, you will be able to figure these factors on the basis of your own body weight. Remember that this is a much more complex process than we have represented here; your figures will only be approximations.

Psychological and Physiological Effects of Alcohol

Immediate Effects

Small differences in blood alcohol concentrations make big differences in our reactions.

Depending on the BAL and drinking history of the drinker, we might commonly see a sense of relaxation, elation, or depression, increased heart rate and blood pressure, slower reaction to stimuli, decreased sexual function, decreased muscular coordination, blurred vision, slurred speech, loss of discrimination among sounds, loss of the sense of odor or taste, lack of balance, mental confusion, decreased sense of pain, altered sense of time and space, unconsciousness, coma, and even death.

In addition, although many people find the sensations of an alcohol high pleasurable for some time within any given period of intoxication, most people who get "drunk," "wasted," "looped," "bombed," or otherwise intoxicated experience a *hangover* sometime later, usually the morning after drinking. No one is exactly sure why hangovers occur. Some people may have an allergic reaction to certain chemicals in alcoholic beverages, while others may experience a dehydration of cerebral tissues. Contrary to some popular beliefs, there is no real cure for a hangover. Indeed, the best cure is prevention. If you decide to consume alcohol, drink only one alcoholic beverage per hour and drink lots of water or other nonalcoholic beverages in between. Never drink alcohol on an empty stomach, and try to combine drinking with eating wholesome foods (*not* salty finger foods, which may actually lead you to drink more alcoholic beverages).

Among the commonly observed effects not listed above are two that may be the most important to those who will use this book. It is generally agreed that alcohol reduces our ability or willingness to be self-critical and releases us from our inhibitions. In addition, for many of us, the drinking of alcohol-containing beverages decreases our natural fears and allows us to more freely engage in risk-taking activities. In short, alcohol has a damaging effect on what we might call common sense or judgment. We will return to this factor later in this chapter.

Long-term Effects

People who are chronic alcohol abusers run a serious risk of developing chronic diseases. One of the most common diseases directly related to alcohol abuse is **cirrhosis** of the liver. Cirrhosis is the last stage in an ongoing destruction of liver cells and can result in death. Alcohol abuse is also a factor in the development of heart and blood diseases. Increased blood pressure and heart rate, irregular heartbeat or loss of heart rhythm, and disruption of blood flow to the heart are all potential results of excessive drinking. Alcohol also makes groups of red blood cells lump together in sticky masses, an effect called *sludging*. Abuse of alcohol has also been shown to be a factor in some kinds of brain damage. Even moderate use of alcohol will result in a decrease in brain size and a loss of some intellectual ability. Finally, long-term abuse of alcohol has been linked to certain types of cancer, particularly those of the gastrointestinal tract (esophagus, stomach, mouth, tongue). Another serious long-term effect of alcohol abuse is represented by fetal alcohol syndrome, discussed in detail later.

It should be noted that alcohol-related physiological damage—like the physiological damage caused by tobacco use and drug abuse—can be partially reversed by adopting lifestyle changes that incorporate good nutrition and abstinence from alcohol consumption. The problem, of course, is to come to terms with and control alcohol dependency. It is an ironic tragedy that many people who develop alcohol dependency also have or eventually develop a dependency on other forms of drugs in addition to alcohol.

Alcohol and Other Drugs

As we discussed in the previous chapter, Americans might be described as a society "on drugs." The comment should not be interpreted to mean that we are all users of illicit drugs; on the other hand, most of us readily use over-the-counter preparations in self-medi-

cation, and many of us are under care for one or more conditions for which drugs have been prescribed. Thus it is safe to assume that those of us who drink alcoholic beverages may be doing so with other drugs already present in our bodies. In addition, it is now an accepted observation that we no longer see abusers who confine themselves to a single drug or class of drugs. The polydrug user or abuser compounds his or her problem, complicating the process of metabolization and often setting up situations of real danger. Table 11.2 spells out some of the dangers of mixing various drugs with alcohol.

Fetal Alcohol Syndrome

Fetal alcohol syndrome (FAS) is a condition found in babies born to women who are heavy users of alcohol. These infants are characterized by low birth weight, small head size, a low nasal bridge, small nose, small midface and short eye openings, and an indistinct groove in a very thin upper lip. This serious condition also includes developmental deficiencies during and after birth, sometimes involving mental retardation and, very often, poor motor development.

In 1990, the NIAAA recommended the use of the term **"Fetal alcohol effect" (FAE)** when some, but not all, of the FAS criteria are present in a child.[3] The NIAAA reported the prevalence of FAS to be between 1 to 3 cases per 1,000 live births. Black and Native American women have the highest incidence of FAS. Some

Consumption of alcohol is particularly problematic for women because they can contribute to various birth defects in their offspring by drinking alcohol when pregnant. Fetal alcohol syndrome (FAS) is the name given to one set of birth defects that result from the consumption of alcohol while pregnant. The federal government has established a Year 2000 National Health Objective to decrease the incidence of FAS.

Year 2000 National Health Objective

The Year 2000 National Health Objectives seek to reduce deaths from cirrhosis of the liver to no more than 6 per 100,000 people. In 1987, there were 9.1 cirrhosis deaths per 100,000 people.

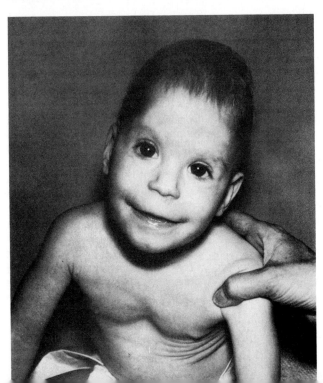

What Could Happen If You Drink While Taking Any of These Drugs

The following chart lists classes of drugs that have been reported to interact with alcohol. Some of the dangers that may result from combining alcohol with the other listed drugs are described. It must be emphasized that this chart, or any other like it, only represents the smallest part of the whole alcohol/drug interaction picture. It is not meant to replace the advice of your family doctor or your pharmacist.

Class	Drug Name	Effects When Combined with Alcohol
Analgesics, Narcotic	Demerol, Darvon, Dilaudid, etc.	When used alone, both alcohol and narcotic drugs cause a reduction in the function of the central nervous system. When used together, this effect is even greater and may lead to respiratory arrest. Death may occur.
Antialcohol Preparations	Antabuse, Calcium carbamide	Use of alcohol with medications prescribed for alcoholic patients to keep them from drinking results in nausea, vomiting, headache, high blood pressure, and possible erratic heartbeat, and can result in death.
Anticoagulants	Panwarfin, Dicumarol, Sintrom, etc.	Alcohol can increase the ability of these drugs to stop blood clotting, which in turn can lead to life-threatening or fatal hemorrhages.
Anticonvulsants	Dilantin, Diphenyl, EKKO, etc.	Drinking may lessen the ability of this drug to stop convulsions in a person.
Antidepressants	Tofranil, Pertofrane, Triavil, etc.	Alcohol may cause an additional reduction in central nervous system functioning and lessen a person's ability to operate normally. Certain antidepressants in combination with red wines like Chianti may cause a high blood pressure crisis.
Antidiabetic Agents/ Hypoglycemics	Insulin, Diabenese, Orinase, etc.	Because of the possible severe reactions to combining alcohol and insulin or the oral antidiabetic agents, and because alcohol interacts unpredictably with them, these medications should not be taken with alcohol.
Antihistamines	Most cold remedies, Actifed, Coricidin, etc.	Taking alcohol with this class of drugs increases their calming effect, and a person can feel quite drowsy, making driving and other activities that require alertness more hazardous.
Sedative Hypnotics	Doriden, Quaalude, Nembutal, etc.	Alcohol in combination further reduces the function of the central nervous system, sometimes to the point of coma or the loss of effective breathing (respiratory arrest). This combination can be fatal.
Sleep Medicines		It is likely that nonprescription sleeping medicines, to the degree that they are effective, will lead to the same kind of central nervous system depression when combined with alcohol as the minor tranquilizers (see below).
Antihypertensive Agents	Serpasil, Aldomet, Esidrix, etc.	Alcohol may increase the blood-pressure-lowering capability of some of these drugs, causing dizziness when a person gets up. Some agents will also cause a reduction in the function of the central nervous system.
Anti-Infective Agents/ Antibiotics	Flagyl, Chloromycetin, Seromycin, etc.	In combination with alcohol, some may cause nausea, vomiting, headache, and possibly convulsions, especially those taken for urinary tract infections.

Class	Drug Name	Effects When Combined with Alcohol
Analgesics, Nonnarcotic	Aspirin, APC, Pabalate, etc.	Even when used alone, some nonprescription pain relievers can cause bleeding in the stomach and intestines. Alcohol also irritates the stomach and can aggravate the bleeding, especially in ulcer patients.
Central Nervous System Stimulants	Most diet pills, Dexedrine, Caffeine, Ritalin, etc.	Because the stimulant effect of this class of drugs may reverse the depressant effect of the alcohol on the central nervous system, these drugs can give a false sense of security. They do *not* help intoxicated persons gain control of their movements.
Diuretics	Diuril, Lasix, Hydromox, etc.	Combining alcohol with diuretics may cause reduction in blood pressure, possibly resulting in dizziness when a person stands up.
Psychotropics	Tindal, Mellaril, Thorazine, etc.	Alcohol and the "major tranquilizers" cause additional depression to central nervous system function, which can result in severe impairment of voluntary movements such as walking or using the hands. The combination can also cause a loss of effective breathing function and can be fatal.
Tranquilizers, Minor	Miltown, Valium, Librium, etc.	Tranquilizers in combination with alcohol will cause reduced functions of the central nervous system, especially during the first few weeks of drug use. This results in decreased alertness and judgment and can lead to household and automotive accidents.
Vitamins		Continuous drinking can keep vitamins from entering the bloodstream. However, this situation changes when a person stops drinking.

Source: National Clearinghouse for Alcohol Information.

Plains Tribe Native Americans have FAS rates as high as 10 per 1,000 live births.

FAS infants studied ten years after their birth demonstrate many development deficiencies. The death rate (from all causes) is more than double that of nonFAS infants. The highest mental functioning children in the group were at what could be considered low normal (IQ = 70–86) with most of the children in the severely retarded group (IQ = 20–57). Recent evidence has shown brain electrophysiological differences even in infants with prenatal exposure to alcohol who do not demonstrate the physical symptoms of FAS as described above. These children also show significant development handicaps ten years later.

Moderate and even light exposure to alcohol by the mother has been shown to affect the fetus. Habituation, or the ability of the infant to "tune out" or stop responding to a repeated stimulus, is indicative of delayed development of the central nervous system. A Seattle-based study demonstrated that the more a mother drank, the longer it took her infant to become habituated.[4] This study also showed a time delay and lack of strength associated with the sucking reflex of infants whose mothers consumed light and moderate amounts of alcohol.[5]

Alcohol appears to act in concert with other factors in the development of alcohol-related syndromes in infants. In a study of 12,000 pregnancies in Cleveland, Ohio, the researchers identified 204 abusive drinkers among the mothers. Yet of the 204 offspring, only 5 babies had physical symptoms of FAS.[6] Clearly, there are other factors which may account for these discrepancies. Some investigators have suggested that the fetus may be particularly vulnerable during the first trimester (the time of most central nervous system development) and that effects upon the infant may be more related to peak alcohol level in the mother during this period rather than overall consumption throughout the pregnancy. This strongly implies that pregnant women may damage their fetus with even one episode of alcohol consumption and that, therefore, the best advice is to abstain.

Using Alcohol Responsibly

In our discussion of the physiological effects of alcohol, we pointed out that responsible drinking requires that you learn how much alcohol you can drink with-

Year 2000 National Health Objective

The Year 2000 National Health Objectives seek to reduce the incidence of fetal alcohol syndrome from the 1987 rate of 0.22 per 1,000 live births to 0.12 per 1,000 live births. However, certain populations have higher than usual fetal alcohol syndrome rates. Consequently, the Year 2000 National Health Objectives designate them as groups who will get special attention in terms of this objective. As such, the objectives seek to reduce the incidence of fetal alcohol syndrome in Native Americans/Alaska Natives from 4 to 2 per 1,000 live births, and in blacks from 0.8 to 0.4 per 1,000 live births.

Exploring Your Health 11.2

The Campus Alcohol Supervisor

Imagine you are given the responsibility of encouraging your college peers campuswide to drink alcohol more responsibly. What changes would you suggest they adopt?

1. _____

2. _____

3. _____

What changes would you want to see the campus administration adopt?

1. _____

2. _____

3. _____

How would you want the campus organizations (such as fraternity or sorority houses, student government) to help?

1. _____

2. _____

3. _____

How would you want community vendors (bar owners, restaurant proprietors) to help?

1. _____

2. _____

3. _____

What would you do to establish yourself as a role model in this area?

1. _____

2. _____

3. _____

Perhaps you, several of your classmates, and your instructor can work together to bring about some of these changes.

out reaching a high blood alcohol level. Using alcoholic beverages responsibly also involves deciding when it is appropriate to drink, drinking in moderation, and showing concern for the health and safety of others.

Guidelines for Serving and Using Alcohol

The following list provides some guidelines that you may find useful when you are serving alcohol in your own home and when you are attending a party or other activity where alcoholic beverages are being served:

- Use alcohol as an adjunct to an activity rather than as the center or focal point of an activity.
- Set a limit on the number of drinks you are going to drink.
- Know your limit and stick to it.
- Respect a person who chooses not to drink.

- Provide alternative beverages at your party.
- Serve food with alcoholic beverages.
- Show displeasure to someone who has drunk too much.
- Do not be insistent about refilling or refreshing someone's drink.
- Make sure alcohol is used carefully in connection with over-the-counter and prescription drugs.
- Take a taxi, ask for a ride, or stay over at a friend's home if you are in no condition to drive, and insist that others for whom you are responsible do the same.

The term "responsible drinking" may be a misnomer. The reduction in our ability to be self-critical, the release of inhibition, and the change of attitude toward risk-taking activity are effects that are observed in many of us after only moderate consumption in a social drinking situation. Therefore, if alcohol has an effect on our "better judgment," it would seem logical to assume that we will have trouble exercising that judgment after we begin to drink. In fact, the statement probably should be *responsibility before drinking,* because that is when you should be deciding who will not drink so that they can drive, what the limit will be and so forth. You cannot make these decisions responsibly after the drinking has started.

The issue of responsibility goes beyond the individual, with most states placing responsibility on the tavern owner, licensee, or bartender not to serve persons who show signs of intoxication. Some states either already have or are considering legislation fixing liability for the acts committed by persons under the influence of alcohol on those who served it, including party hosts. Even though such legislation, if passed and enforced, would act to make us all more responsible in drinking situations, real responsibility rests with you the individual, since the data seem to clearly show that your actions under the influence of alcohol can have serious adverse consequences in your own life and possibly in the lives of others.

Drinking and Driving

Although we have long associated the use of alcoholic beverages with accidents of all sorts—domestic violence, occupational hazards, fire-related deaths, falls, drownings, child abuse, criminal violence including rape, and suicide—for the past several years there has been a special focus on responsible drinking behavior and driving habits.

Drinking, Driving, and Dying The National Highway Safety Administration[7] reports that the leading cause of death among Americans under the age of 35 is traffic accidents. Almost half of these traffic deaths are alcohol related: either the driver or the pedestrian was drunk. In 1989, there were 17,849 fatal crashes in which the driver or the pedestrian was legally intoxicated. Considering only intoxicated drivers, in 1989, 14,644 were involved in traffic accidents that resulted in a death. In addition, 40 percent of all teenage deaths (ages 15 to 19) occur in traffic accidents. And yet, in a U.S. national survey, 6.1 percent of adults responded positively when asked if they had driven "when you've had perhaps too much to drink" during the previous month.[8]

Drinking causes motor vehicle accidents because the driver's judgment is affected. Drivers who lack good judgment are, obviously, more likely to have accidents. However, there are also other effects of alcohol that make one more susceptible to traffic accidents. For example, the eyes are more sensitive to glare; it is more difficult to estimate speed and distance accurately; there is a tendency to feel drowsy and to have reduced attentiveness; peripheral vision is diminished; reaction time is slower; and, in some drivers, there is a tendency to become aggressive.

Table 11.3 lists the psychological and physical effects that alcohol has at increasing levels of blood alcohol concentration. It should be clear from this table that as you drink more, your chances of being involved in an auto accident increase dramatically.

In addition to the shocking weight of the data presented, national organizations are aware that America's attachment to the automobile makes it an obvious focus in programs designed to bring about behavior change. Organizations such as RID (Remove Intoxicated Drivers, P.O. Box 520, Schenectady, New York 12301) and MADD (Mothers Against Drunk Drivers, 669 Airport Freeway, Suite 310, Hurst, Texas 76053) have sponsored programs to draw attention to problems associated with driving while under the influence

How to Reduce Drunk Driving

Former United States Surgeon General C. Everett Koop recommended the following actions to reduce drunk driving:

1. Reduce the definition for intoxication while driving to a blood-alcohol level of 0.04 (instead of the current level of 0.10) by the year 2000. Establish a 0.00 level for drivers under 21 years of age.

2. Increase the excise tax on alcoholic beverages. Tax beer, wine, and distilled spirits based upon their alcohol content.

3. Have each state provide a system to fund driving education programs for those convicted of alcohol-impaired driving.

4. Reduce the availability of alcoholic beverages. Eliminate "happy hours," prohibit the public use of open alcoholic beverage containers, limit the hours and density of places selling alcoholic beverages, and require impaired-driver prevention training for sellers and servers of alcohol.

5. Pass legislation in each state to confiscate on the spot the licenses of drivers found to have blood alcohol levels above the legal limit.

6. Match the level of alcoholic beverage advertisements with an equal number of prohealth and prosafety messages.

7. Reduce certain types of alcohol product advertising and marketing practices, especially those that reach underage youth.

8. Conduct public information efforts based on social marketing, communication strategies, and learning principles.

9. Conduct drinking and driving education within worksites, communities, health-care agencies, and schools.

10. Increase the enforcement of drinking and driving laws and expand the use of sobriety checkpoints.

Source: C. Everett Koop, *Surgeon General's Workshop on Drunk Driving Procedures* (Washington, D.C.: Public Health Service, 1990).

Psychological and Physical Effects of Various Blood Alcohol Concentration Levels[a]

Number of Drinks per Hour[b]	Blood Alcohol Concentration (%)	Psychological and Physical Effects
1	0.02–0.03	No overt effects, slight feeling of muscle relaxation, slight mood elevation.
2	0.05–0.06	No intoxication, but feeling of relaxation, warmth. Slight lengthening in reaction time, slight decrease in fine muscle coordination.
3	0.08–0.09	Balance, speech, vision, and hearing slightly impaired. Feelings of euphoria. Increased loss of motor coordination. Legal intoxication at 0.08 percent in some states.
4	0.11–0.12	Coordination and balance becoming difficult. Distinct impairment of mental facilities, judgment, etc. Legal intoxication at 0.10 percent in many states.
5	0.14–0.15	Major impairment of mental and physical control. Slurred speech, blurred vision, lack of motor skill. Legal intoxication at 0.15 percent in all states.
7	0.20	Loss of motor control—must have assistance in moving about. Mental confusion.
10	0.30	Severe intoxication. Minimum conscious control of mind and body.
14	0.40	Unconsciousness, threshold of coma.
17	0.50	Deep coma.
20	0.60	Death from respiratory failure.

[a] For each one-hour time lapse, 0.015 percent blood alcohol concentration, or approximately one drink.

[b] The typical drink—three-fourths of an ounce of alcohol—is provided by:
• A shot of spirits (1.5 oz. of 50 percent alcohol—100-proof whiskey or vodka).
• A glass of fortified wine (3.5 oz. of 20 percent alcohol).
• A larger glass of table wine (5 oz. of 14 percent alcohol).
• A pint of beer (16 oz. of 4.5 percent alcohol).

Source: From *Drugs: A Factual Account,* 4e, by Dorothy Dusek and Daniel A. Girdano. Copyright © 1987 by Newbery Award Records, Inc. Reprinted by permission of Random House, Inc.

of alcohol. Along with federal and state departments of transportation, automobile clubs, and law enforcement agencies, they have looked at drinking and driving legislation, enforcement, and adjudication, and have helped to keep the issue in the public eye.

Another organization, SADD (Students Against Driving Drunk, Corbin Plaza, Marlboro, Massachusetts 01752), has raised the issue of responsibility while drinking to the newest drivers. High school chapters of SADD have been formed all across the country in the past several years. The main and most powerful part of the SADD program is their "Contract for Life," which is signed by both the student and the parent (see Figure 11.3). In the contract, the student promises not to drive after drinking and not to ride with a driver who has been drinking; the parent promises to either pick up the student or pay the taxi fare for a safe trip home, with no questions asked at that time.

CONTRACT FOR LIFE

A Contract for Life
Between Parent and Teenager
The SADD Drinking-Driver Contract

Teenager   I agree to call you for advice and/or transportation at any hour, from any place, if I am ever in a situation where I have been drinking or a friend or date who is driving me has been drinking.

_____
Signature

Parent   I agree to come and get you at any hour, any place, no questions asked and no argument at that time, or I will pay for a taxi to bring you home safely. I expect we would discuss this issue at a later time.

I agree to seek safe, sober transportation home if I am ever in a situation where I have had too much to drink or a friend who is driving me has had too much to drink.

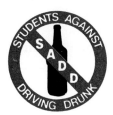

_____
Signature

_____
Date

S.A.D.D. does not condone drinking by those below the legal drinking age. S.A.D.D. encourages all young people to obey the laws of their state, including laws relating to the legal drinking age.

Distributed by S.A.D.D., "Students Against Driving Drunk"

FIGURE 11.3 • SADD's drinking-driver contract. ®
Source: Students Against Drunk Driving, Corbin Plaza, Marlboro, Mass. Reprinted by permission.

alcoholic The term commonly used to indicate an alcohol dependent person.

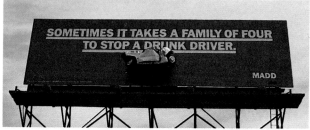

Community groups have gotten together to prevent needless deaths caused by some people driving under the influence of alcohol.

The Tragedy of Alcoholism

Those individuals who do not, or cannot, exercise control over their drinking behavior become problem drinkers. They may ultimately become **alcoholics** if their drinking interferes with or disrupts major areas of

Year 2000 National Health Objectives

The Year 2000 National Health Objectives seek to reduce deaths caused by alcohol-related motor vehicle accidents to no more than 8.5 per 100,000 people. Here, too, certain populations have higher than usual rates and are therefore targeted for special attention. For example, the objectives seek to reduce deaths caused by alcohol-related motor vehicle accidents involving Native Americans and Alaska Natives from the 1987 level of 52.2 to no more than 44.8 per 100,000 people, and in people age 15 to 24 from 21.5 to 18 per 100,000 people.

Furthermore, the Year 2000 National Health Objectives seek to extend to all fifty states legal blood alcohol concentration levels of .04 for motor vehicle drivers age 21 and older and 0.00 for those drivers younger than 21. There are presently no states that have adopted such levels.

A Question of Ethics

Should Colleges Allow Beer Companies to Sponsor Their Events?

Pro Colleges are too often underfunded. The result of this situation is that students are denied services (such as tutoring or counseling) and the amenities they would like during their college years. To remedy this condition, either tuition would have to be raised or, if the college is a public one, taxes would need to be raised. A way of "having your cake and eating it too" is to allow beer manufacturers to sponsor some campus activities for the small price of having their product's name displayed. So rather than the athletic department paying for printing sports teams' schedules, the beer companies would foot the bill and

place their logos in one corner of the program. Concession stands at sports events would give out drinking cups with beer companies' names on them, thereby decreasing the cost to the college of running the concession stand, resulting in greater profit. The effect of allowing beer companies to contribute in this way would be to free some money for other student services.

Con Opponents of this view argue that allowing a beer company to be a visible contributor is a tacit endorsement of its product. Such advertising seems more dangerous when we recognize the number of students who

already abuse alcohol and need help in changing their drinking behavior. Furthermore, in many states, freshmen are too young to purchase alcohol and it would be inconsistent to encourage their buying beer—even if this encouragement was as subtle as their repeatedly seeing the beer company's name displayed at various campus locations. Opponents argue that the price in image and drinking behavior is not worth the benefits of the financial contributions.

What do you think? Should your college accept such contributions?

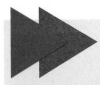

Exploring Your Health 11.3

Who Is Most Likely to Be an Alcoholic?

What is your perception of the person who is likely to have alcohol-related problems? Fill in the blanks below, based only on your personal opinion.

Age: _____

Sex: _____

Ethnic background: _____

Marital status: _____

Employment status: _____

Educational status: _____

Socioeconomic status: _____

Wine drinker: _____

Beer drinker: _____

Hard liquor drinker: _____

Residence (urban, rural): _____

Later in the chapter you'll find a table (Table 11.4) that profiles persons who are and are not most likely to have alcohol-related problems. Compare the table with your responses above.

---

their lives. Each of us, as we read this, probably has someone we know well in mind. Before you read on, complete Exploring Your Health 11.3.

Basic Factors Contributing to Alcoholism

Alcoholism has always been regarded as a serious problem in our society, but only in recent decades have attitudes begun to change regarding the factors contributing to alcoholism. During the nineteenth and early twentieth centuries, most people who opposed alcohol use believed that alcoholics were morally weak. It was this perception that helped to give rise to the prohibition of the sale of alcoholic beverages from 1919 to 1933. Today there is much greater awareness of the complexity of this disorder:

> We now know that alcoholism involves an interplay of biological, behavioral, and cultural components within the individuals who are afflicted. We have come to understand that alcoholism involves biological factors, either as etiological indicators or as biomedical consequences, and that psychological and sociocultural factors enter in as well. The interaction of these components, varying as they do from individual to individual, further deepens the complexity of this disease and makes it quite unlike any other.[9]

Let's take a look at some of the factors that contribute to alcohol-related problems.

Personality Disturbance "The common description of the alcoholic given by those who work in the rehabilitation process is a frustrated, fearful, self-punishing, immature person. *Incidentally,* that person also uses alcohol to excess."[10] The position held by many psychiatrists is that alcohol abuse is a symptom of personality disorder; it is the person's way of seeking relief.

The problem with identifying personality factors that may predispose someone to alcoholism is that we can't easily determine whether those factors are the cause or the effect of alcoholism. For example, we would have difficulty finding out whether an alcoholic's low self-esteem existed before his or her drinking problem developed and led to it, or if the drinking problem led to the alcoholic having less self-esteem.

Despite this difficulty, some researchers[11] have identified traits "associated" with alcoholism. These include a history of antisocial behavior, high levels of depression, and low self-esteem. Some studies have found alcoholics to have certain expectations regarding alcohol. For example, alcohol may be considered a "magic elixir" that enhances sexual pleasure and sexual performance, provides power and aggressiveness, and "loosens" people up so they can function more effectively in social settings such as parties or on dates. In a study of college students, heavier drinkers were found to have greater expectations of positive consequences of drinking than light drinkers.[12] What do you expect alcohol to provide you with?

The personality factors identified as typical of the problem drinker are also characteristics that would cause an individual to experience stress. The conflict between societal and personal goals and expectations, cultural differences that may tend to place a person apart from the immediate population, or attitudes toward drinking may bring about stressful situations from which relief is sought through alcohol.

Physiological Factors Among current studies of the possible physiological determinants of various types of addiction, including alcohol addiction, research concerning the possibility of inherited traits and abnormalities of the endocrine system bears watching. This research focuses on the ability of the body to produce the enzyme necessary for alcohol metabolism. It is well documented that children of alcoholics are more likely to become alcoholics themselves than are children of nonalcoholics. One possible cause of this relationship is a physiologically inherited trait in alcoholism. However, some experts contend that alcoholism runs in families because of the family environment and that therefore alcoholism is sociologically rather than physiologically determined.

Who Drinks?: Sociocultural Correlates

Besides the basic psychological and physiological factors that may lead to alcoholism, there are factors referred to as *sociocultural correlates* that also influence the way a person uses or abuses alcohol. Sociocultural correlates include such factors as age, homelessness, race and ethnicity, gender, and education and income level. These factors, alone or in combination with each other or with the previously discussed psychological factors, may lead to problem drinking and alcoholism. Let's briefly discuss these sociocultural correlates.

Age   Drinking starts for many people at a relatively young age, even before it is legal for them to drink alcohol. A national study of high school students' drug use has been conducted annually since 1978 by Lloyd Johnston. In 1988, Johnston found that 92 percent of high school seniors had tried alcohol at some time.[13] However, as depicted in Figure 11.4, the number of high school seniors who report being either current users or occasional heavy drinkers has been on the decline for several years. Still, in 1988, 64 percent of high school seniors reported they were current drinkers, and 34 percent reported having had five or more drinks in one sitting during the last two weeks (occasional heavy drinkers). And 31 percent of seniors said that most or all of their friends got drunk at least once a week.[14] This figure dropped to 12 percent when asked of 23-to 26-year-olds.

Studies of young adults find that drinking is prevalent among them as well. For example, one study of 17-to 25-year-olds found that about three-fourths were current drinkers, and nearly half (58 percent of the men and 33 percent of the women) were heavy

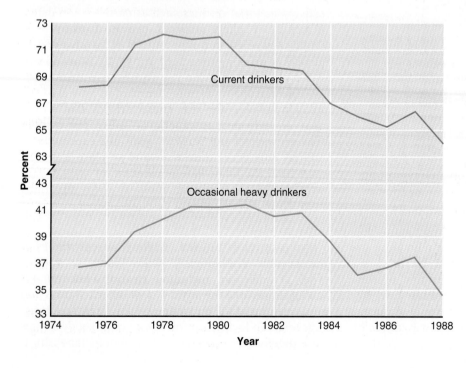

FIGURE 11.4 • Percentage of high school seniors who were current drinkers (used alcohol in the past 30 days) and percentage who were occasional heavy drinkers (took five or more drinks at a sitting during the past 2 weeks), 1975–1988.

Source: Lloyd D. Johnston, P. M. O'Malley, and J. G. Buchman, (1989). *Drug Use, Drinking, and Smoking: National Survey Results from High School, College and Adult Populations, 1975–1988.* DHHS Pub. No. (ADM)89-1638. (Rockville, Md.: Alcohol, Drug Abuse, and Mental Health Administration, 1989).

drinkers who had consumed six or more drinks on at least two occasions during the previous month.[15] Yet, when young heavy drinkers are followed over a number of years, most become social drinkers when they are older. For example, one study[16] found that only half of heavy drinkers identified at age 18 remained heavy drinkers at the age of 31, and 7 percent became abstainers altogether. These researchers found that the reverse pattern also occurred. That is, nearly half of the moderate drinkers became heavy drinkers.

The Homeless   The homeless report high drinking rates. Estimates of the rate of current alcohol abuse or dependence among the homeless range from 20 to 45 percent.[17] Whereas the incidence of alcohol abuse and dependence in the general population is greatest among the young, in the homeless it appears to be highest in the middle years. Making this problem even more significant is the realization that alcohol abuse is often accompanied by mental illness in the homeless. The result is a range of unhealthy consequences.

Race and Ethnicity   Several racial and ethnic groups have been studied to identify their drinking patterns. The following findings of these studies have been reported:

Whites and Blacks   When black men's and women's drinking is studied, similarities as well as differences with white men's and women's drinking patterns emerge.[18] Black men and white men have similar drinking patterns, although black men are somewhat more likely to be abstainers (29 percent versus 23 percent). White men are also more likely to be heavier drinkers. The same is true for white women. Forty-six percent of black women are abstainers compared to 34 percent of white women, and more white women drink heavily.

When drinking is studied by age, significant racial differences are found. White men age 18 to 29 are most likely to be heavy drinkers, with heavy drinking declining with age. For black men, drinking is heavy at ages 18 to 29, but rises even higher among those in their thirties.

Whereas overall drinking rates are lower in blacks than in whites, blacks experience more alcohol-related problems. Blacks, especially males, are more likely to contract cirrhosis of the liver, hepatitis, heart disease, and cancers of the mouth, larynx, tongue, esophagus, and lung. Black alcoholics are also more likely to encounter unintentional injuries and homicide.[19] Generally, blacks experience more social and health problems related to alcohol than do whites, with one major exception: drunk driving. Two and one-half times more whites are apt to drive while drunk than blacks.

Hispanics   Cultural background is certainly related to the consumption of alcohol. However, the culture in which one presently lives is even more important. There is no better example of this than the rates of alcohol consumption among Hispanic populations. For example, Hispanic men living in Spain drink more than five times as much as do Hispanic men living in the United States, and fifteen times more than Hispanic men living in Mexico.[20] Comparable differences also exist among Hispanic women living in different cultures.

However, within the United States there are dramatic differences between male and female Hispanics relative to the consumption of alcohol. Whereas more than 70 percent of U.S. Hispanic women are abstainers or drink less than once a month, almost the same percentage of Hispanic men are drinkers.[21] Heaviest drinking occurs when Hispanic men are in their thirties, and about 18 percent of Hispanic men and 6 percent of Hispanic women experience alcohol-related problems.

Asian Americans   As is the case with Hispanics, Asian Americans are affected by their culture. Consequently, the rates of alcohol consumption differ when the country of origin of Asian Americans is considered. This pertains to Asian Americans with origins in Japan, China, Korea, India, the Phillipines, and Vietnam.[22] Generally, however, alcohol consumption among Asian Americans is the lowest of all major racial and ethnic groups in the United States.[23] As Asian Americans become more acculturated into American society, their drinking levels increase. Other factors related to increased drinking among Asian Americans are their specific ethnic group, place of birth, and their generational status.

Native Americans and Alaska Natives   As with many of the other populations we have discussed, making generalizations about alcohol consumption among such a diverse group as Native Americans is problematic. Rates of alcohol consumption differ significantly among Native American tribal groups. Some tribes almost totally abstain, whereas others are heavy drinkers. Some experience significant problems with alcohol and others do not.[24] However, when conditions typical of alcohol-related problems are studied among both Native Americans and Alaska Natives, these appear to be high. For example, unintentional injuries (accidents), chronic liver disease and cirrhosis, homicide, and suicide are among the ten leading causes of death for Native Americans and Alaska Natives.[25] The rate for unintentional injuries is 2.2 times that found in the general population; the rates of homicide and suicide are approximately 1.7 times as high; and an estimated 75 percent of all traumatic deaths and suicides are alcohol related.[26] Deaths from alcohol-related causes are particularly prevalent among Native Americans between the ages of 25 and 44, and twice as high for men as it is for women.

blackout The loss of memory of what occurred during a bout of heavy drinking; this is an early symptom of alcoholism.

Gender A population that deserves special attention regarding alcohol consumption is women. This is because they make up such a large percentage of the total population, comprise a large percentage of the consumers of alcohol, experience a significant number of alcohol-related problems, and have the potential for affecting their fetuses should they become pregnant. Before 1980 there were few studies of women and alcohol, and it is therefore difficult to compare recent data with a baseline prior to 1980. However, surveys conducted since 1980 have identified subgroups of women subject to alcohol problems.[27] These high-risk women are employed outside the home, are divorced or separated from their spouses or have never married, are in their twenties and early thirties, and have husbands or partners who drink heavily. In addition, it seems that low self-esteem, unemployment, sexual dysfunction, and reproductive problems are associated with drinking problems. However, some of these problems may occur prior to heavy drinking and some as a consequence of heavy drinking. When it comes to drinking and driving, women are quite similar to men. For example, one study[28] of drinking drivers found both men and women to be mostly single and in their twenties and thirties. Driving and drinking is becoming an increasing problem for women. Women accounted for 11 percent of those arrested for drunk driving in 1980 and for 15 percent in 1984.

Education and Economic Level The NIAAA has also reported that educational and socioeconomic levels are important factors in drinking behavior. The higher a group is on those scales, the heavier the drinking.[29] This relationship may be explained by stress and opportunity. More highly educated individuals tend to have jobs involving substantial responsibility and therefore high levels of stress. In addition, they have money to support heavy drinking, as well as many job-related social opportunities to drink. High income itself can be stressful, creating anxiety about maintaining an expensive lifestyle.

Now that you have read about some of the major factors in alcohol abuse, take a moment to study Table 11.4, which gives profiles of those persons most and least likely to have alcohol-related problems. Does your description written in Exploring Your Health 11.3

TABLE 11.4

Profiles of Potential Problem and Nonproblem Drinkers

Profile of Persons with High Rates of Alcohol-Related Problems	Profile of Those Most Likely Not to Have Alcohol-Related Problems
Males at low socioeconomic levels	Persons over 50
Separated, single, and divorced persons	Widowed or married
Persons with no religious affiliation, followed by Catholics and liberal Protestants	Jewish religious affiliation
Those with childhood disjunctions	Rural residents
Beer drinkers, as opposed to hard liquor drinkers	Residents of Southern states
Persons who believe that drunkenness is not a sign of irresponsibility	Wine drinkers
Residents of large cities	Persons with postgraduate education

Source: National Institute of Mental Health.

fit the description of the problem drinker in Table 11.4? What stereotypes of the alcoholic have you found that you hold? Use the discrepancy, if there is any, between your description and Table 11.4 to uncover these stereotypes.

Stages in the Development of Alcoholism

The vast majority of individuals who have trouble handling alcohol arrive at their present stage of drinking behavior after a long period of drinking. Alcoholism is not the type of condition that happens today because of a decision someone did or did not make yesterday, last week, last month, or even last year. It is a gradual process that begins with social drinking and culminates—sometimes decades later—in an addictive drinking pattern that eventually controls most aspects of the individual's life.

As outlined by Dorothy Dusek and Daniel Girdano, and depicted in Figure 11.5, alcoholism generally develops in four phases: the prealcoholic phase, the early alcoholic phase, the true alcoholic phase, and complete alcoholic dependence.[30] During the first three phases, the drinker's tolerance for alcohol steadily increases, whereas it dramatically decreases in stage four.

Prealcoholic Phase
The prealcoholic phase is characterized by social drinking (controlled drinking in social situations, such as parties and eating out). The pattern evolves into drinking occasionally to escape from tension and frustration.

Early Alcoholic Phase
During the early alcoholic phase, drinking itself becomes a more and more important event. The very act of drinking—going to places where drinking takes place rather than to places where one knows it will not, socializing with people who drink rather than with those who do not, planning for the drinking part of a social or recreational event rather than the event itself—becomes a pattern to the point where the drinker is uncomfortable in nondrinking situations and will seek out a drinking situation as a substitute.

One of the most important signs of the early alcoholic phase are **blackouts;** that is, the loss of memory of what occurred while drinking. This loss of memory may or may not be associated with intoxication. The individual may have difficulty remembering who their drinking partners were, where the drinking took place, what events occurred while drinking, who drove, and so forth. These blackouts may be of short or long duration.

True Alcoholic Phase
During the true alcoholic phase, alcohol comes to dominate the drinker's life. Family relationships begin to deteriorate because of the drinking, and family members may try to reorganize their lives in order to avoid confrontations with the alcoholic and to isolate him or her from the family. As a result, the alcoholic is likely to feel self-pity and turn to alcohol for consolation. At this point, the alcoholic generally cannot stop after one drink. It is this element of need or compulsion that separates the alcoholic from other heavy drinkers. The alcoholic feels that drinking is essential, that it is the most important part of life.

Complete Alcoholic Dependence
The final stage, complete alcoholic dependence, is characterized by physiological addiction. If the drinker does not have alcohol, he or she is likely to experience severe withdrawal symptoms. The alcoholic at this stage is physically in danger from poor nutrition and possible liver and brain tissue damage. Without medical and psychological help, the alcoholic may die prematurely.

FIGURE 11.5 • Stages in the Development of Alcoholism

Prealcoholic phase ⟶ Early alcoholic phase ⟶ True alcoholic phase ⟶ Complete alcoholic dependence

Social drinking.

The act of drinking becomes a pattern.

Alcohol comes to dominate the drinker's life.

Alcohol is a physiological addiction. Without medical and psychological help, the alcoholic may die.

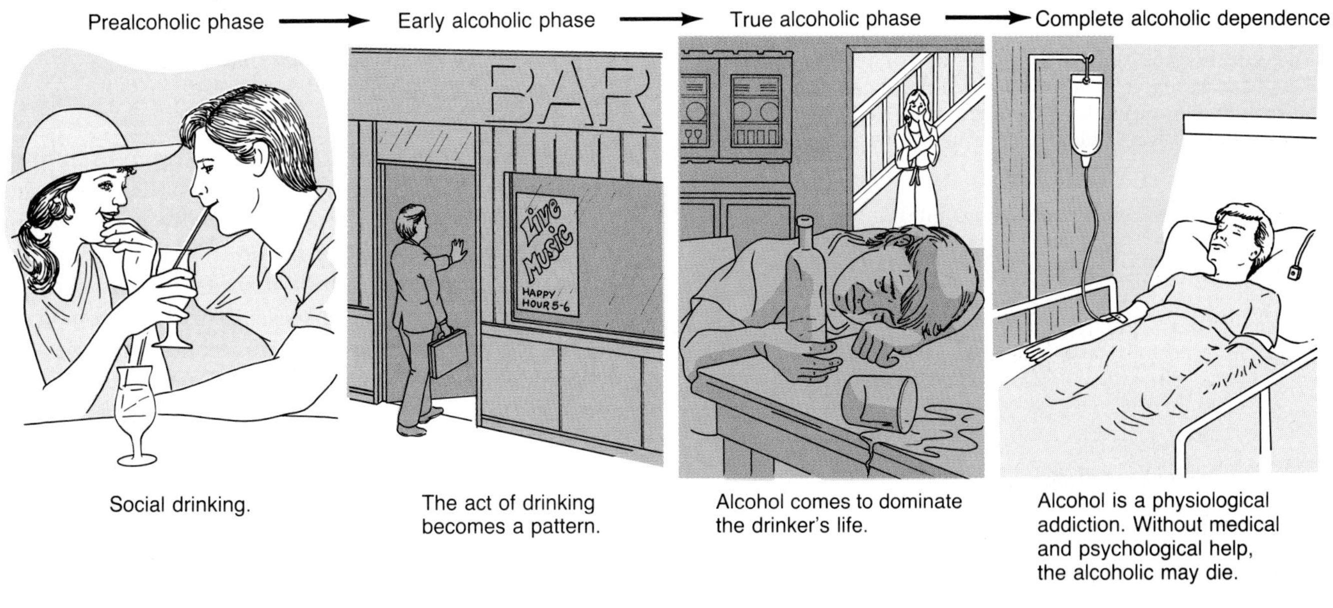

We must reiterate that these stages take several years to unfold and that in most cases they represent such a gradual evolution that they do not spell trouble to the individual, friends, or family. Of course, like everything else in the human dimension, these stages do not apply to every case of alcoholism. Some problem drinkers exhibit the symptoms of later stages in the earliest part of their drinking careers.

If you recognize these signs in yourself or in others, you have arrived at a point where you have to make a health decision. If it is your own drinking behavior that is in question, you will have to seek help. If it is another person's drinking behavior you are concerned about, you will have to consider what role you will play in giving help. There are agencies in your community to provide help. In addition to **Alcoholics Anonymous,** a fellowship of recovering alcoholics dedicated to helping others to recover, your local telephone book will lead you to various mental health and other agencies that will work with you. Not the least among these will be your own physician or health care facility.

This discussion of the progression of alcoholism should help those of you who have no problem with alcohol to see that those who do are ill and that they need understanding and help with their illness. For you, it is a decision of attitude; for those who have the problem, it is a decision of action.

One of the groups with a long history of helping alcohol dependent people to refrain from drinking alcohol is Alcoholics Anonymous. Although not a panacea for all alcoholics, it is an effective treatment for a large number of them.

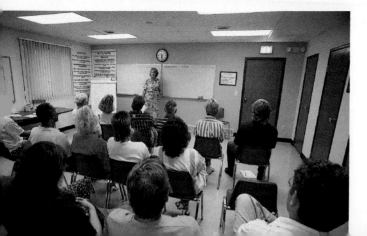

Alcoholism and the Family

You may have firsthand knowledge of the disruption to a family unit in which one member is an alcoholic. Whether the family unit consists only of husband and wife or includes children or other relatives as well, the resulting problems are so great that some authors refer to such units as **coalcoholic.** The family members are so intertwined with the alcoholic that they are unable to escape and feel trapped and helpless. Family members typically experience feelings of guilt, alternately blaming the alcoholic for disrupting the family, and themselves, individually or collectively.

The question of cause and effect is a difficult one. Is the stress of family responsibility or the inability to cope with family life actually the cause of the drinking problem? Or did the problem exist already and become associated with family life simply by virtue of the progressive nature of the disease? No matter which position one takes, it is now common practice to include the immediate family in therapy—that is, to see the alcoholic as a member of a family unit that both affects and is affected by the alcoholic. The reason for this is suggested in the following passage:

> *The fact that alcoholics live with, or in some important way are in contact with, significant others is only one dimension of the rationale for looking to family therapy for help in treating alcoholism. Along more functional dimensions, all aspects of family life are compromised when a member of the family is abusing alcohol. The marital relationships, parents and often the development of the children suffer.*[31]

Separation and divorce are very common in marriages in which one partner is an alcoholic. The result may be difficult for children, especially if the parent who retains custody of the children is the alcoholic.

Are children of alcoholic parents likely to become alcoholic? Whether the disease is actually genetic is debatable. However, children of alcoholic parents are more likely to abuse alcohol themselves. What the experts do agree on is that in many cases it is very difficult for a child to develop normally in an alcoholic home. Children who face aggression, abuse, and rejection from the alcoholic parent and overprotection from

Exploring Your Health 11.4

Signs of Alcoholism

1. Do you occasionally drink heavily after a disappointment, a quarrel, or when the boss gives you a hard time? _____.

2. When you have trouble or feel under pressure, do you always drink more heavily than usual? _____.

3. Have you noticed that you are able to handle more liquor than you did when you were first drinking? _____.

4. Did you ever wake up on the "morning after" and discover that you could not remember part of the evening before, even though your friends tell you that you did not "pass out"? _____.

5. When drinking with other people, do you try to have a few extra drinks when others will not know it? _____.

6. Are there certain occasions when you feel uncomfortable if alcohol is not available? _____.

7. Have you recently noticed that when you begin drinking you are in more of a hurry to get the first drink than you used to be? _____.

8. Do you sometimes feel a little guilty about your drinking? _____.

9. Are you secretly irritated when your family or friends discuss your drinking? _____.

10. Have you recently noticed an increase in the frequency of your memory "blackouts"? _____.

11. Do you often find that you wish to continue drinking after your friends say that they have had enough? _____.

12. Do you usually have a reason for the occasions when you drink heavily? _____.

13. When you are sober, do you often regret things you have done or said while drinking? _____.

14. Have you tried switching brands or following different plans for controlling your drinking? _____.

15. Have you often failed to keep the promises you have made to yourself about controlling or cutting down on your drinking? _____.

16. Have you ever tried to control your drinking by changing jobs or moving to a new location? _____.

17. Do you try to avoid family or close friends while you are drinking? _____.

18. Are you having an increasing number of financial and work problems? _____.

19. Do more people seem to be treating you unfairly without good reason? _____.

20. Do you eat very little or irregularly when you are drinking? _____.

21. Do you sometimes have the "shakes" in the morning and find that it helps to have a little drink? _____.

22. Have you recently noticed that you cannot drink as much as you once did? _____.

23. Do you sometimes stay drunk for several days at a time? _____.

24. Do you sometimes feel very depressed and wonder whether life is worth living? _____.

25. Sometimes after periods of drinking, do you see or hear things that aren't there? _____.

26. Do you get terribly frightened after you have been drinking heavily? _____.

Interpretation Any "yes" answer indicates a probable symptom of alcoholism.

"Yes" answers to several of the questions indicate the following stages of alcoholism:

Questions 1–8—Early stage.
Questions 9–21—Middle stage.
Questions 22–26—The beginning of final stage.

To find out more, contact the National Council on Alcoholism in your area.

Source: Reproduced with permission of the National Council on Alcoholism, Inc.

the nonalcoholic parent may have trouble developing the self-esteem necessary to lead a happy and productive life. For these reasons, experts commonly refer to the children of alcoholics as being *predisposed* to alcoholism.

Treatment of Alcoholism

Alcoholism is a complex problem requiring careful analysis of its development in each individual. Standard treatment regimes can relieve the physical (physiological) problems that are associated with or may accompany the illness. They relieve the symptoms, but they do not eliminate the disease.

Modern treatment programs make a step-by-step analysis of the factors contributing to alcoholism (personality, physiology, and sociocultural correlates), with the aim of helping the alcoholic readjust his or her life to control the need for alcohol. For example, **antabuse**—a drug that causes nausea when alcohol is subsequently ingested—has been used in attempting to control drinking. Individual and group counseling programs and family therapy programs can sometimes offer effective treatment. Programs of in-patient hospital care offer a combination of treatments.

Get Involved!

Insisting on the Responsible Use of Alcohol

Alcohol is considered by many experts to be the most problematic drug in our society. It certainly is the most pervasive and might be described as epidemic on college campuses. However, there are things you can do to improve the health of your immediate environment and the wider society in which you live as it relates to alcohol. For example:

1. Support alcohol-free parties and gatherings on your campus. Suggest several nonalcoholic beverages that could be served instead of beer, wine, or hard liquor. If some alcoholic beverages are nevertheless going to be served, suggest snacks that aren't salty and, therefore, don't increase thirst.

2. Whenever going out with friends to a place where alcohol is served, insist that the person driving not drink. If no one else volunteers to be the designated driver, you assume that role.

3. During discussions by politicians about budget matters—local, state, or national—advocate that revenue be raised by increasing taxes ("sin taxes") on alcohol. That will have the effect of both discouraging the excessive use of alcohol and of placing the responsibility for funding the health care system on a segment of the population that can be expected to use it more often.

4. Encourage campus administrators to meet with local bar owners to educate them about their responsibility for actions by students who become inebriated in their bars. Request that bar owners and bartenders refuse to serve alcohol to someone who has obviously had too much to drink.

5. Educate any pregnant relatives or friends about the potential effects of alcohol consumption on the health of the fetus.

6. Support politicians who advocate sufficient funding for alcohol treatment and alcoholism prevention programs.

We have already mentioned Alcoholics Anonymous (AA), a self-help organization for alcoholics. Since its founding in the late 1930s, this organization —along with groups subsequently patterned on it, Alanon for the family and friends of alcoholics and Alateen for children of alcoholics—has been the single most important factor in the recovery of thousands of alcoholics. The twelve steps of AA describe the approach that is used:

1. We admitted we were powerless over alcohol— that our lives had become unmanageable.

2. Came to believe that a Power greater than ourselves could restore us to sanity.

3. Made a decision to turn our will and our lives over to the care of God *as we understood Him.*

4. Made a searching and fearless moral inventory of ourselves.

5. Admitted to God, to ourselves, and to another human being the exact nature of our wrongs.

6. Were entirely ready to have God remove all these defects of character.

7. Humbly asked Him to remove our shortcomings.

8. Made a list of all persons we had harmed, and became willing to make amends to them all.

9. Made direct amends to such people wherever possible, except when to do so would injure them or others.

10. Continued to take personal inventory and when we were wrong promptly admitted it.

11. Sought through prayer and meditation to improve our conscious contact with God, *as we understood Him,* praying only for knowledge of His will for us and the power to carry that out.

12. Having had a spiritual awakening as the result of these steps, we tried to carry this message to alcoholics, and to practice these principles in all our affairs.

One very important factor to keep in mind: it is generally accepted by those involved in alcoholism therapy that alcoholics do not truly recover from their illness; that is, they can never expect to return to social drinking. Their recovery is dependent on total and continuing abstinence from alcohol.

Conclusion

In the final analysis, we have to think about what kind of family members we are or are going to be. We have to take a close look at how we treat other people, how we respond to the needs of others for security, friendship and understanding. The important question is not how much or even when and how a person drinks, but *why* a person drinks. We have discussed some of the reasons, or at least some of the factors that may lie behind those reasons. By regulating our attitudes and relations to others, each of us may be able to promote those conditions that help people to cope better with their lives and to develop a sound base for growth and development, avoiding the tragedy of alcoholism.

Summary

1. Annual consumption of alcohol has declined somewhat in recent years but still remains at an average of 2.54 gallons of pure alcohol per capita for people age 14 years and older in the United States.

2. The usage of alcohol pervades American society with over 74 percent of Americans reporting alcohol consumption over the past twelve months.

3. Alcohol is the drug most commonly used by high school seniors, with over 91 percent reporting consumption. An alarming 34 percent of these students report that at least once during the past two weeks they have consumed five or more drinks at the same sitting.

4. Only 21 percent of fourth graders believe that wine coolers contain a drug, and only 17 percent believe that daily consumption of wine coolers will cause any harm. A full 42 percent of sixth graders report personal use of wine coolers.

5. Between 35 and 64 percent of the drivers that were involved in fatal automobile accidents had been drinking before the accident. Even though the 16 to 24 age group accounts for only 16.5 percent of the population, over 45 percent of all the single vehicle fatal accidents are accounted for by this group.

6. *Social drinkers* are those who have no serious health consequences from their drinking and can control their consumption. *Alcohol abusers* are drinkers who suffer a variety of social or physical effects of alcohol consumption, but who seem to be able to control their consumption. *Alcohol dependent persons* usually suffer similar but more serious health effects from their drinking, but they are powerless to control their consumption.

7. The media and advertising, social gatherings, cultural rituals, and peer pressure influence drinking behavior.

8. Beer, wine, and wine coolers are *no* less likely to cause intoxication than hard liquor. It is the alcohol that intoxicates, and the alcohol content in a 12 ounce beer is equivalent to that in one shot of an 80 proof whiskey.

9. Once in the bloodstream, between 80 and 90 percent of the alcohol is metabolized by the liver. What is not metabolized will travel to the brain before it is eventually eliminated from the body.

10. Depending upon the amount of alcohol consumed, its effects on the body can range from no overt effects to a sense of relaxation, slower reaction time, impaired judgment, blurred vision, poor motor coordination, coma, and even death.

11. The effect of alcohol is complicated by the presence of other drugs in the body.

12. Alcohol consumed by a pregnant woman is particularly hazardous to the health of the fetus.

13. Alcoholism generally develops in four phases; the prealcoholic phase, the early alcoholic phase, the true alcoholic phase, and complete alcoholic dependency.

14. *Blackout,* the loss of memory while drinking,

may be the single most important predictor of the development of alcoholism later in life.

15. It is generally accepted that alcoholics never recover completely from their illness but rather can enter a *remission.* Because of this they should never expect to be able to return to social drinking.

Questions for Personal Growth

1. Do you consume too much alcohol? Where do you usually drink? When do you usually drink? With whom do you usually drink? Can you get better control over your alcohol drinking behavior by adjusting either where, when, or with whom you drink?

2. What influence did your early childhood and family have on your alcohol drinking behavior? Did others in your family either drink or not drink alcohol? Was alcohol ever discussed in your family? Was alcohol used as a part of family holiday meals? Did you receive education about alcohol in school?

3. What is it you can do to make alcohol less of a problem on your campus? Are you willing to do these things? If so, when will you begin? Who can you get to help you? Maybe you'll want to discuss some of these ideas with your instructor.

4. Have you ever put yourself at risk because of drinking alcohol irresponsibly? If so, what caused you to do that? What did you learn from that experience?

5. If you were responsible for developing national health objectives, what would the alcohol-related objectives be? Why would you choose these objectives? What individuals or organizations would you need to cooperate with you in order to achieve these objectives?

6. What do you think of famous people who have announced that they have a problem with alcohol and have sought treatment? Are you *less* impressed by them because they are alcoholics, or are you *more* impressed by them because of their willingness to admit their problem and then seek help?

7. What should happen to pregnant women who continue to drink alcohol? Should they be confined for the length of their pregnancy? Should their babies be taken from them at birth? Should they be required to pay for any costs associated with a birth defect? What else might be done?

References

1. "Alcohol Use Among Children and Adolescents," *Statistical Bulletin* (New York: Metropolitan Life Insurance, 1987), pp. 2–11.

2. Otis R. Bowen, "Commentary: Just Say No," *Statistical Bulletin, Alcohol Use Among Children and Adolescents* (New York: Metropolitan Life Insurance, 1987), p. 12.

3. U.S. Department of Health and Human Services, *Seventh Special Report to the U.S. Congress on Alcohol and Health* (Washington, D.C.: National Institute on Alcohol Abuse and Alcoholism, 1990).

4. A. P. Streissguth, D. C. Martin, and H. M. Barr, "Maternal Alcohol Use and Neonatal Habituation Assessed with the Brazelton Scale," *Child Development* 54 (1983): 1109–1118.

5. D. C. Martin, J. C. Martin, A. P. Streissguth, and C. A. Lund, "Sucking Frequency and Amplitude as a Function of Maternal Drinking and Smoking," in *Currents in Alcoholism,* Vol. 5, ed. M. Galanter (New York: Grune & Stratton, 1979), pp. 359–366.

6. R. J. Sokol, S. I. Miller, and G. Reed, "Alcohol Abuse During Pregnancy: An Epidemiologic Study," *Alcoholism: Clinical and Experimental Research* 447 (1980), pp. 87–102.

7. National Highway Traffic Safety Administration, National Center for Statistics and Analysis, *Drunk*

Driving Facts (Washington, D.C.: National Highway Traffic Safety Administration, 1988).

8. M. K. Bradstock, J. S. Marks, M. R. Forman, E. M. Gentry, G. C. Hogelin, N. J. Binkin, and F. L. Trowbridge, "Drinking-Driving and Health Lifestyle in the United States: Behavioral Risk Factors Surveys," *Journal of Studies on Alcohol* 48 (1987): 147–152.

9. U.S. Department of Health and Human Services, *Seventh Special Report to the U.S. Congress on Alcohol and Health* (Washington, D.C.: National Institute on Alcohol Abuse and Alcoholism, 1990).

10. L. A. Cappiello, "Prevention of Alcoholism—A Teaching Strategy," *Journal of Drug Education* 7 (1977): 311–316.

11. G. A. Marlatt, J. S. Baer, D. M. Donovan, and D. R. Kivlahan, "Addictive Behaviors: Etiology and Treatment," *Annual Review of Psychology* 39 (1988): 223–252; R. A. Zucker and E. S. L. Gomberg, "Etiology of Alcoholism Reconsidered," *American Psychologist* 41 (1986): 783–793.

12. B. Critchlow, "Brief Report: A Utility Analysis of Drinking," *Addictive Behaviors* 12 (1987): 269–273.

13. Lloyd D. Johnston, P. M. O'Malley, and J. G. Buchman, *Drug Use, Drinking, and Smoking: National Survey Results from High School, College and Adult Populations, 1975–1988.* DHHS Pub. No. (ADM)89-1638 (Rockville, Md.: Alcohol, Drug Abuse, and Mental Health Administration, 1989).

14. Lloyd D. Johnston, P. M. O'Malley, and J. G. Buchman, *Illicit Drug Use, Smoking, and Drinking by America's High School Students, College Students, and Young Adults, 1975–1987.* DHHS Pub. No. (ADM)89-1602 (Rockville, Md.: Alcohol, Drug Abuse, and Mental Health Administration, 1988).

15. B. F. Grant, T. C. Harford, and M. B. Grigson, "Stability of Alcohol Consumption Among Youth: A National Longitudinal Survey," *Journal of Studies on Alcohol* 49 (1988): 253–260.

16. M. T. Temple and K. M. Fillmore, "The Variability of Drinking Patterns and Problems Among Young Men, Age 16–31: A Longitudinal Study," *International Journal of Addiction* 20 (1985–1986): 1595–1620.

17. V. Mulkern and R. Spence, *Alcohol Abuse/Alcoholism Among Homeless Persons: A Review of the Literature. Final Report* (Washington, D. C.: U. S. Government Printing Office, 1984); J. D. Wright, J. W. Knight, E. Weber-Burdin, and J. Lam, "Ailments and Alcohol: Health Status Among the Drinking Homeless," *Alcohol, Health and Research World* 11, 3 (1987): 22–27.

18. D. Herd, "Drinking by Black and White Women: Results from a National Survey," *Social Problems* 35, 5 (1988): 493–505; D. Herd, "The Epidemiology of Drinking Patterns And Alcohol-Related Problems Among U. S. Blacks," in *The Epidemiology of Alcohol Use and Abuse Among U. S. Minorities.* NIAAA Monograph No. 18. DHHS Pub. No. (ADM)89–1435 (Washington, D. C.: U. S. Government Printing Office, 1989).

19. D. Herd, "The Epidemiology of Drinking Patterns" (1989); L. Ronan, "Alcohol-Related Health Risks Among Black Americans," *Alcohol, Health and Research World* 11, 2 (1986–1987): 36–39, 65.

20. R. Caetano, "A Comparative Analysis of Drinking Among Hispanics in the United States, Spaniards in Madrid, and Mexicans in Michoacan," in L. H. Towle and T. C. Harford. *Cultural Influences and Drinking Patterns: A Focus on Hispanic and Japanese Populations.* Research Monograph No. 19. DHHS Pub. No. (ADM)88–1563 (Washington, D. C.: U. S. Government Printing Office, 1988), pp. 273–311.

21. R. Caetano, "Drinking Patterns and Alcoholic Problems in a National Sample of U. S. Hispanics," in *The Epidemiology of Alcohol Use and Abuse Among U. S. Minorities.* NIAAA Monograph No. 18. DHHS Pub. No. (ADM)89-1435 (Washington, D. C.: U. S. Government Printing Office, 1989), pp. 147–162.

22. H. H. L. Kitano and I. Chi, (1986–87). "Asian-Americans and Alcohol Use," *Alcohol, Health and Research World* 11, 2 (1986–1987): 42–47; J. E. Lubben, I. Chi, and H. H. L. Kitano, "Exploring Filipino American Drinking Behavior," *Journal of Studies on Alcohol* 49, 1 (1988): 26–29.

23. D. Sue, "Use and Abuse of Alcohol by Asian Americans," *Journal of Psychoactive Drugs* 19, 1 (1987): 57–66.

24. C. M. Christian, M. Dufour, and D. Bertolucci, "Differential Alcohol-Related Mortality Among American Indian Tribes in Oklahoma," *Social Science and Medicine* 28 (1989): 275–284.

25. Indian Health Service, *Indian Health Service Chart Series Book.* DHHS Pub. No. 1988 0-218-547:QL3 (Washington, D. C.: U. S. Government Printing Office, 1988).

26. E. R. Rhoades, J. Hammond, T. K. Welty, A. O. Handler, and R. W. Amler, "The Indian Burden of Illness and Future Health Interventions," *Public Health Reports* 102, 4 (1987): 361–368.

27. R. W. Wilsnack, S. C. Wilsnack, and A. D. Klassen, "Women's Drinking and Drinking Problems: Patterns From a 1981 National Survey," *American Journal of Public Health* 74 (1981): 1231–1238; R. W. Wilsnack, "Drinking and Drinking Problems in Women: A U. S. Longitudinal Survey and Some Implications for Prevention," in *Addictive Behaviors: Prevention and Early Intervention,* eds. T. Loberg, W. R. Miller, P. E. Nathan, and G. A. Marlatt (Amsterdam: Swets and Zeitlinger, 1987), pp. 1–39.

28. E. R. Shore, M. L. McCoy, L. A. Toonen, and E. J. Kuntz, (1988). "Arrests of Women for Driving Under the Influence," *Journal of Studies on Alcohol* 49 (1988): 7–10.

29. U.S. Department of Health and Human Services, *Second Special Report to Congress on Alcohol and Health.* DHHS Pub. No. 74-124. (Washington, D.C.: U.S. Government Printing Office, 1974), pp. 16–18.

30. D. Dusek and D. A. Girdano, *Drugs: A Factual Account,* 4e (Reading, Mass.: Addison-Wesley, 1987).

31. W. E. Fann et al., *Phenomenology and Treatment of Alcoholism* (New York: SP Medical and Scientific Books, 1980), p. 12.

CHAPTER 12

Tobacco and Health

CHAPTER OBJECTIVES

After reading this chapter, you should understand:

- Why people, especially adolescents, start smoking in the first place and how advertising and other factors encourage tobacco use.

- Basic descriptions of the various forms of tobacco.

- How tobacco affects the human body, the reasons why tobacco is addictive, the various smoking-related diseases, and the economic costs of smoking.

- Two important pieces of antismoking legislation that were passed in the 1980s.

- The dangers of "passive" smoking and the rights of nonsmokers.

- Various methods and programs available to help the smoker kick the habit.

- A specific plan of action for helping a friend stop using tobacco.

- Some of the things being done in the government and private sector to encourage the antismoking movement.

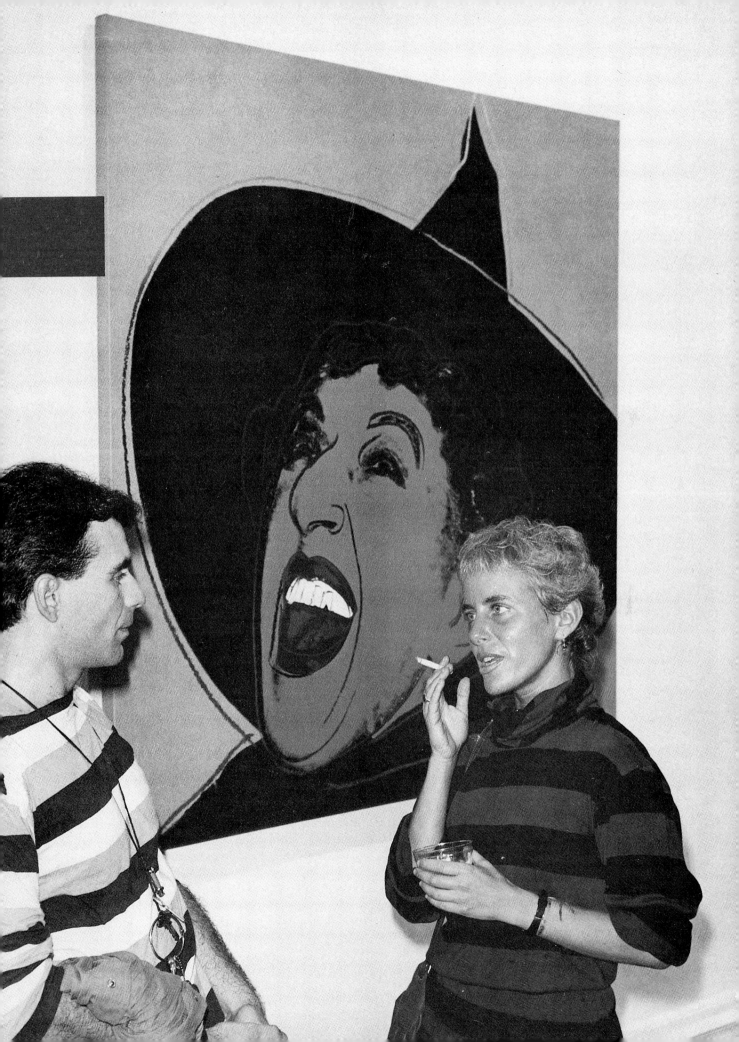

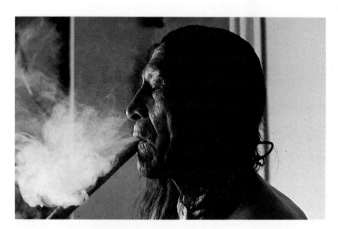

Tobacco holds a special cultural and religious significance for many Native Americans. In addition to smoking a pipe (which members of the white culture have referred to as the "peace pipe"), Native Americans use tobacco for such purposes as sacrificial offerings and as a kind of incense during religious ceremonies.

No less a person than King James I of England wrote of tobacco smoking that it is

> *A custom loathsome to the eye, harmful to the brain, dangerous to the lungs, and in the black stinking fume thereof, nearest resembling the horrible Stygian smoke of the pit that is bottomless.*

> *Counterblaste to Tobacco*

This was written in 1604—obviously long before we had thousands of pieces of hard scientific data indicating the harmful effects of tobacco use. Furthermore, the tobacco smoke that James was writing about was in some ways "healthier" than today's, for in 1604 tobacco did not contain the pesticides and other chemicals that our modern-day tobacco normally contains.

The tobacco plant, of the genus *Nicotiana* of the *Solanaceae* (nightshade) family, was brought to western Europe from the Americas some time after the expeditions of Christopher Columbus. Many Native American peoples used and still use tobacco, though they often reserve its use for religious and cultural ceremonies and for situations that call for demonstrations of good faith. European-American, European, and eventually, Asian peoples came to import, cultivate, and use tobacco for pleasure and recreation. Wherever it was introduced, it became popularly used for smoking or chewing, often amidst claims that it could cure numerous diseases and ailments.

In the United States, the early nineteenth century witnessed considerable opposition to public smoking, with religious groups branding the practice immoral, unhealthy, and improper for "respectable" people. Protective laws were introduced prohibiting minors and women from smoking. Taxation was introduced to curb the practice. Nevertheless, increasing mechanization, invention of the cigarette manufacturing machine for large-scale production, and advances in mass communication ultimately led to an estimated domestic consumption in the United States of more than 600 billion cigarettes annually by 1970. It is fair to say that advertising receives the greater share of the "credit" for such success in tobacco sales.

Today, despite the public outcry of the nineteenth century, only the law forbidding tobacco sales to minors remains on the books. Smoking among perfectly respectable people, including many minors, is widespread. Taxation of tobacco is only regarded as a "sin tax" whose aim is to raise revenue rather than to discourage tobacco use directly. Today, tobacco use, especially cigarette smoking, is the leading cause of preventable death and disability (through lung and other respiratory tract cancers) in the United States.

Why People Smoke

An understanding of the reasons why people smoke is helpful to both smokers and nonsmokers. It represents a very critical first step for the smoker toward eliminating the habit and it provides the nonsmoker with valuable information and insight to help others stop smoking. Take a moment to complete and score the test in Exploring Your Health 12.1. Analyze your scores and those of a smoking friend to determine the basic reasons for smoking and the best approaches to quitting.

Surveys reveal that the majority of smokers give

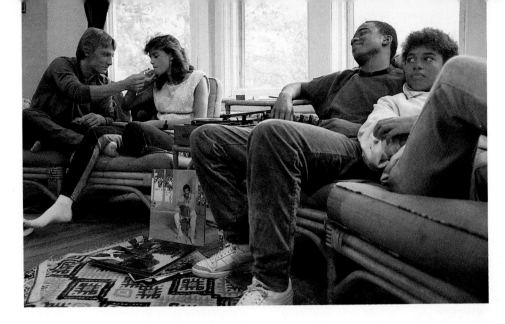

Most young smokers today are aware of the harmful effects of smoking, but they smoke anyway. Why do you think this is so?

several social or psychological reasons for smoking, such as stimulation, pleasure, alleviation of anxiety, relief from tension or anger, satisfaction of a craving for smoke, or merely because it is a habit.[1] Other studies reveal two broad groups of smokers: those motivated by needs (moods, hunger, or solitude) and those motivated by social factors (smoking in a group to gain confidence).

Adolescents generally fall into the category of socially motivated smokers. Recent evidence indicating that the majority (69 percent) of girls ages 12 to 17 prefer to date nonsmokers may influence some male adolescents to avoid the habit. Most young men and women who smoke have parents who smoke now or did in the past. Many of these parents did not object to their children's smoking. The number of high school smokers is twice as high in families in which one or both parents also smoke. Curiosity, impressing peers, and conformity are also factors in smoking among adolescents.

Young adult smokers have a rationale of their own for their behavior. They are very much aware of the harmful effects of smoking but feel that these dangers are exaggerated, that there is an overemphasis on things that are bad for you these days (such as artificial sweeteners, food additives, auto fumes, electrical power lines, and other so-called carcinogens), and that air pollution is as much a cause of lung cancer as are cigarettes. However, studies have revealed that air pollution plays only a minor role in lung cancer and deserves little of the blame for the modern-day epidemic of that disease.[2]

Table 12.1 presents some reasons why male and female teenagers and young women, viewed as a group, do or do not want to smoke. Notice that almost all of the reasons given have a strong element of "social motivation."

The Influence of Advertising

The purpose of cigarette advertising is to sell cigarettes, not to provide people with accurate information for use in decision making. Over $300 million is spent for cigarette advertising each year. This constant barrage of procigarette propaganda rather successfully undermines antismoking efforts. Although the elimination of cigarette advertising on television was an important first step, the cigarette industry has diverted its vast resources to magazines, newspapers, and billboards.

Factors that Encourage Smoking

Numerous political, social, and economic forces almost guarantee the continuance of tobacco smoking in the United States. It is unlikely that any representative sent to Congress from a tobacco-growing state will work toward the abolishment of cigarettes, or that state or federal governments receiving several billion cigarette tax dollars annually will lobby to eliminate smoking. An example of the dilemma is that the Department of Health and Human Services is charged with eliminating cigarette smoking while it and a number of other federal agencies are funded from the $2 billion or more received in cigarette taxes each year. Federal money is provided in the form of agricultural subsidies to tobacco growers, yet at the same time, large sums of money are spent searching for cures for lung cancer when a preventive approach through strong legislation offers an immediate solution. The picture is even more gloomy when considering the tremendous expenditure for advertising, manufacturing, shipping, and distributing involved. The power of the tobacco industry cannot be underestimated. Its insistence that there is no link between smoking and health is evidence of its utter defiance based on vested interest and economic pressures.

Exploring Your Health 12.1

Why Do You Smoke?

Here are some statements made by people to describe what they get out of smoking cigarettes. How *often* do you feel this way when smoking them? Circle one number for each statement.

Important: Answer every question.

If you don't smoke, read through these questions anyway. Perhaps they will help you better understand why other people do smoke.

	Always	Frequently	Occasionally	Seldom	Never
A. I smoke cigarettes in order to keep myself from slowing down.	5	4	3	2	1
B. Handling a cigarette is part of the enjoyment of smoking it.	5	4	3	2	1
C. Smoking cigarettes is pleasant and relaxing.	5	4	3	2	1
D. I light up a cigarette when I feel angry about something.	5	4	3	2	1
E. When I have run out of cigarettes, I find it almost unbearable until I can get them.	5	4	3	2	1
F. I smoke cigarettes automatically without even being aware of it.	5	4	3	2	1
G. I smoke cigarettes to stimulate me, to perk myself up.	5	4	3	2	1
H. Part of the enjoyment of smoking a cigarette comes from the steps I take to light it up.	5	4	3	2	1
I. I find cigarettes pleasurable.	5	4	3	2	1
J. When I feel uncomfortable or upset about something, I light up a cigarette.	5	4	3	2	1
K. I am very much aware of the fact when I am not smoking a cigarette.	5	4	3	2	1
L. I light a cigarette without realizing I still have one burning in the ashtray.	5	4	3	2	1
M. I smoke cigarettes to give me a "lift."	5	4	3	2	1
N. When I smoke a cigarette, part of the enjoyment is watching the smoke as I exhale it.	5	4	3	2	1
O. I want a cigarette most when I am comfortable and relaxed.	5	4	3	2	1
P. When I feel "blue" or want to take my mind off cares and worries, I smoke cigarettes.	5	4	3	2	1
Q. I get a real gnawing hunger for a cigarette when I haven't smoked for a while.	5	4	3	2	1
R. I've found a cigarette in my mouth and didn't remember putting it there.	5	4	3	2	1

Scoring

1. Enter the numbers you have circled in the test questions in the spaces below, putting the number you have circled for question A over line A, for question B over line B, and so on.

2. Add the three scores on each line to get your totals. For example, the sum of your scores over lines A, G, and M gives you your score on *Stimulation;* lines B, H, and N give the score on *Handling,* etc.

TOTALS

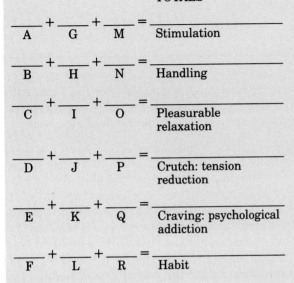

___ + ___ + ___ = _____
A   G   M   Stimulation

11 or above suggests you are stimulated by the cigarette to get going and keep going. To stop smoking, try a brisk walk or exercise when the smoking urge is present.

___ + ___ + ___ = _____
B   H   N   Handling

11 or above suggests satisfaction from handling the cigarette. Substituting a pencil or paper clip or doodling may aid in breaking the habit.

___ + ___ + ___ = _____
C   I   O   Pleasurable relaxation

11 or above suggests you receive pleasure from smoking. For this type of smoker, substitution of other pleasant habits (eating, drinking, social activities, exercise) may aid in eliminating smoking.

___ + ___ + ___ = _____
D   J   P   Crutch: tension reduction

11 or above suggests you use cigarettes to handle moments of stress or discomfort. Substitution of social activities, eating, drinking, or handling other objects may aid in stopping.

___ + ___ + ___ = _____
E   K   Q   Craving: psychological addiction

11 or above suggests an almost continuous psychological craving for a cigarette. "Cold turkey" may be your best method of breaking the smoking habit.

___ + ___ + ___ = _____
F   L   R   Habit

11 or above suggests you smoke out of mere habit and may acquire little satisfaction from the process. Gradually reducing the number of cigarettes smoked may be effective in helping you to stop.

Scores can vary from 3 to 15. Any score of 11 or above is *high;* any score of 7 and below is *low.*

Source: National Clearinghouse for Smoking and Health (USPHS).

TABLE 12.1

Some Reasons Why Male and Female Teenagers and Young Women Do or Do Not Want to Smoke

"I want to smoke because . . ."	"I don't want to smoke because . . ."
"Everybody" smokes anyway.	Only uninformed people smoke.
Health hazards are exaggerated.	I believe the health hazards are true.
My parents don't have a problem with it.	I don't need smoking as a social prop.
All real men/real women smoke.	My whole family smokes and I think it's disgusting.
My best friends smoke. (peer pressure)	It looks to me like most smokers know that it's a bad habit and want to quit.
Everybody in my family smokes.	
I like the way smokers are portrayed in advertising; I want to look that way, too.	I have more self-control than that.
It's antiauthority.	It makes you look ugly.
I'm addicted and can't help myself; it's my "only vice."	I'd never want to date or marry a smoker.
	My friend or relative has a terrible cough/bronchitis/emphysema from smoking and I'm afraid to start.
I'm a young housewife. The work is hard and I'm bored being at home.	I want to have kids and don't want to jeopardize them during my pregnancy or their childhood.
I enjoy it, and it'll be easy for me to give up someday.	I think antismoking regulation is a good thing and I want to set an example for others.
If I quit now, I'll gain a lot of weight.	

Source: United States Department of Health, Education, and Welfare.

Various Forms of Tobacco

When Christopher Columbus arrived in the "New World," Native Americans in North and South America were using the cured leaf of the tobacco plant for smoking, chewing, drinking as a syrup, and sniffing. Most cultures that have since been captivated by tobacco seem to prefer only to smoke or chew tobacco. Nevertheless, there are several forms in which tobacco may be smoked or chewed.

Cigarettes

Cigarettes are the single most popular form of tobacco in the world today. In the United States, cigarettes have been available since the mid-1800s, but in those days three out of four pounds of tobacco grown in the United States became cigars or pipe or chewing tobacco. Since the 1920s, there has been a steady shift to cigarettes. The tobacco used in cigarettes today contains not only nicotine and tar but also hundreds of chemical compounds—many of them from pesticides and other agricultural chemicals—that also find their way into your bloodstream through deep inhalation. To reduce consumer fears about these chemicals, the

cigarette industry has responded over the years with filtered, low-tar and low-nicotine, and clove cigarettes. Let's look briefly at these other kinds of cigarettes.

Low-Tar, Low-Nicotine, and Filtered Cigarettes

Low-tar, low-nicotine, and filtered cigarettes are indirectly promoted as "safe" cigarettes. Although the industry maintains that a less hazardous cigarette with reduced tar and nicotine—T/N—is not harmful to health, research indicates that there is no such thing as a "safe" cigarette. Changing to a low T/N brand, however, does reduce the risk of cancer slightly and may make it easier to quit in the future. Studies show that the mortality of low T/N smokers is about 16 percent less than high T/N smokers, 26 percent lower for lung cancer mortality. Unfortunately, low T/N smokers often change their habits to meet their craving for nicotine. Subjects who are unaware of the brand they are smoking increase the number of cigarettes smoked when using a low T/N brand. Conversely, consumption decreases among subjects smoking a brand high in nicotine. Those smoking nicotine-free brands also tend to "cheat" and substitute their own brand. Although some hazards may be reduced with filters, some filtered brands have been found to deliver more carbon monoxide (associated with heart disease) than unfiltered cigarettes. Unfortunately, a smoker who takes deeper puffs or partially blocks the ventilating holder or channels found in the cigarette filter can turn a 1–5 milligram tar cigarette into a 15–20 milligram tar cigarette.[3]

Clove Cigarettes

Clove cigarettes contain about 60 percent tobacco and 40 percent ground cloves, clove oil, and other flavoring agents. The smoke from these products is actually slightly higher in nicotine, tar, and carbon monoxide than that of most other cigarettes. The numbing effect of this mild sedative to the areas it contacts may result in the user perceiving it as a less hazardous, milder cigarette. Unfortunately, this is not the case and there is no evidence to suggest that clove cigarettes are less of a health hazard than other types. Clove cigarettes also cause more allergic reactions, and like other cigarettes they stimulate the central nervous system, irritate the respiratory membranes, raise blood pressure, and produce sweating, weakness, dizziness, and ringing in the ears in some users.

Cigars and Pipes

Cigars are made from rolled, unshredded tobacco leaves wrapped in a special tobacco leaf. Pipe tobacco is made from shredded leaves and flavored with aromatic substances. Both forms permit nicotine to enter the bloodstream via the mucous tissues of the mouth. The incidence of lip, mouth, throat, larynx, and stomach cancers are higher for cigar and pipe smokers than for cigarette smokers. These risks are present regardless of whether the user inhales or does not inhale. By not inhaling the strong cigar and pipe smoke, the risks of cardiovascular and respiratory diseases are reduced; for those that do inhale, the risks are actually greater than for cigarette smokers.

Smokeless Tobacco

Two popular forms of smokeless tobacco are chewing tobacco and snuff. The trend toward "dipping snuff" is most alarming: tobacco, which has been processed into a course, moist powder, is placed between the cheek and gum. The nicotine and other carcinogens are absorbed directly through the oral tissue. The practice is not only highly addictive but also results in nicotine levels equal to those of cigarette smokers. Chewing tobacco involves placing shredded leaf tobacco or plug from a pouch in the area near the inner cheek. A "chaw" is a golf-ball size quid of leaf or plug tobacco. In both tobacco chewing and snuff use, nicotine is absorbed through the oral membranes.

Evidence indicates that the use of all forms of smokeless tobacco is rising, particularly among male adolescents and young male adults. In 1985, over 12 million people in the United States used smokeless tobacco, half of them on a regular basis. The sight of a professional athlete on national television using smokeless tobacco as an alternative to smoking is common. With cigarette consumption declining, it appears that the tobacco industry is putting more advertising emphasis on smokeless alternatives. Although it is never explicitly mentioned, the industry implies that, unlike cigarette smoking, smokeless tobacco is safe. Studies of fifth graders indicate that the advertising ploy is working; children perceive smokeless tobacco as less of a health risk than smoking cigarettes. It is also not uncommon to see ten- to twelve-year-old boys using snuff or chewing tobacco.

Both snuff and chewing tobacco cause cancer in humans, particularly of the oral cavity. A smokeless tobacco user is several times more likely to acquire oral cancer than nontobacco users. In addition, the risk of acquiring cancer of the cheek and gum reaches nearly fiftyfold among long-term users. Oral carcinoma is among the most common acro-digestive cancers, with the lip the most prevalent site, followed by the tongue and floor of the mouth. Dental caries, receding gums, and increased wear on tooth enamel are also associated with the use of smokeless tobacco. In addition, the sense of taste and smell are depressed, resulting in a need to use more salt and sugar on food.

Physiological Effects of Tobacco Use

Take a moment to complete and score Exploring Your Health 12.2. This activity is aimed primarily at people who smoke, but even if you are a nonsmoker, completing it may give you some valuable insights into the smoker's attitude. Analyze your score and rate your present knowledge in this area.

Concern for the health of the smoker has developed slowly over recent decades. The medical profession started to become concerned over the effects of smoking in the 1930s, and public concern began in the 1950s, when statistics were published showing the rise in the number of cases of lung cancer and other ailments associated with smoking and higher death rates among smokers. An estimated 320,000 deaths annually in the United States alone are attributed to cigarette smoking. The now-famous Surgeon General's Report, released in 1964, substantiated the public's worst fears: "Cigarette smoking is a health hazard of sufficient importance in the United States to warrant appropriate remedial action." Shortly after the report was published, millions of people stopped smoking. Unfortunately, the impact was short-lived, and ten years later, in 1974, 42.2 percent of men over twenty-one and 30.5 percent of women over twenty-one were still smoking.

At present, cigarette smoking is clearly declining in the United States. One of the more negative trends is the tendency for the average smoker to smoke more heavily. Studies indicate that the proportion of adult male smokers who consume twenty-five or more ciga-

Year 2000 National Health Objective

One national health objective strives to reduce smokeless tobacco use by males age 12 to 24 to no more than 4 percent of that age group. Baseline data indicate that 6.6 percent of males age 12 to 17 and 8.9 percent of males age 18 to 24 currently use smokeless tobacco.

nicotine A colorless, odorless chemical compound found in the tobacco leaf. It is an addictive drug, acting first as a stimulant and then as a tranquilizer.

Year 2000 National Health Objective

To reduce the incidence of death from coronary heart disease, cancer, and chronic obstructive pulmonary disease (chronic bronchitis, emphysema, and asthma), a national health objective seeks to reduce cigarette smoking to a prevalence of no more than 15 percent among people age 20 and older. In 1987, 29 percent of people over 20 smoked cigarettes (32 percent for men and 27 percent for women).

Another health objective strives to reduce the initiation of cigarette smoking by children and youth so that no more than 15 percent, rather than the current 20 percent, become regular smokers by age 20.

rettes daily increased from 30.7 percent to 32 percent from 1976 to 1985; and for female smokers from 19 to 21 percent.[4]

Researchers have produced overwhelming and highly conclusive evidence demonstrating that cigarette smoking is a severe health hazard. Most Americans are aware of these health risks, although studies

show that more than 40 percent do not know that smoking causes most lung cancer, 20 percent were not aware that it causes any form of cancer, 30 percent did not know that smoking increases the risk of a heart attack, and 50 percent of female smokers were unaware that smoking during pregnancy increases the risk of stillbirth and miscarriage.[5]

Components of Tobacco Smoke

Cigarette smoke is a heterogeneous and poisonous mixture of gases, uncondensed vapors, and particulate matter. Over one thousand distinguishable chemical compounds have been identified; at least fifteen are known to cause cancer. Tobacco products smolder rather than burn brightly, an incomplete burning that results in a profusion of agents, particles, and chemicals.

Nicotine A colorless, oily compound, **nicotine** produces physical dependence or addiction. Smokers who inhale absorb about 90 percent of the nicotine into the body; noninhalers absorb 25 to 30 percent. Nicotine acts first as a stimulant, then as a tranquilizer. It is a powerful drug that stimulates the cerebral cortex (the outer layer of the brain controlling complex behavior and mental activity) and the adrenal glands. The re-

Besides the basic components of nicotine, tar, and carbon monoxide, tobacco smoke contains many pesticides and other potentially poisonous chemical substances that are used in the processing of tobacco leaves.

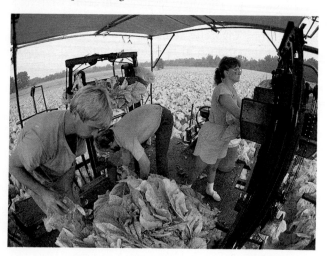

Year 2000 National Health Objective

The surgeon general has promoted the need for education about the risks of smoking by creating a national health objective to establish tobacco-free environments and by including tobacco use prevention in the curricula of all elementary, middle, and secondary schools, preferably as part of quality school health education. In 1988, 17 percent of school districts totally banned smoking on school premises or at school functions; and antismoking education was provided by 78 percent of school districts at the high school level, 81 percent at the middle school level, and 35 percent at the elementary school level.

Exploring Your Health 12.2

What Do You Think the Effects of Smoking Are?

For each statement, circle the number that shows how you feel about it.
Do you strongly agree, mildly agree, mildly disagree, or strongly disagree?

Important: Answer every question.

	Strongly Agree	Mildly Agree	Mildly Disagree	Strongly Disagree
A. Cigarette smoking is not as dangerous as many other health hazards.	1	2	3	4
B. I don't smoke enough to get any of the diseases that cigarette smoking is supposed to cause.	1	2	3	4
C. If a person has already smoked for many years, it probably won't do him or her much good to stop.	1	2	3	4
D. It would be hard for me to give up smoking cigarettes.	1	2	3	4
E. Cigarette smoking is enough of a health hazard for something to be done about it.	4	3	2	1
F. The kind of cigarette I smoke is much less likely than other kinds to give me any of the diseases that smoking is supposed to cause.	1	2	3	4
G. As soon as a person quits smoking cigarettes, he begins to recover from much of the damage that smoking has caused.	4	3	2	1
H. It would be hard for me to cut down to half the number of cigarettes I now smoke.	1	2	3	4
I. The whole problem of cigarette smoking and health is a minor one.	1	2	3	4
J. I haven't smoked long enough to worry about the diseases that cigarette smoking is supposed to cause.	1	2	3	4
K. Quitting smoking helps a person to live longer.	4	3	2	1
L. It would be difficult for me to make any substantial change in my smoking habits.	1	2	3	4

Scoring

1. Enter the numbers you have circled in the test questions in the spaces below, putting the number you have circled for question A over line A, for question B over line B, and so on.

2. Add the three scores across on each line to get your totals. For example, the sum of your scores over lines A, E, and I gives you your score on *Importance;* lines B, F, and J give the score on *Personal relevance;* and so on.

TOTALS

____ + ____ + ____ = _____
A   E   I   Importance

6 or below indicates that you may shrug off evidence available.

____ + ____ + ____ = _____
B   F   J   Personal relevance

6 or below may indicate the "it-can't-happen-to-me" attitude.

____ + ____ + ____ = _____
C   G   K   Value of stopping

6 or below suggests an ignorance of health benefits occurring when you quit.

____ + ____ + ____ = _____
D   H   L   Capability for stopping

6 or below suggests that you feel stopping would be difficult.

Scores can vary from 3 to 12. Any score of 9 or above is *high;* any score of 6 or below is *low.*

Source: National Clearinghouse for Smoking and Health (USPHS).

tar A dark, thick, sticky by-product of burned tobacco leaves; it is poisonous and carcinogenic.

carbon monoxide A poisonous gas found in tobacco smoke. It displaces oxygen in the bloodstream, causing a lack of oxygen in the body.

abstinence syndrome A medical condition experienced by many people who try to give up an addiction to nicotine or any other psychoactive drug. Symptoms include restlessness, changes in heart rate and blood pressure, and a craving for nicotine.

---

sulting bodily changes include increased blood pressure and heart rate, constriction of blood vessels, depression of hunger contractions, interference with the production of urine, and dulling of taste buds. Nicotine is also linked to heart and respiratory disease.

Tar A dark, thick, sticky by-product of burned tobacco, **tar** contains hundreds of chemicals, both poisonous and carcinogenic. These chemicals lodge in the forks of the bronchial tubes in the lungs to produce precancerous changes. Tar also damages the mucus and the cilia in the bronchial tubes, thereby decreasing their ability to remove foreign matter from the lungs.

Carbon Monoxide Another by-product of burned tobacco, **carbon monoxide,** displaces oxygen in the blood and produces shortness of breath. Smoking can result in levels of carbon monoxide in the blood as much as 400 times the safety limit specified by industrial hygienists.

A partial summary of other harmful constituents of tobacco smoke includes acetone (a solvent, carcinogenic agent), acrolain (results in paralysis of ciliated cells), aldehydes (preservative causing paralysis of ciliated cells lining the respiratory tract), ammon (colorless alkaline gas causing paralysis of ciliated cells lining the respiratory tract), arsenic (poisonous element, carcinogenic agent), benzyprane (carcinogenic agent), carbolic acid (powerful poisonous antiseptic, disinfectant, and germicide), formic acid (a blistering agent and counterirritant), methyl alcohol (wood alcohol causing intoxication, blindness, coma, and even death), nitrogen dioxide (a red gas causing paralysis of ciliated cells lining the respiratory tract), hydrocyanic acid (poisonous agent that checks the oxidation process in protoplasm and paralyzes the ciliated cells lining the respiratory tract), phenol (a powerful cocarcinogen), and pyridine (coal tar solvent).

Tobacco and Addiction

Few people think of ordinary cigarettes or tobacco as a potent drug, and probably even fewer view a smoker as a "drug user." In sufficient doses, however, nicotine is every bit as psychoactive as any illicit drug. Any smoker who has tried to quit recognizes that nicotine is addicting. Numerous studies have also identified nicotine as the main dependence-producing substance in tobacco smoke. Approximately thirty to forty million people in the United States are addicted to nicotine. The craving for its effects can be acquired after less than one month of regular smoking and will persist for months after quitting. A person who has a dependence on nicotine (or on any other psychoactive drug, for that matter) and decides to kick the habit may experience what is known as the **abstinence syndrome.** This involves both physical (decreases in resting heart rate and blood pressure, hormone changes, sensations of tingling or numbness, difficulty in sleeping, increased coughing, mild throat irritation, hunger, drowsiness) and temporary, usually short-lived psychological (craving for cigarettes and sweets, nervousness, tension, lack of concentration, loss of creativity, aggressiveness, irritability) withdrawal symptoms. Withdrawal effects may occur after only two hours since the last cigarette, with craving reaching a peak within the first twenty-four hours. This syndrome may be severe and makes quitting difficult even if the dependence is only mild. Nicotine is so addictive that only 2 percent of former smokers report that they can smoke only occasionally; the remaining 98 percent are convinced that even occasional use of tobacco would reestablish this dependence. It is important to recognize that terminating a strong dependence is difficult, regardless of the intensity of the abstinence syndrome.[6]

Smoking-Related Diseases

Smoking-related diseases and disorders are numerous. A discussion of the major health problems associated with smoking follow.

Lung Cancer Research findings in several countries demonstrate that cigarette smoking is the cause of the modern lung cancer epidemic. Approximately 157,000 new cases of lung cancer were reported in 1990, resulting in 142,000 deaths. The American Cancer Society estimates that cigarette smoking is responsible for 85 percent of lung cancer cases among men and 75 percent among women, or more than 83

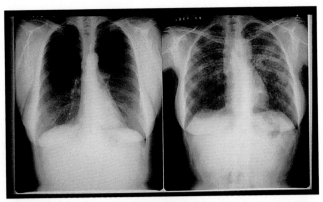

These x-rays show the lungs of a pair of females, both of them 60 years old. The woman on the left is a nonsmoker; her lungs are clean. The woman on the right is a smoker. How can you tell that this is so?

percent overall. The lung cancer death rate for women is steadily rising, and lung cancer is expected to surpass breast cancer as the number-one cancer killer of women.

Although nonsmokers also get lung cancer, it is interesting to note that 75 to 80 percent of all lung cancer in the United States is found among cigarette smokers, who represent less than one-third of the adult population. Even in the most heavily polluted industrial areas or cities, cancer rates are only slightly higher than in rural areas, but very much higher among smokers than nonsmokers in both areas. Among workers exposed to high concentrations of radioactive dust or other carcinogens where the lung cancer rate is much greater than in the general population, the lung cancer rate of smokers is more than 500 percent higher than for nonsmokers.[7]

Lung Cancer and Genes   If smoking is so hazardous, why doesn't everyone who smokes contract lung cancer? This question is all too common from the tobacco industry and the smoking population. Every smoker seems to be able to name one individual who used tobacco for sixty or more years with no ill effects. Finally, researchers appear to have found at least a partial explanation for these exceptions. It is now clear that genes, in addition to smoking, play a central role in who gets lung cancer. Epidemiologists have uncovered a gene, yet to be identified, that greatly increases the risk of lung cancer before the age of 50. A gene that encodes an enzyme that breaks down chemicals in the body has also been studied. The enzyme was found to function more efficiently in some people, increasing the chance of lung cancer sixfold in individuals with its most active form. The enzyme is suspected of turning compounds in cigarettes into carcinogens. But even with good genes, you can develop lung cancer if you smoke long enough. No hereditary protection has been uncovered for other smoking-related diseases, such as heart disease and stroke.

Warning signals of lung cancer include symptoms such as a persistent cough, sputum streaked with blood, chest pain, and recurring attacks of pneumonia or bronchitis. Heavy cigarette smokers with a history of twenty years or more of use are at high risk. Unfortunately, lung cancer is difficult to detect early. When smoking is stopped at the time of early cellular changes, damaged bronchial lining generally returns to normal. Continued smoking, however, results in the formation of abnormal growth patterns that can lead to cancer. Once diagnosed, only 13 percent of all patients in all stages live five years or more. Thirty-six percent of the cases detected in a localized stage survive for five years or more. Approximately one in five new cases are identified this early.

Bladder Cancer   Smoking is the greatest risk factor in bladder cancer. Cigarette smoking doubles the risk and causes an estimated 47 percent of all bladder cancer deaths among men and 37 percent among women. Warning signs include blood in the urine, usually associated with increased frequency of urination. The five-year survival rate is 87 percent when detected at an early stage.

Pancreatic Cancer   Cancer of the pancreas is a silent disease that generally occurs without symptoms. The incidence of pancreatic cancer is more than twice as high for smokers than nonsmokers. Sex, race, and high fat diets are additional risk factors. Only 3 percent of patients live more than five years after diagnosis. The 2 percent of patients contracting cancer in the insulin-producing cells and not its duct cells live longer, with 30 percent surviving for three years after diagnosis.

Oral Cancer   As mentioned previously, smoking and chewing tobacco have also been shown to be contributing factors to various forms of oral cancer, in-

Sigmund Freud, the ''Father of Psychoanalysis,'' suffered terribly from cancer of the palate and jaw in the last years of his life. Is there anything in this picture that helps to explain why?

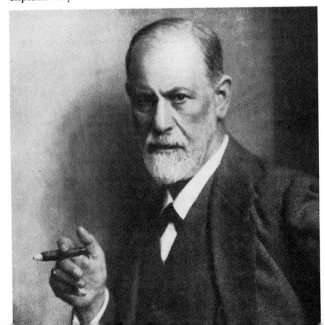

edentulism The loss of the natural teeth; hastened by smoking.

periodontal disease A disease of the gums; aggravated by smoking.

gingivitis A gum inflammation resulting in bleeding gums, pain, and foul mouth odor; aggravated by smoking.

chronic bronchitis A constant cough with the expectorating of mucus, especially upon arising in the morning; aggravated by smoking.

emphysema A serious lung disease characterized by coughing, shortness of breath, and extreme weakness; thirteen times more prevalent among cigarette smokers than among nonsmokers.

cluding cancers of the lip, tongue, and jaw (primarily among pipe smokers) and cancers of the mouth, pharynx, larynx, palate, and esophagus (among cigarette smokers). Most of the 30,500 new cases of oral cancer in 1990—resulting in 8,350 deaths—were related to tobacco use. A very famous and also very sad example of a person who suffered from oral cancer is Sigmund Freud, who lived the last years of his life in extreme pain from cancer of the palate and jaw. The warning signals of oral cancer may include a sore in the mouth that bleeds easily and fails to heal, a lump or thickening, a red or white patch of tissue that doesn't go away, and persistent difficulty in chewing, swallowing, or moving the tongue or jaws. Regular dental exams can sometimes help to detect oral cancer in its early stages. The five-year survival rates vary depending on the location of the cancer, from 35 percent for cancer of the pharynx to 92 percent for cancer of the lips.[8]

Other Oral Problems In addition to oral cancer, there are several other serious oral problems that smokers experience with much greater frequency than nonsmokers, including (1) **edentulism,** or loss of teeth; (2) **periodontal disease (pyorrhea),** a disease of the gums, spreading to the sockets containing the teeth and resulting in the destruction of the supportive structure of the teeth; (3) the delayed healing of tooth sockets after extraction; and (4) **gingivitis,** a gum inflammation resulting in bleeding gums, pain, and foul mouth odor. It is interesting to note that cigarette smoke is slightly acid and its nicotine does not penetrate mouth tissues. Pipe and cigar smoke and smokeless tobacco, however, are alkaline and permit nicotine to enter the bloodstream via the mucous tissues of the mouth. Mouth, lip, and tongue problems are therefore more common in pipe, cigar, and smokeless tobacco users.

Chronic Bronchitis and Emphysema Cigarette smoking is the most important predisposing cause of both **chronic bronchitis** and **emphysema.** Constant coughing and expectorating of mucus, particularly upon rising in the morning, are common symptoms of chronic bronchitis. While other causative factors may exist, cigarette smoking is the most com-

mon cause of inflammation of the bronchial tubes and their subdivisions and of the production of excessive mucus.

Emphysema is thirteen times more prevalent among cigarette smokers than among nonsmokers. The irritants in cigarette smoke reduce the lung's effectiveness as an oxygenating organ, making it more susceptible to disease.

With cessation of smoking, mild bronchitis will improve, although severe damage to the lungs (emphysema) cannot be repaired. Take a moment to test your ability to summon air to blow out a match held six inches from the mouth. Open your mouth and generate the air without puckering your lips as you normally would to blow out candles on a birthday cake. This is not a difficult task for the normal individual but is often impossible for an emphysema victim. Avoidance of cigarette smoking and keeping fit through regular aerobic exercise (see Chapter 9) offer the best protection against chronic bronchitis and emphysema.

Coronary Artery Disease, Heart Attacks, and Stroke Cigarette smoking is a major factor in the high death rate from circulatory diseases, heart attacks, and strokes (see Figure 12.1). It contributes to an estimated 325,000 deaths each year in the United States alone. Between the ages of forty-five and fifty-four, the death rate for male smokers from coronary heart disease is three times higher than the rate for nonsmoking males and two times higher than the rate for nonsmoking females. Research findings link nonfatal heart attacks to cigarette smoking independently of any other causative factors. Experimental evidence has also demonstrated the damaging effects of smoking on the heart and coronary arteries. Moderate to advanced thickening of the coronary arteries is more common in heavy smokers. Numerous autopsy studies show increased atherosclerosis in the coronary arteries of smokers. In addition, strokes and arterial disease of the leg are related to cigarette smoking.

Smoking and the Woman

Many early studies of the effects of tobacco use concentrated on male populations. The adverse health ef-

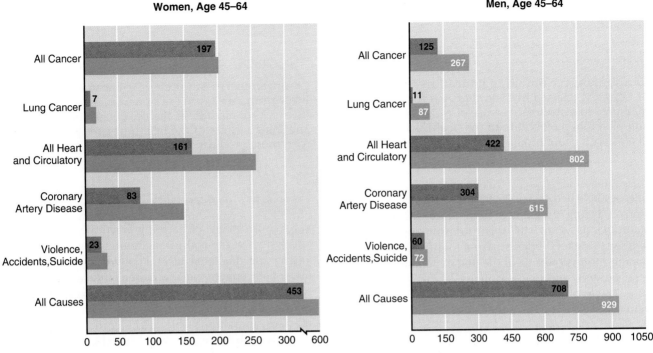

Women, Age 45–64

Men, Age 45–64

Note: Scales for Men and Women Are Different

FIGURE 12.1 • Death rates of cigarette smokers versus nonsmokers by selected diseases related to smoking (rates per 100,000 person-years).

Source: U.S. Department of Health, Education, and Welfare. *Chart Book on Smoking, Tobacco, and Health.*

fects of smoking for men are fairly well known and many of these effects—such as the increased risk of heart disease and lung cancer—apply to women also. However, more recent studies have shown that women face several unique health risks by using tobacco.

All smoking women face the prospect of bone density loss leading to osteoporosis. However, the woman who smokes and uses or intends to use the birth control pill or who is or intends to become pregnant faces other special health problems. Although the use of oral contraceptives by itself is no longer considered a heart disease risk factor, the combination of using birth control pills and smoking tobacco does pose a serious threat of heart disease for women by increasing the risk of blood clot formation, which increases the risk of heart attack and stroke.

Women who decide they want to become pregnant pose other risks to their own health and, eventually, to the health of their unborn children by smoking. One study has shown that women smokers who become pregnant have a 40 percent greater risk of a tubal pregnancy (see Chapter 6) than nonsmoking women. Ironically, this study also found that tubal pregnancy is less common in women who smoke heavily than in women who smoke lightly; the researchers believe that this finding reflects the fact that women who smoke heavily have a much lower chance of becoming pregnant in the first place (perhaps because nicotine

may decrease the levels of female reproductive hormones).[9]

Smoking during pregnancy poses dangers to both the mother and the fetus. Smoking results in the absorption of carbon monoxide and reduction in the supply of oxygen to the mother and the unborn baby. Smoking one pack of cigarettes per day can reduce oxygen supply to the unborn fetus by 20 percent or more. In addition, smoking elevates fetal heart rate and blood pressure, constricts blood vessels, and impairs breathing.

While no direct cause-and-effect relationship has

Year 2000 National Health Objective

To reduce the health hazards to the fetuses of smoking mothers, the federal government has established a national health objective to increase smoking cessation during pregnancy so that at least 60 percent of women who are cigarette smokers at the time they become pregnant quit smoking early in pregnancy and maintain abstinence for the remainder of their pregnancy. Approximately 39 percent of white women age 20 to 44 quit at some time during pregnancy in 1985.

Comprehensive Smoking Education Act An Act of Congress enacted in 1984 that calls for various measures to discourage the use of cigarettes, cigars, and pipe tobacco because of the health hazards connected with those products.

Comprehensive Smokeless Tobacco Health Education Act An Act of Congress enacted in 1986 that seeks to discourage the use of chewing tobacco and snuff because of the health hazards associated with those products.

been established, it has been found that women who smoke during pregnancy have more stillbirths and spontaneous abortions than nonsmoking pregnant women. Smokers' infants have a higher mortality rate during the first month of life and experience retarded fetal growth, and twice as many of them are premature. Traces of nicotine have been found in the milk of smoking mothers, which will affect the nursing infant.

Other Health Problems

Tobacco is capable of harming practically every organ and system in the body. In addition to various cancers, gastric and duodenal ulcers, pulmonary tuberculosis, lower body weight, and decreased physical fitness have been linked to tobacco smoking. Heavy cigarette smoking has even been correlated with deep wrinkling in the face, most noticeable at the corners of the eyes. There is evidence suggesting that smoking heavily can result in a facial appearance that is ten to fifteen years beyond one's chronological age.

The Economic Cost of Cigarette-Induced Major Illnesses

Since the release of the 1964 Surgeon General's Report on Smoking and Health, the American people have incurred more than $930 billion in medical costs for cigarette-induced major illnesses (see Table 12.2). Experts feel that this is a conservative figure that would be much higher if ailments other than cancer, cardiovascular disease, and chronic lung disease were included. Both smokers and nonsmokers bear the cost. Nonsmokers support public welfare programs that provide benefits to individuals who are disabled by smoke-related diseases and to their survivors, pay higher insurance premiums and increased prices for consumer goods due to the high work absenteeism of smokers.

TABLE 12.2

Costs to American Economy for Cigarette-Induced Major Illnesses, 1964–1983

Health-care costs for cigarette-induced cancer	56,200,000,000
Productivity lost because of cigarette-induced cancer	186,300,000,000
Subtotal: Cancer	$242,500,000,000
Health-care costs for cigarette-induced cardiovascular disease	108,300,000,000
Productivity lost because of cigarette-induced cardiovascular disease	265,600,000,000
Subtotal: Cardiovascular Disease	$373,900,000,000
Health-care costs for cigarette-induced chronic lung disease	120,000,000,000
Productivity lost because of cigarette-induced chronic lung disease	195,400,000,000
Subtotal: Chronic Lung Disease	$315,400,000,000
Total Cost	$931,800,000,000

Source: National Interagency Council on Smoking and Health, "American Council on Science and Health Bills Tobacco Industry," *Smoking and Health Reporter* 1, 4 (July 1984): 1. Copyright © 1984 National Interagency Council on Smoking and Health. Used with permission.

Tobacco and the Law

Since 1984, two very important pieces of legislation were passed to help the public make wise choices concerning the use of tobacco.

1. **The Comprehensive Smoking Education Act,** signed by President Ronald Reagan on October 12, 1984, has been labeled one of the most important pieces of antismoking legislation ever passed by Congress. The new act contains three provisions: (1) replacement of the current health warning on cigarette packages, advertisements,

and billboards with four much stronger and more visible disease-specific warnings, (2) the requirement that all companies disclose to the secretary of Health and Human Services a complete list of all chemicals and other ingredients added to cigarettes during the manufacturing process, and (3) the creation of a statutory mandate for the federal Office on Smoking and Health and a new federal interagency council to coordinate and oversee federal and private research efforts dealing with the health hazards of smoking.

Under the new law, the following four warning signals began to be rotated quarterly on all cigarette packages and advertisements beginning October 1985:

SURGEON GENERAL'S WARNING: Smoking Causes Lung Cancer, Heart Disease, Emphysema, and May Complicate Pregnancy.

SURGEON GENERAL'S WARNING: Quitting Smoking Now Greatly Reduces Serious Risks to Your Health.

SURGEON GENERAL'S WARNING: Smoking by Pregnant Women May Result in Fetal Injury, Premature Birth, and Low Birth Weight.

SURGEON GENERAL'S WARNING: Cigarette Smoke Contains Carbon Monoxide.

Standards also exist for the size of these warnings on cigarette ads to make them more visible.

2. **The Comprehensive Smokeless Tobacco Health Education Act** was passed by Congress in February 1986. The Act requires manufacturers of chewing tobacco and snuff to include health warning labels on packages. The Law also banned radio and television advertising of these products and requires manufacturers to reveal to the U.S. Department of Health and Human Services what additives and flavorings they contain.[10]

Rights of Nonsmokers

Characteristics of Nonsmokers

While not all nonsmokers can be grouped in a single category, several characteristics are common to this group. Some nonsmokers are very religious, respectful of authority, and turned off by the lack of moral values.

Issues in Health

Is the Smoking Data Released by the Cigarette Industry Accurate?

According to the cigarette industry, most Americans hear and read only one side of the issue—that of the surgeon general of the United States and a few scientific studies that draw conclusions unwarranted from their data. Researchers find a statistical link between tobacco use and disease, it is argued, and then make the very large jump to cause-and-effect. A significant relationship between tobacco use and lung cancer, for example, provides no proof that tobacco actually caused the cancer. In fact, statements by the tobacco industry suggest that there is absolutely no evidence of a cause-effect relationship between cigarette smoking and any type of disease, including heart disease and cancer. The dangers of secondhand or passive smoke and smokeless tobacco (plug, leaf, and snuff) have been called ridiculous. Some evidence generated by the cigarette industry also suggests that it would require considerably more cigarettes than any human could ever smoke to produce cancer.

Nor has any study, according to the industry, demonstrated that smokeless tobacco causes cancer of the lip, mouth, tongue, or other body part, or any other ailment. It is therefore unjust to ban smoking in public, eliminate TV advertisements, restrict advertisements aimed at specific groups, and force the use of health warning labels.

The tobacco industry spends large sums of money to buy ads and sends speakers across the country to refute the scientific evidence that smoking is the major cause of preventable death in the United States. This strategy plants seeds of doubt in smokers' minds through a complete distortion of facts. The truth is that there is no controversy about the association between smoking and disease and death. Practically all scientists who conduct the research and experts who read and interpret it are convinced that the data are accurate and that tobacco use, in any form, constitutes a serious health hazard. Numerous studies that uncovered

these findings were actually funded by the cigarette industry. According to many experts, the data are so convincing that its conclusions are not even worthy of debate.

Is the evidence concerning the health hazards of tobacco use accurate or nothing more than a conspiracy? Is this giant industry merely being unjustly attacked? Certainly, this industry is important for the U.S. economy because of the tax revenues it generates. What is the motivation behind the attacks if no health hazards exist? Is the data released by the tobacco industry nothing more than irresponsible propaganda aimed at selling their product at any cost? Is the tobacco industry interested in the health or merely the wealth (the industry's own profit!) of the nation?

What do you think?

passive smoking Inhaling tobacco smoke that comes from the cigarettes, cigars, and pipes of other people. The smoke from these sources is known as second-hand smoke.

Others share many of the same values as smokers but feel that by not smoking they will be more in control of their lives. Nonsmokers are likely to be concerned about nicotine addiction and to emphasize physical fitness and health. In recent years nonsmokers have been increasingly vocal about insisting on certain rights that they believe are essential to preserving the health, comfort, and safety of everyone.

Passive Smoking

As we mentioned earlier, tobacco smoke contains about 1,000 chemical compounds, including 15 known carcinogenic (cancer-causing) substances. When someone smokes, these poisons are released into the air, which is inhaled by other people in the area. Whether these other people like it or not, when they inhale "secondhand smoke," they engage in **passive smoking.** Secondhand smoke consists of two kinds of smoke: (1) *mainstream smoke,* which the smoker pulls into the mouth and lungs and exhales through the mouth and nostrils, and (2) *sidestream smoke,* which goes directly into the air from the burning tobacco. Like the smoker, the nonsmoker breathes in carcinogenic substances from both kinds of smoke when she or he is in a smoker's presence. Every nonsmoker should be aware that *there is twice as much tar and nicotine and three times as much carbon monoxide (which robs the blood of oxygen) in sidestream smoke as in*

Year 2000 National Health Objective

In recognition of the dangers of secondhand smoke, the federal government has established a national health objective to reduce to no more than 20 percent the proportion of children age 6 and younger who are regularly exposed to tobacco smoke at home. In 1986, there was a cigarette smoker in 39 percent of households with one or more children age 6 or younger.

mainstream smoke. In addition, there is more cadmium in the smoke that drifts off burning ends of cigarettes than in the drag the smoker takes. Cadmium has been related to hypertension, chronic bronchitis, and emphysema. Smoke from the idling cigarette also contains more tar and nicotine than inhaled smoke. The amount of carbon monoxide in the blood of nonsmokers doubles in a poorly ventilated room filled with cigarette smoke and this carbon monoxide remains in the body for three to four hours.

The realization that clean air in the United States is everyone's right is now widespread. Unfortunately many nonsmokers still tolerate smoke pollution. The "Nonsmoker's Bill of Rights" shown in Figure 12.2 emphasizes the need for nonsmokers to speak out and act on their own behalf.

Local, state, and federal governments are also in-

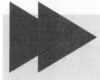

Exploring Your Health 12.3

Secondhand Smoke and Heart Rate

The next time you are in an automobile or an enclosed room, sit quietly for five to ten minutes before taking your radial pulse. To take your pulse, place the index and middle fingers of your right hand in the small hollow just below your left thumb. Count the beats for thirty seconds and record that number for future reference. Do the same thing with your breathing rate. Stand before a mirror and count the number of times your chest rises or sit quietly and count the number of times you breathe for one minute. Record this on the same note pad. Repeat these two procedures immediately after an individual or group of individuals have smoked in your presence in an enclosed room or automobile. Compare the two heart and breathing rates. What did you find? Does secondhand smoke affect your body?

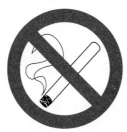

Non-Smoker's Bill of Rights

NON-SMOKERS HELP PROTECT THE HEALTH, COMFORT AND SAFETY OF EVERYONE BY INSISTING ON THE FOLLOWING RIGHTS:

THE RIGHT TO BREATHE CLEAN AIR
NON-SMOKERS HAVE THE RIGHT TO BREATHE CLEAN AIR, FREE FROM HARMFUL AND IRRITATING TOBACCO SMOKE. THIS RIGHT SUPERSEDES THE RIGHT TO SMOKE WHEN THE TWO CONFLICT.

THE RIGHT TO SPEAK OUT
NON-SMOKERS HAVE THE RIGHT TO EXPRESS – FIRMLY BUT POLITELY – THEIR DISCOMFORT AND ADVERSE REACTIONS TO TOBACCO SMOKE. THEY HAVE THE RIGHT TO VOICE THEIR OBJECTIONS WHEN SMOKERS LIGHT UP WITHOUT ASKING PERMISSION.

THE RIGHT TO ACT
NON-SMOKERS HAVE THE RIGHT TO TAKE ACTION THROUGH LEGISLATIVE CHANNELS, SOCIAL PRESSURES OR ANY OTHER LEGITIMATE MEANS – AS INDIVIDUALS OR IN GROUPS – TO PREVENT OR DISCOURAGE SMOKERS FROM POLLUTING THE ATMOSPHERE AND TO SEEK THE RESTRICTION OF SMOKING IN PUBLIC PLACES.

National Interagency Council on Smoking and Health, 419 Park Ave. So. Room 1301, New York, NY 10016

FIGURE 12.2 • Nonsmoker's Bill of Rights
Source: American Cancer Society.

volved in the effort to help nonsmokers. The majority of states now have laws limiting or banning smoking in public places, including the work place. Hundreds of cities and towns have ordinances covering smoking at work. A growing number of states and communities are proposing legislation to restrict smoking in public places, and smoking has been banned on all air flights of two hours or less. The antismoking movement is nationwide and growing. A complete ban on smoking in public areas is not too far in the future.

Smokers no longer have the social edge; 70 percent of Americans are now nonsmokers. The realization by both groups that secondhand smoke is harmful and that both smokers and nonsmokers have rights is leading to nationwide regulations that will improve the health of millions of Americans.

How Nonsmokers Can Deal with Smokers

Even with the law and the number of citizens on the side of the nonsmoker, it is not easy for some people to be assertive enough to say "yes" when asked, "Do you mind if I smoke," to move to another area in a public place if a nonsmoking area does not exist, or to ask an individual to stop smoking. New laws and smoking and nonsmoking sections in public places are making it easier to avoid secondhand or passive smoke; however, there will still be times when only you can change the situation. Perhaps it is important to remember that you have the right to do so. Figure 12.3 features several other specific ways that nonsmokers can deal with smokers in various settings.

The Benefits of Not Smoking

The obvious benefits of not smoking are improved health and vitality, reduced risk of the chronic and degenerative diseases discussed in this chapter, healthier offspring, improved performance in exercise, and a longer life. There are additional advantages. For example, there is strong speculation that smoking and sexual performance are related. It is known that carbon monoxide reduces the blood oxygen level and impairs hormone production. There is also evidence that nicotine constricts blood vessels and may inhibit sexual ex-

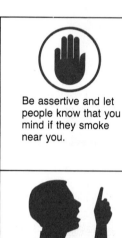 Be assertive and let people know that you mind if they smoke near you.	Be obvious; wear buttons and use stickers and signs in your home, car, and office.	Use body language; wave away smoke, grimmace and take defensive postures.	Keep informed; know the no-smoking regulations in your community.
Help uphold the law; speak up when the law is broken.	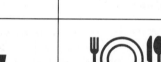 **NO SMOKING** Be firm, but polite; use courteous appeals for cooperation, not put-downs.	*Smoking on patio only* Protect your home and friends; disallow smoking or designate a special area for smokers.	**SMOKING PROHIBITED** Protect the work place; many state superior courts have granted the right to a smoke-free work place.
Propose no-smoking resolutions at organization and club meetings.	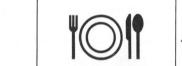 Request seating in a non-smoking area when dining; suggest a survey to owners on the subject if there are no restricted areas.	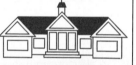 Seek a total ban on smoking in schools, including teachers' lounges, and . . .	Support legislation about your desire for more non-smoking areas in public places.

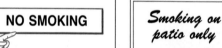

FIGURE 12.3 • Suggestions from the American Lung Association to Help You Deal with Smokers in Various Settings

Source: American Lung Association, *Facts and Figures for Nonsmokers and Smokers* (1982).

citement and, in men, the physiological capability for a full erection. For some individuals, a low level of fitness due to sedentary living, obesity, and smoking can reduce stamina and the ability to continue intercourse for as long as they'd like. Whether discolored teeth and smoking breath make one less sexually attractive or desirable depends upon the partner; they are apparently much less offensive when both partners are smokers.

Another advantage to the nonsmoker is cost. For the heavy smoker or a family with two or more smokers, the habit can be quite expensive. In addition, a number of life, accident, and disability insurance companies provide discount rates for nonsmokers. Studies clearly demonstrate that nonsmokers live longer, have fewer automobile accidents, and are less likely to become disabled. Depending upon the state, the nonsmoker may pay 5 to 20 percent less in insurance premiums. Middle-age smokers will also spend an average of $59,000 each in extra medical bills and lost earnings during their lifetime. Quitting at any time would reduce this cost.

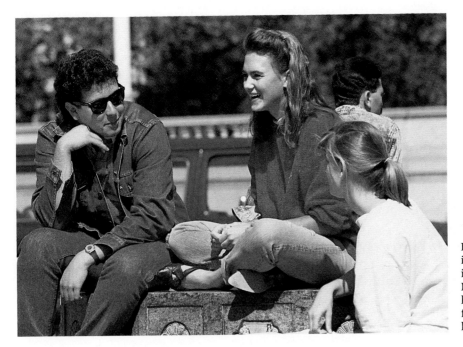

Even with all the data to tell us so, it is clear to most of us that not smoking is obviously better than smoking. Nonsmokers enjoy fewer health risks, higher levels of stamina and overall fitness, and, possibly, better sexual lives than smokers!

Kicking the Tobacco Habit

The single most important factor in eliminating any habit is motivation. Complete and score Exploring Your Health 12.4 to determine your motivation or the motivation of a friend to quit smoking.

According to the American Cancer Society, over twenty-five million people in the United States (two million per year, one in five adult men) have kicked the smoking habit. Approximately 85 percent of the smoking population have indicated that they would like to quit. The four most common reasons for giving up cigarette smoking are: (1) concern over the effects on health; (2) desire to set an example; (3) esthetics, or the unpleasant aspects of smoking; and (4) the desire for self-control.

Smokers express a number of reasons for continuing the smoking habit. Table 12.3 summarizes the most common excuses of smokers in the United States. The success rate is higher among light smokers (less than one pack per day). Cessation programs are based on eliminating dependence on nicotine. Breaking the dependence may involve supportive social or psychological measures or a pharmacological approach aimed toward changing the smoker's behavior.

Health Education Programs

Although it would seem logical to assume that a smoker, when presented with the medical facts, would change his or her smoking behavior, this rarely occurs. The high failure rate of traditional educational pro-

grams aimed at helping people to stop smoking is explained by the following:

- Nicotine dependence can be very intense and can counter one's desire to quit smoking.
- Peer pressure can negate educational efforts.
- A link between the message (harmful effects of smoking, benefits of stopping) and the personal well-being of the smoker must be established. The smoker must associate the information with *his or her* life and health. The concept that cessation of smoking now will allow an individual to live until age 72 instead of age 65 is meaningless to a 16-year-old.

Experiencing the physical, social, emotional, and psychological changes that result from several weeks of abstinence from smoking is much more effective than merely hearing what life would be like without smoking. Programs in which smokers volunteer to give up the habit for a few weeks have a higher success rate than traditional educational programs that merely provide smokers with antismoking information.

It is very difficult to get "hardened" smokers to quit, but some programs do work. A "group spirit and peer pressure program," for example, produced a 45 percent success rate, with 99 of 222 volunteers still not smoking after one year.[11] The names of those who remained in the program were published monthly in a local newspaper. Social pressure appears to have been the strong motivator for program continuance.

Weight Problems for Quitters

More than 75 percent of smokers who quit are puffing away one year later. Besides nicotine addiction, a

Exploring Your Health 12.4

Do You Want to Change Your Smoking Habits?

For each statement, circle the number that most accurately indicates how
you feel. For example, if you completely agree with the statement, circle 4,
if you agree somewhat, circle 3, and so on.

Important: Answer every question.

	Completely Agree	Somewhat Agree	Somewhat Disagree	Completely Disagree
A. Cigarette smoking might give me a serious illness.	4	3	2	1
B. My cigarette smoking sets a bad example for others.	4	3	2	1
C. I find cigarette smoking to be a messy kind of habit.	4	3	2	1
D. Controlling my cigarette smoking is a challenge to me.	4	3	2	1
E. Smoking causes shortness of breath.	4	3	2	1
F. If I quit smoking cigarettes it might influence others to stop.	4	3	2	1
G. Cigarettes cause damage to clothing and other personal property.	4	3	2	1
H. Quitting smoking would show that I have willpower.	4	3	2	1
I. My cigarette smoking will have a harmful effect on my health.	4	3	2	1
J. My cigarette smoking influences others close to me to take up or continue smoking.	4	3	2	1
K. If I quit smoking, my sense of taste or smell would improve.	4	3	2	1
L. I do not like the idea of feeling dependent on smoking.	4	3	2	1

Scoring:

1. Enter the numbers you have circled in the test questions in the spaces below, putting the number you have circled for question A over line A, for question B over line B, and so on.

2. Add the three scores across on each line to get your totals. For example, the sum of your scores over lines A, E, and I gives you your score on *Health;* lines B, F, and J give the score on *Example,* and so on.

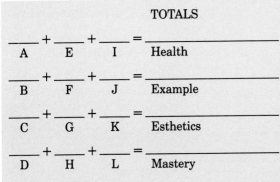

TOTALS

___ + ___ + ___ = _____	A	E	I	Health
___ + ___ + ___ = _____	B	F	J	Example
___ + ___ + ___ = _____	C	G	K	Esthetics
___ + ___ + ___ = _____	D	H	L	Mastery

9 or above suggests the harmful effects of smoking may be enough for you to want to quit smoking.

6 or less indicates you are probably not interested in giving up cigarettes to set an example for others.

9 or above suggests you are disturbed enough by some of the unpleasantness of smoking to give up the habit.

9 or above suggests you are aware that you are not controlling your desire to smoke and may want to challenge your self-control and give up smoking.

Scores can vary from 3 to 12. Any score of 9 or above is *high;* any score of 6 or below is *low.*

Source: National Clearinghouse for Smoking and Health (USPHS).

TABLE 12.3

Excuses for Smoking/Reasons for Quitting

For many smokers, smoking has become such a deeply ingrained habit and has worked itself so thoroughly into their daily behavior patterns that they have developed many excuses for continuing to smoke. Some of these excuses are in the smoker's conscious mind, some may be unconscious—and all have little or no basis in fact.

"If I Quit Smoking, I'll Gain Weight."
This is a common fear: According to the U.S. Public Health Service, 60 percent of women and 47 percent of men say they continue to smoke because they're afraid of gaining weight. Studies have indicated, however, that most smokers do *not* gain weight when they quit. "On the average, only about one-third of ex-smokers gain weight, one-third remain about the same, and one-third actually lose weight because they incorporate their quitting into a total self-improvement program."

"But I Really Enjoy Smoking. I Like the Taste."
The question here is, how many moments are truly enjoyable—and how many are just so-so? Is it real enjoyment the smoker is getting—or just satisfaction for the physical craving? After a day of particularly heavy smoking, almost every smoker can remember cigarettes tasting terrible the next morning.

"If I Quit Smoking, I'd Be Too Nervous. Smoking Helps Me Relax."
The truth here is that nicotine is actually a stimulant, not a depressant; it is not a substance that tends to make people relax. After the first few days of trying to quit, when ex-smokers may find themselves feeling nervous because they have nothing to do with their hands, most people find they have better self-control and are actually *less* nervous than they were when they smoked.

"I Have to Smoke in Order to Perform/Produce/Create/Study."
Here we're looking at that problem of habit again. For a long time, the individual may have *associated* smoking with writing, studying, dealing with coworkers, or whatever the performance behavior in question is. Actually, once they quit, ex-smokers may find they spend more of their time productively. As a plus, their bodies will function more efficiently now that the excess carbon monoxide from inhaled smoke is no longer displacing oxygen in their bloodstreams.

"I'll Quit When I Have to—When My Health Is Threatened."
As we noted in our discussion of lung cancer, the symptoms of many smoking-related diseases don't show up until after the disease is well established. Moreover, many of those diseases result in a long, painful death.

"It's Too Late to Quit. I've Been Smoking Too Long."
It's *never* too late, as long as you quit before a serious disease has developed. After you quit, your chances of dying from smoking-related diseases gradually decrease till they're close to those of people who have never smoked.

"The Air Is Polluted Anyway—I Might as Well Smoke."
In fact, even in a heavily polluted urban area, the concentrations of pollutants in the air are *tiny* in comparison with the concentrations in the cigarette smoke the smoker breathes in and out.

"I Can't Afford to Join a Stop-Smoking Program."
Most approaches to quitting cost nothing. But if you think paying to join a formal program is the only way you can succeed, you should take into account how much money you'll be saving by not buying cigarettes.

Source: U.S. Department of Health and Human Services, "Helping Smokers Quit: A Guide for Physicians" (NIH Publication No. 79-1825).

major reason for this relapse is weight gain. About one-third of all smokers put on up to thirty pounds soon after they quit. However, the other two-thirds either stay the same weight or actually lose weight (see Table 12.3). This smoking-weight connection seems to be more pronounced in women. This may also be one reason why teenage girls, a particularly weight-conscious group, are the fastest-growing group of cigarette smokers. It appears from laboratory studies that nicotine intake decreases the consumption of sweet foods. In the absence of nicotine, the amount of sweet foods consumed increases in proportion to the rise in weight. Early research indicates that it may be important to restrict the type, not the quantity, of food accessible to the ex-smoker if weight gain is to be prevented.

Nicotine Substitutes and Nicotine Gum

Programs employing nicotine substitutes (which do not produce dependence), drugs having drying effects on the mucous membranes, sedatives to manage psychological withdrawal problems, and metallic salts, which produce an unpleasant taste during tobacco inhalation, have been relatively ineffective. However, programs using a combination of nicotine substitutes (administered both orally and by injection), sedation, group therapy (including positive suggestion therapy), and aversion therapy have had a higher success rate.

Nicotine chewing gum and other substances containing nicotine have been only about 25 percent effective in helping smokers to quit, because relapse tends to occur when the supply of nicotine is cut off. The substances should not be given to children, because they are likely to produce nicotine dependence in youngsters who do not use tobacco and may turn to it later. Programs attempting to replace smoking-induced nicotine with chewing gum, snuff, or chewing tobacco all have one serious limitation—nicotine dependence is left untreated.

Cold Turkey

"Cold turkey," or quitting all at once, is effective for some smokers and not for others. It may be the best approach for the heavily addicted, whereas gradual withdrawal may be less painful and more effective for those only mildly addicted.

The Five-Day Plan

Seventh-Day Adventist medical doctors and ministers have been successful in helping people give up smoking through their "Five-Day Plan." Five consecutive two-hour sessions, using proven principles to overcome the craving for nicotine, are scheduled. Plans are held wherever there is a Seventh-Day Adventist medical institution or a Seventh-Day Adventist church of sufficient size. About 85 percent of smokers remaining with the program for the entire five days are likely to break the habit. For information on such a program in your area, write: Five-Day Plan, Hinsdale Sanitarium and Hospital, 120 North Oak Street, Hinsdale, Illinois, 60521.

Other Programs

Pacifiers (noncombustible plastic cigarettes) to keep the mouth and fingers occupied, mild electroshock to the hands (to create a negative association), hypnosis, acupuncture, herbal nicotine substitutes, and various behavior modification programs have been tried. The success rate has been rather low for all these approaches.

Year 2000 National Health Objective

The national health objectives place emphasis on smoking cessation programs by attempting to increase to at least 50 percent (currently the figure is 34 percent), the proportion of cigarette smokers age 18 and older who stop smoking for at least one day during the preceding year.

vousness, and grouchiness. Point out that these are positive signs of recovery.

Setting the Q-Day

Your quit list should provide you with all the basic information you'll need as well as a few strategies for overcoming any defensiveness or defeatism on your friend's part when you approach her about quitting. Now it's time to put your plan into action. A good way to do this has been put forth by the American Cancer Society. It's called *Q-Day.* The "Q" stands for "quit," and Q-day is the day that the smoker is supposed to quit smoking—forever. The basic approach involves four steps, to which we will add a fifth for purposes of "follow up":

1. Help your friend set an exact date (one to four weeks in advance) for Q-Day, the day that the smoking will stop *completely.*

2. As Q-Day approaches, your friend should gradually reduce smoking on a daily or weekly basis.

3. As Q-Day approaches, have your friend pick and use any of the following suggestions that will work for her:

- Smoke only one cigarette per hour.
- Avoid smoking between 9:00 and 10:00 A.M., 11:00 and 12:00 P.M., or 3:00 and 4:00 P.M., extending the nonsmoking time by a half hour, an hour, two hours.
- Smoke exactly half as many cigarettes the first week and half this amount again each week until Q-day arrives.
- Inhale less and with less vigor, avoiding deep inhalation.
- Smoke each cigarette only halfway before discarding.
- Remove the cigarette from your mouth between puffs.
- Smoke slowly.
- Smoke brands with low nicotine and tar content.
- Make it difficult to locate a cigarette by leaving yours at home, not carrying pocket change, and so forth.
- Place unlighted cigarettes in your mouth when you have the urge to smoke.
- Switch to a brand you dislike.

4. Your friend should maintain a daily record of her smoking habits. Be sure that you check this record with your friend on a regular basis during the specified period before Q-day. Note should be made of the smoker's thoughts and feelings as she reduces tobacco consumption; this information will be especially valuable in uncovering the

Helping a Friend Stop Using Tobacco

Now that you know about some of the techniques and programs available to help people who smoke or chew tobacco give up this extremely unhealthy addiction, you should also know that there is much that you can do on your own to help a friend, family member, or fellow student to quit using tobacco. The fact is, most smokers can and do quit on their own, without entering a special program. Nine out of ten smokers indicate that they do want to give up smoking. The question is whether the individual smoker possesses the necessary willpower to make the decision to quit *now. If you are a smoker, get a friend to read through the following information and help you to stop using tobacco!*

Making a Quit List

Before you actually approach a smoker about giving up smoking, make a "quit list" consisting of these four elements:

1. The things that make your relationship to this person meaningful or special.

2. How smoking tends to make the relationship stressful for you.

3. Specific things the smoker can do to overcome the addiction.

4. Specific things that you are willing to do to help the smoker quit smoking permanently.

Applying the Quit List: An Example   Let's say, by way of example, that the first smoker you want to

FIGURE 12.4   •   Helping a Friend Stop Using Tobacco

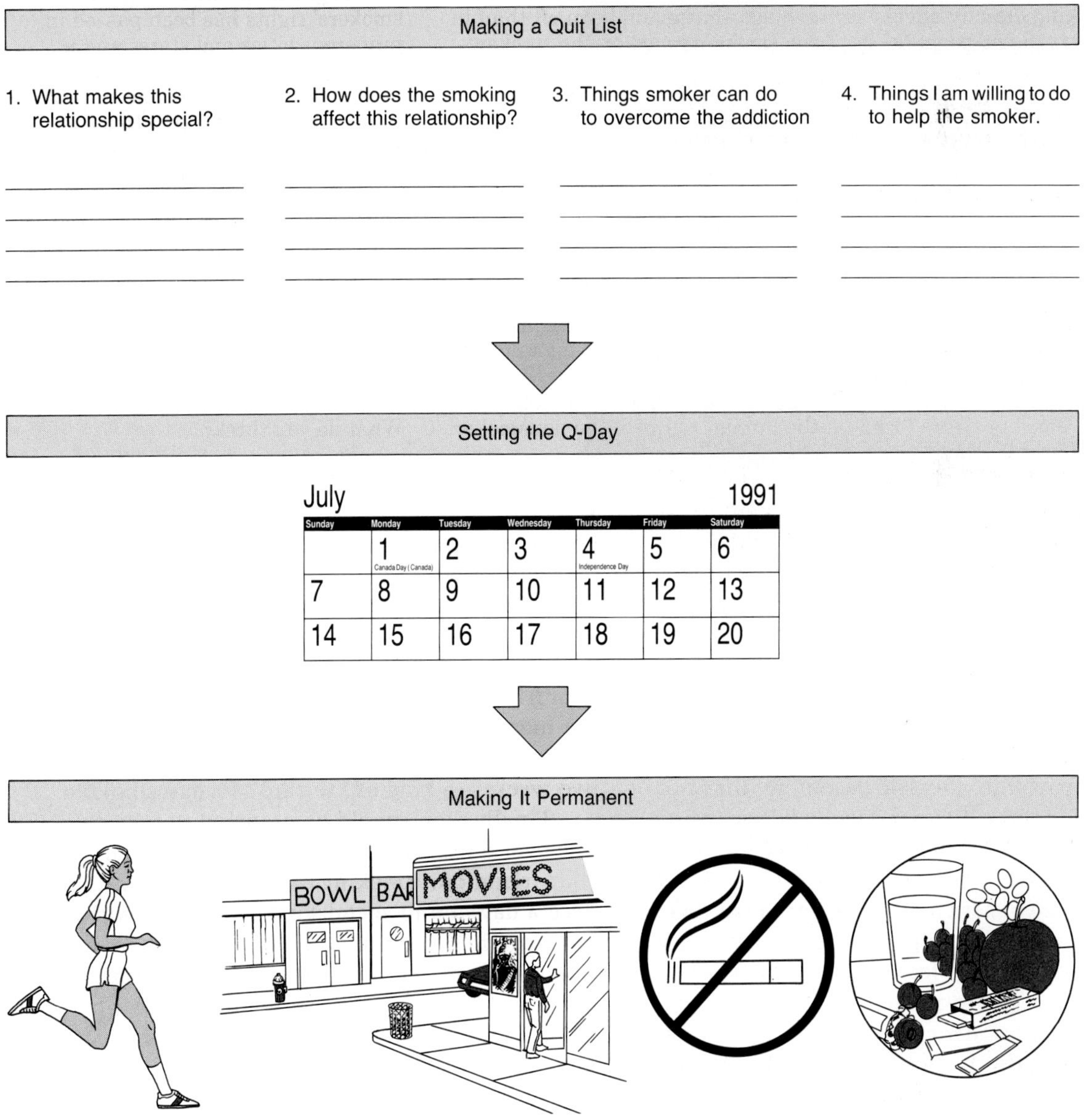

A Question of Ethics

Should Smokers Be Required by Law

Advocates of nonsmokers' rights argue that smoking directly affects the lives of others. Some people's eyes, nose, and throat are sensitive to smoke; some people are offended by the odor or sight of smoke; and some object on moral or religious grounds. Secondhand smoke is dangerous to the nonsmoker. It causes a number of physiological changes in the nonsmoker in a closed, poorly ventilated room or vehicle, including an increase in heart rate and blood pressure, and a rise in carbon monoxide levels in the blood. In addition, the nonsmoker's system takes in by-product poisons, such as cadmium (related to high blood pressure, bronchitis, and emphysema), and these

poisons are actually hig
exhaled smoke and bur
the smoke inhaled by t
Smoke from an idling c
off more tar and nicotii
smoker consumes from
level of carbon monoxic
smoker's blood can dou
upon room ventilation.
approximately 34 milli
sensitive to smoke, and
lion of them suffer smo
asthma attacks. Lung i
the children of parents
twice that found in nor
ilies. All these health h
argued, make smoking
the human rights of th

help quit is your best friend, with whom you've shared some wonderful experiences. Put some of those experiences down on paper and think about what they have meant to you. This will allow you to help your friend remember how "important" you are to her.

Now, write down the ways that your friend's smoking affects your relationship. Have you avoided visiting your friend because you don't want to breathe smoky air? Do you find yourself becoming angry or upset when you go out with your friend and she insists on lighting up? When you speak to your friend, be sure to express yourself as calmly and as considerately as possible, otherwise your friend may become defensive. For instance, instead of saying "You make me angry when you smoke," say, "I feel uncomfortable when you smoke because you're important to me and you and I both know how dangerous smoking is." You could also include in this section of your quit list a simple chart, which you and your friend could fill out to-

Get Involved!

Working for a Smoke-Free Society

The association between tobacco use and disease has been strongly established. The controversy is over: Tobacco use in any form is without a doubt the leading cause of preventable death and disability in the United States. Unfortunately, many American teenagers and adults continue to smoke or use smokeless tobacco. A little earlier, you learned a way to help a friend quit using tobacco. How can you help your community and society become smokeless?

1. Adopt a smoke-free lifestyle and set an example for your friends, colleagues, and fellow students.
2. Join the movement to discourage tobacco use in the United States. Make your dormitory, apartment, or house completely smoke-free by eliminating ash trays, matches, and "designated" smoking areas. If you work for a private company, ask your human resources or personnel department to encourage antismoking programs and to eliminate cigarette machines and ashtrays in the workplace. Discourage individuals from smoking in every way possible.
3. Organize free informational programs to help people stop smoking through your church or temple, fitness or wellness club, school, or workplace. You could use some of the techniques and suggestions you learned about in the "Helping a Friend Stop Using Tobacco" section of this chapter.
4. Work with young people in group sports, day camps, or other activities, such as Girl Scout and Boy Scout groups, and encourage them to discourage the use of tobacco among their families, friends, and communities.
5. Effectively use the power of peer pressure to encourage friends and family to stop smoking. Get friends, siblings, parents, and other relatives to express their concern directly to the smoker about her or his tobacco use.
6. Actively support programs and legislation aimed at monitoring and discouraging tobacco advertising.
7. Support the American Lung Association, the American Cancer Society, and the American Heart Association. These organizations offer effective programs to help people stop using tobacco. Check your phone book for their addresses and phone numbers.

Discuss these activities with your friend the day before Q-day and have any necessary items on hand by the beginning of Q-day: fresh ginger root, (sugarless) gum, fresh fruit and vegetables, and so on.

Finally, we must include a word of caution. The agony of giving up cigarettes is much the same as that of dieting. It passes quickly after the first three or four days. Unfortunately, the majority of dieters and would-be ex-smokers give up during this initial period. If your friend fails in the first attempt to quit smoking, by all means express your disappointment to him or her, but don't be cruel about it. Let the smoker know that you are still interested in helping whenever he or she feels ready to try to quit again.

Epilogue: The Struggle for a Tobacco-Free Society

Spearheaded by the Office of the Surgeon General of the United States and the desire for a smoke-free America by the year 2000, the federal government has launched a massive antitobacco educational campaign that already has produced positive results. The number of smoking restrictions enacted is steadily increasing in spite of the counterefforts of the tobacco industry. In addition, states are raising cigarette taxes and using this revenue to encourage smokers to quit. Smoking has also been banned by the Department of Transportation on domestic airflights of less than two hours, and some states are banning smoking on other modes of public transportation. In spite of these efforts, it is not always easy to determine whether the federal government is for or against tobacco. While the Surgeon General's Office fights for a smoke-free America, the government controls and subsidizes the growing of tobacco, allowing over 180,000 farms in twenty-three states and Puerto Rico to grow tobacco. It actually lends farmers money against the value of their crops to do so. These subsidies cost the U.S. government over $1 billion annually.

Although attempts have been unsuccessful to date, litigation is increasing in an attempt to make the tobacco industry responsible for damage done by tobacco. An appeals court ruling preventing smokers from suing for damages from cigarettes smoked after 1966, when mandated health warnings first appeared, is currently protecting the cigarette industry. The court indicated that, at this point, smokers became both aware of and responsible for the risks of smoking. This decision is being challenged. On the other hand, the number of product liability suits against the tobacco industry is also rising. A 1988 case ruled that Liggett Group, Inc., was responsible for the death of a smoker who died of lung cancer. A small award of $400,000 was granted to the widow. This precedent is almost certain to influence the several hundred similar cases now pending. Numerous national and international conferences on smoking have been sponsored by groups such as the World Health Organization (WHO),

and professional associations are combining their efforts to ban smoking in hospitals and to encourage health care professionals to set an example by not smoking.

The antismoking movement in the United States and throughout the world is strong; however, so is the financial power of the tobacco industry. Countercampaigns and advertising on their behalf can be expected to increase in years to come. For years, the tobacco industry has been diversifying their interests, realizing that the antismoking movement is gaining momentum and may eventually eliminate their product. It may be a good sign that the industry is preparing for a tobacco-free environment. Hopefully, it will not be too far in the future.

Conclusion

The decision to smoke is generally made during the early teens. In spite of the evidence with regard to the dangers of smoking, 32.6 percent of the adult population continue to subject their bodies to the harmful effects of tobacco. The sidestream smoke (secondhand smoke) that can be inhaled by those in close proximity to the smoker also poses health hazards to the nonsmoker. A controversy has arisen over an individual's

right to smoke and the nonsmoker's right to breathe clean air. If you smoke, you can decide to give up the habit at any time. Depending upon your level of addiction, the habit can be stopped by motivation and willpower alone or through one of the smoking cessation programs discussed in this chapter. After several weeks of abstinence from cigarettes, you will discover some pleasant changes in your body.

Summary

1. Adolescent smoking behavior is encouraged by poor influence, rebellion, curiosity, and advertising.

2. The efforts of the tobacco industry to promote smoking and to minimize the harmful effects of smoking is certain to increase in the future to counter the powerful worldwide antismoking movement. Programs that continue to educate our nation's youth must, therefore, also reduce the number of new smokers in our society and increase the number of ex-smokers.

3. Practically all cigarette smoking starts in the teenage years and eventually becomes a lifelong habit.

4. If you must smoke, switching to a low tar, filtered cigarette may reduce your chances of getting cancer and help you break the smoking habit later. Some low T/N cigarettes, however, have been shown to deliver more carbon monoxide than cigarettes with normal tar and nicotine levels.

5. Although clove cigarettes contain only 60 percent tobacco, they are a dangerous alternative and may actually be more of a health hazard than regular cigarettes.

6. Cigars and pipes permit nicotine to enter the bloodstream via the mucous tissues of the mouth, increasing the risk of lip, mouth, throat, larynx, and stomach cancer.

7. Evidence linking the use of smokeless tobacco, such as snuff and chewing tobacco, to lip, tongue, mouth, and throat cancer is increasing.

8. Cigarette smoke contains several substances that are harmful to both the smoker and nonsmoker.

9. Smoking has declined among the adult population and increased among the nation's youth, particularly among teenage girls and young women.

10. Cigarette smoking is associated with cancer of the bladder, esophagus, lung, and pancreas. It contributes to oral disease, chronic bronchitis, emphysema, coronary artery disease, heart attack, stroke, pulmonary tuberculosis, and facial skin wrinkling.

11. A genetic link has been uncovered that may explain why a few individuals can smoke most of their lives and not develop lung cancer. The gene may also place some smokers at six times the risk of developing lung cancer.

12. The combined use of oral contraceptives and smoking increases the risk of blood clot formation, heart attack, and stroke in women.

13. Smoking during pregnancy poses dangers to both the mother and unborn fetus, increasing the risk of miscarriage tenfold. It increases bone density loss leading to osteoporosis, decreases estrogen levels, and makes conceiving more difficult.

14. Cigarette smoking is the largest preventable cause of death in America.

15. The Comprehensive Smoking Education Act of 1984 and the Comprehensive Smokeless Tobacco Health Education Act of 1986 require manufacturers of tobacco products, including smokeless tobacco, to include health warning labels on packages of their products.

16. Breathing in secondhand smoke from others' cigarettes, pipes, and cigars poses a health hazard for nonsmokers.

17. Nonsmokers have the right to breathe uncontaminated air in public places.

18. Nonsmokers tend to be more health conscious and feel more in control of their lives than do smokers.

19. Many smokers want to terminate their dependency on nicotine.

20. Weight gain is a common problem for ex-smokers, who tend to consume more sweets after quitting. Approaches are available to modify eating habits during this period to reduce this effect.

21. Approaches to help people quit smoking include health education programs, pharmacological programs, the cold turkey treatment, the Five-Day Plan, mild electroshock, hypnosis, and behavior modification programs.

22. You can increase the success rate of "smoking cessation" programs by providing organized individual support to a friend or family member. Such support is an important part of most programs.

Questions for Personal Growth

1. In spite of the obvious health hazards of cigarette smoking, including an unpleasant death, people continue to smoke. Why do you think people take such serious risks with their health? List the things you consider effective in getting people to stop smoking. List those factors that you consider counterproductive.

2. Prepare a plan in writing to help a friend or family member quit smoking. Plan to become a major support person for that individual for several months.

3. Identify five ways the tobacco industry encourages people to smoke. Evaluate the information presented in ads and other media for accuracy. Are consumers led to believe that smoking is attractive, sexy, sporty, and savvy?

4. List the five most dangerous health hazards of cigarette smoking. Observe smokers carefully in a social setting for some overt indications of negative health that may be caused by smoking. Are any of your smoking friends or family members exhibiting any symptoms of future illness?

5. Arrange a meeting with the Parent Teachers Association in a middle school or high school. Encourage a program for parents, teachers, athletes, and other students on the dangers of smokeless tobacco. Develop a program, in writing, to help athletes stop using smokeless tobacco.

6. The antismoking movement in the United States is gaining momentum, yet there is much to be done. What additional steps do you think are needed to eliminate the use of tobacco? How can you as a private citizen provide further support to this movement?

References

1. American Cancer Society, *World Smoking and Health* 1 (Summer 1977).
2. American Cancer Society, *Cancer Facts and Figures* (1990).
3. Ibid.
4. Ibid.
5. Ibid.
6. Jonas Hartelius and Lita Tibbling, "Nicotine Dependence and Smoking Cessation Programs: A Review," *World Smoking and Health* 2 (1) (Summer 1977): 4–10 (an American Cancer Society Journal).
7. *Cancer Facts and Figures.*
8. Ibid.
9. "Smoking boosts risk of tubal pregnancy," *Science News* 139, 11 (March 16, 1991): 175.
10. Stephen Barrett, "Smokeless Tobacco Is Dangerous," *Healthline* (December 1986).
11. Hartelius and Tibbling, "Nicotine Dependence," 4–10.

CHAPTER

13

Infectious and Noninfectious Diseases

CHAPTER OBJECTIVES

After reading this chapter, you should understand:

- The infectious disease-causing agents, or pathogens, and how they cause disease in the human body.

- How nonspecific and specific forms of immunity defend the body against attack by infectious diseases.

- Currently available treatments and preventive measures for infectious diseases.

- The difference between infectious and noninfectious diseases, and how you can reduce your risk of developing certain noninfectious diseases through lifestyle changes.

- The symptoms and treatments of diabetes and three of the better-known disorders of the nervous system.

- Several genetic diseases, and why some people are more likely than others to develop certain diseases.

- How infectious and noninfectious lung diseases develop, and what can be done to prevent and control them.

CHAPTER OUTLINE

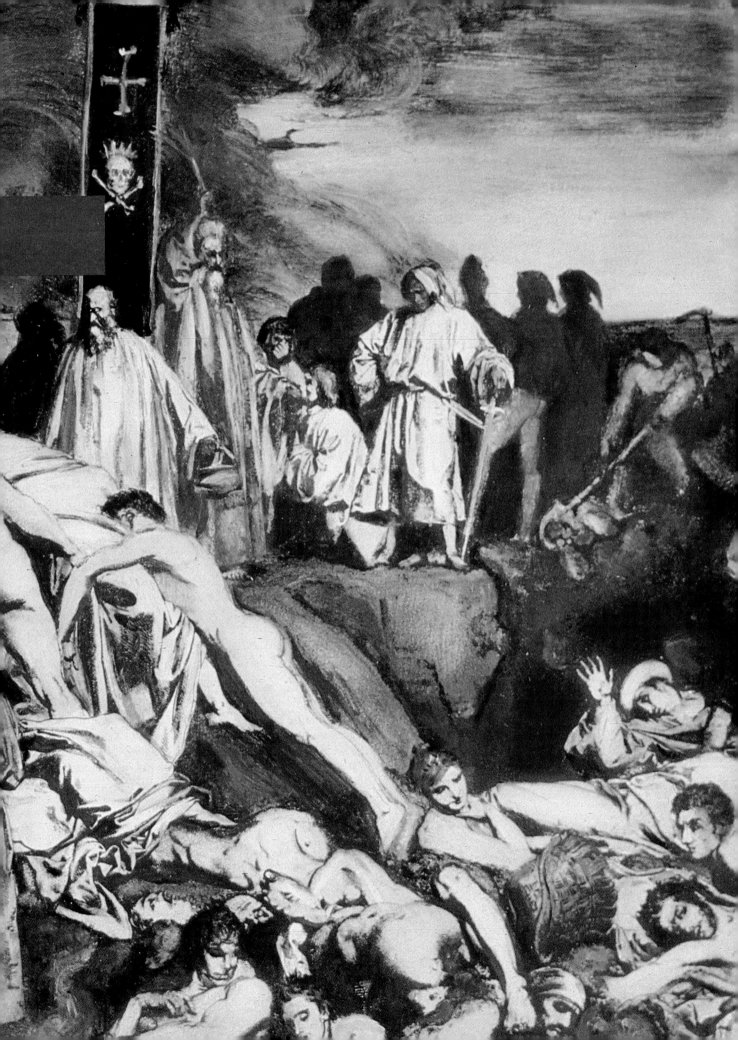

pathogen Any disease-causing agent, such as a bacteria, a virus, or a toxin.

bacteria Microscopic, single-cell organisms; plantlike in some characteristics. Some bacteria cause disease; others are beneficial. They are often classified by shape.

botulism A serious food-poisoning disease caused by the botulism bacteria.

tetanus A serious blood-poisoning disease caused by the tetanus bacteria.

viruses Minute parasitic agents that live and reproduce inside living cells; viruses cause many diseases, including the common cold and serious, often fatal, illnesses.

All living creatures have suffered from infectious and noninfectious diseases since the beginning of recorded history. Infectious diseases such as plague, smallpox, tuberculosis, and polio were once common throughout the world. Now these diseases occur mainly in developing countries. However, infectious diseases such as AIDS and other sexually transmitted diseases (STDs) have come forward to wreak havoc on Americans, the industrialized nations, and other peoples throughout the world. In addition, although Americans enjoy a relatively high level of hygiene and standard of living, they nevertheless experience a very high level of pain and death from noninfectious diseases such as cardiovascular disease, stroke, and cancer. With the exception of AIDS, most of the infectious diseases Americans experience are not life-threatening, due to advanced medical diagnosis and treatment. However, cardiovascular disease (including stroke) and cancer are the leading causes of death in the United States today.

We will consider AIDS and other sexually transmitted diseases in detail in Chapter 14, and Chapters 15 and 16 will feature detailed discussions of cardiovascular disease and cancer respectively. In this chapter, we will discuss several other infectious and noninfectious diseases that are common in the United States. For the sake of clarity, we have divided the chapter into two distinct parts:

I. Infectious Diseases
II. Noninfectious Diseases

Your instructor may wish you to read Chapter 14 on (infectious) STDs in conjunction with the first section, and Chapters 15 and 16 on (noninfectious) cardiovascular disease and cancer in conjunction with the second section of this chapter.

I. Infectious Diseases

Infectious diseases are transmitted from an infected object, animal, or person to an uninfected individual through agents that include bacteria, viruses, fungi, and animal parasites. Some infectious diseases are spread from one "host" to another and are said to be *communicable*, or *contagious*. Some of these communicable infectious diseases, such as rubella (German measles) and influenza (the "flu"), are highly contagious, while others—certain types of pneumonia, for example—are much less contagious. *Noncommunicable* or *noncontagious* infectious diseases are acquired from the environment but do not spread from one host to another even though they are caused by infectious agents. Tetanus, for example, is an acute bacterial infection transmitted to a body wound by spores in soil.

Relatively long-lasting vaccines and treatments have been developed for a number of communicable and noncommunicable infectious diseases. Most children, for instance, are vaccinated for diseases such as polio and rubella. Other infectious diseases require repeated vaccinations, or have no vaccines and only limited treatments. For example, a person can contract the "common" cold several times in a year. Similarly, the flu can be contracted many times in one's life despite the availability of yearly flu vaccinations.

In this section, we will examine how infectious diseases are spread, some of the mechanisms the body uses to defend against infection, and how infectious diseases can be controlled and prevented.

Agents of Infection

By practicing a healthy lifestyle, avoiding substances like tobacco, drugs, and alcohol that can compromise your health, and by maintaining good general health, you will reduce your chances of being attacked by disease-causing agents, which are called **pathogens.** However, when your immune system is weakened or when you make contact with a virulent pathogen, even if your immune system is healthy, the risk of disease is increased. What are the pathogens that can cause infectious diseases and where do they come from?

Bacteria

Bacteria are microscopic single-celled organisms, plantlike in some characteristics, that can be classified by shape. *Cocci* are spherical, *bacilli* are cylindrical, and *spirilla* and *spirochetes* are spiral. Some bacteria reproduce by dividing into two cells. The time between divisions is referred to as the *generation time* and is the key to how quickly a disease spreads through the body. Still other bacteria reproduce by creating spores that are inactive and highly resistant to dryness and heat. Under favorable conditions, these bacteria become active, as is the case with **botulism** (serious food poisoning) and **tetanus** (an infectious disease causing spasm of muscle groups). Many harmful bacteria grow on surfaces or between cells and do not actually invade the cell.

Most kinds of bacteria originating within the body are not harmful and are actually vital to our existence, like the bacterium *Escherichia coli,* which lives in our intestines. Still other bacteria help to ward off foreign infectious organisms. When our own endogenous bacteria get out of hand, problems, such as acne, pyorrhea, urinary tract infections, and other conditions, may result.

Staphylococcal Infections

Staphylococci are bacteria that can be present on the skin without causing serious infection ("staph" infection). But once infection begins, the bacteria multiply and produce various toxins and enzymes that allow it to spread to the bloodstream, causing *bacteremia,* or bacteria in the blood. In the central portion of the lesion, the tissue dies and is used to nourish the bacteria. Thus, an abscess is formed, leading to breakage at the point of least resistance (skin), or to internal drainage of abscess contents in deep tissue infections. You may have seen a dog suffering from an abscess acquired in a fight with a cat. Or you may have had a group of staph-infected hair follicles (pimples) appear on your cheeks and chin just in time to embarrass you for a Saturday night date. The pus pockets forming in response to the infections should be drained, flushed with an antibiotic, and allowed to continue draining to promote healing.

Staph organisms are everywhere and can be transmitted by contact with contaminated material (for instance, blankets) or in the air (sneeze droplets). Newborn babies are particularly at risk and can develop an infection if skin breaks due to diaper chafing.

Toxic Shock Syndrome *Toxic shock syndrome (TSS)* was first recognized as a disease in 1978, although it was not until June 1980 that an association was made between TSS and the continuous use of tampons by young women throughout their menstrual periods. TSS victims experience flulike symptoms in the early stages: fever (102°F or higher), vomiting, diarrhea, sore throat, and in some cases headache and muscle ache. These symptoms later disappear and are replaced by a sunburnlike rash and shock involving a rapid decrease in blood pressure, kidney failure, and heart irregularities.

TSS is more common in menstruating women, although nonmenstrual TSS does occur. The cause appears to be a *Staphylococcus,* which spreads through the body. Blood-soaked tampons in the vagina provide a fertile haven for these bacteria. After the initial infection, the bacteria produce a strong toxin that causes the serious symptoms of TSS. Nonmenstrual TSS also appears to be caused by *Staphylococcus aureus,* which grows in wounds, surgical incisions, or other body openings.[1]

A woman has about 15 chances in 100,000 (less than 0.5 percent) of contracting TSS. This low incidence has prompted the Centers for Disease Control in Atlanta to state that it seems "unwarranted to recommend the use of tampons be discontinued." Many women, however, feel that any risk is too high. To reduce the chances of contracting TSS, the following suggestions are offered:

- Select your tampon very carefully. Avoid the superabsorbent tampons, and use the traditional cottonlike materials until further evidence is available. Sea sponges, which some women use as tampons, may be contaminated with ocean pollutants and are suspected in several cases of TSS.
- Avoid changing the tampon too often. Repeated insertion and removal may irritate the vagina and provide additional entry points for TSS bacteria.
- Switch to maxipads at bedtime and minipads as the flow tapers; avoid continuous use of tampons throughout menstruation.
- If you use maxipads, avoid those with superabsorbent fibers.
- Avoid using tampons to absorb nonmenstrual secretions or to disguise vaginal odor.

Streptococcal Infections

Streptococci cause sore throats, ear infections, nasopharyngitis, tonsillitis, impetigo, and bacterial endocarditis and can lead to rheumatic fever and tooth decay. Infection in wounds (skin abrasions or surgical wounds) is caused by Group A streptococci, as are many sore throats and ear infections. Impetigo is a Group A skin infection, usually prevalent among children, and is extremely infectious. Gymnasts and wrestlers can contract the disease after exercising on contaminated mats. Like staph infections, strep infections respond well to antibiotic treatment.

Viruses

Viruses are minute parasitic agents that live and reproduce inside other living cells. They consist of a core of genetic material surrounded by a protective protein membrane and have no metabolic activity of their own. They do, however, control the metabolism of the cell in which they live and direct it to produce many hundreds of new viruses. The cell eventually becomes engorged with new viruses and breaks apart, spewing its contents in all directions. Each new virus can then enter another cell and repeat the cycle. Viruses cause

interferon A protein released by body cells infected with a virus that works with body membranes to prevent and fight viral infection.

fungi Plantlike organisms that obtain nutrition by growing on the tissue of other organisms. Fungi cause some diseases in humans.

rickettsia Now believed to be a very small form of bacteria, rickettsia cause the diseases of typhus and Rocky Mountain spotted fever in humans.

vector An organism or some other object that carries a disease-causing agent from one organism to another.

protozoa Single-cell animals that live in or on other organisms, sometimes causing disease.

parasitic worms Multicelled animals that live in or on other organisms, sometimes causing disease.

disease The destructive processes found during an illness that lead to noticeable symptoms of pain and discomfort.

---

such diseases as yellow fever, measles, mumps, rabies, poliomyelitis, smallpox, warts, fever blisters, chicken pox, and the common cold.[2]

Unfortunately, viruses are unaffected by antibiotics, and drugs neither combat nor cure a viral infection. The body itself, however, produces a protective substance known as **interferon.** Interferons are proteins released from body cells that are infected with a virus. Interferons can help protect the body against certain other types of viruses. Interferons interact with cell membranes to block viral invasion. Not all viruses trigger the production of interferons, but certain synthetic chemicals and bacteria have been found to stimulate interferon production.

Fungi

Fungi, yeasts, and molds are many-celled organisms. They must live on other plants or animals because they contain no chlorophyll and cannot manufacture their own food. Fungi generally form filaments called *hyphae* and are blown to new locations in great numbers through the release of spores or seedlike cells. In humans, fungi usually affect the external body parts such as the skin, scalp, or nails. Dermatomycoses is an example of a fungus responsible for skin infections. Common ringworm is spread from animals or from other humans. Athlete's foot fungus is spread from person to person in showers, locker rooms, and so forth. Some generalized fungal infections, usually from the soil or vegetation, attack the lungs and the meninges of the brain.

Fungi require an environment of high humidity and warmth and are therefore more common in tropical climates. Fungal infections are rarely serious and can be controlled by topical application of fungicides. Proper personal hygiene (regular bathing, clean clothes, drying properly, and avoiding the use of other people's shoes, socks, and clothes) prevents fungal infections. Since practically all antibiotics are extracted from soil fungi, they are of little help in fighting fungal diseases and may actually destroy harmless bacteria in the body that help restrain the growth of these dis-

eases. The trend toward overuse of antibiotic therapy (see A Question of Ethics in this chapter) may be contributing to the increase in fungal diseases.

Rickettsia

Once considered to be a kind of virus, **rickettsia** is now believed to be a small form of bacteria. Rickettsia need an insect acting as a **vector** (carrier) in order for disease to be transmitted to humans. There are two common types of rickettsial disease: *typhus,* carried by the tick or flea, and *Rocky Mountain spotted fever,* carried by the tick. Symptoms for both diseases include fever, rash, general weakness, and eventually coma. Both are potentially life-threatening. Rickettsia produce toxins within small blood vessels that block the flow of blood and cause tissues to die. It is important to realize that you don't actually have to be bitten by a tick or flea to be infected with rickettsia. Infection may also result if an insect vector deposits excrement on any small or large skin wound.

Animal Parasites: Protozoa and Parasitic Worms

Animal parasites, including the single-celled **protozoa** and the multicelled **parasitic worms,** live on or inside another living organism (host). Many animal parasites live part of their life on one animal and part on another, with both hosts essential to the life cycle of the parasite. Generally, the development of a fertilized egg to the larva stage occurs in the first host, with the adult form living on the second. Typically, offspring are produced in one animal and growth occurs in another. To ensure survival, large quantities of eggs are produced (the beef tapeworm lays more than 1 million eggs per day). Parasitic worms vary from 1 inch to 60 feet long and are not a major health problem in the United States. Pinworms, flukes, and tapeworms are examples of common parasitic worms found in humans.

Some major diseases, most common in tropical areas with poor sanitation, are caused by protozoan parasites. The *Plasmodium* protozoan parasite causes

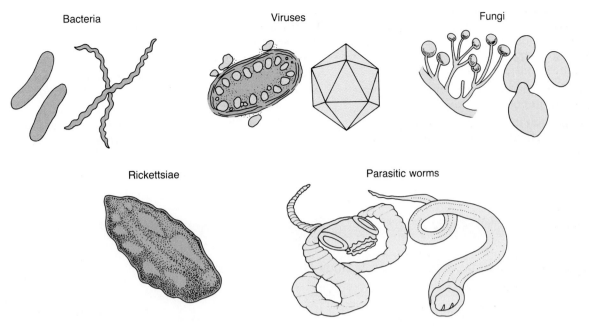

Figure 13.1 • Examples of the various pathogens that cause diseases in humans. Most pathogens are microorganisms, so that you can only see them with a microscope. However, some parasitic worms can grow to lengths of several meters.

malaria. African sleeping sickness, transmitted by the tsetse fly, and amebic dysentery are other protozoan diseases common outside the United States. Trichomoniasis, caused by *Trichomonas,* is a common vaginal infection in women in the United States. Drugs are effective in the treatment of protozoan diseases.

Figure 13.1 features depictions of the various pathogens that cause disease in humans.

Defenses Against Infectious Diseases

Now that we know something about pathogens, we must examine exactly how these agents are able to take hold in the body and how the body defends itself against them.

Setting the Stage for Infection

Generally speaking, infection occurs when a microorganism (1) successfully penetrates the host's defense barriers and (2) multiplies. When microorganisms have destroyed tissue or used large quantities of host nutrients in sustaining their growth and causing infection to such an extent that a person senses noticeable discomfort, fever, and malaise, we use the term **disease** to characterize the symptoms. As normal, healthy humans, we all carry infections around with us continually. For instance, more than 90 percent of throat cul-

tures taken at random contain streptococcal bacteria. Such low-level infections, however, are not sufficiently debilitating to cause discomfort.

There are six factors that set the stage for debilitating infectious diseases in humans. Here are these factors in summary: (1) A pathogen (live virus or bacteria) must be present, and the pathogen must be able to (2) live in, (3) multiply in, and (4) escape from a place where it has settled ("a reservoir"). Then the pathogen must (5) contract and enter an appropriate host (in this case, a human), and (6) the host must receive the pathogen. These six factors, along with explanations of what they are and how they operate, are located in Table 13.1. Please read through this table now. If all of these six factors are met, a pathogen may be able to cause disease.

Non-Specific and Specific Defenses

When we speak about the body's defenses against disease, we usually refer to *non-specific* and *specific* defenses. We will discuss each of these in detail.

Non-Specific Defenses: Defense Mechanisms

Non-specific defenses, which help prevent infection from spreading when microorganic pathogens enter your body, include the skin, the respiratory tract (mucous membranes of the nose, throat, and lungs), the gastrointestinal tract (oral cavity, esophagus, stomach, and alimentary tract), the urogenital tract (bladder, ureters, penis, vagina), the eyes, and the ear canals. These defenses represent a first line of defense against disease.

immunity The ability of the human body, or another organism's body, to recognize and defend itself against specific infectious agents.

antigen A specific outside agent that upon entering the body promotes antibody formation.

antibody Specific protein complexes that are produced by a body to defend against, destroy, or neutralize antigens.

lymphocytes White blood cells formed in the bone marrow that produce antibodies to battle specific disease-causing agents.

toxin A poison formed by antigens; toxins stimulate an immune response in the body, causing antibodies to the toxin to be formed.

vaccination The injection or ingestion of a vaccine in order to stimulate an immune response to a specific antigen.

TABLE 13.1

Six Factors Necessary to Produce Infectious Disease in Humans

Factor	Interpretation	Examples	Comments
A causative agent	A living organism (pathogen) must exist that is capable of invading the body and causing disease.	Viruses, bacteria	Viruses and bacteria that cause disease are in the environment at all times.
A reservoir	The pathogen must have a place to live and multiply until it is passed on to a host, such as a human being.	Humans: infected human or someone who is a carrier and is not affected; or an animal, insect, or bird.	Animal diseases that are transmitted to humans are generally not transmitted from human to human.
A means of escape	The pathogen must have a means of escape from the reservoir.	Through the respiratory tract (nose, throat, lungs, bronchial tree via coughing, sneezing, or breathing); the digestive tract (feces, saliva, vomitus, contaminated items); open sores, wounds, and lesions.	Each disease has a period when the pathogen is most likely to escape (infectious period) and infect another human. Quarantine during this period reduces the risk of spreading the disease.
A means of transmission	The pathogen must have a means of contacting a host.	Body to body (kissing, touching, sexual contact); animals and insects; inanimate objects (clothing, eating utensils, tissues, toilet articles).	Pathogens that can survive outside a host pose the greatest threat to humans.
A means of entry	The pathogen must have a way to enter the host.	Respiratory tract (breathed in), digestive tract (swallowed), breaks in the skin (cuts, abrasions), or mucous membranes (lining of the mouth, nose, eyes, vagina, anus).	Hand-to-mucous membrane contact is a common way the pathogen enters the human body.
A host that is susceptible to the pathogen	The host must receive the pathogen.	Strong body defenses or immunity can fight off the pathogen before the disease occurs.	The period between entry of the pathogen and the disease's first symptoms is called the incubation period. It is easier to eradicate the disease during this period than during subsequent stages of the disease.

After the pathogen penetrates the body's external defenses, it encounters a second line of defense. Various enzymes and other compounds in blood can kill an infectious organism by causing it to break open, destroying its cell wall, or preventing it from multiplying. Special white blood cells, called *phagocytes,* engulf and digest bacteria. Larger phagocytic cells, called *macrophages,* are contained in the body's tissues, and these too fight off bacteria so that the offending organism may never be able to establish itself.

If the invader does become established, the body then resorts to a third line of defense in which tissue fluids and antibacterial proteins accumulate. You will recall from our discussion of viruses that, in the case of a viral (rather than bacterial) infection, *interferons* are released from body cells that are infected with the virus. Interferons work in two ways: they can keep viruses from multiplying in infected body cells or they can keep viruses from entering healthy body cells. The body's fight to repel the disease becomes evident through inflammation of the infected area and accompanying discomfort. Fever is also a sign that the body is fighting infection.

Once the third line of defense is penetrated, the infection may spread through the body tissues and perhaps into the bloodstream. If this happens, the infection becomes serious. If the infection remains localized, an abscess may form as more and more tissue in the infected area is destroyed. An *abscess* is a cavity filled with fluid, white cells battling the disease microbe, and *pus* (dead white cells). The body returns to normal only when enough of the infectious organisms are killed or rendered inactive so that the disease and its symptoms disappear.

Specific Diseases: The Immune Mechanism

Many specific kinds of infectious agents require the body's specific defenses. Specific defenses make up the body's immune mechanism. **Immunity** refers to the body's ability to recognize and defend itself against specific infectious agents. When the body recognizes a specific harmful outside agent, called an **antigen,** the body produces specific proteins, called **antibodies,** to battle this specific agent. This process is called the *immune response.* Antibodies are produced by **lymphocytes,** white blood cells formed in the bone marrow. *B lymphocytes,* or *B cells,* play the primary role in manufacturing antibodies. Antibodies are found primarily in the blood but are also present in mucous membranes in the respiratory, urogenital, and gastrointestinal tracts. They are very important in preventing both initial infection and the subsequent spread of infectious agents. Another kind of lymphocyte, *T-lymphocytes* or *T-cells* (also called T-suppressor or T-helper cells) circulate in the bloodstream, either suppressing or helping the general immune responses of other lymphocytes.

Let's look at an example of how the specific immune response works. A practical example of an antigenic stimulus is **toxin,** produced during a bacterial infection. Your immune system recognizes the toxin (antigen) as foreign, and antibodies produced in response to the toxin (by plasma cells), either in the past or during the present infection, combine chemically with the toxin. The resulting aggregation of toxin and antibodies is engulfed by immune cells, metabolized, and excreted. Thus the primary role of antibodies is to combine with a specific antigen and aid in the clearance of antigens from your body. Once you have been exposed to an antigen, you retain the ability to respond to it for a period of months or years.

Primary and Secondary Immune Responses

The first time you are infected with a virus—influenza, for example—you react immunologically to antigens produced by the virus. A virus is usually inhaled in mucus droplets from an infected person (for example, after a sneeze); it is absorbed in the mucous layer of the respiratory tract, penetrates susceptible cells in the nose, bronchi, or lungs, and multiplies. While infection is continuing, macrophages in the infected area are engulfing virus particles. Macrophages then present some form of the virus protein to a B lymphocyte that is predetermined to produce an antibody to that antigen. The B lymphocyte then produces an antibody (IgM) to influenza virus.

Up to this point, the virus has had one to two days to incubate in the respiratory tract. During this time, you may have chills, aching muscles, and fever. Fever may continue for several days. As soon as enough virus is present to be detected by your immune cells, you begin your defense against the infection. Within twenty-four hours after immune cell recognition of the viral antigen, you may produce some specific IgM. Within seven days after antigen recognition, you have a high level of IgM in your blood, and some IgG, another antibody, is being produced. Within two weeks after antigen recognition, you have a high level of IgG in your blood; it is this IgG that can protect you from subsequent influenza virus infections. This is your primary immune response.

When infected a year later with similar influenza, you have an antibody present in your blood that can react with the virus (and macrophages) to aid in ridding your body of the virus. At this time, some of your plasma cells, which were previously committed to making the specific antibody to influenza A virus, recognize the antigen of this year's virus (A group). These committed cells are now ready to commence production of IgG directly, and do so immediately. The second dose of natural influenza virus antigen acts like a vaccination that stimulates your immune cells to produce an influenza-specific antibody. This is your secondary immune response.

Treatment of Infectious Diseases

Vaccination

The term **vaccination** is derived from the word *vaccinia,* or cowpox. Edward Jenner performed the first vaccination against smallpox in 1798. He noted that

vaccine A pharmaceutical preparation made from specific antigens that, when injected or ingested by an individual, stimulates the production of antibodies against that antigen, causing either a partial or complete immune response to that antigen.

active immunity When a body can produce antibodies against a specific antigen, causing a long-term immune response to that antigen and its associated disease.

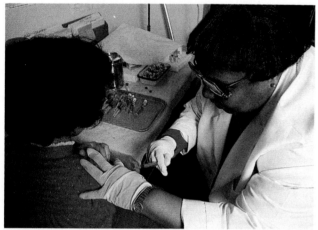

Inoculation against measles and other diseases is a valuable part of maintaining public health.

milkmaids rarely contracted smallpox and wondered why this was so. He found that milkmaids did contract a related disease from cows (cowpox), but that the illness was not serious and left no disfiguring marks. He prepared an inoculum from the pustule of a milkmaid with cowpox, inoculated susceptible humans, and found that these vaccinated individuals did not contract smallpox even when exposed to virulent smallpox virus.

Since Jenner's time, medical professionals have prepared vaccines against many different infectious agents. A **vaccine** is a preparation of an antigen or antigens from an infectious agent that, when injected into a normal, susceptible body, initiates an immune response against a subsequent infection by the organism. A vaccine may consist of live organisms that retain their antigenic properties and can replicate in the body but will not cause severe illness; killed organisms that retain antigenic properties but will not replicate in the body and will not cause severe illness; or pure antigens.

Many successful vaccine preparations have been developed over the years, particularly to combat virus infections. Some of these are polio, rubella (German measles), measles, mumps, adenovirus, smallpox, and influenza. Table 13.2 indicates the principal vaccines used to prevent human viral diseases. Use Exploring Your Health 13.1 to trace your vaccination record.

The vaccines most commonly used to protect against bacterial infections are diphtheria, pertussis, and tetanus toxoid (the latter to protect against infection by *Clostridium tetani,* the causative agent of lockjaw). Although there are thousands of strains of bacteria, only a few bacterial vaccines have been developed because most bacterial infections are readily controlled through the use of antibiotics. In contrast, most viral infections cannot be controlled by drugs; therefore, immunization by vaccination is of more benefit.

Active and Passive Immunity When your body is capable of producing its own antibodies to fight off specific disease-causing organisms, you possess what is called **active immunity.** Active immunity can develop naturally in your body or it can be acquired "artificially" from a vaccination. Once you have active im-

Year 2000 National Health Objective

Several national health objectives have been established to decrease the incidence of infectious diseases. One objective seeks to reduce cases of vaccine-preventable diseases to zero. These diseases include diptheria and tetanus for all people and polio, measles, and rubella for people age 25 and younger. Other objectives seek to improve immunization levels as follows:

- Increase the basic immunization series for children under age 2 to at least 90 percent, up from 80 percent in 1989;

- Increase the basic immunization series for children in licensed care facilities and for young people in kindergarten to post-secondary education programs to at least 95 percent, up from 94 percent in 1989.

- Among noninstitutionalized high-risk populations, increase immunization for pneumococcal pneumonia and influenza to at least 60 percent, up from the 1985 levels of 10 percent and 20 percent, respectively.

- For hepatitis B, increase overall immunization rates among high-risk populations, including infants with antigen-positive mothers, occupationally exposed workers, homosexual men, and IV drug users in treatment programs.

TABLE 13.2

Principal Vaccines Used in Prevention of Human Virus Diseases

Disease	Source of Vaccine	Condition of Virus	Route of Administration
Recommended Immunization for General Public (in U.S. and Other Developed Countries)			
Poliomyelitis	Tissue culture (human diploid cell line, monkey kidney)	Live	Oral
Measles[a]	Tissue culture (chick embryo)	Live	Subcutaneous[b]
Mumps[a]	Tissue culture (chick embryo)	Live	Subcutaneous
Rubella[a,c]	Tissue culture (duck embryo, rabbit, or dog kidney)	Live	Subcutaneous
Immunization Recommended Only Under Certain Conditions (Epidemics, Exposure, Travel, Military)			
Smallpox	Lymph from calf or sheep (glycerolated, lyophilized); choorioallantois, tissue cultures (lyophilized)	Active	Intradermal: multiple pressure, multiple puncture, or (with specially prepared vaccine) by jet injection
Yellow Fever	Tissue cultures and eggs (17D strain)	Live	Subcutaneous or intradermal
Influenza	Chick embryo allantoic fluid (formalized or UV-irradiated, concentrated by various processes)	Inactive	Subcutaneous
	Highly purified or subunit forms recommended where available	Inactive	Subcutaneous
Rabies	Duck embryo treated with phenol or ultraviolet light	Inactive	Subcutaneous
Adenovirus[d]	Monkey kidney tissue cultures (formalinized)	Inactive	Intramuscular
	Human diploid cell cultures	Live	Oral, by entericcoated capsule
Japanese B encephalitis[d]	Mouse brain (formalinized), tissue culture	Inactive	Subcutaneous
Venezuelan equine encephalomyelitis[e]	Guinea pig heart cell culture	Live	Subcutaneous
Eastern equine encephalomyelitis[d]	Chick embryo cell culture	Inactive	Subcutaneous
Western equine encephalomyelitis[d]	Chick embryo cell culture	Inactive	Subcutaneous
Russian spring-summer encephalitis[d]	Mouse brain (formalinized)	Inactive	Subcutaneous

[a] Available also as combined vaccines.
[b] With less attenuated strains, gamma globulin is given in another limb at the time of vaccination.
[c] Neither monovalent rubella vaccine nor combination vaccines incorporating rubella should be administered to a postpubertal susceptible female unless she is not pregnant and understands that it is imperative not to become pregnant for at least three months after vaccination. (The time immediately postpartum has been suggested as a safe period for vaccination.)
[d] Not available in the United States except for the Armed Forces or for investigative purposes.
[e] Available for use in domestic animals (from the U.S. Department of Agriculture) and for investigative purposes.
Source: E. Jarvetz, J. L. Melnick, and E. A. Adelberg, *Review of Medical Microbiology,* (Los Altos, Calif.: Lange Medical Publication), p. 323. Used by permission.

passive immunity The injection or ingestion of pharmaceutically produced antibodies against a specific antigen in order to boost the immune system and provide short-term immunity to a disease.

antibiotic A pharmaceutical, such as penicillin,

which will destroy bacteria and other microbes that cause disease.

influenza (flu) A viral infection of the upper respiratory tract causing severe coldlike symptoms. There are several strains of flu and various vaccines are manufactured to combat them. Influenza can lead to pneumonia or death in weak or aged people.

Exploring Your Health 13.1

Your Vaccination Record

Which diseases have you been vaccinated against? Consult your family physician or your university health service to obtain access to your medical file.

Vaccinations	Dates Vaccinated	Vaccinations	Dates Vaccinated	Vaccinations	Dates Vaccinated
1. _____ _____		5. _____ _____		9. _____ _____	
2. _____ _____		6. _____ _____		10. _____ _____	
3. _____ _____		7. _____ _____			
4. _____ _____		8. _____ _____			

---

munity against certain infectious diseases, you seldom need to worry about being infected by them.

Sometimes, however, your active immunity might be threatened by unusual health circumstances, or it might be reduced by sickness or by chemotherapy for cancer (see Chapter 16). During times when your body's immune mechanism is especially weak, it may need an extra boost in the form of antibodies taken from another person or animal. The result of this extra boost is called **passive immunity.** Produced from *gamma globulins* taken from donors' blood, passive immunity antibodies tend to be short-lived, but they will get your immune mechanism through difficult periods. Mother's milk is a good source of passive immunity for newborns, which is one of the most important reasons why breastfeeding is preferable to bottle formula feeding.

Antibiotics

Chemicals had been used to combat infectious diseases for hundreds of years before Paul Ehrlich made chemotherapy a science. In 1903, he developed Salvarson, a drug containing arsenic, which is effective against the causative agent of syphilis. In 1929, Sir Alexander Fleming discovered that a compound (later shown to be penicillin) produced by a fungus could inhibit the

growth of certain bacteria. In 1940, Chain and Florey reported that penicillin could be used to treat humans with bacterial infections. Meanwhile, Domagk, in 1935, discovered sulfonamides and their inhibitory action on bacterial multiplication. Once these compounds had been discovered, advances in antimicrobial chemotherapy were rapid. **Antibiotic** (*anti*—against; *bios*—life) was originally a term used to mean natural products of microorganisms, but it now includes synthetic compounds (for example, synthetic penicillin, ampicillin) as well.

Antibiotics can successfully control several major bacterial diseases, such as strep and staph infections, bacterial pneumonia, and many of the sexually trans-

Year 2000 National Health Objective

The federal government has established a national health objective to reduce epidemic-related pneumonia and influenza deaths among people age 65 and older to no more than 7.3 per 100,000 per year. Between 1980 and 1987, an average of 9.1 deaths per 100,000 occurred per year.

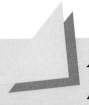

mitted diseases. However, these drugs cannot treat viruses. Although antibiotics have made a vital contribution, some problems are associated with their use, including allergic reactions and the development of strains resistant to the drugs.

Common Infectious Diseases

The Common Cold

The *common cold* is an infection of the membrane lining the upper respiratory tract, including the nose, the sinuses, and the throat. Contrary to popular belief, you cannot "catch" a cold from a draft, wet feet, a chill, or going out without a hat in inclement weather. The infection can, however, be transmitted by direct contact, such as handshakes or kissing, through mucus droplets coughed or sneezed into the air, and through contact with soiled tissues used by an infected person. There is currently no known means of preventing, curing, or shortening a cold, but the symptoms can be treated with aspirin (for headache, fever, and body aches); a humidifier; saltwater gargle or lozenges (for sore throat); limited use of nasal decongestants; and fluids, such as juice, tea, or soup. Antibiotics are ineffective in treating a cold virus, and the value of taking massive doses of vitamin C to prevent or cure a cold is debatable.

Colds are more prevalent during the winter months, when people spend more time indoors. Preventive measures including avoiding carriers (particularly during the first twenty-four hours of symptoms, when the virus is most contagious), avoiding handshakes, avoiding contact with the mucous membranes, and practicing proper hygiene (washing hands and face frequently).

Influenza

Influenza (flu) (viral infection of the respiratory tract) is caused by three types of viruses (A, B, and C), and each has several strains that tend to change slightly from year to year. Type A occurs in epidemic cycles every ten to twelve years and is the most serious. Type B produces a milder virus but can also reach epidemic proportions. Epidemics of Type C virus do not occur. Because so many different strains of flu exist, a vaccine must be repeated annually and may not offer protection unless the specific type of flu virus is identified. The elderly and the chronically ill whose resistance is lower may benefit from vaccination against Type A virus.

Treatment involves bed rest until body temperature is back to normal, along with symptomatic treatment similar to that described for the common cold. If complications develop, such as earache, sinus pain, persistent cough, or sore throat, a physician should be consulted.

measles A highly infectious disease caused by the measles virus.

encephalitis An inflammation of the brain. Encephalitis is sometimes a complication of measles.

infectious mononucleosis A viral infection like the common cold, but lasting much longer; occasionally there are serious complications.

infectious hepatitis (type A hepatitis) A common disease characterized by an inflammation of the liver, caused by a virus. Contracted usually through fecal contamination of food; usually not a severe disease.

serum hepatitis (type B hepatitis) A serious disease characterized by an inflammation of the liver, caused by a virus. Transmitted through the blood, semen, and saliva of infected people; it is much less common than infectious hepatitis.

jaundice A yellowing of the skin and the whites of the eyes, caused by an inflammation of the liver.

Measles

Measles is a highly contagious disease caused by measles virus. The airborne virus enters the upper respiratory tract, where it replicates and is spread via blood, mucus, or secretions throughout the respiratory tract. A red rash appears in the mouth and on the skin. The rash is caused by serum seepage from the blood and dead or dying cells forming discrete spots on the skin.

Measles is a serious disease and, under certain circumstances, can lead to inflammation of the brain, or **encephalitis.** It is a common disease: more than 80 percent of individuals over age 20 have an antibody to the virus. A measles vaccine is now available for children and adults; infants are usually protected by the maternal antibody until 6 months of age and should be vaccinated at 15 months.

Approximately 5 percent of young adults are susceptible to measles. Some of these individuals were never vaccinated and others received a vaccine that did not offer lifetime protection. Individuals who were born after 1956 should be protected by live vaccine. Revaccination should also be considered for those who received the live vaccine before age 1 and those who received the killed measles vaccine during the years 1963–1967. Those who are allergic to eggs or the antibiotic neomycin, pregnant women, and those with impaired immune responses should not be vaccinated.

Mumps

Mumps virus exists in only one form. After inhalation of the virus, infection may proceed in the outer layer of cells of the respiratory tract or through the oral cavitiy into the parotid glands, located in the tissue in the floor of your mouth to either side of the tongue. Once virus replicates and enters the blood, it can localize in salivary glands, reproductive organs (testes and ovaries), pancreas, thyroid, and brain.

The incubation period is twelve to thirty-five days, and the disease is characterized by swelling of the parotid glands, fever, and general malaise. In adults, the reproductive glands can be affected: 20 percent of males around the age of puberty develop a swelling of the testes, but this does *not* generally lead to sterility.

You may have heard that if only one side of your face swells during mumps infection, you could contract mumps again. This is not true. Once you have had mumps virus infection in one or both parotid glands, with or without swelling of the reproductive glands, you are protected against a future mumps infection.

Rubella

Rubella is generally a disease of childhood. It is often referred to as "German measles" because it was closely studied in Germany in the nineteenth century. The rubella virus infects the outer layer of cells of the upper respiratory tract but may replicate in the cervical lymph nodes. The virus appears in the blood about a week after infection and persists for an additional two weeks. A characteristic skin rash develops when the antibody appears in the blood. Once you have contracted the rubella virus, you are generally immune. However, reinfection may occur in some cases, due to inadequate levels of antibody.

Rubella infection may have serious effects if contracted during early pregnancy. Infection during the first ten weeks of pregnancy can lead to birth defects in the fetus.

Children are generally given the combined measles, mumps, and rubella vaccine at fifteen months. Adults may be immunized at any time, although the great majority of adults are already immune, even if they have no history of the disease. If a woman is pregnant and there are unimmunized children in the household, those children should be vaccinated, as they are the most likely rubella carriers. Table 13.3 indicates the recommended schedule for immunization of infants and children against a number of viral diseases.

Mononucleosis

Infectious mononucleosis can be transmitted in the saliva during kissing or in a manner similar to the common cold. The highest rate of occurrence is in the 15 to 19 age range, followed by the 20 to 24 age range. Symptoms appear from two weeks to two months after exposure: fever, sore throat, enlargement of the spleen

TABLE 13.3

Recommended Schedule for Active Immunization of Normal Infants and Children

Recommended Age	Immunization(s)	Comments
2 months	DTP,[1] OPV[2]	Can be initiated as early as 2 weeks of age in areas of high endemicity or during epidemics.
4 months	DTP, OPV	2-month interval desired for OPV to avoid interference from previous dose.
6 months	DTP (OPV)	OPV is optional (may be given in areas with increased risk of poliovirus exposure).
15 months	Measles, Mumps, Rubella (MMR)[3]	MMR preferred to individual vaccines; tuberculin testing may be done.
18 months	DTP,[4,5] OPV[5]	
24 months	HBPV[6]	
4–6 years[7]	DTP, OPV	At or before school entry.
14–16 years	Td[8]	Repeat every 10 years throughout life.

[1]DTP—Diphtheria and tetanus toxoids with pertussis vaccine.
[2]OPV—Oral, poliovirus vaccine contains attenuated poliovirus types 1, 2, and 3.
[3]MMR—Live measles, mumps, and rubella viruses in a combined vaccine.
[4]Should be given 6 to 12 months after the third dose.
[5]May be given simultaneously with MMR at 15 months of age.
[6]*Haemophilus* B polysaccharide vaccine.
[7]Up to the seventh birthday.
[8]Td—Adult tetanus toxoic (full dose) and diphtheria toxoid (reduced dose) in combination.

and other lymph glands, headache, and fatigue. Serious complications occur in only a small percentage of cases, but the disease is debilitating and requires several weeks to months for full recovery.

Treatment is similar to that for a common cold; the course of the disease is not altered. Bed rest may be required in the early stages. There is currently no known prevention, although a vaccine is under development.

Hepatitis

Hepatitis is essentially an inflammation of the liver that is caused by a number of different viruses, although two well-known viruses are the culprits in most cases. There are two basic types of hepatitis. **Infectious hepatitis,** or **type A hepatitis,** is caused by fecal contamination of food or the environment and is easily preventable by proper hygiene. Type A hepatitis is more common and usually much less severe than **serum hepatitis,** or **hepatitis type B,** which accounts for only 10 percent of all hepatitis cases. Hepatitis B is transmitted through the blood, semen, and saliva—but not the fecal matter—of infected people. Sexual transmission is common for hepatitis B, especially among homosexual men, as is transmission by the sharing of used hypodermic needles among IV drug

users. Occasionally hepatitis B is also transmitted by tattooing, ear piercing, and breastfeeding by an infected nursing mother.

Common symptoms for both types of hepatitis include fever (possibly mild or absent in hepatitis B), general weakness and fatigue, loss of appetite, nausea, abdominal discomfort in the upper right quadrant, and sometimes **jaundice** (yellowing of the skin and eyes).

Year 2000 National Health Objective

Recognizing the numerous preventable causes of viral hepatitis, several national health objectives strive to reduce the incidence of hepatitis B (HBV) from 63.5 to 40 per 100,000, hepatitis A from 31 to 23 per 100,000, and hepatitis C from 18.3 to 13.7 per 100,000. Specific types of HBV cases have been targeted. Reductions per 100,000 being sought are intravenous drug abusers (30,000 to 22,500), heterosexually active people (33,000 to 22,000), homosexual men (25,300 to 8,500), children of Asians/Pacific Islanders (8,900 to 1,800), occupationally exposed workers (6,200 to 1,250), infants (3,500 to 550), and Alaska Natives (15 to 1).

Onset of the disease is usually sudden for hepatitis A and gradual for hepatitis B. Recovery can be very slow for both types of hepatitis, and some cases require as much as several months. Unlike hepatitis A, hepatitis B can remain in the bloodstream for many years following general recovery from its symptoms. Hepatitis B also greatly increases the risk of developing liver cancer and cirrhosis of the liver. The disease is fatal to approximately 1 percent of those afflicted.

It is possible to receive temporary protection or immunity against hepatitis through an injection of gamma globulin. A new vaccine has been developed for hepatitis B. It is costly (three treatments costing a total of $100) but recommended for high-risk groups including homosexual males, IV drug users, patients of kidney dialysis, hemophiliacs, morticians, and some health care workers.

Herpes Simplex, Type 1

Herpes simplex is a virus that occurs in two types: Herpes, type 1, causes cold sores and fever blisters; herpes, type 2, is a sexually transmitted disease and will be discussed in the next chapter.

Although cold sores may disappear rapidly, the type 1 herpes virus remains in a dormant state until triggered to reappear at a lesion site. You may have had a cold sore on your lip and recall that it hurt and looked unsightly, and you were quite relieved when it was gone. The bad news is that it isn't really gone. The virus is still with you in a latent or dormant form, just waiting for the proper stimulus (sunburn, nervous tension, hormone imbalance) to reappear as a lesion. Infection recurs in spite of high levels of antibody and good cell-mediated immunity because the virus leads a relatively sheltered existence in a part of your nervous system where antibody and immune cells can't reach it. Your immune system can only act against the virus after your skin has been traumatized.

Lyme Disease

Some infectious diseases are carried by a *vector*, which is any animal or insect that transmits a disease-producing organism from a host to a noninfected animal or human. One vector-borne bacterial infection that has

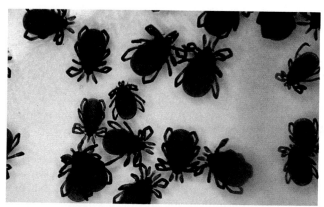

The deer tick *(Ixodes dammini),* a vector of Lyme disease, is about the size of a pinhead.

held popular attention for the last few years is **Lyme disease,** which was identified in Lyme, Connecticut, in 1975. In 1982, Willy Burgdorfer of the National Institutes of Health laboratory in Montana discovered the actual agent of infection, a type of bacteria previously unknown *(Borrelia burgdorferi).* The insect vector for this bacteria is the deer tick *Ixodes dammini,* which feeds on small wild mammals in addition to deer. Humans and domestic animals bitten by the poppy seed-sized deer tick can be infected with Lyme disease.

Although symptoms of Lyme disease vary, in about 50 percent of the cases a "bull's-eye" rash develops within a few days where the bite occurred.

If you are bitten by a deer tick, you might develop, after two to thirty days, the "bull's-eye" rash that is a characteristic symptom of Lyme disease.

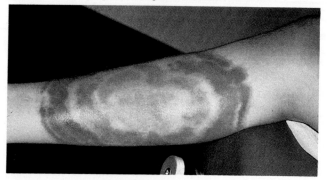

Other symptoms may include flulike symptoms, fever, chills, dizziness, and fatigue. If left untreated, bouts of severe headache, stiffness in the neck and joints, arthritic pain, and even cardiac and neurological problems may occur. Eventually, these problems can become much worse, to the point where people who are already ill or at risk in some other way may die.

Lyme disease can be treated with antibiotics, but the best treatment for the disease is prevention. Are you planning a camping trip or hike through the woods? Don't change your plans because of Lyme disease! Wear tightly-woven, light-colored long trousers (with the legs tucked into your socks) and long-sleeve shirts. Check your clothing often for ticks. Be sure to check places on your body where ticks can easily hide, such as your scalp and in the genital area. If you must wear light clothing, shorts, and short-sleeve shirts, use insect repellent at least on your legs, socks, and footwear. If you do find a tick firmly stuck in your skin, don't panic! Using tweezers, grasp the tick firmly as close to its head as possible and slowly pull it out. Make sure you have removed the entire tick. If you develop any of the symptoms discussed above after a few days, seek medical help.

Infectious Lung Diseases

Fungus Infections

The air contains many spores (fungi) or moldlike substances that enter the lungs without producing disease. Unfortunately, some fungi produce TB-like symptoms. *Histoplasmosis* is caused by tiny spores that float in dusty air and flourish in warm, moist dark places, such as old chicken houses, pigeon lofts, barns, and under trees where birds roost. The inhaled spores may enter the air sacs and multiply in the lymph nodes. The infection may remain in the lungs where it can be effectively treated, or it may spread throughout the body producing a fatal reaction. *Coccidioidomycosis* (valley fever) is caused by inhaling dust contaminated by spores. Most people exhibit no symptoms; others develop a fever 1 to 3 weeks after the spores invade the lungs and body, followed by a measlelike rash, sores on the shins, and joint pain. Within several months symptoms disappear.

Skin tests, blood tests, chest x-rays, and tests of body fluids can detect fungus infections. Modern drugs generally offer effective treatment.

Pneumonia

Acute lung inflammations, called **pneumonia,** are caused by bacteria, viruses, fungi, aspiration of food or fluid, inhalation of poisonous gases, and other factors. Common symptoms include fever, coughing, shortness of breath, chest pains, blood in the phlegm, and a bluish tinge in the skin. *Double pneumonia* involves an inflammation in both lungs. *Bronchial pneumonia* refers to an inflammation in the bronchi or air tubes and the lungs. *Walking pneumonia* is a mild form of pneumonia that does not require hospitalization or confinement.

Bacterial pneumonia is a major killer among older Americans, directly causing over 50,000 deaths and contributing to 200,000 other deaths each year. The severe pneumonia (infection with group A streptococcus bacteria) that killed Muppets' creator Jim Henson is a rare complication from a common bacteria. This bacteria causes a variety of infections and most are mild, such as sore throat and impetigo. A vaccine that is 60–75 percent effective is available that protects against the 23 types of bacterium *Streptococcus pneumoniae,* which accounts for about 90 percent of all cases of bacterial pneumonia. Unfortunately, less than 15 percent of the high-risk population have been vaccinated. Some experts feel that all healthy Americans over the age of 50 should receive the vaccine.

Tuberculosis

Tuberculosis (TB) is a highly contagious disease that produces symptoms similar to those of other lung disease or of no particular disease at all. Anyone experiencing chronic cough, fatigue, weakness, unexplained weight loss, loss of appetite, or spitting of blood should see a physician immediately. Most individuals who develop TB have had the germs in their bodies for long periods of time. They may have had contact with a TB patient years ago, breathed in the germs, and fought them off with the body's defenses. Instead of killing the germs, the body may have walled them up in tiny hard capsules (the "tubercles" of tuberculosis). Years later, when resistance is low and when the immune system is not functioning properly, the germs break out of the capsules, spread, and do their damage. It is estimated that 15 million Americans have TB germs in their body: they are infected and prime candidates for coming down with TB. Although a simple tuberculin test would reveal the presence of the germ, most people do not know they are infected.

Treatment to prevent TB involves medication for

Year 2000 National Health Objective

Because of a rise in the incidence of tuberculosis in the United States, the federal government has established a national health objective to reduce the incidence per year to no more than 3.5 cases per 100,000 people. In 1988, 9.1 cases per 100,000 people occurred.

noninfectious diseases Chronic and degenerative diseases.

diabetes A disease of the metabolic system caused by an insufficient amount of the hormone insulin, which is produced by the pancreas.

insulin A hormone produced by the pancreas that is used by the body to metabolize glucose to provide energy for bodily functions. It may be administered as a medication to treat diabetes.

Exploring Your Health 13.2

Your Infectious Disease Pattern

List the infectious diseases you have contracted since birth. Indicate the month and year you contracted each disease. Separate childhood and adult diseases. Summarize the severity of your symptoms.

What infectious diseases are you still exposed to that you did not have as a child? How serious is it to contract these diseases as an adult? What can you do to avoid contracting these diseases? Is there a pattern in the diseases you have contracted?

Childhood Disease/Date Symptoms/Severity	Adult Disease/Date Symptoms/Severity
1.	1.
2.	2.
3.	3.
4.	4.
5.	5.

List the common childhood infectious diseases you have not contracted and state the possible symptoms and effects these might have on you as an adult.

1.
2.
3.

---

approximately one year to kill the walled-up germs that may break free years from now. Treatment to cure TB involves a tuberculin test, chest x-ray, laboratory tests, and outpatient treatment with regular medication. Thanks to new drugs, patients can usually continue with their present job and family activities and avoid long hospital stays and surgery. Combinations of several drugs are usually administered for about nine months.

Before moving on to a consideration of noninfectious diseases, briefly test your knowledge of infectious diseases in Exploring Your Health 13.2 by charting the occurrence of infectious diseases in your own life.

II. Noninfectious Diseases

As Americans' life spans continue to increase, chronic and degenerative diseases—or **noninfectious diseases**—become more common. All aging body systems exhibit signs of wear and tear. Diseases of the skeletal and muscular system, such as arthritis and

dental disease; malfunctions of the endocrine system, such as diabetes; disorders of the nervous system, such as multiple sclerosis; respiratory system problems, such as allergies; and problems with the circulatory system, such as heart disease and stroke, are now common among the middle-aged and older populations in the United States. In addition, a number of serious genetic diseases still occur in our country. The rest of this chapter examines some of the most common noninfectious diseases and discusses various ways you can reduce your risk and help others reduce their risk of falling prey to them in the future.

Diabetes Mellitus

Diabetes is caused by insufficient production of the hormone **insulin** in the pancreas. All carbohydrates must be transformed into glucose before they can be used as energy, and lack of insulin interferes with the body's ability to use carbohydrates. When the body can no longer use glucose efficiently, the blood sugar level

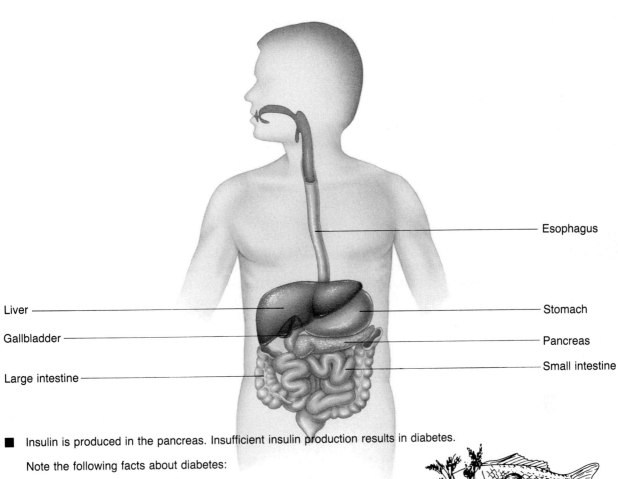

Esophagus

Liver

Stomach

Gallbladder

Pancreas

Small intestine

Large intestine

■ Insulin is produced in the pancreas. Insufficient insulin production results in diabetes.

Note the following facts about diabetes:

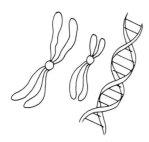

There is a genetic tendency to develop diabetes.

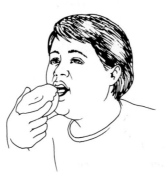

Obesity is the single most common nongenetic factor in developing diabetes.

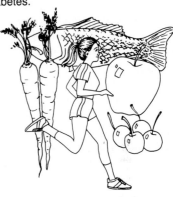

Healthy eating habits and regular exercise are very important in controlling diabetes.

Diabetics should not smoke at all.

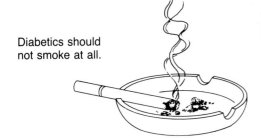

Diabetics should wear an identification bracelet that can be noticed easily

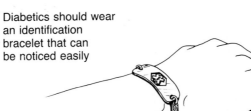

FIGURE 13.2 • Diabetes: Causes and Management

insulin shock A medical condition in a diabetic individual who is suffering from low blood sugar due to excessive insulin administration. The condition can be relieved by giving the person something sweet to eat or drink.

becomes extremely high (a condition called *hyperglycemia*). Without proper control, serious complications may develop. Some of the more common problems of untreated diabetes include vascular disease leading to heart attacks, heart pain, heart failure, strokes, senility, gangrene of the feet, blindness resulting from damage to the arteries in the retina, liver and kidney damage, nerve damage, foot and leg ulcers, and susceptibility to infections.

With insufficient insulin in the blood, generally aggravated by excessive ingestion of carbohydrates, *diabetic coma* may occur. The victim may have a fever, appear extremely ill, complain of intense thirst, and vomit. An acetone odor may be present on the breath. It is imperative that you call an ambulance or a doctor. The victim should be kept lying down flat and covered with a blanket until a physician arrives. Fluids may be given to a conscious victim, providing they do not contain sugar or starches.[3]

With too much insulin in the blood, **insulin shock** may occur. The diabetic becomes very weak, skin is moist and pale, and tremors or convulsions may occur. Sugar (orange juice, soft drinks, granulated sugar on the tongue) can be given if the diabetic is conscious; sugar cubes can be rubbed on the tongue of the unconscious victim.

Diabetes may occur in childhood or adolescence (juvenile diabetes); the average age is ten to twelve years. Juvenile diabetes is caused by a severe deficit in the synthesis of insulin by the pancreas. Adult diabetes

People who develop diabetes early in life are usually dependent on regular injections of insulin.

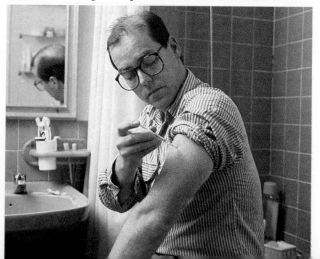

is common in obese individuals over the age of 40. This form is caused by insufficient insulin rather than lack of insulin and is rarely as severe as juvenile diabetes.

Some of the more easily recognized symptoms of diabetes include excessive thirst and urination, unexplained weight loss, slow healing of cuts and bruises, excessive hunger, low energy level, intense itching, changes in vision, chronic skin infections, and pain in the extremities. If you possess any of these symptoms, see your physician immediately. Urinalysis will determine whether further tests are needed.

Factors in Developing Diabetes

There is a genetic tendency to develop diabetes. One of every four people is a carrier of this tendency. The individual carrier does not have and will not develop diabetes. Being a carrier of the diabetic trait means that some close relative has or had diabetes. Possessing the diabetic trait means that at some time in one's life, some evidence of diabetes may develop. The genetic pattern can be predicted:

- If both parents are diabetic, all their children will have the diabetic trait. If both parents are nondiabetic, none of their children will have the diabetic trait.
- If one parent is diabetic and the other is a carrier, the probability that any one child will have the diabetic trait will be one in two.
- If both parents are carriers, the probability that any one child will have the diabetic trait will be one in four.
- If one parent is nondiabetic and the other is a carrier, it is unlikely that any of the children will have the trait.
- If one parent is diabetic and the other is nondiabetic, the probability that any one child will have the trait will be one if four.

Possessing the diabetic trait is not the only determining factor. In studies of identical twins, researchers have noted that one may acquire diabetes much sooner than the other. Prevention centers on a number of factors. Because obesity is the single most common non-

Issues in Health

If Nothing Can Be Done to Prevent or Cure a Fatal Disease, Is There Any Point in Knowing If You Will Acquire It Later in Life?

Genetic counseling has acquired general acceptance as a means of preventing the birth of many babies with serious inherited physical and mental birth defects (more than 250,000 such American babies are born each year). Counseling also helps prospective parents understand the odds of an offspring acquiring a serious genetic disease. Based upon test results and probabilities, parents make decisions about pregnancy and abortion. Unfortunately, not everyone seeks genetic counseling, nor is everyone aware of the genetic diseases in their family, so thousands of babies are both each year at risk of developing a serious disease. Many of these diseases are not evident at birth, and symptoms appear at varying ages in different children: cystic fibrosis and Tay-Sachs disease (birth to six months), sickle-cell anemia (from 6 months on), Duchenne muscular dystrophy (2 to 4 years), glaucoma and Huntington's disease (late thirties on). For fatal genetic diseases such as Huntington's (25,000

total cases) with symptoms not appearing until the third or fourth decade (patients eventually become bedridden, exhibiting uncontrolled rapid muscular movements and extreme mental confusion), one has to wonder if screening after birth is more harmful than helpful to patients and family.

Opponents of after-birth testing argue that information contained in the genes should remain a secret. Since the disease cannot be prevented or cured, there is no point in knowing. Knowledge of impending disease will only reduce one's quality of life and disrupts the entire family. In addition, no one can accurately predict exactly how they will handle the information. People at risk may feel that they can cope with the dreaded news that they will definitely develop a serious disease, and later find themselves totally incapable of adjusting. Tests are also expensive and predict with less than 100 percent accuracy. The probability, however remote, of receiving inaccu-

rate information does exist. It would be better, it is argued, to enjoy life to the fullest without knowing if or when such a disaster will occur.

Some at-risk people cope better by securing as much information as possible. Certain knowledge of their fate reduces their anxiety levels and helps them cope with the future. Such advance knowledge may change the way they want to live their lives, both personally and economically. It also allows ample time to plan for those who will be left behind. Certainly, knowing approximately when loss of function will occur is an advantage. Also, no disease is entirely hopeless. Research into the cause and treatment of Huntington's disease has made steady progress. Discovering whether you will develop the disease offers opportunities to participate in recent research and benefit from new treatment that may eventually halt the disease.

The decision is a tough one. What do you think? What would you do?

---

genetic factor, weight control is essential. In addition, infectious illnesses, accidental wounds, surgery, psychic stress, and emotional shock frequently seem to trigger diabetes in individuals who have the trait. Healthy eating habits and regular exercise aid in prevention by using calories and decreasing the need for insulin, preventing obesity, and lowering blood fat levels.

Managing Diabetes

Once a diagnosis of juvenile diabetes is confirmed, a few changes are needed immediately, but there is no reason why one's life must be drastically altered. Although there is no special diabetic diet, it is necessary to eat well-balanced meals with all the essential vitamins and minerals. Obesity must be eliminated, and this may erase many or all of the symptoms. The diet should be designed by a physician or a registered dietitian. Regular exercise is important in regulating body weight and blood fat levels and in decreasing the body's need for insulin.

Diabetics should stop smoking tobacco immediately. They are already prone to heart disease and

should avoid the added risk. In addition, smoking stimulates blockage of circulation in the legs.

Diabetics should wear an identification bracelet that can be noticed easily. A bracelet with a warning phrase will guarantee proper diagnosis or treatment. In case of diabetic coma, the inscription can list the medicines one is taking, including the amount of insulin.

Year 2000 National Health Objective

To help prevent and control diabetes, the federal government has established three health objectives: (1) to reduce diabetes-related deaths per year to no more than 34 per 100,000 people (from 38 per 100,000 in 1986); (2) to reduce the incidence of the most severe complications of diabetes, such as end-stage renal disease, blindness, lower extremity amputation, perinatal mortality, and major congenital malformations; and (3) to reduce the incidence of diabetes to no more than 2.5 per 1,000 people per year and a prevalence of no more than 25 per 1,000 people (these figures were 2.9 and 28 per 1,000, respectively, in 1987).

epilepsy A disease of the central nervous system that causes seizures; various causes exist.

aura A certain feeling which to an epileptic is a warning that a seizure is impending.

multiple sclerosis (MS) A disease of unknown origin, possibly caused by a virus, that attacks the myelin sheaths of nerves. MS can lead to difficulty with motor control of the body and to paralysis.

Disorders of the Nervous System

There is much to be learned about the functioning of the brain and nervous system. Disorders of the nervous system are difficult to diagnose and treat. In addition, the causes of many disorders remain elusive. This section covers three known disorders.

Epilepsy

In the Middle Ages, people who experienced recurrent physical convulsions and other such disturbances were often considered to be possessed by demons. Later, and until about the turn of this century, people with these symptoms were usually regarded as mentally ill or feebleminded. Unfortunately, even though we understand it better today, many people still fear epilepsy. This fear is simply not necessary. Before reading on, test your knowledge of epilepsy in Exploring Your Health 13.3.

Recurrent seizures from any cause can be termed **epilepsy.** This condition affects approximately 0.5 percent of the population. The exact causes are unknown, although some factors have been identified. Seizures of unknown cause generally appear from age 3 to 15. Seizures before age 2 may be related to developmental defects, birth injuries, or metabolic diseases affecting the brain. Seizures appearing for the first time after age 25 generally are a result of cerebral trauma, tumors, or organic brain disease.[4]

Epileptic Attacks   Three general types of epileptiform attacks can be distinguished, each with unique traits and symptoms. The *grand mal* (major epilepsy) attack may begin in one part of the body and gradually move upward to other body parts. A so-called **aura,** referred to as a warning of an oncoming seizure, is actually part of the seizure. The aura directs attention to the portion of the brain where the attack originates. Loss of consciousness may or may not occur with this type. The typical grand mal may involve a cry, loss of consciousness, falling, and contractions of the muscles of the arms, legs, trunk, and head. The attack lasts between two and five minutes and may be followed by a deep sleep, soreness, and headache. Attacks can occur at any age and are often associated with organic brain disease.

Attacks of *petit mal* (minor epilepsy) usually involve some clouding of consciousness for one to thirty seconds, after which the patient recovers rather rapidly. Petit mal attacks are more common in children and often outgrown by midadolescence. Attacks may occur several times daily, generally when at rest. Seizures during exercise are rare.

Psychomotor attacks are usually minor seizures of one to two minutes in duration. The patient may stagger around and perform automatic movements, make unintelligible sounds, lose contact with the environment, and suffer mental confusion for a short period after the seizure ends. Psychomotor attacks are associated with brain damage and can occur at any age.

Treatment varies with specific type of attack and may take the form of (1) eliminating the causative or precipitating factors (infections, endocrine abnormalities), (2) proper care during a convulsion, (3) maintaining emotional balance by leading a normal life, and (4) drug therapy.

Some advances have been made in the prevention and treatment of epilepsy. Researchers believe that women can do much during pregnancy to help prevent epilepsy from developing in their children. Avoidance of people with infectious diseases and of tobacco, alcohol, and all drugs, as well as good medical care throughout pregnancy may greatly decrease the likelihood of epilepsy. In general, use of protective head equipment in vehicles and in sports, avoidance of poisonous substances, and regular medical checkups are also sound preventive measures. Treatment centers around proper medical care to eliminate infections and endocrine abnormalities, proper care during a convulsion, and drug therapy.[5]

Multiple Sclerosis

Both the cause and the cure of **multiple sclerosis (MS)** are unknown, although recent findings suggest that a delayed-action virus may be the cause. The disease affects the myelin sheath of the nerves. This

Exploring Your Health 13.3

What Do You Know About Epilepsy?

Epilepsy victims suffer considerable discrimination from a misinformed public. Mark each question True or False to rate your knowledge of this illness.

	True	False
1. Epilepsy, if untreated, will lead to insanity.	T	F
2. A bystander should place an object between the teeth of a victim of convulsions in order to prevent the tongue from being swallowed.	T	F
3. It is important to prevent or restrain the jerking and rigidity of muscle groups that can occur during a seizure.	T	F
4. The best thing for a bystander to do for a person suffering a seizure is nothing.	T	F
5. Bystanders should attempt to make a person "walk it off" after suffering a grand mal seizure.	T	F
6. All seizures are indicative of epilepsy.	T	F
7. Epilepsy cannot occur after age eighteen.	T	F
8. Epilepsy is inherited.	T	F
9. In most instances, epileptic seizures cannot be controlled.	T	F

Answers

1. False. This myth developed many years before modern medicine determined what epilepsy is. Epilepsy will not lead to insanity.

2. False. It is difficult to open the jaws of a person having a grand mal seizure, and an object could damage the interior of the mouth. It is also impossible to swallow the tongue.

3. False. The more a person is restricted, the greater the chance of a repeat seizure of greater magnitude.

4. True. You need only protect the victim from being injured by objects in the room and from other well-meaning bystanders.

5. False. It is best to allow the victim to sleep as long as he or she desires and avoid talking about the seizure unless the victim initiates the discussion.

6. False. Factors such as illness and poison contribute to seizures.

7. False. Epilepsy can occur at any age; however, among adults it is often brought on by a head injury.

8. False. The likelihood that any epileptic will have a child who will become epileptic is very slim.

9. False. Medication greatly reduces the incidence of seizures.

---

sheath insulates nerve fibers and prevents the overflow and loss of nerve impulses. Many different (multiple) parts of the nervous system are attacked and scarred (sclerosis).

Some minor symptoms may appear and disappear months or years before the disease is recognized. Minor visual disturbances, stiffness or fatigue in a limb, occasional dizziness, and mild emotional disturbances are some of the early warning signs. After diagnosis, the disease progresses differently from individual to individual; it is slow in some and more rapid in others; attacks are frequent in some, infrequent with many remissions in others. In the more advanced stages, the victim may experience partial or complete paralysis, numbness, double vision, slurring of speech, general weakness, loss of bowel control, and difficulty in swallowing. Life expectancy is shortened, although it is difficult to predict how the disease will progress in different individuals.

There is no known "cure" for MS, but medications can be used to control its symptoms. It is important that psychological counseling and stress management strategies be made available to MS patients.

The public playing career of the brilliant young English cellist Jacqueline du Pré ended shortly after she was diagnosed with MS in 1973. Nevertheless, du Pré continued an active teaching schedule until her death in 1987.

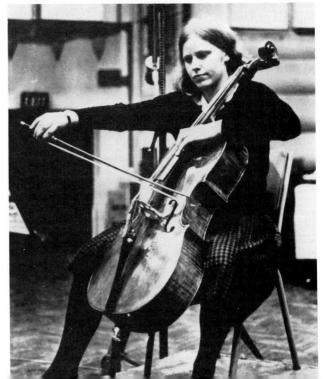

cerebral palsy A disease of the central nervous system characterized by uncontrolled muscular contractions.

sickle-cell anemia A genetically transmitted blood disease that becomes manifest in one out of every four hundred African-American people.

muscular dystrophy A genetically transmitted disease that disables the muscles.

Down's syndrome A genetically transmitted disease that results in some facial and body abnormalities and in mild to severe mental retardation.

amniocentesis A medical test in which amniotic fluid is drawn from the uterus of a pregnant woman to determine the health of the unborn fetus.

Tay-Sachs disease A serious genetically transmitted disease that is found primarily in Jewish families from Eastern Europe.

Cerebral Palsy

There are 500,000–700,000 victims of **cerebral palsy** in the United States. The exact cause of this disease is unknown; however, some factors have been isolated. Among known factors are rubella when contracted during the first three months of pregnancy, birth trauma, *anoxia* (lack of oxygen), Rh factors, and possibly heredity.

Symptoms of the disease may be present from birth. In less severe cases, symptoms may not appear until the child fails to perform certain developmental tasks, such as sitting, crawling, walking, or talking. The *spastic* and *athetoid* types of cerebral palsy represent about 80 percent of cases. Spastics experience muscle tenseness and excessive muscle contractions, which in turn make coordinated movements difficult. Symptoms of the athetoid type include slow, involuntary movements. A third type, *ataxia,* is characterized by difficulty with balance and frequent falls. Mixtures of the three basic types are common.

A number of preventive techniques are possible today. Researchers believe that pregnant women can decrease the chances of cerebral palsy affecting their unborn children through the following: (1) routine testing for the Rh factor, (2) immunization within 72 hours after the pregnancy terminates to prevent adverse consequences of blood incompatibility in a subsequent pregnancy, (3) exchange transfusion in a baby to prevent blood incompatability if the woman has not been immunized, and (4) the use of neonatal intensive care units for high-risk infants. Newborn babies with jaundice can be treated by phototherapy. Additional programs focus on reducing the exposure of pregnant women to viral and other infections; eliminating unnecessary exposure to x-rays, drugs, and medications; and controlling diabetes, anemia, and other nutritional deficiencies.

Genetic Diseases

Diseases are passed on through the genes in one of four patterns: *dominant inheritance* (harmful gene is dominant and can be transmitted by only one parent), *recessive inheritance* (harmful gene is recessive and two genes, one from each parent, are necessary to transmit the gene), *sex-linked inheritance* (the female X chromosome carries the bad gene and the male child is affected), and *polygenic (multifactorial) inheritance* (the interaction of several genes, with or without the influence of environmental factors, causes the defect). Some inherited diseases are evident at birth (PKU or cystic fibrosis); others show up during infancy (Tay-Sachs), during the teenage years (familial hypercholesterolemia), or in adulthood. There are more than 300 inherited diseases. Most are considered inborn errors of metabolism or chemical mistakes. Some of the more common inherited disorders follow.

Sickle-Cell Anemia

Approximately two out of every twenty-five African-American people carry the trait for **sickle-cell anemia,** although only one out of every four hundred actually has the disease. When both parents are carriers, the probability is that, of every four children, one will possess sickle-cell anemia, two will be carriers, and one will have neither the disease nor the trait. The Sickledex test lends itself to mass-screening methods. A positive reaction to the test means the person either carries the trait or possesses the disease. Further tests are then needed to confirm the disease.

In sickle-cell anemia, the abnormal structure of the hemoglobin causes red blood cells (oxygen carrying) to pucker and assume a sickle shape. These cells have difficulty passing through capillary walls and at times pile up to block the flow of blood to body tissues. In addition, because these cells possess a life span of 30 to 40 days, rather than the normal 120 days, they are easily destroyed. New cells are not produced as fast as old cells are destroyed, and anemia results. The so-called sickle-cell crisis results when blood flow to normal tissues is hampered from a blockage and excessive cell destruction occurs, causing severe pain, anemia, weakness, nausea, and jaundice.

Treatment methods have improved tremendously in past years. The disease is most severe in the young and much less so after adolescence. Most therapy focuses upon treating the symptoms. Patients should avoid high altitudes and unpressurized planes because lower oxygen tension increases the sickling tendency.

Muscular Dystrophy

Approximately 200,000 persons (half of them between the ages of 4 and 15) are afflicted with some form of **muscular dystrophy.** The causes have not been discovered to date. The pattern of inheritance is sex-linked and recessive. In one form, affecting only boys and involving pelvic-girdle weaknesses, symptoms of the disease tend to appear as the child starts to walk. Waddling, toe-walking, frequent falling, and difficulty in getting up occur at this stage, with symptoms progressing until adolescence, when the patient is usually confined to a wheelchair. In another form, affecting both sexes, the disease starts later in life, generally during adolescence. Progression of symptoms is slower and more variable from one patient to another. Some become disabled, whereas others are barely aware of symptoms throughout life. Because there is no known drug therapy, treatment focuses on physical therapy.

Down's Syndrome

One in 600 American babies born each year has **Down's syndrome.** This condition is caused by chromosome abnormality in which the individual possesses 3 instead of the normal 2 twenty-first chromosomes. Down's syndrome is much more common in children born to women over the age of 40 than it is in children born to younger women. For example, the risk of a woman's giving birth to an infant with Down's syndrome is about 1 in 3,000 before age 30, 1 in 300 at age 35, 1 in 60 at age 40, and about 1 in 40 over age 45.

Individuals with Down's syndrome exhibit such physical defects as slanted eyes, facial deformities, and short legs and torso. Mild to severe mental retardation occurs.

Down's syndrome can be detected by **amniocentesis,** in which amniotic fluid is extracted from the pregnant woman's uterus and analyzed. This procedure is recommended for all pregnant women over the age of 35.

Tay-Sachs Disease

The massive accumulation of fat lipids in the brain that occurs with **Tay-Sachs disease** leads to mental retardation, blindness, and death at the age of 3 or 4. Approximately 85 percent of the victims are from Jewish families of Eastern European origin. Prevention through genetic counseling has proven effective. Blood tests on both parents determine whether one is a carrier. If both parents are carriers, each pregnancy is monitored by amniocentesis.

Familial Hypercholesterolemia

Familial hypercholesterolemia (FH) strikes about 1 in every 500 people in the United States, making it one of the most common genetic diseases. FH occurs in all segments of the population.

Most genetic diseases are recessive; a bad gene must be inherited from both parents before it is transmitted to the offspring. FH is a dominant genetic disease, requiring only one FH gene to transmit the disease to an offspring. If both parents are carriers, the victim receives a double dose. FH victims are born with a cholesterol count five to twelve times the normal level. The molecules at fault are *low-density lipoprotein* (LDL) receptors. LDL receptors act as cellular gatekeepers and transmit needed cholesterol into the cell. If a cell is deficient in LDL receptors, it cannot remove the cholesterol it needs from the bloodstream and therefore makes its own. The liver cells, also suffering from the same genetic deficiency, receive no signal to stop production and therefore continue to produce and circulate cholesterol. The entire cycle burdens the blood with excess cholesterol it can't get rid of. FH homozygotes (both parents carried the gene) may show signs of the disease by age 5: yellowish lumpy areas loaded with cholesterol develop in the knees, elbows, heels, and between the fingers. The combination of diet and exercise has little effect on the cholesterol level of homozygotes, and symptoms of heart disease may appear before the age of 10 or in the teens. Few victims live beyond age 20. The prognosis for FH heterozygotes (one parent carried the gene) is much better because they have half the normal LDL receptors. Signs of early heart disease may appear by age 20 to 29, with the first heart attack normally occurring in the 30s or 40s. Few victims live into their sixties.

Current research is focusing on genetic counseling and early screening. Drugs, careful diet, and altered lifestyles are then utilized in an attempt to lower the risk of heart attack to a normal level.

Noninfectious Lung Diseases

Over 75 million children and adults suffer from some form of chronic respiratory disease such as asthma, chronic bronchitis, emphysema, and occupational lung disease. Respiratory distress syndrome is also the number-one killer of newborn children in the first 27 days of life, causing more than 12,000 infant deaths. Acute respiratory distress accounts for more than one-half of all school absenteeisms in the United States.[6] Although some of these lung diseases are genetic, most are caused by what we breathe into the lungs, such as cigarette smoke, pollens, and indoor and outdoor pollutants. As a result, lung problems can often be prevented and controlled. After reading this section, you might find it helpful to review the section on Infectious Lung Diseases, presented earlier in this chapter.

acute bronchitis A short-term severe inflammation of the bronchial tubes.

chronic bronchitis A long-term inflammation of the bronchial tubes, resulting in weeks or months of coughing, phlegm production, and labored breathing.

emphysema A chronic disease of the lungs resulting in restricted breathing, general debilitation, and death.

pneumoconiosis Usually an occupational or environmental lung disease caused by deposition of particulate matter in the lungs, such as black lung or asbestosis.

allergy A hypersensitivity to a specific substance (such as food, pollen, or dust) or condition (such as cold or heat) that in similar amounts would appear to be harmless to most people.

allergens Substances that induce an allergic reaction.

Chronic Bronchitis

Bronchitis refers to an inflammation of the lining of the bronchial tubes, which connect the windpipe with the lungs. Inflamed or infected bronchial tubes produce a heavy mucus or phlegm and cause air flow to and from the lungs to become labored. **Acute bronchitis,** which produces fever, coughing, and spitting, may occur with a severe cold. When coughing and spitting continue for months, return annually, and last longer with each bout, the individual is said to be suffering from **chronic bronchitis.** The condition is nearly always associated with heavy cigarette smoking and air pollution. Initial irritation could also be caused by bacteria or a disease such as inflamed or infected tonsils.

Although chronic bronchitis is not a killer disease, early treatment is important to prevent permanent lung damage or heart failure later in life. Antibiotic drugs along with the elimination of all sources of irritation and infection in the nose, throat, mouth, sinuses, and bronchial tube usually provide effective treatment. Patients must quit smoking, eliminate their exposure to dust and fumes at work and in the home, reduce their exposure to colds and flu, and improve their general health and fitness through proper nutrition and regular aerobic exercise.

Emphysema

Emphysema is a gradually occurring late effect of chronic infection of the bronchial tubes, which connect the windpipe with the lungs. The tubes, called bronchi, look like branches of a tree that become smaller and smaller, eventually forming a cluster of tiny air spaces in the lung (alveoli). Oxygen enters the blood through the alveoli as oxygen is inhaled and carbon dioxide is exhaled. When irritation occurs, some airways may be obstructed and trap air in the lungs, or the walls of the air spaces may tear. As small blood vessels disappear, there is less and less contact between blood and air. With continued irritation, the lungs may enlarge and become much less efficient in exchanging oxygen for carbon dioxide. Interference with the pas-

sage of blood through the small blood vessels of the lungs also forces the heart to work harder. A serious complicating factor for many people is chronic bronchitis, described previously. The heart enlarges under the strain and congestive heart failure may result (see Chapter 15). More than 2,400,000 Americans suffer from emphysema, causing approximately 13,000 deaths each year.

A typical emphysema patient is a 50 to 70-year-old adult who has been smoking heavily for many years and lives in an area with polluted air. In 3 to 5 percent of patients, emphysema occurs due to a genetic defect resulting in severe alpha-1-antitrypsin deficiency. These individuals are much more likely to develop emphysema in their twenties and thirties rather than middle or old age. A blood test can identify this high-risk group in the first month of life.

Early symptoms include a shortness of breath on exertion in the morning or evening. Although emphysema cannot be cured, modern treatment improves the quality of life. Preventive techniques include absence of smoking, keeping physically fit, avoiding influenza and pneumococcal pneumonia, avoiding polluted air, and obtaining proper physician care for colds and other respiratory infections.[7]

Occupational Lung Disease

Exposure to air containing cotton fibers, coal dust, asbestos, and a number of other substances can produce lung diseases.[8] **Pneumoconiosis** is a general term applied to the various types of occupational lung diseases. *Black lung,* or coal worker's pneumoconiosis, is caused by heavy exposure to coal dust over many years. Over one-half million miners and their dependents have received benefits under the Federal Black Lung Program. *Asbestosis* is caused by inhaling asbestos fibers that irritate lung tissue and produce thickening of the walls of the air sacs. Symptoms may not develop for thirty years or more after exposure. Lung cancer is also much more common among asbestos workers. *Beryllosis* is caused by inhaling dust from the metal beryllium, which is used in nuclear reactors and missile systems. Symptoms often do not appear for years after exposure. *Silicosis* is caused by breathing silica dust. It is found among workers in rock, granite, and marble industries; miners; coal workers; and those who make china and pottery. Additional less common dust diseases are caused by sugar cane dust or fungal spores found in moldy hay.

Allergies*

An **allergy** is any hypersensitivity to a specific substance (such as food, pollen, or dust) or condition (such as cold or heat) that in similar amounts appears harmless to most people. Allergies affect approximately one out of every seven people in the United States today. Some 17 million Americans suffer from hives, hay fever, eczema, or some other hypersensitivity reaction. In addition, about 15 million people suffer from *asthma,* a chronic disorder characterized by coughing, wheezing, difficulty in breathing, and a suffocating feeling. Asthma is usually, but not necessarily, related to allergic hypersensitivity, and "asthma attacks" can be triggered by the presence of certain **allergens** (substances that induce an allergic state or reaction).

*This section was prepared by G. E. Rodriguez, M.D., Director Pediatric Chest-Allergy-Immunology, Medical College of Virginia, Virginia Commonwealth University, Richmond, Virginia.

Allergies do not often kill, but they certainly make life miserable. It is estimated that at least half of the people affected are not aware of their condition and that these people are probably only about 60 percent successful in alleviating allergic discomfort. Yet in the great majority of cases, excellent allergic control can be achieved.

The term "allergy" was introduced in 1939 by C. von Pirquet, a pediatrician, to represent the concept of changed or "altered" reactivity as a result of contact with a foreign substance. Harmful allergic reactions are called *allergic hypersensitivity reactions.* Four different classes of hypersensitivity reactions have been identified. Some involve antibodies that "recognize" a particular foreign material and cause the cells of the body to react to it. Other reactions seem to involve only cells and foreign material. We will describe the most common form of allergy: *atopy.*

Common Allergies In *atopy,* target cells (in the nose for hay fever or in the lung for asthma) are coated with reaginic antibodies made elsewhere and interact with an allergenic foreign substance *(allergen).* The chemical response that is initiated results in the liberation of pharmacologically active substances *(mediators)* by the target cells. These chemical mediators are

FIGURE 13.3 • Before and During an asthma attack.

II. During an asthma attack:

Detail of branching bronchial airways

Lungs

Muscles around airway contract,

Membranes around airway swell,

Bronchial airway in an asthma attack

Mucus forms in airway,

Resulting in a narrowed airway and difficulty breathing

I. Signs before an asthma attack:

Coughing
Labored breathing
Wheezing
Suffocating feeling

Normal bronchial airway

III. If attack continues, these signs may develop:

Rapid pulse
Sweating
Blueness in skin
Coldness in extremities

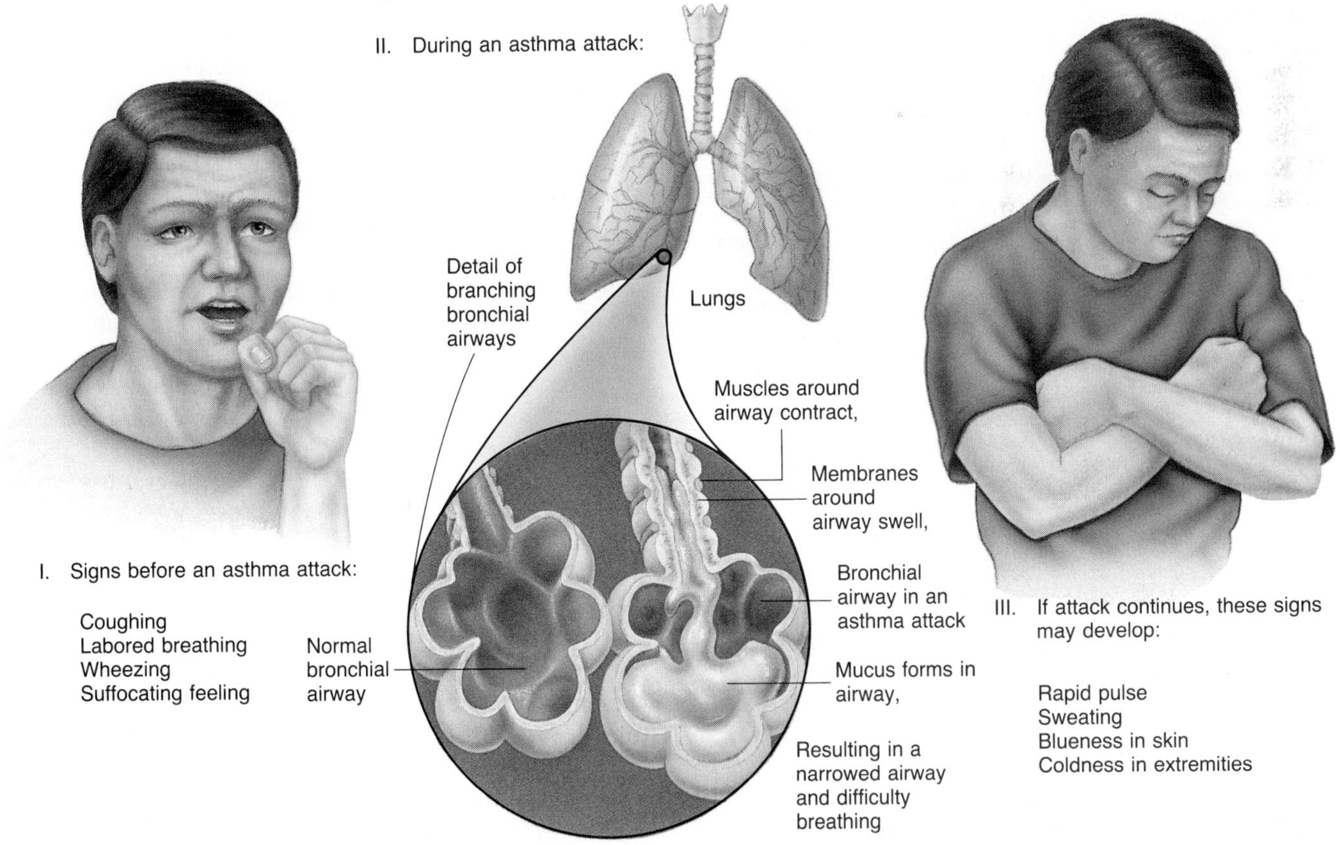

hay fever Also called *allergic rhinitis,* hay fever is a commonly found allergic hypersensitivity reaction to house dust, pollen, mold, or spores.

hyposensitization A treatment of allergies that employs small doses of the allergen over a period of time in order to desensitize the patient to the allergen and thereby to lessen the allergic reaction.

immunotherapy A term used synonymously with *hyposensitization* to describe a therapy which desensitizes a patient to a particular allergen.

arthritis A disease in which there is a degeneration of the joints and connective tissues, leading to inflammation and pain.

Exploring Your Health 13.4

Do You Have an Allergy?

Check those items below that apply to you. Over the past twelve-month period, have you had:

1. Three or more colds and sore throats?
2. Chronic, croupy cough?
3. Frequent runny nose?
4. Night cough?
5. Coughing bouts after exercising or laughing?
6. Repeated attacks of shortness of breath, wheezing, or itchy nose and palate?
7. Frequent sneezing attacks?
8. Itchy eyes?
9. Dark circles under your eyes?
10. Recurrent skin eruptions?

If you have had some of these symptoms, you may have an allergy. This can be confirmed by an examination of your nose, skin, and chest by a doctor, who will also order appropriate laboratory tests.

Year 2000 National Health Objective

One national health objective seeks to reduce asthma morbidity in terms of asthma hospitalizations per year to no more than 160 per 100,000 asthma sufferers by improving the total environment, including the air. In 1987, 188 per 100,000 asthma sufferers were hospitalized. An additional objective strives to reduce to no more than 10 percent the proportion of people with asthma who experience activity limitation. (This figure was 21.9 per 2,000 during the period 1986 to 1988.)

Because a number of diseases are related to our environment, the federal government has also defined a national health objective to establish and monitor, in at least thirty-five states, plans to define and track sentinel environmental diseases (lead poisoning; other heavy metal poisoning, such as from cadmium, arsenic, and mercury; pesticide poisoning; carbon monoxide poisoning; heatstroke; hypothermia; acute chemical poisoning; methemoglobinemia; and respiratory diseases, such as asthma, that are triggered by environmental factors).

responsible for the symptoms of atopic allergy. For example, in the case of a skin test done on a ragweed-sensitive patient, ragweed introduced into the skin interacts with reaginic antibodies fixed to tissue mast cells *(target cells).* As a result of this interaction, mediators such as histamine and slow-reacting substances of anaphylaxis are released from the mast cells. The pharmacologic action of histamine and anaphylaxis on the blood vessels in the skin is responsible for the swelling and redness observed in the positive skin test. Hives occur in the same way, but in multiple areas of the skin at the same time.

In **hay fever,** also known as allergic rhinitis, allergens such as house dust, plant pollen, or mold spores blow through the air and collect on the mucous membranes of the nose and eyes, where they are absorbed. In a sensitized individual, reaginic antibodies on tissue mast cells combine with the allergens and cause the release of histamine and other chemical mediators. The result is swelling and congestion of the mucous membranes, leading to such unpleasant symptoms as sneezing, itching, runny nose, and watering and swelling eyes.

Factors in Allergic Reactions Heredity seems to be very important in the development of an allergy. Other known factors include allergen concentration, time of exposure and of reexposure to allergens, quality and quantity of reaginic antibody present, and the nonspecific stimulation threshold required to induce symptoms. This last point, non-specific stimulation threshold, means that a particular organ such as the nose can be stimulated by mediators to a certain point before symptoms are experienced. The degree of sensitivity in various organs of an allergic person determines what symptoms will occur.

Most children with asthma also have other allergies. Allergies, however, are only one way in which symptoms can be triggered. Other factors, such as weather changes, stress, air pollution, colds, and exercise, are nonallergic inducers of nasal symptoms or expiratory wheezing. Most adults have nonallergic asthma, although in some, allergic triggers are also important. Nonallergic hives, rhinitis, and eczema often occur in response to stress.[9]

Treatment of Allergies Treatment of allergic conditions has two objectives: elimination or avoidance of the specific or contributory factors, and a change in the degree of sensitivity to them, usually accomplished by hyposensitization injections. Sometimes, treatment with drug therapy is also required. Complete elimination of the offending allergen from the environment or diet is the ideal therapeutic method, because it makes further treatment unnecessary. However, complete avoidance is possible in only a few instances, such as removing a feather pillow or cat from the home. It is virtually impossible to avoid house dust, plant pollens, and atmospheric molds. Nonetheless, certain precautionary measures can significantly decrease the degree of exposure. All items that collect dust, such as rugs, drapes, old mattresses, upholstered furniture, and books, should be removed from the bedroom. Air filters, air conditioners, and zippered casings for the mattress and pillow are also very helpful in decreasing the dust and mold concentration.

Any food that is known to cause symptoms should be avoided. Although most people usually do this, they may not realize that other food products can also contain the allergen. Therefore, it is important to read all labels before using new food products. **Hyposensitization,** or **immunotherapy,** is a specific form of treatment using an extract of the allergen to which the patient is reacting. Gradually increasing amounts of the specific allergens are injected until the maximum tolerated dose is reached, resulting in lessened sensitivity. It takes several years of immunotherapy before all sensitivity is lost. The similarity of allergic reactions allows similar medicines or combinations of medicines to be employed in treating most patients. These are bronchodilators, corticosteroids, and antihistamines.

Managing Noninfectious Lung Diseases

Because most lung problems produce a cough, phlegm, or wheezing, and arise from irritation of the bronchial tubes, management involves keeping the tubes as open as possible. The following general suggestions are provided to avoid irritation of the lungs caused by smoking, infections, dusts, fumes, chilling, nasal discharge, allergies, and emotional tension:[10]

1. Consume adequate fluids to remain hydrated and to help loosen phlegm in the bronchial tubes.
2. Breathe correctly—slowly and gently through your nose before pausing, and then exhaling gently and slowly; the chest and abdomen should relax and the air should come out naturally.
3. Avoid overbreathing.
4. Synchronize your breathing in a rhythmic manner; avoid holding your breath.
5. Do not force coughing.
6. Keep you nose, throat, and teeth clean; avoid blowing your nose hard, wash your nose with warm salt water in the morning and at night if you have been advised to do so, and brush your teeth regularly.
7. Continue or begin a regular exercise program.
8. Follow your physician's treatment if you experience esophageal reflux; elevate the head of your bed about eight inches with blocks; avoid lifting heavy objects or bending over; avoid coffee, colas, cigarettes, alcohol, chocolate, and fatty foods; avoid eating for two to three hours prior to bedtime, and take prescribed antacids before going to bed.

To help you understand the difficulty lung diseases places on breathing, complete Exploring Your Health 13.5 and write down your reactions.

Other Noninfectious Diseases

Arthritis

Arthritis in some form afflicts more than 17 million people in the United States. Degenerative arthritis is common among older people. An estimated 4.5 million people suffer from *rheumatoid arthritis*—a disease of the connective tissue occurring when certain antibodies behave like antigens, causing the body to produce other antibodies, resulting in chronic inflammation of the joints. Women are three to four times more likely than men to develop this condition.

Treatment and management of arthritis are directed at controlling the symptoms, relieving discomfort, and preventing or correcting deformity. Drugs may be prescribed to relieve pain, and physical therapy and sometimes surgery can help to correct deformities.[11] In addition, individuals should strictly adhere to their physician's advice, apply heat (to relax muscles temporarily, especially before exercise) and cold (for the temporary relief of pain and soreness), avoid abusing the joints by maintaining a balanced routine of rest and exercise, improving posture (sitting, standing, and

dental caries Tooth decay or cavities, usually occurring on tooth surfaces that are in contact with other teeth.

periodontitis (pyorrhea) The most common form of periodontal disease in which the gums gradually become detached from the teeth.

periodontosis A rare form of periodontal disease in which some of the bone around the roots of molar and upper incisor teeth has been destroyed; afflicts adolescents and young adults and has few symptoms.

Exploring Your Health 13.5

The Effects of Lung Diseases on Breathing

Secure a small straw with an opening of approximately one-eighth of an inch. Place the straw in your mouth. Pinch your nose with one hand to eliminate all inhaled air and breathe through the straw for a total of 30 seconds.

How difficult was it to breathe? How labored was your breathing? Could you have continued to breathe through the straw for hours?

You have just experienced the breath-by-breath drama of people with severe lung disease, including children with severe asthma. Although relaxation and breathing techniques can improve air flow slightly, the struggle is ever present. Individuals who fail to protect their lungs from the various health hazards discussed in this chapter could face this hardship later in life.

sleeping), and exercising daily for short periods (beginning slowly and increasing gradually).

Arthritis is often extremely painful, and as a result many sufferers are susceptible to the lures of quacks who promise miracle treatments. We'll discuss such quackery in Chapter 19.

Dental Diseases

Dental diseases are quite prevalent as the following data suggest:

- It is estimated that 95 percent of Americans will at some time have dental decay.
- Nearly 23 million people in the United States have lost all of their teeth.
- At least 34 percent of Americans between the ages of twelve and seventeen have a gum disease.

Health scientists have identified the cause of dental diseases and have developed methods of preventing most of them.[12]

Dental Caries   **Dental caries** refers to tooth decay or cavities. Cavities usually occur in crevices, fissures, and surfaces that are in contact with other teeth, because these are the most difficult areas to keep clean.

Year 2000 National Health Objective

Recognizing that tooth loss is generally preventable at all ages, the federal government has established national health objectives to increase to at least 45 percent the proportion of people age 35 to 44 who have never lost a permanent tooth due to dental caries or periodontal disease (31 percent of employed adults had never lost a permanent tooth for any reason in the years 1985 to 1986. Additional health objectives are to reduce to no more than 20 percent the proportion of people age 65 and older who have lost all of their natural teeth (the figure was 36 percent in 1986), to reduce the prevalence of gingivitis among people age 35 to 44 to no more than 30 percent (42 percent in 1985–1986), and to reduce destructive periodontal diseases to a prevalence of no more than 15 percent among people age 35 to 44 (24 percent in 1985–1986).

Periodontal (Gum) Disease   A condition frequently seen in both youths and adults, *gingivitis* is actually an early stage of most *periodontal disease*. You may recall from the last chapter that gingivitis, periodontal disease, and many other dental and mouth problems are associated with tobacco use. In all cases of gingi-

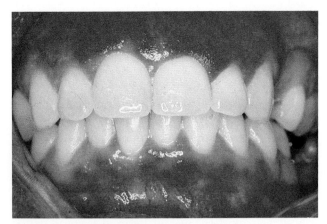

Gingivitis is common among young adults who do not brush their teeth and use dental floss regularly.

vitis, there is at first a mild inflammation and swelling of the gum tissue around one or more of the teeth. Later, the redness and swelling become more pronounced, and the gums tend to bleed easily. Bleeding while toothbrushing is one of the earliest signs of gum disease. During these changes, the gums may or may not feel tender. Thus there may be no warning that disease is present. If the inflammation is not con-

trolled, it usually progresses to the more severe condition called periodontitis, which includes bone destruction.

Periodontitis (pyorrhea) is the most common form of destructive periodontal disease. The gums gradually become detached from the teeth, and pockets develop, sometimes progressing to a depth of one-half inch or more. As the gums recede, some of the roots of the teeth are exposed. Eventually, the connective-tissue fibers that fasten the teeth to bone are destroyed, and much of the bone socket gradually disintegrates. The tooth loosens and is eventually lost.

Periodontosis is a more rare and puzzling condition that afflicts adolescents and young adults. Little inflammation or discomfort is associated with it. The first sign of trouble is loose teeth. X-rays reveal that some of the bone around the roots of the molar teeth and upper incisors has been destroyed. Yet the mouth appears healthy, and the teeth are undamaged. Current treatment for this condition is surgery with antibiotic supplementation.

Acute necrotizing gingivitis is an acute infection in which the tissue is ulcerated and dying. This disease is associated with the presence of two specific types of bacteria. The condition is usually painful, and the in-

Get Involved!

Preventing Infectious and Noninfectious Diseases

It is well known that, among other factors, our own behavior affects the level of risk we face in contracting both infectious and noninfectious diseases. Consequently, there is much you can do to reduce your own risk as well as that of family, friends, and other people.

1. By maintaining a high level of general health, you will help to set an example for other people. Your lifestyle should include a solid schedule of aerobic activity, sound nutrition, a complete absence of illicit drugs and tobacco, avoidance of alcohol, and regular medical and dental care. Do not use crash or "yo-yo" diets because these will depress your immune system.

2. How many unhealthy behaviors—smoking, careless use of alcohol, lack of regular exercise—can you identify among your family and friends? Make a list of the infectious and noninfectious diseases associated with each behavior. Try to encourage at least one behavior change for each person who engages in unhealthy behaviors. Don't use "scare" tactics or pushiness, but let the person know that you care and that his or her behavior could be dangerous to that individual's health in terms of disease.

3. Do you have a friend or relative who has a noninfec-

tious disease like epilepsy, hypercholesterolemia, or chronic bronchitis? If you would feel comfortable doing so, go to that person and discuss the disease with him or her. Learn as much as you can about the disease and how this person copes with it. This will not only increase your understanding of and compassion for people with this disease, but it will also enable you to offer help and information to other people who have or are in some way affected by this disease.

4. Become informed about the cause, prevention, and treatment of allergies. This will help you reduce your own risk of developing an allergy problem later in life, and it will increase your sensitivity to the needs of friends and family members who suffer from allergies.

5. Develop a proposal for a "Reducing Your Risk" disease-awareness day on your campus. Focus the program on health behaviors that can reduce or prevent the risk of serious disease. Discuss your proposal with personnel at your college or university student health office in order to develop a strategy for advertising and implementing your program, which can be as simple as a series of posters or as elaborate as a series of speeches or brief seminars by faculty or student health service representatives.

plaque A sticky, colorless layer of harmful bacteria that is constantly forming on teeth.

calculus (tartar) The hardened mineralized deposit made up of plaque that has not been properly removed from the teeth.

Year 2000 National Health Objectives

With regard to dental health care, the Year 2000 National Health Objectives stress education and prevention, especially during the childhood years. Among other things, the objectives seek (1) to increase to 90 percent the proportion of all children entering school programs for the first time who have received oral health screening and follow-up (66 percent in 1986); (2) to increase to 50 percent the proportion of children and adolescents who have received protective sealants on the chewing (occlusal) surfaces of permanent teeth (9 percent in 1986); and (3) to reduce the proportion of children and adolescents with untreated dental caries (cavities) to 17 percent (25 percent in 1986).

flamed, tender gums make eating a problem. It is likely to develop in times of severe stress and often occurs in students and soldiers. Dentists find that removal of the bacteria and dead tissue, good nutrition, rest, hygiene, and sometimes a short course of an antibiotic usually control this type of periodontal disease.

Causes and Prevention The cause of dental caries and most periodontal disease is **plaque.** Plaque is a sticky, colorless layer of harmful bacteria that is constantly forming on your teeth.

If plaque is not removed from the teeth, within twenty-four hours it will become a hard, mineralized deposit known as **calculus** or **tartar.** Calculus makes the removal of plaque from the teeth much more difficult and therefore increases the risk of periodontal disease.

Dentists suggest that the daily removal of plaque by brushing and flossing, as well as periodic professional cleaning to remove calculus, will prevent most dental disease. Limiting the number of times you snack each day and eating sugary foods only with meals will also help. Also, fluoridation has a profound effect on dental decay. *Fluorides* (mineral salts) in your water supply (one part per million) can significantly reduce dental decay. In their absence, topical fluoride applied to your teeth by a dentist can help.

Some experts feel that raising the pH level in the mouth is one way to help prevent tooth decay. Flossing the teeth after eating, regularly brushing the teeth with toothpaste containing baking soda after each meal, using fluoridated water, chewing sugarless gum, and eating certain foods, such as cheddar, gouda, brie, blue, and Swiss cheese, remove plaque or raise the pH in the mouth.

Conclusion

Although there is no guarantee of a lifetime free from infectious and noninfectious diseases, you can (1) greatly reduce your risk of contracting an infectious disease and (2) lessen the effects of both infectious and noninfectious diseases by pursuing healthy lifestyle practices.

The body is capable of warding off and preventing many infectious diseases through non-specific and specific defense mechanisms, even though there is no known prevention for some infectious diseases like the common cold or some types of flu. The body prevents many specific kinds of disease through its immune mechanism. Active immunity to specific antigens is achieved naturally or through vaccinations, while vaccination with extra antibodies when the immune system is weakened can provide valuable short-term passive immunity.

Noninfectious diseases afflict millions of people. Improved understanding of these diseases over the years has shown that lifestyle indeed plays a major role in both the incidence and severity of these ailments. The majority of nongenetic diseases and disorders can be prevented, delayed, or managed through regular exercise, proper nutrition, regulation of body weight and fat, cessation of tobacco use, moderate use of alcohol, and by using the proper medication. The best protection against passing on harmful genetic traits is genetic screening.

Summary

1. Infectious diseases are transmitted from an infected object, animal, or person to an uninfected individual through agents that include bacteria, viruses, fungi, rickettsia, and animal parasites.

2. Communicable infectious diseases are spread from one host to another, while noncommunicable infectious diseases, even though they are caused by infectious agents, are acquired from the environment rather than from a host.

3. Bacteria are single-celled organisms, plantlike in nature, that can produce infection.

4. One well-publicized bacterial infection is toxic shock syndrome (TSS), which appears to be caused by staphylococci bacteria that spread from a local infection throughout the body. TSS victims are generally menstruating women who use superabsorbent tampons.

5. Viruses are even smaller than bacteria and have an amazing ability to survive and reproduce.

6. Certain factors must exist for an infectious disease to occur in humans (see Table 13.1): a pathogen (a live virus or bacteria) must be present; the pathogen must be able to live, multiply in, and escape from a reservoir; the pathogen must then contract and enter a host (human); and the host must receive the pathogen.

7. The body's non-specific defense mechanisms generally fight off potentially harmful microbes before serious infections occur.

8. In order to ward off severe infections, the body's immune system manufactures specific antibodies in response to specific, potentially harmful outside agents (antigens).

9. Vaccination can prevent several infectious diseases of childhood, including polio, measles, mumps, rubella, and diptheria.

10. Active immunity to specific antigens is achieved naturally or through vaccinations, while vaccination with extra antibodies when the immune system is weakened can provide valuable short-term passive immunity.

11. Antibiotic therapy has no effect on viral infections; it does control many secondary bacterial infections that penetrate the body's defense mechanisms.

12. There is still neither a prevention nor a cure for the common cold, and despite available vaccinations, influenza outbreaks are a common recurring epidemic.

13. Measles, mumps, and rubella (German measles) are examples of infectious diseases that were fairly common until the development of reliable, long-lasting vaccines.

14. There is no known prevention for infectious mononucleosis, which is spread in a manner similar to the common cold.

15. Hepatitis is essentially an inflammation of the liver that is caused by a number of different viruses, although two well-known viruses are the culprits in most cases. Infectious or type A hepatitis is more common and usually much less severe than serum hepatitis or type B hepatitis.

16. Most people who were healthy just prior to infection can be treated effectively for infectious lung diseases like fungus infections, pneumonia, and tuberculosis.

17. As Americans' life spans have increased, noninfectious (chronic and degenerative) diseases become more common.

18. Diabetes mellitus can be prevented and managed through healthy eating habits, regular exercise, and the control of body weight and fat.

19. Diseases of the nervous system are difficult to diagnose and treat, and their causes are often unclear. Epilepsy, multiple sclerosis, and cerebral palsy are three of the better-known nervous system disorders.

20. Genetic diseases are passed on through dominant inheritance, recessive inheritance, sex-linked inheritance, or polygenic (multifactorial) inheritance. Of the more than 300 hereditary diseases, most are considered inborn errors of metabolism or chemical mistakes.

21. Rheumatoid arthritis affects about 4.5 million Americans. Women are three to four times more likely than men to get arthritis.

22. Over 75 million Americans suffer from some form of chronic respiratory disease such as asthma, chronic bronchitis, emphysema, and occupational lung disease. Although some of these diseases are genetic, most are caused by what we breathe into our lungs.

23. One of every seven people in the United States suffers from some type of allergy. Asthma usually results from a complication of allergic

reactions. Allergy treatment consists of eliminating the contributing factors and changing the degree of sensitivity to these factors through hyposensitization injections.

24. Dental diseases can be prevented through proper care of the teeth and gums and through proper nutrition.

Questions for Personal Growth

1. Cold and flu season is particularly troublesome to busy college students who are faced with periodic deadlines, examinations, and other pressures. One less cold could mean greater learning and higher grades. It is possible to reduce your risk of getting a cold or flu virus. List five behaviors you could follow to reduce your chances of contracting a virus this semester. What specific behaviors could you avoid? What new behaviors could you add?

2. Examine your dormitory room, apartment, or house, and workplace for dust, chemicals, poor ventilation, and other potential lung irritants. What changes could be made to reduce the irritation? What areas could you request be changed in the workplace? What could be done in your dormitory room, apartment, or house?

3. Check with your parents or guardians to make certain you received the active immunizations for infants and children shown in Table 13.3. Record each infectious disease you have contracted. Did you receive the proper immunizations? What natural immunities have you developed? Are there any special precautions needed to prevent the contraction of any of the childhood diseases during your adult years?

4. Do any specific diseases, infectious or noninfectious, run in your family? Does your family have the tendency to develop a specific disease? If so, list the steps you can take now to reduce your risks.

5. Do you visit your dentist at least twice annually? How carefully do you care for your teeth and gums? Do you brush correctly on a regular basis? Do you use dental floss at least once every 24 hours? How healthy are your gums? If you are still getting new cavities or if your gums bleed from time to time, take more time to brush and floss and make certain that you are doing both procedures correctly.

6. One of the keys to good health is the maintenance of a healthy immune system. This requires proper nutrition, regular aerobic exercise, and regular physician care. How do you rate yourself in these three areas? Do you eat three meals daily and avoid skipping a meal? Do you avoid fasting and unsafe dieting? Do you exercise daily using some form of aerobic program? Do you see your physician at least once a year?

7. You can reduce your risk of contracting many infectious and noninfectious diseases by practicing a healthy lifestyle. What unhealthy behaviors do you engage in that may predispose you to disease? What is the single most important change you could make in your life to increase your chances of a disease-free adult life?

8. Does anyone in your immediate family have diabetes? What factors do you think place you at risk for developing adult-onset diabetes in the future? Identify the three most important changes you could make now to prevent diabetes in the future.

References

1. K. N. Shands, et al., "Toxic Shock Syndrome in Menstruating Women," *New England Journal of Medicine* 303, 25 (1980).

2. Lawrence K. Altman, "Infections Still a Big Threat," *New York Times* (July 20, 1983): C2.

3. American Diabetes Association, *Complications of Diabetes,* 1989.

4. Epilepsy Foundation of America, *Questions and Answers About Epilepsy,* 1989.

5. Epilepsy Foundation of America, *Children and Seizures: Information for Babysitters,* 1989.

6. American Lung Association, *Facts in Brief About Lung Disease,* 1985.

7. National Jewish Center for Immunology and Respiratory Medicine, *Understanding Emphysema,* 1989.

8. National Jewish Center for Immunology and Respiratory Medicine, *Healthy Breathing,* 1989.

9. National Jewish Center for Immunology and Respiratory Medicine, *Understanding Asthma,* 1989.

10. National Jewish Center for Immunology and Respiratory Medicine, *Management of Chronic Respiratory Disease,* 1985.

11. Arthritis Foundation, *Arthritis: Basic Facts-Answers to Your Questions,* 1986.

12. National Institute of Dental Research, *Periodontal (Gum) Diseases* (Washington, D.C.: Department of Health, Education, and Welfare, Pub. No. 76-1142).

CHAPTER

14

Sexually Transmitted Diseases

CHAPTER OBJECTIVES

After reading this chapter, you should understand:

- What sexually transmitted diseases are and how our perception and understanding of them has changed through history.

- How STDs are transmitted, what effects they have on the body, and how they can be treated.

- Some strategies for coping with STDs in terms of individual emotions as well as individual responsibility with regard to society.

- Several basic strategies to prevent STDs, including the most effective strategy: abstinence.

- What acquired immune deficiency syndrome (AIDS) is, the number of Americans who are infected with it, and how it is spread. Also, what treatments are available for AIDS patients and the social and political implications of AIDS.

CHAPTER OUTLINE

"VD" to "STD"

Gonorrhea, Syphilis, Herpes Genitalis

Chlamydia, Nongonococcal Urethritis (NGU)

Pelvic Inflammatory Disease (PID)

Trichomoniasis, Moniliasis or Yeast Infection

Genital Warts, Pubic Lice, Scabies

Other STDs

Coping with STDs

Prevention of STDs

Acquired Immune Deficiency Syndrome (AIDS)

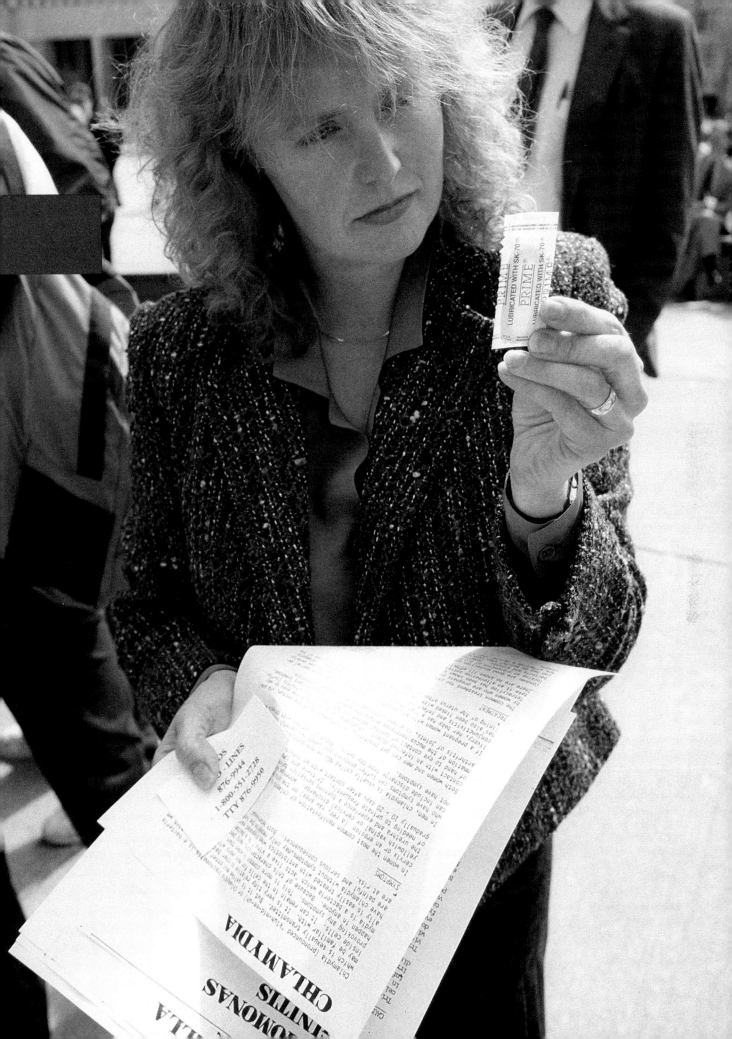

sexually transmitted diseases (STDs) Bacterial, viral, and parasitic diseases that are transmitted through sexual contact, which usually affect the genital areas and may cause serious disease complications throughout the body.

Some diseases are primarily spread through sexual contact. We will soon discuss several of these diseases in detail, but first let's see how much you already know about these diseases and what misconceptions you may possess about them. To do so, complete Exploring Your Health 14.1 before reading further.

"VD" to "STD"

Sexually transmitted diseases (STDs) are bacterial or viral infections that attack the genital areas and may cause serious complications elsewhere in the body. The

Exploring Your Health 14.1

Test Your Knowledge About STDs

Complete the true-false test below to discover how much you know about sexually transmitted diseases. Circle either T or F and score your test from the answers below.

	True	False
1. Syphilis can be acquired by coming in contact with a contaminated toilet seat.	T	F
2. Pubic lice can be transmitted only through sexual contact.	T	F
3. Gonorrhea is easily eradicated through the use of penicillin.	T	F
4. STDs cannot be transmitted from one partner to another unless one or both reach orgasm.	T	F
5. Some people have developed an immunity to STDs and need not take precautions.	T	F
6. Gonorrhea is easily detected in the female.	T	F

7. Syphilis can be transmitted by kissing an infected person.	T	F
8. STDs are uncommon and there is generally no need for precautionary measures.	T	F
9. If one partner is infected with gonorrhea or syphilis, the other partner has only a slight chance of acquiring the disease during sexual contact.	T	F
10. Acquired immune deficiency syndrome (AIDS) can be spread by mosquitoes.	T	F

Answers

1. False. Highly unlikely and nearly impossible.
2. False. Pubic lice are commonly spread through use of contaminated towels, clothing, or bed linen.
3. False. Some strains of gonorrhea are extremely resistant to penicillin

and very difficult to eradicate with other antibiotics.
4. False. Reaching orgasm has nothing to do with the spread of STDs.
5. False. One cannot develop a natural immunity to STDs.
6. False. Gonorrhea in the female is difficult to detect and may exist for months before any symptoms become noticeable.
7. True. A person with a chancre sore on the mouth could transmit syphilis to a partner through kissing.
8. False. STDs are quite common among all socioeconomic and age groups.
9. False. The probability of acquiring an STD from an infected partner is quite high.
10. False. It would take too many bites to transfer enough blood to cause infection.

Scoring: 9–10 correct—Excellent, 7–8 correct—Good; 5–6 correct—Poor; fewer than 5 correct—Very poor.

organisms thrive on warm, moist body surfaces, such as the mucous membranes that line the reproductive organs, mouth, and rectum. STDs are transmitted via sexual contact. However, evidence suggests that some STD—such as trichomoniasis, pubic lice, and scabies—can be contracted from clothing, bedding, or other items worn or used by infected people.

Until the 1970s, these infections were called venereal diseases or "VD" (named for Venus, the Roman goddess of love). Recently, however, the term "sexually transmitted diseases" has come into use because it is thought to be more descriptive. Medical knowledge about STDs has increased dramatically in recent years. In the past, venereal disease referred to five types of infections, the most important being syphilis and gonorrhea. Today, however, it is known that more than twenty different organisms are linked to STDs.

Historical Background

Sexually transmitted diseases were mentioned in the Old Testament as early as 1500 B.C. The first epidemic of venereal disease was blamed on Christopher Co-lumbus's crew, who were said to have brought the diseases back from the New World. However, some authorities discount this theory. In fact, there is no evidence to make a conclusion either way. In the modern era, the first worldwide epidemic of gonorrhea took place during and after World War I. With the introduction of sulfa drugs in the 1930s and penicillin in the 1940s, both gonorrhea and syphilis seemed to have been checked and appeared headed for eradication. This apparent victory resulted in reduced research dollars, less emphasis on prevention, and lack of follow-up on the sexual partners of treated patients. As a result, hundreds of thousands of people infected with STDs unknowingly transmitted the diseases to others.

Several social factors contributed to the growing incidence of STDs, which by the 1960s had begun to reach epidemic proportions. The introduction of birth control pills and IUDs decreased the use of condoms, which had provided good protection against some STDs. Changing sexual standards meant that people were engaging in sex at younger ages and with more partners than in the past. Many people felt complacent about contracting an STD because they assumed that the disease could be easily treated. Others were reluctant to seek treatment, fearing the social stigma associated with STDs. In addition, strains of gonorrhea appeared that were resistant to treatment with penicillin. Even in strains that responded to penicillin, larger dosages of the drug were required. Since the 1950s, an injection four times more powerful in men and ten times more powerful in women has been required to effect a cure. And even though new antibiotic treatments are being explored, experts are concerned that

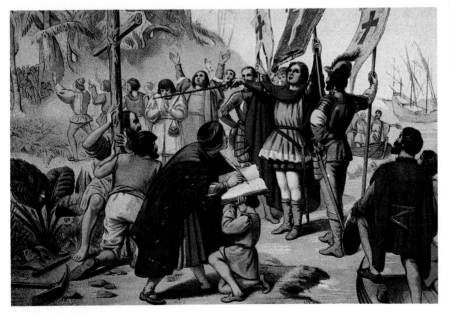

There is some debate as to whether Christopher Columbus's crew brought back STDs to Europe. In any case, the first worldwide epidemic of gonorrhea didn't take place until during and after World War I.

gonorrhea An STD that is caused by a bacterium. Although the disease can be treated with antibiotics, if left untreated it can lead to serious complications, including bladder and kidney disease and diseases of the pelvic and genital areas.

syphilis A serious STD caused by a spirochete; untreated syphilis has very serious complications and is eventually fatal. Treatment includes the use of antibiotics, but some strains of syphilis are resistant to treatment.

chancre A painless sore on the penis, mouth, anus, or in the vagina where the spirochete that causes syphilis has entered the body.

strains might develop that are resistant to these treatments.

We will discuss several of the more common sexually transmitted diseases: gonorrhea, syphilis, herpes genitalis, nongonococcal urethritis, chlamydia, acquired immune deficiency syndrome (AIDS), pelvic inflammatory disease, trichomoniasis, moniliasis, genital warts, pubic lice, and scabies; as well as chancroid, lymphogranuloma venereum, and granuloma inguinale.

Gonorrhea

Gonorrhea, popularly known as the "clap," the "drip," and many equally descriptive names, is caused by the *Neisseria gonorrhoeae* bacterium. It is increasing in incidence—more than one million cases are reported in the United States per year, with the actual incidence estimated to be four times that amount—and is one of the most prevalent communicable diseases.

Gonorrhea is transmitted by intercourse and by oral-genital and anal-genital contact. Since the *Neisseria gonorrhoeae* needs the warmth and moisture provided by the mucous membranes of the vagina, mouth, or anus, it is unlikely (though not impossible) that you could acquire gonorrhea from using someone else's

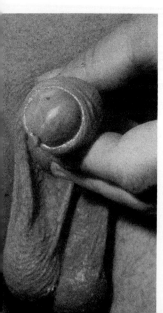

It is important to recognize gonorrhea before it has a chance to cause further damage. This is easier done in males where the signs are more obvious than in women, where the signs may appear as a common vaginal infection.

towel or from sitting on a public toilet seat unless the bacterium has just been deposited there and the area is warm and moist. A male exposed to *Neisseria gonorrhoeae* bacteria through coitus has about a 20 percent chance of developing gonorrhea, whereas a female likewise exposed has about an 80 percent chance of contracting gonorrhea. The difference is due to the vaginal environment which is conducive to the growth of the *Neisseria gonorrhoeae* bacteria.

Effects and Treatment of Gonorrhea

Gonorrhea affects the urogenital tract in both sexes—the urethra in males and the urethra, vagina, and cervix in females. There is no way to acquire immunity to the gonorrhea-causing bacterium, neither by vaccine nor by having contracted gonorrhea previously.

The symptoms are somewhat different in men and women. The early symptom in men is a milky, bad-smelling discharge from the penis. Beginning three to eight days after exposure, urination may become compelling and be accompanied by a burning sensation. If the infection goes untreated, it can cause swelling of the testicles and can damage the prostate gland, resulting ultimately in sterility. Further complications may include bladder or kidney conditions.

Whereas infected men are usually aware that something is wrong with them, women may not notice the early signs of gonorrhea. The symptoms are similar to those in common vaginal infections—a slight burning sensation in the genital area and a mild discharge from the vagina. It is estimated that 80 percent of women who have gonorrhea are unaware of it until the disease has become more severe. If left untreated, gonorrhea invades the uterus, fallopian tubes, and ovaries. Pelvic infection may result, causing sterility or requiring surgical removal of the pelvic organs.

Gonorrhea can be passed from an infected mother to her infant as it passes through the vaginal canal during delivery, often resulting in blindness. To prevent this from occurring, the eyes of newborns are routinely treated with silver nitrate.

Diagnosis of gonorrhea is not as simple as it is for syphilis. It requires laboratory examination of a sample taken from the infected area with a cotton swab or growing the bacteria under laboratory conditions. The disease usually responds to penicillin treatment or, if the victim is allergic to penicillin, to tetracycline drugs. As mentioned earlier, researchers have recently uncovered a new strain of penicillin-resistant gonorrhea. This development has prompted interest in using tetracycline drugs rather than penicillin in the initial treatment of gonorrhea.

Those treated for gonorrhea are advised to return for follow-up examination about ten days after treatment is concluded to be certain that the medication has actually eradicated all the bacteria and that a reinfection will not occur. During treatment, the individual should refrain from sexual intercourse and other sexual activities that can transmit the bacteria. To help prevent gonorrhea in the first place, sexually active people should use a condom. Some experts even suggest that sexually active people be screened for gonorrhea on a regular basis (perhaps every six months or so).

Syphilis

Known in the past as the "great pox" or the "great imposter" because people thought is resembled smallpox, **syphilis** now is often referred to as just "the syph." Syphilis is caused by the *Treponema pallidum*, a corkscrewlike organism that resembles bacteria and which is part of a group of such organisms called spirochetes.

Because *Treponema pallidum* can survive only in the warmth and moisture provided by the mucous membranes of the human body, it quickly dies outside the body. For this reason, syphilis cannot usually be contracted from a toilet seat (unless the spirochete has recently been deposited there just prior to someone else with an open sore sitting on the seat, the chances of which are extremely remote). Syphilis is transmitted during sexual intercourse, oral-genital or anal-genital contact, or by kissing a person who has a syphilitic sore in the mouth. These activities provide the spirochete with a route of entrance to the body.

Effects and Treatment of Syphilis

The disease progresses through four stages. In Stage 1 (primary stage) a painless sore, called a **chancre** (pronounced "shanker"), appears three to four weeks after the spirochete enters the body. The chancre looks like a pimple or wart and appears where the spirochete entered the body, often on the penis, the lips, or the vaginal wall. The chancre may go unnoticed in women or may be ignored in men, because it is painless and disappears in a few weeks without treatment.

Stage 2 (secondary stage) occurs about six weeks after contact. Symptoms may include a rash over the entire body, welts around the genitals, low-grade fever, headache, hair loss, and sore throat. These symptoms also disappear without treatment. However, if the symptoms are noticeable, most victims see a doctor at this time. Thus, it is uncommon for cases of syphilis in the United States to progress to the third stage.

Stage 3 (latency stage) begins about two years after contact (up to five years in some people). After one year, the victim cannot transmit the disease to anyone else. The only exception is that a pregnant woman can transmit the disease to her fetus through the placental wall. Latency may last for forty or more years. During this time, the organism infects and irreparably damages the heart, brain, and other organs. By Stage 4 (tertiary stage), the disease may lead to heart failure, blindness, other organ damage, and finally death.

Syphilis can be detected by means of a simple blood test. Because it is such a potentially dangerous disease and can be transmitted to unborn babies, most states require a blood test for syphilis before marriage and, in pregnant women, during the prenatal period. Syphilis generally responds well to penicillin or, in some cases, to other antibiotics. Because no immunity

Syphilis is usually easier to identify than gonorrhea because the chancre forms on the external genitalia and is obvious to the naked eye.

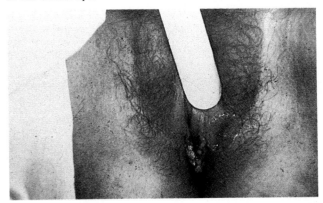

genital herpes An STD that is caused by the herpes simplex, type 2 virus. The disease is incurable. Carefully treated it is not a serious disease, but its spread to the rest of the body can result in serious complications. It has been linked to the onset of cervical cancer.

prodrome An itching or tingling sensation that develops near the site where the herpes simplex, type 2 virus enters the body.

autoinoculation The spread of a disease from one part of the body to another because of poor hygiene habits.

develops to the disease, prompt diagnosis and treatment after any possible exposure are essential.

When syphilis is passed from the mother to the fetus prior to birth, it is known as congenital syphilis. Until the sixteenth week of pregnancy, the fetus is protected from spirochetes by a membrane called Langhan's layer. However, after the sixteenth week, spirochetes can pass through the placental barrier and enter the fetus's bloodstream, causing a number of birth defects such as mental retardation or physical abnormalties.

Once syphilis is contracted, the individual should refrain from all sexual activity that can transmit the spirochete. Treatment should also consist of follow-up examinations to determine if antibiotics have been effective in eliminating the spirochete. As with gonorrhea and the other sexually transmitted diseases, since the disease-causing organism needs a route of entry into the body, the use of a condom can help prevent the spread of syphilis.

Recent data on syphilis infection in the United States present a somewhat disturbing history. Between 1979 and 1982, the incidence of primary and secondary syphilis infection rose from approximately 11 cases per 100,000 to 15 cases per 100,000. A decrease in this rate between 1982 and 1984 to 12 cases per 100,000 may be attributed in part to improved federal funding for syphilis education and testing.

The latest statistics, however, paint an alarming picture. In 1989, the syphilis rate skyrocketed to 18.4 per 100,000 population—the highest rate since 1949! There were 37,000 new cases of syphilis reported in 1989; more than double the 16,000 reported just four years earlier. Although the rate of syphilis rose 60 percent for the country as a whole, it affected different populations of Americans differently. For blacks, the rate had risen 132 percent since 1985 to 122 per 100,000; whereas for whites the rate had actually fallen to 2.6 per 100,000. Researchers explained these rates as a function of increased abuse of cocaine in inner-city minority populations that led to the practice of exchanging drugs for sex. In addition, the lack of funding to treat syphilis victims and to trace their sexual partners has affected these rates. As a result, 1989 infection rates since 1985 for black women had jumped 176 percent and for black men, 106 percent.

Herpes Genitalis (Herpes Simplex, Type 2)

Genital herpes is a viral infection caused by the virus herpes simplex, type 2. The virus related to herpes simplex, type 1, causes cold sores or fever blisters. Whereas type 1 herpes affects the mouth region, type 2 herpes affects the genital region and is transmitted through sexual contact. Herpes, type 2, now rivals gonorrhea as one of the most common sexually transmitted diseases in this country. The Centers for Disease Control estimates that more than 20 million Americans have been exposed to herpes, type 2, with 500,000 new cases reported each year.

Effects and Treatment of Herpes

Approximately two to ten days after the virus enters the body, some symptoms such as sores and swollen glands (around the groin), flulike symptoms (fever, muscle aches, and a sick feeling), and pain in the genital area during urination or intercourse may occur. Other symptoms may include fatigue, swelling of the legs, and watery eyes. The disease progresses through four stages:

1. **Prodrome stage.** An itching or tingling sensation **(prodrome)** develops near the site where the virus invaded the body, with the skin turning red and becoming sensitive; prodrome is also an early symptom of a recurrent infection or outbreak.

Year 2000 National Health Objective

The Year 2000 National Health Objectives seek to reduce primary and secondary syphilis to no more than 10 cases per 100,000 people; and for blacks specifically, to 65 cases per 100,000 people. Further, the objectives seek to reduce congenital syphilis to an incidence of no more than 50 cases per 100,000 live births.

2. **Blister stage.** A sore or cluster of sores appears; fever, swollen glands, and other symptoms may occur; after two to ten days, the sores break open (on future outbreaks, fever and swollen glands usually do not occur).

3. **Healing stage.** Sores shrink; scabs form; pain, swollen glands, and fever subside (scabs fall off by the end of the second week).

4. **Inactive stage.** The virus retreats to nearby nerve cells; stress and poor health may cause the virus to reemerge.

Symptoms can be alleviated by soaking the genital area in hot water, then keeping it clean and dry. The drug acyclovir may also be effective. In case of severe outbreaks, a doctor should be consulted. Recurrences are much less painful and much shorter than the initial bout. Also, future outbreaks are not as frequent as people believe and may occur several times monthly in some and rarely in others. Approximately one-third of those with the disease never have a recurrence and another one-third have outbreaks only rarely.[1]

Herpes has potentially more harmful effects on women than on men. It has been found that women who have type 2 herpes are eight times more likely to develop cervical cancer than noninfected women.

Unlike gonorrhea, herpes is a virus, and antibiotics cannot cure it. Once the virus is in the body, it remains there, and outbreaks can occur periodically,

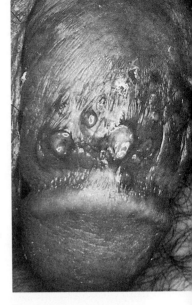

Genital herpes results in a sore or cluster of sores that eventually shrink and form scabs. Once the scabs leave, the disease is in its inactive stage.

spreading the disease. The most severe, painful outbreak is generally the first episode. It appears that the disease can be transmitted only through direct sexual contact when the disease is active; it is unlikely that it can be transmitted when dormant.

Living with Herpes

Learning to live with herpes involves special care of the body and the need to protect others. **Autoinoculation** (spreading the virus to other parts of the body)

Issues in Health

Should Minors Who Have a Sexually Transmitted Disease Be Treated Without Parental Consent?

In most states, minors who have a sexually transmitted disease can be treated without the consent of their parents. There is considerable debate over the merits of this situation, and legislation has even been introduced that would require parents to be notified.

Pro Advocates of treatment without parental consent feel that such an approach encourages youngsters to seek treatment if they have an STD. If parental consent is required, minors are less likely to seek treatment, so they may delay treatment until the disease has progressed. During the delay, symptoms of some STDs (such as herpes) may disappear, and the unknowing child may believe the disease has gone away. Needless to say, such delays can result in serious health problems.

Children also have the right of privacy, particularly in this intimate area of their lives. Furthermore, it is imperative that each of the minor's sexual partners be notified of their own potential risk. This is unlikely to happen if the minor has to inform his or her parents. Finally, if parents must be notified, there may be serious emotional consequences for the child, especially if the parental response is judgmental rather than supportive.

Con Those who argue for parental consent believe that parents have the right to know if their child has a health problem, particularly a problem related to sexual behavior. Contracting an STD obviously indicates that the minor is having sexual relations, and this is an area where parental counseling is imperative. If

parents are not informed, they may remain unaware that their child is behaving in a manner that may be detrimental to health and emotional well-being.

A minor's contracting an STD can provide an opportunity to open lines of communication and pave the way toward improved parent-child relationships in the future. Family problems may worsen if parents discover the problem months after treatment. Until a child reaches the age of majority, it is argued, parents have the obligation and responsibility to be informed and aware of all the child's problems. Most parents want to be involved and are deeply hurt when they are not consulted.

What do you think?

chlamydia A common STD caused by a viruslike bacterium; can lead to sterility, inflammation in the reproductive and urinary tracts, and pelvic inflammatory disease. Treated with antibiotics.

urethritis An infection of the urethra.

nongonococcal urethritis (NGU) An STD caused by some organism other than the *Gonococcus* bacterium and which causes urethritis.

pelvic inflammatory disease (PID) A dangerous and difficult to diagnose disease that afflicts women; not necessarily an STD.

trichomoniasis A disease that invades the vagina, causing vaginitis and other complications; not necessarily an STD.

vaginitis A disease that causes inflammation in the vagina; not necessarily an STD.

Year 2000 National Health Objective

One national health objectives seeks to reduce the annual number of first-time consultations with a physician for genital herpes from the 1988 rate of 167,000 to 142,000 by the year 2000.

Year 2000 National Health Objective

In 1985, there were 215 cases of nongonococcal urethritis per 100,000 people. The Year 2000 National Health Objectives seek to reduce that rate to 170 per 100,000 people.

can be dangerous. If spread to the eye, for example, serious damage and blindness can result. Secondary infections are also possible should bacteria enter the body through open sores caused by the herpes virus. Keeping the area clean and dry; avoiding the rubbing, scratching, picking, or touching of sores; washing hands with soap if a sore is accidentally touched; and avoiding the use of saliva to wet contact lenses help prevent further infection. You can also help prevent recurrences by maintaining good health habits (eating a balanced diet, getting sufficient rest, avoiding drugs and alcohol, managing stress, practicing good personal hygiene) and avoiding tight-fitting clothing, synthetic underwear, and friction that irritates skin tissue.

To prevent spreading the disease to others, additional precautions are necessary. If a pregnant woman has an outbreak of herpes at the time her child is delivered, she runs a one-in-four risk that the newborn child will contract the disease and suffer damage or even die. Thus, the wisest course of action for pregnant women with herpes is to obtain delivery by Caesarean section unless it is obvious that delivery can occur in

the absence of herpes symptoms. Infants can also contract herpes after birth if kissed by someone who has active oral herpes. It is also important to learn to recognize the prodrome that precedes outbreaks. One should not engage in sexual intercourse or any other type of sexual activity that might spread the virus from the onset of the prodrome until sores have completely healed (use of a condom is not a guarantee that the virus will not be spread). It is good practice to wear pajamas to bed to reduce the chance of body contact.

Chlamydia

Caused by a viruslike bacterium called *Chlamydia trachomatis,* **chlamydia** has recently been recognized as a prevalent and fast-growing sexually transmitted disease. It is estimated that 4 million new cases of chlamydia occur each year and as many as 500,000 progress to pelvic inflammatory disease.[2] It is reported to be up to ten times more prevalent than gonorrhea and is present in an estimated 4 percent of all pregnant women. In women, chlamydia can cause vaginitis and pelvic inflammatory disease and, in extreme cases, can lead to infertility. In men, it can cause inflammation of the urinary and reproductive tracts, and in extreme situations, sterility. In women, symptoms include vaginal discharge, but as many as 70 percent of female chlamydial infections go undetected until more serious problems (such as pelvic inflammatory disease) develop.[3] The most common symptom in men is a mild burning during urination, followed by a thin, watery, clear discharge. Chlamydia is usually treated by administering tetracycline for one week.

Year 2000 National Health Objective

The Year 2000 National Health Objectives seek to reduce chlamydia trachomatis infections to no more than 170 cases per 100,000 people, from a 1988 baseline of 215 per 100,000 people.

Nongonococcal Urethritis

Urethritis refers to an infection of the urinary tract. **Nongonococcal urethritis (NGU)** is urethritis that is caused not by the *Gonococcus* bacterium but by some other organism. It has been found that about half of the cases of NGU are caused by the organism *chlamydia trachomatis.* In males, NGU causes a discharge, as in gonorrhea, but in females there may be no symptoms. As a result, many cases go undiagnosed.

Most patients treated for NGU are young, white, single, sexually active, and affluent. NGU is probably the most common form of urethritis seen in student health centers and by private physicians. Whereas gonorrhea usually responds to treatment with penicillin, NGU responds to other antibiotics (usually tetracycline). Often NGU is recognized in cases where gonorrhea has been ruled out as the problem or when penicillin treatment for gonorrhea proves ineffective.

Pelvic Inflammatory Disease

With the exception of AIDS (covered later in this chapter), **pelvic inflammatory disease (PID)** is the most dangerous and the most difficult to diagnose of all the sexually transmitted diseases affecting women. Unless the disease is promptly diagnosed and treated, scar tissue forms inside the Fallopian tubes, which can result in infertility by partially or totally blocking the tubes to prevent the egg from entering the uterus. Scar tissue also increases the risk of *tubal pregnancy* (in which the fertilized egg becomes implanted inside the Fallopian tube rather than the uterus).

Symptoms of PID include abdominal pain or tenderness, increased menstrual cramps, lower back pain, pain during intercourse, profuse bleeding during menstruation, irregular menstrual cycles, vaginal bleeding at times other than menstruation, nausea, loss of appetite, vomiting, vaginal discharge, burning sensation during urination, chills, and fever. Diagnosis is based on medical and sexual history, a pelvic examination, and laboratory tests. PID can usually be treated effectively through antibiotic therapy on an outpatient basis.

PID may be caused by a number of organisms and conditions, certain sexually transmitted diseases, and the use of an intrauterine device for birth control. To avoid reexposure, it is important for all sex partners to be examined and treated.

Trichomoniasis

Trichomoniasis vaginalis (or *Trichomonas)* is a one-celled organism that burrows under the vaginal mucosa to cause **trichomoniasis,** or "trich," a vaginal infection **(vaginitis).** According to the United States Centers for Disease Control, the estimated incidence is 600,000 to 1,000,000 or more cases annually. The common mode of transmission is through sexual intercourse, but trichomoniasis can be contracted by prolonged exposure to moisture (for example, wet bathing suits, towels, or other clothing). Women who are pregnant or who use an oral contraceptive may be more prone to trichomoniasis infections. These women have high levels of progesterone, which increases the alkalinity in the vagina, creating a hospitable environment for the *Trichomonas* organism. The main symptom of trichomoniasis is an odoriferous, foamy, white or yellow discharge that irritates the vagina and vulva. Frequently, trichomoniasis is accompanied by urethritis. A microscopic examination of a sample of the discharge will reveal the causative agent.

Because the infection can be passed back and forth between partners (the ping-pong effect), both partners should be treated when trichomoniasis is confirmed in a woman. The man may harbor the disease organism but be asymptomatic. Metronidazole, trade name Flagyl, is the only effective systemic drug used. Some topical agents are sometimes prescribed. Both partners are administered the drug. Consumer advocates have suggested that metronidazole is linked with cancer, because cancer appeared in laboratory animals given massive doses of the drug. Others argue that much greater doses than those used in treating trichomoniasis were administered to these laboratory animals and that no danger exists for humans. However, an increased risk of cancer of the cervix does exist in women with a history of trichomoniasis infections.

Moniliasis, or Yeast Infection

The second most common form of vaginitis, **moniliasis,** also called monilia or *yeast infection,* is caused by the fungus *Candida albicans.* This fungus normally lives

Year 2000 National Health Objective

The Year 2000 National Health Objective for PID states its goal in terms of hospitalization rate rather than total reported incidence (as did the corresponding 1990 objective). That is because trends in hospitalization are more readily obtainable and are more reliable. Consequently, this Year 2000 objective seeks to reduce hospitalizations for PID from the 1988 rate of 311 per 100,000 women to 250 per 100,000 women age 15 to 44.

moniliasis A common form of vaginitis caused by the fungus *candida albicans;* not necessarily an STD.

genital warts An STD of the genital and perineal areas of both men and women caused by a virus; linked to an increased incidence of cancer.

pubic lice A parasite that prefers to live in the genital areas of both men and women, often (but not always) transmitted through sexual contact.

scabies A parasite of the genital and other areas often (but not always) transmitted through sexual contact.

chancroid An STD that results in sores very similar to the chancre sores of syphilis.

lymphogranuloma venereum (LGV) An STD, usually of tropical areas, which exhibits pimplelike sores on the genitalia.

---

in the vagina, because it grows well in the alkaline environment. It is also known to be present in the mouths and intestines of many men and women. Women normally have lactobacilli in the vagina, where they are necessary to maintain a healthy condition. They protect against a variety of infections, particularly those caused by bacteria in the urinary tract and the colon. When these lactobacilli are reduced in number, the yeast multiply and overgrow other vaginal organisms. The protective lactobacilli can be reduced by general poor health or lowered resistance, too frequent douching, and taking antibiotics (which can kill the lactobacilli as well as the bacteria causing the disease for which the antibiotic is prescribed).

Oral contraceptives and deodorant sprays also alter the vaginal environment, making it more susceptible to fungus growth. Wearing tight jeans and nonabsorbent nylon under and outer clothing and prolonged exposure to wet, synthetic bathing suits prevent air from circulating around the vulva and keep normal discharges in contact with vaginal tissues, contributing to yeast growth. In addition, if material from the bowel is carried to the vagina, the person becomes more susceptible to moniliasis, because the bowel harbors the *Candida* fungus.

When the normally acid environment is changed, the yeast multiply and overgrow other vaginal organisms, resulting in a white and curdy discharge. Examination reveals a whitish plaque around the vagina and on its walls. Itching, frequently associated with a rash or redness of the vulva, is common. In advanced cases, intercourse is painful, and burning and discomfort occurs during urination.

Clothes should serve as a means for absorbing normal discharges. Good hygiene and wearing cotton or cotton-crotch underclothing will go far toward offering protection. For women with confirmed yeast infections, mycostatin tablets inserted high in the vagina twice a day for a few weeks is the standard treatment, although vaginal suppositories or creams can also be used.

Genital Warts

Genital warts, the result of a viral infection, occur in most areas of the genitals and anus. In females, the warts appear in the lower area of the vagina; in males, they appear on the glans, foreskin (if uncircumsized) and shaft of the penis, and in homosexual males in the anal area as well. It is estimated that there are about 200,000 to 400,000 cases of genital warts in the United States annually. University health centers report genital warts are quite prevalent on college campuses.

Interest in—and fear of—genital warts has increased in recent years because of the relationship established between genital warts and cevical cancer. *Human papillomavirus (HPV),* the family of viruses identified as the causative agent of genital warts, may have up to sixty-five different strains, twelve of which have

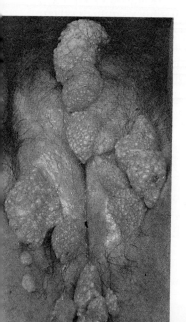

Genital warts are quite prevalent among college students. Since the standard treatment does not kill the virus causing the warts, they will reappear periodically.

***Year 2000
National Health Objective***

The National Health Objectives seek to reduce the annual number of first-time consultations with a physician for genital warts from 451,000 visits in 1988 to 385,000 visits annually by the year 2000.

been liked to cervical cancer. The incubation period for HPV is approximately three months after contact with an infected person. Some lesions are moist and some are dry; the moist lesions respond well to treatment. Large warts should be biopsied for cancerous cell growth. Genital warts have a high recurrence rate; that is, they often reappear in people who have been treated before. Diagnosis is made by the appearance of the warts. In moist areas of the body, they tend to be white, pink, or white to gray; in dry areas they are hard and yellow-gray.

The usual treatment is the drug podophyllin, an irritant that causes the outer skin in the area containing the virus to be sloughed off. Thus, the drug does not kill the virus; it removes the infected tissue. Podophyllin is applied to each lesion by the health practitioner; it dries and then is washed off four hours later by the patient. Sometimes an antibiotic ointment is prescribed as well to treat infection at the site and to help keep the wart moist. The podophyllin is usually applied once a week for five or six weeks or for the time it takes to control the infection. Surgery may be needed for persistently resistant warts.

Pubic Lice

Pubic lice, commonly referred to as crabs, are parasites. Actually, there are three different kinds of lice, and each seems to prefer its own habitat. *Pediculus corporis* is a body louse; *Pediculus capitus* is a head louse; and *Pediculus pubis* is the louse of the pubic area. Pubic lice are usually transmitted from person to person by sexual contact. The organism grips the pubic hair and feeds on tiny blood vessels of the skin.

Female crabs live for one to two months and lay up to ten eggs a day. As they feed on the human skin and blood, they irritate the skin, causing itching and occasionally swelling of the glands in the groin. The nits, or eggs, stick to the pubic hair with a thick substance. Aided by body warmth, the eggs hatch and the new lice perpetuate the cycle of feeding on the human before dropping off. They can live for about a day off the body and are visible to the naked eye on clothing and bedsheets. Two different preparations are effective: A-200 Pyrinate, an over-the-counter preparation, and Kwell (gamma benzene), available only by prescription. Either one is applied to the pubic hair. Directions should be followed carefully. One dose is usually curative, but sometimes the nits, though inactive, will adhere to the pubic hair for weeks after treatment unless removed. A fine-toothed comb dipped first into vinegar and then into water, and combed through the pubic hair will dissolve them. And, of course, clothing and bed linen used before treatment should be washed.

Scabies

Scabies is caused by a tiny mite that can barely be seen. The organism generally lives for up to two months. The female burrows under the skin at night, probably due to warmth of the human host, and the result is intense itching and the formation of pus. There is a characteristic distribution pattern of scabies. It is seen most commonly on the wrists, in the spaces between the fingers, under the breasts, and on the buttocks. Nodular scabies (raised lesions) can last up to one year. The mites lay two to three eggs a day, and in two to three weeks the new cycle begins. Because the incubation period is four to eight weeks, one individual can transmit scabies to another before being aware of its existence. Close contact that is usually, but not exclusively, sexual can transmit the mite. Scabies is rarely contracted from clothing, bedding, or toilet seats.

To diagnose scabies, a physician scrapes a burrow and puts the scraping on a slide, often with mineral oil to make the swimming mite more readily visible. Kwell is the medication used to treat scabies, as well as crabs. It must be applied very judiciously, because it can be toxic for some people. In particular, there is concern about the safety of using Kwell with women who are pregnant.

Other STDs

Less common sexually transmitted diseases are chancroid, lymphogranuloma venereum (LGV), and granuloma inguinale.

Chancroid

Chancroid is a sexually transmitted disease that results in sores very similar to the chancre sores associated with syphilis. It is caused by the bacterium *Hemophilus ducreyi.* Since this bacterium does not exist in temperate climates such as that in the United States, cases of chancroid are rarely found here; more commonly, it occurs in tropical climates. Differentiating chancroid from syphilis requires taking either a biopsy or a culture from the sores. Treatment consists of administration of the antibiotic sulfonamide.

Lymphogranuloma Venereum (LGV)

Also more prevalent in tropical climates, **lymphogranuloma venereum** is a venereal disease exhibiting pimplelike sores on the genitalia. LGV is caused by an organism that resembles both a virus and a bacterium, *Chlamydia trachomatis,* and, if left untreated, can

granuloma inguinale An STD, usually of tropical areas, which exhibits painful sores and blisters on the genitalia.

result in various infections and possibly pelvic inflammatory disease. However, usually there are no complications from LGV, and all that results is swelling of the lymph nodes. Treatment consists of the administration of the antibiotic tetracycline.

Granuloma Inguinale

This is another sexually transmitted disease that is rare in the United States since the bacterium that causes **granuloma inguinale,** *Calymmatobacterium granulomatis,* needs a tropical climate to survive. Symptoms include painful sores or blisters on the genitalia that have the potential to rupture, thereby causing secondary infections somewhere on the body (for example, the anus). Treatment consists of the administration of either tetracycline or erythromycin.

Coping with STDs

A person's first priority when she or he is diagnosed with a sexually transmitted disease is to obtain treatment. That may mean taking an antibiotic or some other medication, refraining from sexual contact for a period of time, applying a salve or ointment, or having surgery if the STD has been left untreated and has caused secondary damage (such as pelvic inflammatory disease).

Another part of coping with an STD is behaving responsibly and ethically. This means, as difficult as it may be, communicating with previous sexual partners so they can be tested for the disease, and refraining from sexual contact that might pass the disease to someone else.

Being diagnosed with an STD can be devastating, and the devastation may be greater from the accompanying emotional reactions than from physical health concerns. Feelings of guilt and shame are not unusual. Anger and resentment, sadness and depression, and feelings of stress and lowered self-esteem may also occur. For some the emotional trauma is too much to bear. Most individuals work through these feelings on their own or with their families, although support

groups consisting of others who are afflicted can be of enormous help.

The danger of extreme emotional reactions may be more harmful than the actual disease. Anger toward the opposite sex, loss of self-confidence resulting in changes in personal and professional behavior, and the conviction of lost health, attractiveness, or ability to be loved may be signs that an individual is not coping.

These reactions often vary with the nature of the disease. For example, the social stigma associated with trichomoniasis is quite different than that associated with syphilis and gonorrhea. Curable diseases also convey a different emotional reaction than do noncurable ones. For example, even though syphilis and gonorrhea may evoke strong emotional reactions, these may be temporary because these diseases can be cured and need not be coped with over one's lifetime. However, genital herpes is a different story. It will periodically flair up, necessitating a change in behavior; it requires medication, and its signs and symptoms are observable to others who see the genitals.

There is still another difference in the degree of reaction to an STD like AIDS that is fatal and to a disease that is not. Knowing the STD will result in death can have dramatic changes in one's life. It may require coming to grips with one's mortality, sharing feelings of death and dying with others, expressing anger about having contracted the disease, and maintaining constant vigilance for secondary infections and other signs of the disease's progression.

Lastly, how the disease was contracted may affect the emotional reaction to it. One need only imagine the guilt and shame accompanying an STD contracted through an extramarital sexual liaison as compared with an STD contracted through a blood transfusion or in utero. In one instance, the disease resulted from one's free choice of behavior, and the more socially unacceptable the behavior, the more guilt and shame can be expected. In other instances, the disease resulted "innocently" from a normal medical procedure (such as a blood transfusion) or through an action taken by someone other than the victim (as in the case of a baby born to a woman with an STD).

Regardless of the disease, the social stigma associated with it, or the manner in which it was acquired,

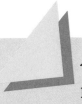

there are people and groups ready and willing to help. There are family and clergy; local community health departments, health providers, and hospitals; and support groups to offer both medical advice and emotional support. If you contract an STD you need not feel alone. Take advantage of the resources available to help you. Perhaps a good place to start is your campus health center.

Prevention of STDs

The most effective way to prevent contracting a sexually transmitted disease is to abstain from sexual activity. That means more than just refraining from coitus; it means not having any contact with someone else's genitalia altogether because organisms that cause sexual disease can be transmitted through any

FIGURE 14.1 • Abstinence is the best way to prevent contracting a sexually transmitted disease. For people who choose not to remain abstinent, the use of a condom, proper hygiene (such as washing the genitals after sex), and limiting the number of sexual partners can provide some protection.

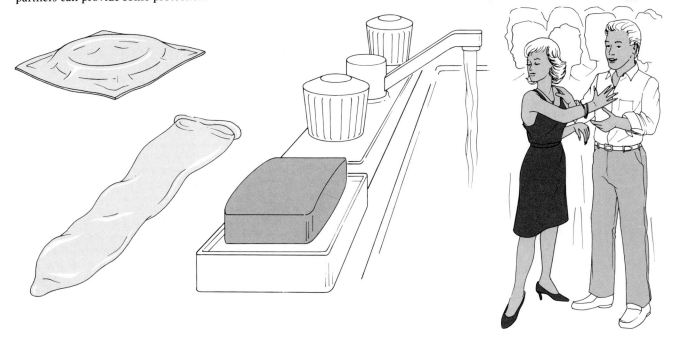

acquired immune deficiency syndrome (AIDS)
An STD that weakens the human immune system leading to serious opportunistic diseases; usually fatal in the long run.

AIDS-related complex (ARC) A medical condition which is an STD, wherein the HIV virus that causes AIDS is contracted by the patient, but the patient does not develop a full-blown case of AIDS, although the immune system is weakened.

opening in the skin. Obviously, oral-genital sex involves an opening to the body (the mouth), and manual contact can provide the organism a route into the body through a sore or a cut on the hand.

Short of abstinence—which many people are not willing to accept as a lifestyle—a sexually monogamous relationship with someone who is STD-free or using a condom can be effective in protecting against STDs. The condom—synthetic rubber (latex) rather than lambskin—protects against small openings in the skin of the penis or vagina that develop from the friction caused by thrusting movements. Refer to Chapter 6 for instructions on using the condom correctly.

The more sexual partners one has, the greater is the chance of exposure to a sexually transmitted disease-causing organism. Therefore, if you are not willing to remain abstinent and are not able to establish a monogamous relationship, it is recommended that you limit the number of sexual partners to as few as possible.

Hygiene can also be helpful in STD prevention. Women and men should wash their genitals before and after sexual contact. And because STDs can be transmitted to a fetus or to a newborn, prenatal screening for women is also important.

If you have sexual relations with several partners, you should have periodic screening for STDs. This is especially important if you experience any persistent symptoms. If you do have an STD, it is essential that your sexual partners be notified and that they receive screening and, if necessary, treatment.

Acquired Immune Deficiency Syndrome (AIDS)

In 1979, it was noticed that homosexual men in San Francisco and New York were developing a rare form of cancer called Kaposi's sarcoma. By 1981, it was discovered that the cause of this situation was that these men suffered from ineffective immunological systems that were unable to ward off infections, cancers, and pneumonias. A virus that causes a condition known as

acquired immune deficiency syndrome (AIDS) was found to be responsible. That virus has come to be known by various names: *human T-lymphotropic virus type III (HTLV-III)*, and *lymphadenopathy associated virus (LAV)*. Another name for AIDS virus, *human immunodeficiency virus (HIV)*, is the name scientists are now using.

AIDS-Related Complex (ARC)

AIDS is a condition that decreases the body's ability to fight off otherwise controllable infections—called *opportunistic infections* because they wait for the "opportunity" provided by a weakening of the body's immune system to attack the body. In terms of the ways in which it is transmitted and the ways in which it might be avoided, AIDS is similar to many other sexually transmitted diseases. However, there is one major difference between AIDS and other STDs: All the people who have developed full-blown cases of AIDS to date have died or are expected to die of the disease.

However, researchers are simply not yet sure whether everyone who is infected with HIV is doomed. Some people apparently remain well after infection with the AIDS virus; others develop a condition called **AIDS-related complex (ARC),** and still others develop a full-blown case of AIDS. ARC patients have milder symptoms than AIDS patients. They may experience loss of appetite, weight loss, fever, night sweats, skin rash, diarrhea, tiredness, lack of resistance to infection, or swollen lymph nodes. The number of people with ARC that will eventually develop AIDS is unknown, but conservative estimates range as high as over 50 percent.

AIDS in America

By 1991, there were 174,893 known cases of Americans who had contracted AIDS. There were also 110,530 AIDS-related deaths. AIDS is now one of the leading cause of death in the United States. The government estimated that between 800,000 and 1.3 mil-

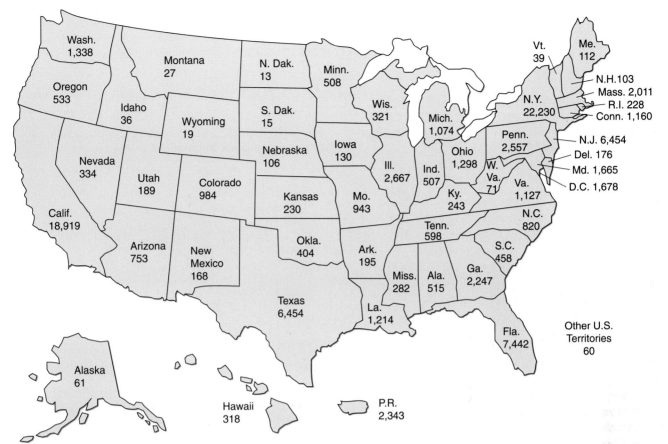

FIGURE 14.2 • Number of AIDS cases by state as of 1990.

lion additional Americans are infected with the AIDS virus. In 1990 alone, physicians diagnosed 55,000 new cases of AIDS. Could AIDS affect you? For every 500 students on your campus, there is approximately one case of an AIDS-infected student. This means that for a campus of 10,000 students, there are about 20 students who are infected with the AIDS virus.[4] Table 14.1 shows U.S. cities with the most AIDS cases and Figure 14.2 depicts the incidence of AIDS for each state. Although it seems from these data that rural areas are not nearly as hard hit by AIDS as urban areas, it should be noted that the National AIDS Commission warned in September 1990, of a 37 percent increase in rural AIDS cases over the previous year, as compared with a 5 percent increase in urban areas. No community is safe from AIDS.

How Is AIDS Spread?

AIDS is spread through contact with bodily fluids, predominantly blood and semen. The primary methods of transmission are sexual, blood, and congenital (see Figure 14.3):

1. Deposit of semen in the vagina, rectum, or

Cities with the Most Cases of AIDS*

City	Number of Cases
New York	32,167
Los Angeles	11,406
San Francisco	10,117
Houston	5,194
Washington, D.C.	4,946
Miami	4,795
Newark	4,670
Chicago	4,255
Atlanta	3,634
Philadelphia	3,630

* As of April 1991 (Centers for Disease Control, HIV/AIDS Surveillance Report, May 1991)

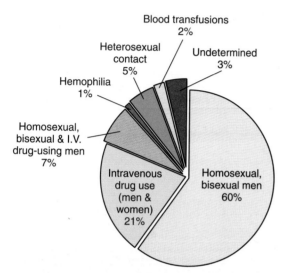

FIGURE 14.3 • Methods of Transmission for AIDS cases reported through May 1990

mouth. Anal intercourse is a primary mode of transmission because it causes the rectum to tear, allowing the virus a route of entry into the body, and because there are many blood vessels near the surface in the rectum.

2. Sexual intercourse involving microscopic tears in the vagina and penis to permit passage of the virus.

3. Blood transfusion with infected blood. All blood is now tested for the HIV virus and screened before being added to the blood supply.

4. Sharing infected needles, a common practice among intravenous drug users.

5. Accidental contamination by medical personnel pricking themselves with needles used to remove blood samples from AIDS patients.

6. Mothers infecting babies in utero (prior to birth).

Homosexual men, intravenous drug users, and people who engage in sexual intercourse with numerous sexual partners or who participate in anal intercourse and do not protect themselves by using a condom are those at most risk (see Figure 14.4). Although AIDS started out as a disease in the homo-

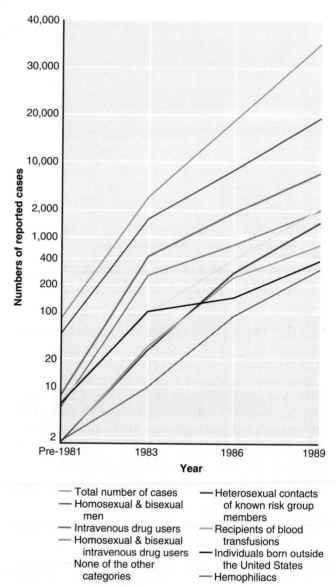

FIGURE 14.4 • Reported AIDS cases by risk category.
Source: Centers for Disease Control.

sexual community, it has since permeated the heterosexual community. No one who engages in high-risk behavior is protected from AIDS. Short of sexual abstinence or a monogamous sexual relation-

How to Talk about Condoms with a Resistant, Defensive, or Manipulative Partner

If the partner says:	You can say:	If the partner says:	You can say:
"I'm on the Pill, you don't need a condom."	"I'd like to use it anyway. We'll both be protected from infections we may not realize we have."	"What kinds of alternatives?"	"Maybe we'll just pet, or postpone sex for a while."
"I *know* I'm clean (disease-free); I haven't had sex with anyone in X months."	"Thanks for telling me. As far as I know, I'm disease-free, too. But I'd still like to use a condom since either of us could have an infection and not know it."	"This is an insult! Do you think I'm some sort of disease-ridden slut (gigolo)?"	"I didn't say or imply that. I care for you, but in my opinion, it's best to use a condom."
"I'm a virgin."	"I'm not. This way we'll both be protected."	"None of my other boyfriends uses a condom. A *real* man isn't afraid."	"Please don't compare me to them. A real man cares about the woman he dates, himself, and about their relationship."
"I can't feel a thing when I wear a condom; it's like wearing a raincoat in the shower."	"Even if you lose some sensation, you'll still have plenty left."	"I love you! Would I give you an infection?"	"Not intentionally. But many people don't know they're infected. That's why this is best for both of us right now."
"I'll lose my erection by the time I stop and put it on."	"I'll help you put it on—that'll help you keep it."	"Just this once."	"Once is all it takes."
"It destroys the romantic atmosphere."	"It doesn't have to be that way."	"I don't have a condom with me."	"I do," or "Then let's satisfy each other without intercourse."
"Condoms are unnatural, fake, a total turnoff."	"Please let's try to work this out—an infection isn't so great either. So let's give the condom a try. Or maybe we can look for alternatives."	"You carry a condom around with you? You were planning to seduce me!"	"I always carry one with me because I care about myself. I have one with me tonight because I care about us both."
		"I won't have sex with you if you're going to use a condom."	"So let's put it off until we can agree." or "OK, then let's try some other things besides intercourse."

Adapted from the article "Cutting the Risks for STDs" by Alan Grieco, PhD., which appeared in the March 1987 issue of *Medical Aspects of Human Sexuality.*
Prepared by the editors of *Medical Aspects of Human Sexuality* in collaboration with Reed Adams, PhD., Emanuel Fliegelman, DO., and Alan Grieco, PhD.

ship in which both partners are AIDS-free, the latex condom is the best protection against HIV. See the boxed insert to learn what to say to a sexual partner who is resistant to using a condom.

AIDS cannot be contracted through casual contact such as shaking hands, sharing food, towels, cups, razors, toothbrushes, or kissing. Although HIV has been found in saliva (though in very small amounts), "deep" kissing or "French" kissing is considered safe since too little HIV is present in saliva to result in AIDS.

Treating AIDS Patients

Although there is no cure for AIDS, there are a number of experimental drugs that can slow the disease's progress or relieve some of the disturbing symptoms. Among the most effective of these is **zidovudine** (for-merly referred to as **azidothymidine** or **AZT**), which was approved by the Food and Drug Administration (FDA) for distribution in March 1987. AZT users find they develop fewer infections, gain weight, show a more effective immunological system (a greater number of T cells), and live longer (fewer than 30 percent of men diagnosed with AIDS in New York City lived longer than 18 months; on AZT over 60 percent have lived that long[5]). However, some people develop severe anemia on AZT and cannot tolerate it for very long. The FDA cut the recommended dosage in half in 1989 after it was found to be just as effective in the lower dosage. This should help many AIDS patients who are not strong enough to tolerate the larger dosage. Another disadvantage of AZT is that it is very costly—$3,000 to $9,000 per patient annually, depending on how often it is needed.

Other drugs are available, but they are not as effective as a general AIDS treatment as AZT is. One of

Year 2000 National Health Objectives

The Year 2000 National Health Objectives devote a priority area to HIV infection. Several of the objectives cited include these recommendations:

1. Confine the annual incidence of diagnosed AIDS cases to no more than 98,000 cases.
2. Confine the prevalence of HIV infection to no more than 800 per 100,000.
3. Increase to at least 80 percent the proportion of HIV-infected people who have been tested for HIV infection. (An estimated 15 percent had been tested in publicly funded clinics by 1989.)
4. Provide HIV education for students and staff in at least 90 percent of the nation's colleges and universities.
5. Increase to at least 90 percent the proportion of cities with populations over 100,000 that have outreach programs to deliver HIV risk reduction messages to drug abusers.

Get Involved!

Controlling Sexually Transmitted Diseases

Given the national and worldwide concern for the control of sexually transmitted diseases, this is an appropriate area in which you can get involved in the health of the community around you and your society in general. The following suggestions can provide a vehicle for you to accomplish this goal:

1. Design a poster to educate people about some aspect of STDs. For example, one that advocates the use of latex condoms. Display the poster in a dormitory, dining hall, place of work, or some other place frequented by lots of people.
2. Read up on STDs and volunteer to be interviewed on the campus radio station or a local community radio station.
3. Volunteer to work for an organization that educates people about STDs. An organization such as Planned Parenthood would be appropriate.
4. Write to the World Health Organization and ask how you could contribute to the control of STDs. They might suggest a charitable fund to which you could contribute, or politicians to whom you could write concerning advocacy for STD research funding.
5. Enroll for internship credit at your school and use that course to teach about STDs at a local school district, at a local community center, or at a local hospital.
6. Organize a "Condom Awareness Program." Such a program could include demonstrations of the correct manner in which to use a condom, the distribution of free condoms, and education about the effectiveness of condoms in preventing conception and in preventing STDs. Inflating condoms as balloons might be a good attention-getter for those in attendance.
7. Volunteer at a treatment facility for AIDS patients.

these medications is *r-erythropoietin,* which treats the AZT-induced anemia. Another is *dideoxyinosine (DDI),* an antiviral drug that helps restore the immune function. In late 1989, the FDA recommended DDI for patients who cannot tolerate AZT or for whom AZT is ineffective. DDI results in patients showing improved blood counts and weight gain. However, it too may be accompanied by undesirable side effects.[6]

Two other drugs approved by the FDA in 1989 were *aerosal pentamidine* and *ganciclovir.* These drugs treat complications of AIDS. Aerosal pentamidine is effective in preventing a form of pneumonia (pneumocystis carinii pneumonia) that can cause the death of people whose immune systems are weakened by AIDS. Ganciclovir is used to treat eye infections, which can cause blindness in AIDS patients.

With these new medications and new knowledge about treating AIDS, the view has changed from considering AIDS a short-term terminal illness to considering it a long-term manageable disease. Thus, although there is still no cure for AIDS, it is possible both to prolong the life of AIDS patients and to treat the accompanying conditions and symptoms more effectively than ever before.

Pro There are some people who believe the AIDS scare to be so serious that the only way to wipe it out and protect those not yet infected is to identify people who have the disease. Once people know they have the disease, they can be instructed in how to prevent its spread to others. For example, once they know they test positive to the AIDS virus, people might decide to not marry, to not donate blood, to maintain regular medical examinations, or to alert others with whom they come into contact of their condition (such as health workers who may need to draw blood or work with blood products). In addition, they may then be held accountable for behavior that purposely spreads the disease; some people with AIDS who knowingly engaged in sexual intercourse and transmitted the disease to others have been charged and held legally liable for that behavior. Lastly, in order for the government to effectively respond to the AIDS crisis, the extent of the spread of the disease must be known.

Con There are others, however, who believe AIDS testing is inappropriate. They argue that those who test positive will be subjected to such discrimination and ostracism that it would be better to leave their condition undisclosed. For example, health insurance companies might exclude them from their plans, leaving AIDS sufferers unable to pay for their medical care. The government would have to pay for their care, and taxes would have to be raised to finance that type of expenditure. In addition, since AIDS is prevalent amongst homosexual men, it is feared that identifying those testing positive would stigmatize them as homosexuals. Lastly, the test most often administered for AIDS is not 100 percent accurate. False positive results would be devastating. The devastation of hearing one tested positive when later tests show different results can be avoided. Aside from the test's accuracy is the question of cost. Who would pay for the tests?

If you were the nation's public health officer, would you order people to be tested for AIDS? Would you test everyone or select populations of people; for example, school teachers or food handlers? If select populations, which ones? Would you require people applying for marriage licenses to be tested? Immigrants to our country? Would the testing be mandatory or voluntary?

What do you think?

During the later phases of AIDS, hospitalization is required. The cost of hospitalization—estimated to be between $60,000 and $70,000—is overwhelming to patients who may have previously gone through their savings and lost their qualifications for health insurance in treatment prior to being hospitalized. How to humanely and effectively treat AIDS patients and still maintain fiscal responsibility is a major societal issue. When tax dollars are used to support the care of AIDS patients, that money must be diverted from other programs. Which programs these should be is a matter of great debate.

Social and Political Implications of AIDS

There are many societal issues related to AIDS other than the cost of hospitalization. One of the major issues that people faced early in the AIDS crisis was how to treat AIDS patients. There were some people who, realizing AIDS was a function of voluntary sexual behavior, argued that societal resources should not be used—at least not in any significant amounts—for AIDS treatment. The belief that AIDS was predominantly a "gay disease" strengthened this point of view.

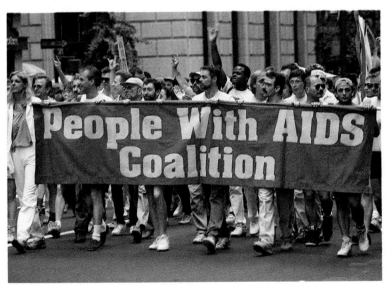

AIDS affects every segment of our society, regardless of age, ethnicity, culture, or sexual preference. We should, therefore, all be concerned, even if for selfish reasons, about preventing the spread of AIDS and about scientists' efforts to find a cure.

After all, some people argued, homosexuality is sinful as well as antisocial. This view became less vocalized as it soon was realized that AIDS affects heterosexuals as well as homosexuals and that it can even be transmitted through nonsexual contact (for example, through blood transfusions).

However, a debate still rages regarding the amount of federal dollars that should be spent on AIDS treatment, prevention, education, and research. AIDS affects a lot of people, but its impact pales in comparison to the numbers affected by heart disease, stroke, cancer, and many other conditions. In fact, AIDS is merely the eleventh leading cause of death in the United States. How much federal money should be diverted from research on these other medical conditions? Is it right to spend more money to research AIDS alone than to research all these other conditions combined?

Even if there was agreement regarding the amount of federal dollars that should be devoted to AIDS, there would still be arguments about where those funds should go. For example, should they be designated for educational campaigns to prevent AIDS from developing in the first place? Or should they go to research facilities seeking a cure for AIDS or a vaccine to prevent its occurrence? Or should it be used to treat people who have already contracted AIDS—to pay for their hospital bills, their medications, their living requirements after they have used up all their savings, their burials?

Given this societal debate, it is understandable that groups and individuals concerned with AIDS have organized to lobby for funds to be spent as they believe best. They have become involved in the political campaigns of legislators who support their causes, and they

For More STD Information

1. U.S. Public Health Service AIDS Hotline

   (800) 342-AIDS
2. National Sexually Transmitted Diseases Hotline
   American Social Health Association
   (800) 227-8922
3. SIDA Hotline
   (in Spanish)
   (800) 344-7432
4. TTY/TDD
   (for Deaf Callers)
   (800) 243-7889

have organized letter-writing campaigns to legislators already in office. They have made their concerns known to the public through marches on Washington, D.C., and in local communities, they have organized AIDS Awareness Weeks. In a national effort a quilt was made with the names of people who died of AIDS boldly emblazoned on its patches. In addition, they have conducted candlelight ceremonies in honor of those who have died of AIDS in order to confront the public with the need to invest compassion, political action, and money in the AIDS issue.

We expect that, as more and more people die of AIDS, the societal debate will flame brighter and the issues become even more complex. As a citizen of this society, you have the responsibility to stay informed about the AIDS debate and to express your viewpoint on this issue through your vote or other means.

Conclusion

Organisms causing sexually transmitted diseases are extremely fair: they do not discriminate by socioeconomic status, education, family background, age, or gender. If you are sexually active, you are at risk to contract an STD. There are several preventive measures you can take, though, which will either decrease your chances of contracting an STD or increase your chances of recovering if you do contract one. For example, establishing a monogamous relationship or limiting the number of sexual partners, and using a latex condom can help decrease the chances of your contracting a sexually transmitted disease. In addition, early detection and treatment can prevent the disease from progressing into serious medical complications.

Therefore, knowing the early signs and symptoms of STDs will allow you to identify a problem early on and get treatment promptly.

Sexually transmitted diseases, and particularly AIDS, can be life-threatening. They should not be taken lightly. You should actively attempt to prevent them as well as seek treatment for them as soon as possible if you become infected.

Summary

1. Sexually transmitted diseases (STDs) are diseases that are primarily spread through sexual contact. STDs can be caused by bacteria or viruses.

2. Organisms that cause sexually transmitted diseases thrive on warm, moist body surfaces, such as mucous membranes that line the reproductive organs, mouth, and rectum.

3. Sexually transmitted diseases were previously called "venereal diseases" ("VD") named after Venus, the Roman goddess of love. Because these diseases are passed sexually, and because love may or may not be a factor, the term "venereal disease" has been replaced with "sexually transmitted disease," a more descriptive name.

4. Sexually transmitted diseases were mentioned in the Old Testament as early as 1500 B.C.

5. Several social factors are suspected of contributing to the growing incidence of STDs in the 1960s: the introduction of the birth control pill and IUDs decreased the use of condoms; changing sexual standards meant more people were engaging in sex at younger ages and with more partners than in the past; attitudes that STDs could be easily treated led to carelessness; and sufferers were reluctant to seek treatment because of the social stigma attached to contracting an STD.

6. The more common sexually transmitted diseases include gonorrhea, syphilis, herpes genitalis, nongonococcal urethritis, chlamydia, acquired immune deficiency syndrome (AIDS), and pelvic inflammatory disease.

7. Gonorrhea, popularly known as "clap," is caused by the *Gonococcus* bacterium. Symptoms in men include a milky, bad-smelling discharge from the penis, painful urination, and swelling of the testicles. Symptoms in women include a slight burning sensation in the genital area and a mild discharge from the vagina. However, it is common for gonorrhea in women to be initially asymptomatic.

8. Syphilis is caused by a spirochete. It develops progressively in four stages. Stage 1 includes the development of open sores called "chancres" about three or four weeks after infection. Stage 2 (secondary stage) of syphilis occurs about six weeks after infection. Stage 2 symptoms include a rash over the entire body, welts around the genitalia, a low-grade fever, headache, hair loss, and a sore throat. Stage 3 syphilis (the latency stage) begins a couple of years after initial infection and may last up to forty or more years, causing various kinds of organ damage. Stage 4 (the tertiary stage) may lead to heart failure, blindness, other organ damage, and finally death.

9. Herpes genitalis (herpes simplex, type 2) is a viral infection that is one of the most common sexually transmitted diseases in the United States. Symptoms include sores, swollen glands, flulike symptoms, and pain during urination or sexual intercourse. Herpes genitalis progresses through four stages: the prodrome stage, the blister stage, the healing stage, and the inactive stage. Although there is no cure, symptoms can be relieved by soaking the genital area in hot water and/or administering the drug acyclovir.

10. Chlamydia affects about 5 to 10 million North Americans and causes up to 50 percent of the cases of pelvic inflammatory disease. In men, chlamydia can cause inflammation of the urinary and reproductive tracts, leading eventually to sterility. In women, it can cause vaginitis and pelvic inflammatory disease and, in extreme cases, can lead to infertility.

11. Nongonococcal urethritis (NGU) refers to an infection of the urinary tract caused by some organism other than the one that causes gonorrhea. In males, symptoms include a discharge from the penis, but in women, there may be no recognizable symptoms. Treatment usually consists of administration of the antibiotic tetracycline.

12. Pelvic inflammatory disease (PID) can lead to scar tissue being formed inside the Fallopian tubes, resulting in infertility. Symptoms of PID include abdominal pain or tenderness, increased menstrual cramps, lower back pain, pain during

intercourse, nausea, vaginal discharge, a burning sensation during urination, and fever.

13. Coping with any STD involves seeking treatment, behaving responsibly and ethically, and dealing successfully with emotional reactions to the disease.

14. The chances of contracting a sexually transmitted disease can be reduced by limiting the number of sexual partners, using a condom, and washing genitalia with soap and water after coitus.

15. Acquired immune deficiency syndrome (AIDS) is caused by human immunodeficiency virus (HIV), resulting in the immunological system's loss of effectiveness in fighting off infection. As a result, AIDS patients die of opportunistic infections. For every 500 college students, there will be approximately one student infected by HIV. AIDS can best be prevented by sexual abstinence. Alternatives are a sexually monogamous relationship where each partner is AIDS-free and the use of condoms.

16. AIDS-related complex (ARC) is a condition that is a precursor for AIDS in many people. Symptoms include loss of appetite, weight loss, fever, night sweats, skin rash, diarrhea, tiredness, lack of resistance to infection, and swollen lymph nodes.

Questions for Personal Growth

1. If you contracted a sexually transmitted disease, would you be embarrassed to tell people? Whom would you be most embarrassed to tell? Why?

2. Assume you just learned you had contracted a sexually transmitted disease. What would you say to the person(s) from whom you suspect you contracted the STD? What would you say to those to whom you think you might have passed the STD?

3. If you were fearful you might have contracted an STD, where would you go for testing? If you were found to actually have an STD, where would you go for treatment?

4. Who is the person you would least suspect to have a sexually transmitted disease? Why would you be surprised to learn that person contracted an STD? Is it because of that person's behavior; that is, was he or she not sexually active? Or is it because you perceive that person to be "clean," "healthy," or "moral"? (Of course, you know by now that it is the behavior and not the outward appearance of a person that subjects him or her to STDs.)

5. How would you feel in the presence of a person who had AIDS? Would you feel comfortable touching that person? Eating at the same table? Drinking from the same water fountain? If you would feel some discomfort engaging in these activities, would you share your feelings with the person with AIDS? Why or why not? With whom else would you share these feelings?

6. If you had children of school age, would you allow them to attend school if they shared a classroom with a child who had AIDS? If not, why not? If so, what precautions would you insist that the school take?

7. Which STD would you guess is the most prevalent on your campus? How could you find out if you're right? What can be done to decrease the number of new cases of this and other STDs at your school?

References

1. *Herpes Simplex* (South Deerfield, Mass.: Channing L. Bete, 1983).

2. William Hines, "Beyond AIDS, a Threat from Other Diseases Spread by Sexual Contact," *Washington Post* (July 11, 1989): 7–8.

3. David Fletcher, "Chlamydia," *Medical Self-Care* (November-December 1986): 34–38.

4. "Study Reports College HIV Rate of 1 in 500," *Washington Post* (November 29, 1990): 1A.

5. Bruce M. King, Cameron J. Camp, and Ann M. Downey, *Human Sexuality Today* (Englewood Cliffs, N.J.: Prentice-Hall, 1991).

6. T. P. Cooley, et al., "Once-Daily Administration of 2', 3'-Dideoxyinosine (DDI) in Patients with the Acquired Immunodeficiency Syndrome or AIDS-related Complex," *New England Journal of Medicine,* 322 (1990): 1340.

CHAPTER 15

Cardiovascular Disease

CHAPTER OBJECTIVES

After reading this chapter, you should understand:

- The causes and symptoms of, and treatments for, the major types of cardiovascular disease, such as arteriosclerosis and atherosclerosis, heart attack, and stroke.

- Many of the controllable and uncontrollable risk factors for cardiovascular disease, and how individuals can lessen their chances of developing heart and artery illnesses even in the face of uncontrollable risk factors (such as heredity).

- Several strategies for preventing cardiovascular disease beginning right now —in the college years.

- Medical solutions to cardiovascular illnesses when the damage has been done.

CHAPTER OUTLINE

Major Cardiovascular Diseases

Risk Factors in Cardiovascular Disease

Strategies for Preventing Cardiovascular Disease

Medical Solutions to Cardiovascular Disease

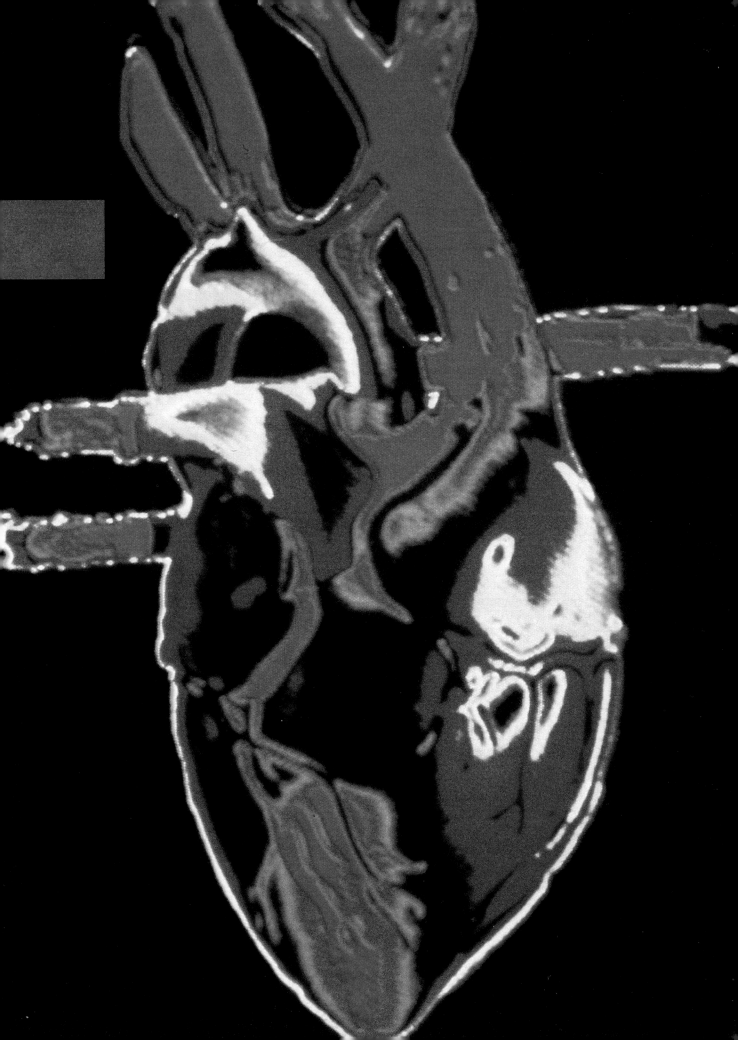

cardiovascular disease A general term used to describe heart disease, stroke, high blood pressure, and other diseases of the circulatory system.

arteriosclerosis The thickening and hardening of the arteries, a process that normally occurs as a person ages.

atherosclerosis The buildup of plaque on the inner lining of arteries; a major cause of cardiovascular disease.

plaque Material that builds up on the inner lining of arteries during the process of atherosclerosis; plaque is composed of fatty substances, cholesterol, cellular waste products, calcium, and the clotting material fibrin.

Cardiovascular disease—heart disease, stroke, and related disorders—account for nearly as many deaths as all other causes of death combined, including cancer, accidents, pneumonia, and influenza. More than 63 million people, one in four, in the United States, suffer from some form of these diseases, and almost one in two Americans eventually die of cardiovascular disease, one every 32 seconds. One in five men and one in seventeen women will die of a heart attack prior to the age of 60.[1]

Evidence suggests that lifestyle is a significant factor in many forms of these diseases. As a result, numerous Americans have altered their lifestyles: they no longer smoke, they exercise regularly, control their blood pressure and blood fat levels, manage their diets more carefully, maintain proper weight, and stay informed of recent medical advances. The number of deaths caused by cardiovascular disease is declining. Survival rates for those who have had a heart attack are also increasing. Research suggests that the future may be even brighter.

This chapter focuses on specific behavioral changes that can influence the pattern of cardiovascular disease. Major emphasis is placed upon increasing your understanding, clarifying the various theories about the causes, and helping you to make wise decisions to prevent cardiovascular disease.

Major Cardiovascular Diseases

The major diseases of the cardiovascular system include coronary artery disease, heart rhythm disorders, diseases of the heart valves, high blood pressure, atherosclerosis, stroke, diseases of the heart muscle, congenital defects, congestive heart failure, and varicose veins. Coronary artery disease has reached epidemic proportions in Western countries and is responsible for over one-half of all cardiovascular deaths, with strokes accounting for approximately one-fifth. Increasing evidence supports the hypothesis that coronary artery disease can be delayed or prevented with early changes in lifestyle.

Arteriosclerosis and Atherosclerosis

People sometimes confuse the terms arteriosclerosis and atherosclerosis. **Arteriosclerosis** is a general term referring to the thickening and hardening of the arteries, a condition that occurs normally as a person ages. **Atherosclerosis** refers to a type of arteriosclerosis characterized by a buildup of **plaque**—deposits of fatty substances, cholesterol, cellular waste products, calcium, and the clotting material fibrin—in the inner lining of an artery (see Figure 15.1).

Although the process of atherosclerosis becomes more advanced and prevalent with increasing age, it is incorrect to think of atherosclerosis as something that

Year 2000 National Health Objectives

Because of scientific data indicating that even small changes in blood serum cholesterol reduce the incidence of heart attacks and strokes, five national health objectives have been established: (1) to reduce the mean serum cholesterol level among adults to no more than 200 milliliter per decaliter (1976–1980 data revealed mean readings of 211 for men and 213 for women age 20 through 74); (2) to reduce the prevalence of blood cholesterol levels of 240 milliliter per decaliter or greater to no more than 20 percent among adults (29 percent of women and 25 percent of men exceeded these guidelines in 1976–1980); (3) to increase to at least 60 percent the proportion of adults with high blood cholesterol who are aware of their condition and who are taking action to reduce their blood cholesterol to recommended levels (currently only 11 percent of all people age 18 and older, and an estimated 30 percent of people with high blood cholesterol, were aware of their high levels in 1988); (4) to increase to at least 90 percent the proportion of adults who have had their blood cholesterol checked within the preceding 5 years (59 percent of people age 18 and older had "ever" had their cholesterol checked in 1988); and (5) to increase to at least 90 percent the proportion of clinical laboratories that meet the recommended accuracy standard for cholesterol measurement (53 percent met this standard in 1985).

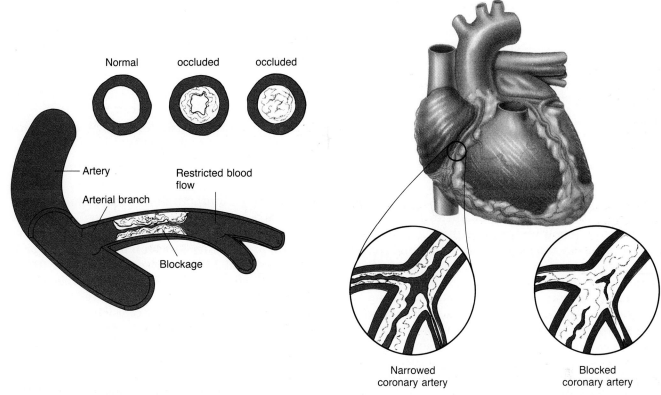

FIGURE 15.1 • Coronary Artery Blockage Leading to Heart Attack

only happens to older people. As early as age 3, fatty streaks are noticeable in the walls of larger arteries. By the late teens and early twenties, substantial fatty cholesterol deposits may develop. Progressive buildup of plaque may eventually obstruct or completely block the flow of blood to the body's vital organs, such as the heart and brain. If one of the major coronary arteries or its branches are involved, a heart attack can occur. If blood vessels supplying the legs are involved, the attack is called *claudication*. If the carotid arteries or their branches in the upper body are involved, the attack is called a *stroke*.

Exploring Your Health 15.1

Is Your Blood in Tune?

Ask your family physician to check your serum cholesterol. This can be performed with a small amount of blood from a simple finger prick. Analyze the results by comparing your readings to the information below.

Total Cholesterol:

Total Cholesterol is less than 200: No further evaluation, recheck in five years.

Total Cholesterol is more than 200: Recheck in 1–8 weeks. If two values are within 30 milligrams per decaliter, average these two values.

Total Cholesterol is 200–239 (border-line high cholesterol): Evaluate risk factors. If not a high risk, active treatment is not necessary. Follow the American Heart Association diet and recheck in one year.

Total Cholesterol is above 240 (high cholesterol): Analyze lipoproteins that measure "fasting" total cholesterol, HDL, triglycerides, and LDL.

If a lipid profile is obtained, answer the following questions:

Is your total cholesterol no more than 4.5 × HDL cholesterol?

_____ Yes _____ No

Is your cholesterol/HDL ratio at least 5:1?

_____ Yes _____ No

Is your HDL reading above 35?

_____ Yes _____ No

Is your LDL cholesterol less than 160? _____ Yes _____ No

If the answer to the above questions is "yes," your lipid profile is good.

List the key changes you could make to lower your total cholesterol and increase your HDL cholesterol over the next 12-month period:

low-density lipoproteins (LDL) A type of cholesterol that is considered harmful because it promotes fatty deposits on the inner lining of arteries.

high-density lipoproteins (HDL) A type of cholesterol that is considered beneficial in certain amounts because it lubricates the inner linings of arteries.

myocardial infarction (MI) Commonly called a "heart attack," myocardial infarction occurs when a restricted blood flow to the heart (ischemia) causes tissue death in a part of the heart.

coronary thrombosis A blood clot in the coronary artery, frequently the cause of myocardial infarction.

coronary occlusion A complete blockage of the coronary artery caused by a blood clot.

collateral circulation The development of small arteries called arterioles that bypass a blockage in a main artery.

Fat and Cholesterol: A Major Risk of Atherosclerosis The exact cause of atherosclerosis is not known, but it is now well accepted that a high number of fats (lipids) in the bloodstream, a condition called *hyperlipidemia*, is a major risk in the development of the disease. The more fatty particles in the blood, the greater the tendency for the accumulation of plaque on the arterial walls. According to this *lipid infiltration theory*, blood fats penetrate the innermost layer of the artery (*endothelium*) and slowly build up until a partial or complete obstruction of blood flow occurs. Researchers also feel that the process is enhanced when the artery linings are damaged by tobacco use or high-fat diets.

Where does this fat come from? The fatty particles that increase the tendency toward atherosclerosis are called lipoproteins, which consist of fat (triglyceride), a blood protein (to make the fat soluble in the water portion of the blood), and cholesterol. Blood measurements of triglycerides and cholesterol provide an index of fatty particles in the bloodstream. Although some heart disease patients have elevated triglycerides, a clear association between triglyceride levels and cardiovascular disease has not been established. The real culprit in cardiovascular disease appears to be cholesterol, which is found in foods of animal origin and is also manufactured by the liver. Although both are important factors, total cholesterol is affected more by the consumption of saturated fat, which stimulates the liver to produce cholesterol, than by the amount of cholesterol-containing foods you eat. The average American consumes one and a half to three times the recommended daily consumption of 300 milligrams of cholesterol and nearly twice the recommended amount of saturated fat (17–18 percent of total calories).

Because of our dietary habits, high cholesterol levels above the recommended 200 milliliter per decaliter blood for adults and 175 milliliter per decaliter blood for children are common. Approximately 50 percent of elementary school children exceed the 175 reading, 25 percent have readings higher than 200. By the late teens and early twenties, the cholesterol levels of American youth commonly climb to 225 to 230 and increase the risk of cardiovascular disease.

Low-Density and High-Density Lipoproteins Your total blood cholesterol reading is only part of the picture. There are actually five families of lipoproteins of which **low-density lipoproteins (LDL,** the "bad" cholesterol) and **high-density lipoproteins (HDL,** the "good" cholesterol) have the most influence on cardiovascular disease. HDLs are produced in the liver and released into the bloodstream where they carry some of the LDL cholesterol away and possibly provide a protective layer of grease to help prevent plaque buildup on artery walls. The LDL cholesterol that remains circulates in the bloodstream and promotes fat deposits on artery walls.[2] It is recommended that HDL levels exceed 35 for adult men and 45 for adult women, and that LDL levels remain less than 165.

Individuals with high amounts of HDL have a decreased risk of cardiovascular disease. A total cholesterol/HDL ratio of 5:1 (20 percent of total cholesterol is of the HDL variety) begins to provide some protection.[3] Table 15.1 estimates the risk of cardiovascular disease based on these ratios. The second column of Table 15.1 converts the ratio to the percentage of HDL. Individuals at high risk should consult their physician and

TABLE 15.1

Correlation of C-V Risk and HDL Ratio

Cholesterol: HDL Ratio	Equivalent HDL %	Estimated Risk
6:1	16	Very high risk
5:1	20	Some protection
4:1	25	Good protection
3.5:1	28	Excellent protection
3:1	33	Excellent; ratio present in very few

consider reducing dietary saturated fat and cholesterol intake, and they should also initiate an aerobic exercise program to improve their ratio. Another way to check your risk is to multiply your HDL cholesterol times 4.5. If this figure exceeds your total cholesterol, you are not currently at risk.

Heart Attack

Heart attack is the leading cause of death in America, causing more than 524,000 deaths each year; over 300,000 victims die before reaching the hospital. In addition, 4,940,000 people have a history of heart attack, chest pain, or both. Approximately 5 percent of

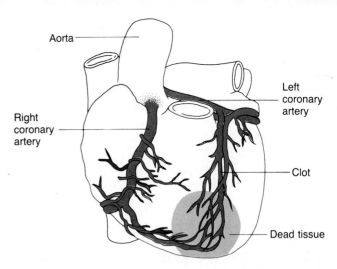

FIGURE 15.3 • Clot or blockage in a branch of the coronary artery.
Source: National Heart, Lung and Blood Institute. National Institutes of Health.

all heart attacks occur in individuals under age 40, and 45 percent occur in individuals under age 65.[4]

An explanation of the function of the heart, shown in Figure 15.2, will help you understand how and why a heart attack occurs. The heart receives nourishment from blood that passes through two main coronary arteries that branch off the aorta, the largest artery in the body and the one that supplies blood to the rest of the body. The right coronary artery branches into smaller and smaller arteries that penetrate the back wall of the heart, eventually branching into tiny capillaries that supply oxygen and nutrients to the heart and its electrical conduction system. The left coronary artery is divided into two parts, which nourish the front and the left side of the heart. Through these coronary arteries, the heart maintains its own nourishment. Unfortunately, these arteries are highly susceptible to the buildup of fat deposits, which result in diminished blood flow.

Wherever blood flow to body tissues is diminished (a condition called *ischemia*), the tissues are deprived of needed nutrients and tissue death or *infarction* occurs. If blood flow to the heart muscle, or *myocardium,* is severely reduced, **myocardial infarction** or **M.I.** ("heart attack") occurs.

Coronary Thrombosis and Occlusion

A typical heart attack results from **coronary thrombosis,** a clot in a coronary artery. If coronary thrombosis leads to complete blockage, or **coronary occlusion,** in the larger sections of a coronary artery, the resulting reduction in blood supply to the heart muscle could result in a heart attack (see Figure 15.3).

In some instances, particularly in individuals over 60 years of age, however, the body naturally avoids or delays a heart attack through **collateral circulation,**

FIGURE 15.2 • Your heart and how it works. The heart is hollow. Its tough, muscular wall (myocardium) is surrounded by a fiberlike bag (pericardium) and is lined by a thin, strong membrane (endocardium). A wall (septum) divides the heart cavity down the middle into a "right heart" and a "left heart." Each side of the heart is divided again into an upper chamber (atrium or auricle) and a lower chamber (ventricle). Valves regulate the flow of blood through the heart and to the pulmonary artery and the aorta.

The heart is really a double pump. One pump (the right heart) receives blood that has just come from the body after delivering nutrients and oxygen to the body tissues. It pumps this dark, bluish-red blood to the lungs, where the blood gets rid of a waste gas (carbon dioxide) and picks up a fresh supply of oxygen that turns the blood a bright red again. The second pump (the left heart) receives this "reconditioned" blood from the lungs and pumps it out through the great artery (aorta), to be distributed by smaller arteries to all parts of the body.

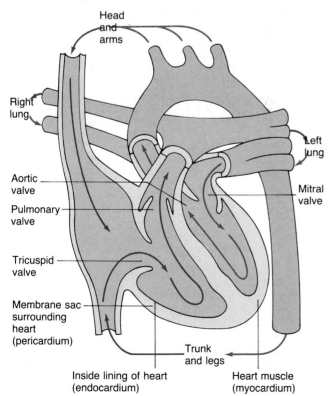

angina pectoris A common symptom of heart disease, angina pectoris is chest pain caused by ischemia, a reduced blood supply to the heart.

cerebrovascular accident (CVA) The severe reduction of blood flow to a portion of the brain, often caused by a blood clot, causing a part of the brain to be damaged; commonly called a stroke.

embolus A stroke caused by a blood clot that travels from another part of the body to the brain; only about 10 percent of strokes occur in this way.

transitory ischemic attack (TIA) A mild stroke caused by a temporarily inadequate supply of blood to the brain; although permanent damage may not result, it is a sign of serious cardiovascular disease.

hemiplegia A paralysis on one side of the body; a classic finding in cases of stroke.

aphasia Speech and language difficulties, often occurring with left-sided hemiplegia, a common finding in cases of stroke.

which occurs when tiny arteries called *arterioles* develop near a blockage in a large artery and actually bypass the clogged area. These naturally occurring "detours" around blocked portions of arteries help maintain a constant flow of blood to the heart muscle and help to prevent a heart attack. Although everyone has collateral vessels, at least in microscopic form, considerable enlargement of these vessels occurs in some people with *coronary artery disease* or *coronary heart disease*.

Angina Pectoris

A common symptom of heart disease is **angina pectoris,** or chest pains. Angina pectoris, often referred to as angina, is caused by ischemia (reduced blood supply) to the heart muscle. The angina victim may experience a tightness or pressure in the chest and pain that radiates to the shoulders or arms. It is estimated that 2,470,000 Americans suffer from angina and that over 300,000 new cases are reported each year.[5] In addition, between 3 and 4 million Americans are suffering from a painless form of angina called *silent ischemia*. People with silent ischemia may even experience a heart attack without knowing it.

If angina pectoris is confirmed, a physician's care and certain lifestyle changes can often prevent a heart attack. It is interesting to note that 70 percent of ischemia occurs in situations where physical activity is minimal but where mental activity is high, such as in committee meetings, when driving a vehicle, and during interviews and conversations.

Symptoms of Heart Attack

For the male over thirty years old and the female over 50, any chest pain is often regarded as a sign of a heart attack. In actuality, however, apparent pain in the chest may be occurring in the chest wall (muscle, ligament, rib, or rib cartilage), the lungs or outside covering, the gullet, diaphragm, skin, or other organs in the upper part of the diaphragm. It is not easy to distinguish between chest pain associated with heart attack and other pains. Table 15.2 identifies the signals of a heart attack.

Anyone who experiences heart attack symptoms should be transported immediately to the hospital by ambulance, and his or her blood pressure, breathing, and heart rate should be monitored.

Stroke

Stroke is the third largest cause of death (147,000 each year) in America after diseases of the heart and cancer. The risk of stroke increases steadily with age in both men and women (see Figure 15.4). Stroke is also a major cause of disability and accounts for one-half of all patients hospitalized for acute neurological disease.

TABLE 15.2

What You Should Know About Heart Attack		**The Signals of Heart Attack**
An estimated 65,980,000 Americans have one or more forms of heart or blood vessel disease. As many as 1.5 million may have a heart attack this year; about 524,000 will die—300,000 of them before they reach the hospital. Many thousands of these might have been saved if the victims had heeded the signals.	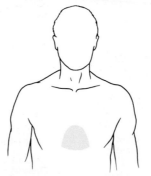	Uncomfortable pressure, fullness, squeezing, or pain in center of chest lasting two minutes or more.
		Pain may spread to shoulders, neck, or arms.
		Severe pain, dizziness, fainting, sweating, nausea, or shortness of breath may also occur.
Delay spells danger. If symptoms persist for more than two minutes, an ambulance should be called.		Not all of these signals, however, are always present.

Intensity and location of pain

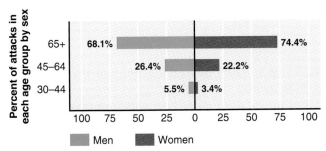

FIGURE 15.4 • Age/sex distribution of stroke incidence.
Source: Framingham Heart Study, 24-year followup.

The estimated annual cost of stroke-related health care in 1987 was 12.8 billion dollars.

The good news is that mortality rates from stroke in the United States are steadily declining. From 1972 to 1984, stroke-related deaths decreased by 47.77 percent. The debate continues over how much of this reduced mortality can be attributed to better medical care for stroke victims and how much to the occurrence of fewer strokes.[6]

Like the heart, the brain must be continuously nourished. When blood supply to any portion of the brain is greatly reduced or cut off completely, nerve tissue in the brain is unable to function, and body tissue controlled by this nerve tissue also ceases to operate. This occurrence is known as a **cerebrovascular accident (CVA)** or *stroke.* Depending on the portion of the brain affected, a victim may experience loss of speech, loss of memory, or partial paralysis. The four ways in which a stroke occurs are shown in Figure 15.5. Fewer than 10 percent of strokes are caused by an **embolus,** or small clot from another body part. A much more frequent cause is atherosclerosis. The same fatty deposits that cause heart attacks also block the arteries supplying the brain.

A mild stroke occurs when the brain is deprived of adequate blood supply for a short period (ischemia). A **transitory ischemic attack (TIA)** often results in moments of paralysis, vision problems, or inability to

FIGURE 15.5 • Causes of a stroke.

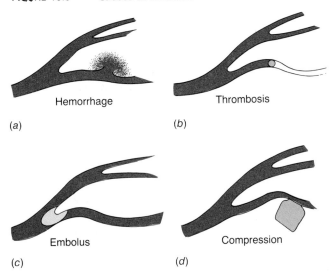

Hemorrhage

(a)

Thrombosis

(b)

Embolus

(c)

Compression

(d)

speak. Generally, the deeper brain cells are not permanently damaged, although repeated episodes can bring about personality changes. TIAs are warning signs of insufficient blood supply to the brain. Careful diagnosis and prompt action can prevent a stroke from occurring. Some 80 percent of victims survive the first stroke, with the likelihood of death increasing with age. However, more than 20 percent of those who recover have a second stroke within two years, and over half of the survivors eventually die of a heart attack.

The most visible sign of a stroke is paralysis on one side of the body, or **hemiplegia.** Paralysis of the right side (*right hemiplegia*) indicates injury to the left side of the brain, whereas left-side paralysis (*left hemiplegia*) indicates right-brain injury. Left-brain injury produces speech and language difficulties (**aphasia**) and results in slow, cautious, and disorganized behavior when the victim is confronted with an unfamiliar problem. Right-brain damage causes difficulty with spatial-perceptual tasks (judging distance, size, position, rate of movement, form, and the relation of parts to wholes). Many stroke patients also experience "visual field cuts," producing vision similar to what you would see if you wore goggles with tape across half of each lens. Right hemiplegics tend to have right field cuts, and left hemiplegics left field cuts. Patients learn to turn their heads to compensate, although not everyone makes this adjustment. Any patient who has suffered a stroke will show evidence of brain damage. Loss of memory, short attention span, difficulty with new learning, inability to generalize learning to new situations, and *emotional lability* (loss of emotional control) may occur.

Practically all spontaneous recovery of intellectual abilities will occur in the first three to six months after the stroke. A stroke will not affect all areas of the brain equally, nor will all aspects of intellectual functioning be affected equally. Patients will behave differently depending on the portion of the brain that has been injured, the severity of the injury, and the recency of the stroke.

Dealing with Stroke Patients   Each stroke patient and his or her family have unique problems. Although a complete cure is unlikely, many stroke patients can adapt successfully with a doctor's care, good nursing, special exercises, a healthy diet, and the

Major Cardiovascular Diseases   •   395

tachycardia A very rapid beating of the heart.

sudden cardiac death A sudden malfunctioning of the heart that causes it to behave chaotically and finally stop beating, causing death.

heart murmur A sound audible on listening to the heart.

functional heart murmur A murmur occurring in a normal heart.

valvular or rheumatic heart disease Damage to the valves of the heart caused by a bacterial infection, commonly a streptococcal infection that begins in the throat or tonsils and leads to rheumatic fever.

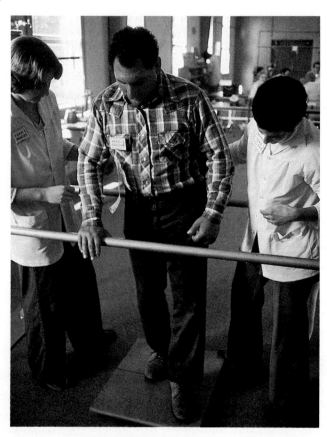

Complete recovery from most strokes is unlikely, but the majority of stroke patients can adapt to their new health situation through a combination of physical therapy and the patience and love of family and friends.

love, patience, and understanding of family and friends. People commonly feel uncomfortable in the presence of a stroke victim and say and do things that may be harmful. The National Easter Seal Society offers these suggestions for those who care for or visit stroke patients:

- Never talk about the stroke patient in the patient's presence. Failure to answer does not necessarily mean failure to understand.
- Speak in your natural voice; shouting won't help the patient understand.
- Don't talk for a patient who has trouble speaking. Ask questions that can be answered by a nod or shake of the head.

- Don't interrupt when the patient tries to speak. Give your whole attention.
- Don't correct mistakes made in speech or writing. Say what you think the patient is trying to say and ask if you understand correctly.
- Don't confuse the patient with too many people around at one time. Make visits short and cheerful. Encourage trips outside the home, but do not push.
- Don't forget to stand on the "good" side if a patient had a loss of half of the visual field. Place yourself where you can be seen easily.
- Don't be alarmed, embarrassed, or afraid if the patient cries, acts depressed, or swears. Be casual about such behavior; be courteous and resourceful.

Other Cardiovascular Problems

Sudden Cardiac Arrest Each year, approximately 330,000 people experience sudden cardiac arrest and die. In 80 to 90 percent of the cases, a torrent of electrical impulses suddenly disrupt the rhythm of the heart, producing a condition known as **tachycardia** (overaccelerated arrhythmia) that may degenerate into a chaotic state in which the heart can only twitch instead of pump. The large majority of victims are middle-age and older people. Studies indicate that 15 to 20 percent of **sudden cardiac death** victims have no detectable coronary atherosclerosis; the remaining 75 to 80 percent possess one or more symptoms of heart disease. The exact cause of sudden cardiac death is unknown. Researchers feel that a temporary, but preventable, malfunction occurs that is sometimes referred to as an electrical accident. Evidence suggests that fear, depression, and isolation may play a part, particularly in those with diseased, vulnerable hearts.[7]

Heart Valve Defects Irregular blood flow results in a **heart murmur**, which is also a heart rhythm disturbance. The difficulty may be an impaired valve that fails to close completely or valve orifices that are narrowed and slow the flow of blood. In the case of valve defects, a greater load is placed on the heart, heart walls may increase in size, and tension increases inside them. In effect, the heart is less efficient and, in a sense, has to pump the same blood twice.

In what are termed **functional heart murmurs,** no structural defect is evident to account for the abnormal rhythm. In children, most heart murmurs are not indicative of disease or physiological impairment.

Rheumatic fever is a leading cause of **valvular** or **rheumatic heart disease.** Generally regarded as a disease of children and young people, it accounts for approximately 95 percent of all heart disease in patients under 20 years of age and results in an estimated 6,900 deaths each year. The condition involves damage to heart valves by a disease that begins with a strep throat (streptococcal infection). The most common symptoms of strep throat are the sudden onset of a sore throat, accompanied by painful swallowing; fever; tender, swollen glands under the jaw; headache; nausea and vomiting. The first symptom of rheumatic fever is high fever lasting from ten to fourteen days. Symptoms indicating that the heart has been affected include shortness of breath, chest pains, fatigue, poor eating habits, and pale skin color. At this point, a physician may detect an abnormal heart murmur or an enlarged heart. Inflammation also occurs in several areas of the body, especially the joints, lungs, brain, and endocardium (lining of the heart). When the inflammation is in the heart, granular nodules develop on the cusps of the heart valves, with permanent connective tissue forming around the injured valve during the healing process.

Rheumatic heart disease is largely preventable. When severe sore throat persists for more than a few days, the individual should have a throat culture to determine whether there is a strep infection. If the infection exists, antibiotic therapy can prevent rheumatic fever and secondary valve damage.[8]

Congestive Heart Failure   In some individuals, a heart that has been damaged lacks the strength to keep blood circulating normally throughout the body. The original heart damage may have been caused by hypertension, a heart attack, atherosclerosis, congeni-

A Question of Ethics

The Case of Baby Fae

In early November 1984 a 12-day-old girl, called "Baby Fae" to protect her family's privacy, received a heart transplant. Heart transplants were nothing new in 1984, but this case was different for at least one major reason: The heart Baby Fae received was taken from a baboon.

As the world watched, Baby Fae's immune system began to attack the heart that was keeping her alive. Additional drug therapy, kidney dialysis, and closed-heart massage failed to save her life. Barely three weeks after her transplant, Baby Fae's life ended. For society, however, Baby Fae's highly publicized operation and death represented the beginning of a new set of ethical questions that remain as perplexing today as the questions posed by the use of artificial hearts in humans (see the Question of Ethics box in Chapter 18 for a discussion of that problem).

In the eyes of some, the three-week life extension was a real sign of medical progress and indicated that the technique is definitely feasible. For Baby Fae, suffering from hypoplastic left-heart syndrome (the main pumping chamber failed to develop adequately), and others of all ages who, like her, are days, perhaps

hours away from death with no human heart available, such an approach offers hope. It is estimated that 15,000 patients each year are in need of a new heart. This far exceeds the number of human hearts available for transplants. Animal hearts can fill the void. Even short-term success may be long enough for a compatible human heart to be found. In the future, drug therapy may be successful in preventing rejection and providing a permanent means of survival for such patients. Only the patient can decide whether the extended life is worth the suffering. In addition, it is argued that the medical profession has the responsibility to maintain life by any means when a chance for success exists. The heart transplant procedure, like its predecessor, kidney transplants, was one labeled a useless, experimental approach; now, it is considered a valuable life-extension procedure.

Opponents argue that the use of animal hearts for human transplants is not ethical at this stage and is nothing more than "heroics," causing tremendous expense, physical discomfort, and trauma with very little chance for success. In fact, it is argued, physicians knew that the

baboon heart could not grow sufficiently to accommodate a human being as the years passed. The three-week survival period provides no conclusive evidence of the value of the procedure, since this is about how long it typically takes for a rejection crisis to take hold. Professor Norman Scotch of the Boston University School of Public Health labeled similar techniques a "melodrama" that distracts from more important but less glamorous medical efforts. According to Dr. Thomas J. Ryan, president of the American Heart Association, the three major breakthroughs in cardiac care over the next fifteen years are going to be prevention, prevention, and prevention.

What is your view? Should the medical profession continue to pursue modes of treatment like the one attempted in Baby Fae's case? Or should our energy and finances be devoted mostly toward prevention? Could Baby Fae's problem have been "prevented"? What do you think you would do if a child born to you and your spouse had a similar problem?

congestive heart failure A condition in which the heart is not strong enough to keep the blood circulating properly, causing the blood to back up as it returns to the heart.

veins The vessels through which the blood returns to the heart from other parts of the body.

varicose veins Permanently distended veins resulting from an improper functioning of valves within the veins.

hypertension An excessive amount of blood pressure within the arteries and veins of the body; this common condition has many causes and is a major component of cardiovascular disease.

tal heart defect, rheumatic fever, primary disease of the heart muscle (cardiomyopathy), infection of the heart valves or heart muscle (endocarditis or myocarditis), or high blood pressure in the lungs. This inadequate blood flow causes the blood to back up as it returns to the heart through a system of veins, causing congestion in the tissues and, ultimately, **congestive heart failure**. *Edema* (swelling) is common in the legs and ankles. Fluid may also collect in the lungs, interfere with breathing, and cause shortness of breath. In addition, the kidneys become unable to eliminate sodium and water, which increases the edema. Most cases of congestive heart failure can be treated successfully with rest, proper diet, reduced daily activity, and medication.

Congenital Heart Disease

Inborn heart defects, known as congenital heart disease, fall into four major groups: (1) narrowing or constriction of a blood vessel or a heart valve; (2) abnormal holes between the two blood vessels, in the muscle, or in the septum that separates the two chambers of the heart; (3) combination of (1) and (2); and (4) abnormal connections of the blood vessels leading to or from the heart. Approximately 25,000 babies are born with heart defects each year, resulting in 6,100 deaths; more than 500,000 victims are living.[9] In most cases, the exact cause of these congenital abnormalities is unknown. One known disease that can interfere with the normal heart development of the baby is German measles (rubella), when contracted by a mother during the first three months of pregnancy. Congenital heart defects are sometimes detected at birth by an unusual sound, a murmur, with each beat. A bluish-tinged skin color (cyanosis), difference in blood pressure between an arm and a leg, and slow pulse rate also provide clues to the presence of heart defects. Using x-rays (that can show an enlarged heart and congested lungs), echocardiogram (use of echoes from pulses of high-frequency sound waves to produce a sonar picture of the heart), and cardiac catheterization (insertion of a catheter through an artery into the chambers of the heart to measure blood pressure and the amount of oxygen in the blood) are other ways that heart defects can be detected. In most cases, these defects can be corrected through surgery. Although it cannot repair the defect, medication is some-

times used to prevent complications, relieve symptoms until surgery can be performed or throughout a patient's life.

Varicose Veins

Blood flows away from the heart through arterial blood vessels and returns to the heart through vessels called **veins.** Blood flows through veins at a much lower pressure than through arteries. Because there is less pressure, veins are not equipped with the same strong, elastic muscular walls of arteries. In fact, very little muscle tissue exists in veins. A system of valves spaced irregularly along the inside walls open as blood flows upward toward the heart, and close to prevent blood moving backward toward the feet. When these valves are not working properly, a condition referred to as **varicose veins** develops. Deep inner veins are imbedded in muscles which help support the blood that flows from the ankle to the heart. The contraction of muscles produced by walking and moving provides support to the veins and helps force the blood upward. Veins near the surface of the skin are connected to the deep veins by communicating veins. It is these surface veins with little muscular support that become varicose when valves or walls weaken. Weak walls can give way under pressure of blood and sag outward at the site of the valves. Valves now cannot close tightly, which further increases pressure. As pressure increases, more and more of the valves are affected. Some individuals are born with weak veins or valves; others may acquire a weakened condition through diseases such as phlebitis, producing inflammation of the veins, or through injury. Tiny, purple veins visible just under the skin, referred to as the "spider burst" type, are not related to varicose veins and do not require treatment. The presence of varicose veins and spider bursts appears to be hereditary.

Medical treatment involves use of elastic stockings and elastic bandages to provide support to the veins and reduce swelling. Stockings should reach the knee and provide the greatest pressure at the foot, with gradually diminishing pressure up the leg. Physicians may choose to close off portions of a vein or veins or strip damaged veins and reroute blood flow to the deep veins. Patients are encouraged to elevate their feet

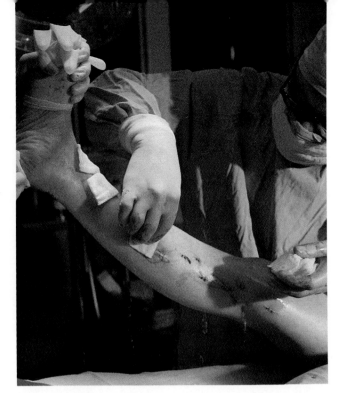

There are many reasons why people may develop varicose veins, and there are many ways—surgical and nonsurgical —to control the condition.

when sitting, exercise regularly, sleep with their feet raised slightly above the level of the heart or raise the bed with a six-inch block placed under the foot posts, avoid garters and elastic girdles, lie down occasionally during the day, and avoid standing and sitting for long periods of time.

Risk Factors in Cardiovascular Disease

Several factors have been linked with a high risk of cardiovascular disease. Among the factors that cannot be controlled are sex, race, age, and heredity. Controllable factors include hypertension, obesity, inactivity, hyperlipidemia, smoking, and diabetes. With normal blood pressure and cholesterol levels and in the absence of smoking and diabetes, the chances of a male having a heart attack before age 65 are fewer than one in twenty. With one of these risk factors, the risk doubles; with two, the chances become one in two, or 50 percent.

Men have a higher incidence of cardiovascular disease than women, across all age groups. Although the rate of heart attacks in women increases after menopause—presumably because of hormonal changes, there is evidence that women are developing cardiovascular disease at an earlier age than in the past. Black Americans have a much higher risk of developing hypertension and are likely to suffer strokes at an earlier age than whites. Older people suffer more heart attacks than young people.

↑ blood fat level

Hereditary Traits

The genetic tendency to develop atherosclerosis early in life greatly increases the risk of early cardiovascular disease. Although a small percentage of individuals apparently develop little plaque buildup regardless of living habits, others develop large amounts very early in life. In the past decade, several professional athletes between 23 and 39 years of age suffered serious heart attacks. Diagnosis by autopsy or by arteriography revealed advanced atherosclerosis. Apparently, these young adults possessed the hereditary tendency to acquire plaque and hardening of the arteries. There is also some evidence that a tendency toward high blood pressure or hypertension is inherited. A history of early heart disease in your family is a signal for you to form healthy living habits and receive periodic physical examinations. This is especially important for individuals from families in which one or more parents or grandparents suffered a heart attack or stroke before age 60.

Hypertension

The condition known as **hypertension,** or **high blood pressure,** forces the heart to work harder than normal and places the arteries under strain. Eventually, this condition contributes to heart attacks, strokes, and atherosclerosis. Arteries and arterioles become scarred, hardened, and less elastic later in life.

Measuring blood pressure is an easy, painless test that uses an instrument called a sphygmomanometer. After being placed around the arm above the elbow, a rubber cuff is inflated with air. This places pressure on a major artery in the arm (the brachial artery) and temporarily stops the flow of blood. The blood pressure measurement consists of determining how much pressure is necessary for the inflatable cuff to stop the blood flow in the brachial artery.

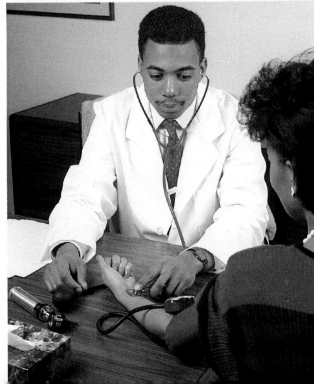

Exploring Your Health 15.2

Does Your Exercise Program Improve Cardiovascular Endurance?

In Chapter 9, you learned how to determine your target heart rate (THR). You also learned that protection from heart disease appears to occur only when your exercise program elevates your heart rate to the target level and maintains that level for twenty to thirty minutes three to four times weekly. The next time you exercise, stop in the middle of your routine (after fifteen minutes) and take your radial pulse (just below your thumb) for ten seconds and multiply this number by six to determine your beats per minute. Add 10 percent to that figure to estimate your actual exercise heart rate before you stopped to take your pulse (heart rate begins to drop immediately after cessation of exercise). An individual whose pulse rate is 25 for ten seconds, for example, records 150 beats per minute before adding 10 percent (15) for an estimated exercise heart rate of 165 beats per minute.

Is your exercise program doing the job? Compare your THR to your exercise heart rate. Are you at or above your THR? Are you too far above your THR? Adjust your exercise intensity and determine your exercise heart rate again.

Year 2000 National Health Objective

Recognizing the importance of controlling high blood pressure in the prevention of numerous diseases and disorders, the federal government has established the following national health objectives involving medical care and dietary, smoking, and exercise behaviors: (1) to reverse the increase in end-stage renal disease (requiring maintenance dialysis or transplantation) to no more than 13 per 100,000 people (13.9 per 100,000 were identified in 1987); (2) to increase to at least 50 percent the proportion of people with hypertension whose blood pressure is under control (only 24 percent of people age 18 and older had their blood pressure under control in 1982–1984); (3) to increase to at least 90 percent the proportion of people with hypertension who are taking action to help control their high blood pressure (79 percent of aware hypertensives age 18 and older were taking action in 1985); and (4) to increase to at least 90 percent the proportion of adults who have had their blood pressure measured within the preceding 2 years and can state whether their blood pressure was normal or high.

This arterial damage can lead to damage of the heart, brain, kidneys, and other organs by restricting the oxygen and nutrients needed to function properly. Hardened or narrowed arteries also increase the risk of a blood clot.

In 90 percent of high blood pressure cases (referred to as *essential hypertension*), the causes of the condition are unknown. In the remaining 10 percent (referred to as *secondary hypertension*), the condition is a symptom of problems such as kidney abnormality, tumor of the adrenal gland, or a congenital defect of the aorta. Unfortunately, many cases of hypertension have few or no symptoms. You can have dangerously high blood pressure and feel just fine. Knowledge of a number of risk factors can help you decide how often you should have your blood pressure checked. Family history of high blood pressure, obesity, Type A personality, use of a birth control pill, pregnancy, and race (black men and women are more susceptible to high blood pressure than whites) are all risk factors and necessitate relatively frequent blood pressure checks (perhaps once every 6 months; certainly at least once a year).

A nine-member group sponsored by the National High Blood Pressure Coordinating Committee has been

Classifications of Blood Pressure

Systolic Pressure (mm Hg)	Category*
140 or less	Normal
140–159	Borderline isolated systolic hypertension
160 and above	Isolated systolic hypertension

Diastolic Pressure (mm Hg)	Category*
85 or less	Normal
85–89	High normal
90–104	Mild hypertension
105–114	Moderate hypertension
115 and above	Severe hypertension

*A classification of borderline isolated systolic hypertension or isolated systolic hypertension takes precedence over a classification of high normal blood pressure when both occur in the same individual. A classification of high normal blood pressure takes precedence over a classification of normal blood pressure when both occur in the same person.

working on a redefinition of normal and abnormal blood pressure based on recent research linking hypertension with heart attack and stroke. Previously accepted normal ranges of 110–139 (systolic) and 60–90 (diastolic) are now considered too lenient. The new classification of blood pressure shown in Table 15.3 provides a scheme for categorizing arterial pressure in individuals age 18 years or over.[10]

People suffering from mild hypertension can, under a physician's supervision, treat their own condition with exercise and dietary changes. People with more severe hypertension may need antihypertensive medications such as *diuretics* to eliminate excess fluids and salt, *beta blockers* to reduce heart rate and cardiac output, *sympathetic nerve inhibitors* to inhibit the ability of nerves from the brain to constrict or narrow blood vessels, or *ACE inhibitors* that interfere with the body's production of *angiotensin*, a chemical that causes the arteries to constrict.

Obesity or Overweight

Excess weight places added strain on the heart and adversely influences blood pressure and blood cholesterol. Studies indicate that individuals who have gained more than 20 pounds since age 18 double their

risk of heart attacks. Obesity is also linked to diabetes. The location of the fat on the body may also be important. A waist/hip ratio greater than 1.0 for men and 0.8 for women indicates an increased risk. In other words, a man's waist measurement should not exceed his hip measurement and a women's waist should not be more than 80 percent of her hip measurement.

Hyperlipidemia

This refers to high blood lipid levels. See our discussion of fat and cholesterol earlier in this chapter and in Chapter 7 on nutrition.

Inactivity

Inactivity appears to contribute to early cardiovascular disease in a number of ways. Lack of exercise is often associated with obesity, high cholesterol levels, and plaque accumulation (see the next section on preventing heart disease). In addition, numerous studies have found an inverse relationship between coronary artery disease and physical fitness levels—that is, the lower the level of physical fitness, the higher the risk of coronary artery disease (see Figure 15.5). Regular aerobic exercise may also help eliminate mild hypertension, keep blood pressure normal, aid in plaque reversal when combined with aggressive nutrition changes, increase the size of the lumen or the opening of the coronary arteries (to allow more blood to pass through), increase HDL cholesterol, reduce LDL cholesterol, and reduce triglycerides. A number of studies confirm the value of aerobic exercise in reducing the risk of coronary disease, although it is important to be aware that highly fit individuals, such as runners, are not immune to heart disease and atherosclerosis.

Cigarette Smoking

The use of tobacco in any form, particularly cigarette smoking, is associated with a much higher incidence of heart disease, peripheral vascular disease (claudication), and stroke. The risk increases with the number of cigarettes smoked and heavy inhalation. Women who smoke and also use oral contraceptives have a ten times higher risk of cardiovascular disease than women who do neither. Even nonsmokers who live with smokers have a higher risk of dying from heart disease.

Birth Control Pills

The use of the contraceptive pill has been associated with a higher incidence of both heart attack and stroke in some studies and not in others. The association is stronger among those who use the pill and also smoke. Women who have used the pill for ten years or more may benefit from physician screening for symptoms of cardiovascular disease.

Diabetes

Because diabetes affects cholesterol and triglyceride levels and may damage blood vessels, it is extremely important to control other risk factors. Changes in eating and exercise habits, weight loss, and drugs (if necessary) are needed to control diabetes to avoid significant increases in the risk of heart attack and stroke.

Type A Personality

The idea that personality is an important factor in the development of heart disease was first advanced by Meyer Friedman and R. H. Rosenman in their research

Hypertension forces the heart to work harder than normal and places the arteries under strain. Many "Type A" people, who seem to thrive under stressful conditions, may actually be placing themselves at risk of damaging their hearts.

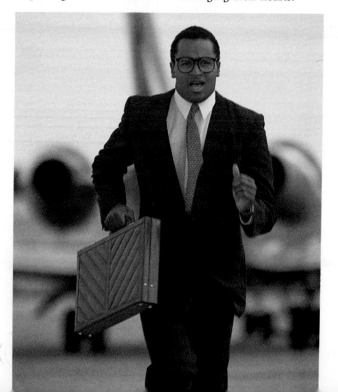

on Type A and Type B personalities. As was described in Chapter 3, the Type A individual is typically in a hurry, pressed for time, competitive, aggressive, impatient, and, beneath the surface, hostile. The Type B individual is typically unaggressive, not overly concerned with job advancement, not concerned with time pressures, more interested in family than career.

In a revised edition of their book. Friedman and Rosenman expanded their description of Type A and Type B behavior patterns. In addition to having the characteristics mentioned above, a significant number of Type A individuals eat a high-fat diet (including a high-cholesterol breakfast), have abnormally high blood cholesterol and high blood pressure, and smoke more than twenty cigarettes a day. The Type B individual is more likely to be of normal weight and blood pressure, and a nonsmoker.

This revised description of the two behavior patterns suggests that Type A behavior, in combination with other risk factors, increases the chances of early heart disease.[11] You can get an idea of your own personality behavior type by completing Exploring Your Health 15.3.

Risk Factors for Stroke

In addition to those discussed previously, several other risks exist for stroke: (1) a moderate to marked increase in the red blood cell count increases the thickness of the blood and makes clots more likely, (2) transitory ischemic attacks (TIAs precede strokes in about 10 percent of the cases and are strong predictors of stroke), and (3) asymptomatic carotid bruit, an abnormal sound heard when the stethoscope is placed over the carotid artery, which indicates atherosclerosis and is considered a serious risk factor. Drugs that inhibit clot formation and thin the blood are effective treatments for both high red blood cell counts and TIAs.[12]

Risk Reduction Strategies for Cardiovascular Disease

The college years and the third decade of life is a critical health period characterized by good-to-excellent general health. Unfortunately, it is also a time when si-

Exploring Your Health 15.3

Are You Type A or Type B?

Instructions: Opposing behavior patterns are presented in the left- and right-hand columns with a horizontal line between. Place a vertical mark across the line where you feel you belong between these two extremes. For example, most of us are neither the most competitive nor the least competitive person we know; we fall somewhere in between. Your task is to make a vertical line where you feel you belong between the two extremes.

1. Never late.	_____	Casual about appointments.
2. Not competitive.	_____	Very competitive.
3. Anticipates what others are saying.	_____	A good listener, hears others out.
4. Always rushed.	_____	Never feels rushed, even under pressure.
5. Takes things one at a time.	_____	Tries to do many things at once, thinks about what to do next.
6. Emphatic speech (may pound desk).	_____	Slow, deliberate talker.
7. Wants a good job recognized by others.	_____	Only cares about satisfying self no matter what others think.
8. Fast (eating, talking, etc.).	_____	Slow doing things.
9. Sits on feelings.	_____	Expresses feelings.
10. Easygoing.	_____	Hard driving.
11. Many interests.	_____	Few interests except work.
12. Satisfied with job.	_____	Ambitious.
13. Can wait patiently.	_____	Impatient when waiting.
14. Goes "all out."	_____	Casual.

Scoring Using a ruler, one point is scored for each $\frac{1}{16}$ inch you fall from the non-Type A behavior end of the $1\frac{1}{2}$-inch line to the point marked. Points are summed for all 14 questions. Items 2, 5, 10, 12, and 13 are measured from the *left* of the line to your mark; items 1, 3, 4, 6, 7, 8, 9, 11, and 14 are measured from the *right* of the line to your mark.

Type B average score: 178.21
Type A average score: 211.51

Source: Reprinted with permission from R. W. Bortner, "A Short Rating Scale as a Potential Measure of Pattern A Behavior," *Journal of Chronic Disease* 22. Copyright © 1969, Pergamon Press, Ltd.

lent health changes occur that may go unnoticed for another decade or two; changes that will eventually bring on early cardiovascular disease. Although it is never to late to change, the earlier in life you practice sound health, the later in life symptoms of cardiovascular disease develop. It is also important to remember that cardiovascular disease has no single cause, and therefore no single mode of prevention or cure. Although adopting one or two techniques to reduce the risk of heart disease will be helpful, a total approach is needed.

Lifestyle Changes and Medical Care

A healthy lifestyle that includes regular aerobic exercise, no tobacco or other drugs, a monitoring of the use of oral contraceptives (avoiding use altogether if you smoke), and healthy eating habits will reduce your risk of cardiovascular disease.

By scheduling regular medical checkups you can identify contributing factors to cardiovascular disease such as diabetes, high blood pressure, EKG abnormalities, compression of the arteries in the neck, and high

Exploring Your Health 15.4

Risk Factor Analysis: The Game of H-E-A-L-T-H

Carefully complete the following form to determine your risk of heart attack. Tabulate your points and compare your score with those below to secure your rating. Keep in mind that a high score does not mean you will develop heart disease; it is merely a guide to make you aware of your potential risk. Because no two people are alike, an exact prediction is impossible without carefully individualized evaluation.

	1	2	3	4	6
Heredity	No known history of heart disease	One relative with heart disease over 60 years	Two relatives with heart disease over 60 years	One relative with heart disease under 60 years	Two relatives with heart disease under 60 years
Exercise	1 Intensive exercise, work, and recreation	2 Moderate exercise, work, and recreation	3 Sedentary work and intensive recreational exercise	5 Sedentary work and moderate recreational exercise	6 Sedentary work and light recreational exercise
Age	1 10–20	2 21–30	3 31–40	4 41–50	6 51–65
Lbs.	0 More than 5 lbs below standard weight	1 ± 5 lbs standard weight	2 6–20 lbs overweight	4 21–35 lbs overweight	6 36–50 lbs overweight
Tobacco	0 Nonuser	1 Cigar or pipe	2 10 cigarettes or fewer per day	4 20 cigarettes or more per day	6 30 cigarettes or more per day
Habits of eating food	1 0% No animal or solid fats	2 10% Very little animal or solid fats	3 20% Little animal or solid fats	4 30% Much animal or solid fats	6 40% Very much animal or solid fats

Your risk of heart attack: 4–9   Very remote   16–20   Average   26–30   Dangerous
                              10–15   Below average   21–25   Moderate   31–36   Urgent danger—reduce score!
Other conditions—such as stress, high blood pressure, and increased blood cholesterol—detract from heart health and should be evaluated by your physician.

cholesterol. Mass screening of elementary school-age children, as well as high school and college students, in the areas of blood pressure and blood lipid levels would greatly assist early identification and management of heart disease. Your new lifestyle should help control borderline and moderately high risks of heart disease. Aggressive treatment, which includes medication, may be needed to control the high levels of blood pressure

Does Aspirin Prevent Heart Disease?

Can a painkiller that has been available as an over-the-counter drug for over 90 years actually help prevent death from heart disease, the nation's leading killer? A number of medical studies say yes and draw some interesting conclusions: (1) if aspirin is taken soon after the onset of symptoms of a heart attack, the chances of death from a heart attack in the ensuing months are reduced; (2) the risk of having a stroke due to clotting is reduced by taking aspirin on a regular basis; (3) the risk of a second heart attack occurring is reduced in heart attack patients who take aspirin on a daily basis; and (4) aspirin may improve the immune system. Proponents of aspirin use point out that blood clots that become attached to fatty deposits in arteries and cut off blood supply cause heart attacks and strokes. These clots are caused in part by the clumping of blood cells called platelets. Aspirin inhibits platelets from clumping by reducing the *prostaglandins* responsible for the platelets' stickiness. As a result, the risk of a heart attack is reduced. Advocates of regular aspirin use emphasize the importance of consulting a physician before going on an aspirin regimen.

Opponents of the aspirin therapy point out that too much medical "hype" stirs up the American public who will "jump on the aspirin bandwagon" without consultation with a physician. The results could be dangerous. Already, the Food and Drug Administration has threatened legal action and forced the drug industry to remove aspirin advertisements that promote its use for preventing heart attack from the media. Too much aspirin interferes with blood clotting and increases the risk of internal bleeding. Studies have found a higher risk of stroke from brain hemorrhage in individuals who took only one aspirin tablet daily. Although aspirin may help in one area, the drug may be harmful in another and pose certain risks. For individuals with angina or a family history of heart disease, the benefits may outweigh the risks. For others, however, the risks may be too high. The best way to prevent heart disease, it is argued, is to change unhealthy habits, not to rely on aspirin to counter their effects.

What do you think? Should aspirin be used as preventive medication for all adults? Should the use of aspirin be restricted to those in the high-risk group?

---

or blood serum cholesterol. With an aggressive approach, for example, research shows that you can actually reverse some of the damaging plaque buildup in your arteries.[13]

Nutrition and Diet

As we indicated in Chapter 7, a diet low in saturated fat, cholesterol, salt, and calories, which provides adequate nutrition and maintains an ideal weight, will help regulate blood cholesterol and perhaps slow plaque buildup in key arteries. Having two to three meatless meals weekly, avoiding red meats, increasing consumption of fish high in omega-3 fatty acids (anchovies, herring, mackerel, sablefish, salmon, fresh tuna, mullet, ocean perch, pollack, rainbow trout, sea trout, smelt, and oysters), increasing the intake of complex carbohydrates, and eliminating alcohol are also important factors in the prevention of cardiovascular disease.

Aerobic Exercise

Aerobic exercise three to four times weekly for 20–30 minutes at a level of intensity above your target heart rate (see Chapter 9) produces numerous changes that may help prevent cardiovascular disease. In addition to reducing some of the most critical coronary risk factors (see Table 15.4), aerobic exercise increases the diame-

TABLE 15.4

Exercise and Coronary Risk Factors

Risk Factor	Effect of Regular Physical Exercise
Obesity and overweight	Reduction of body fat, return to ideal weight.
High lipid levels	Reduction of atherogenic fatty particles in the blood.
Hypertension	Aid in the control of blood pressure.
Tension and stress	Increased tolerance of stress, release of tension and nervous or emotional energy.
Lack of physical activity	No longer a risk factor for the exercising person.
Genetic history	No change.
Smoking	Changes in smoking habits are likely to take place.
Age	Slows aging process.

ter of the arteries to allow more space for blood flow. It also lowers resting heart and breathing rate, and improves the general efficiency of the cardiorespiratory system. Evidence indicates that men and women who

Get Involved!

Getting to the Heart of Risk Reduction for Cardiovascular Disease

Some health care professionals predict an end to cardiovascular disease for those born after the year 2025. However, these professionals are not predicting a magic cure by then, but rather a comprehensive change and a general improvement in lifestyles, eating and exercise habits, and fitness and nutrition education. Whether you realize it or not, you are a part of this comprehensive change and improvement—by reading this textbook and participating in this health course, as well as by making smart health choices in your own life. Become an even more active participant in your own and other peoples' cardiovascular health by implementing some of these suggestions:

1. Arrange a "fast food night" within the university and secure speakers from the fast food industry, the health education department, the school of medicine, and the department of nutrition. Fast food eating is here to stay for college students. Build the program around the prudent use of fast food and the selection of sound food items that are reasonably low in calories, salt, saturated fat, and cholesterol.

2. In cooperation with your instructor, meet with the department of health and physical education in your university to discuss bulletin board displays on healthy heart eating and special programs for the entire student body on preventing heart disease.

3. Master the art of food label reading and teach your new-found skills to friends and family. Wise food purchasing of items low in fat, cholesterol, salt, and calories is an important first step in the prevention of cardiovascular disease.

4. Identify area restaurants that include heart healthy foods on their menu. Prepare a list of these restaurants for the university community.

5. Ask your university dietitian to speak to your class about the food served in the cafeteria. Students are quite uninformed about the nutritional soundness of university meals, and are often unaware of the careful planning involved in providing balanced, healthy meals to the student body.

stay within the *good-to-excellent* category on the 1.5 mile test (see Chapter 9) for their age group have a lowered incidence of cardiovascular disease at all ages.[14]

Medical Solutions to Cardiovascular Disease

Thanks to numerous medical advances, heart disease can be successfully treated with drugs, balloon angioplasty, bypass surgery, and human and artificial heart transplants.

Drug Therapy

Immediate treatment with drugs called "clotbusters" while a heart attack or stroke is in progress can partially stop the heart attack and significantly reduce damage to the heart muscle or brain by dissolving clots that form on fatty plaques. This recent breakthrough in drug therapy highlights the importance of seeking medical attention as soon as any symptoms of cardiovascular disease appear. To be effective, treatment must be initiated promptly after symptoms appear.

Drug therapy is also available to lower blood pressure, increase cardiac output in congestive heart failure, relieve the pain of angina, and control arrhythmias.

Coronary Bypass

More than 200,000 bypasses are performed in the United States annually, with a mortality rate of approximately 2 percent.[15] Portions of a vein from the patient's leg are grafted onto one or several coronary arteries to detour blood around blocked areas. Studies indicate that some bypass surgery is unnecessary and is not much more effective in prolonging the life of patients with mild to moderate angina (except those with significant obstructions in the left main artery) than drug therapy and lifestyle changes. In approximately 80 percent of bypass patients, the grafts develop blockages within 10 years. For individuals with left main artery clogging or severe clogging in multiple arteries, bypass surgery may be the only alternative.

FIGURE 15.6 • Angioplasty

1. A small tube (called a catheter) is inserted into an artery in the arm or leg and gently guided to an area of blockage.

2. A smaller tube topped with a balloon is then threaded through the catheter until it is in place at the blockage.

3. Then the balloon is slowly inflated several times, flattening fatty plaque deposits against artery walls, which widens the passage for increased blood flow.

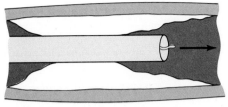 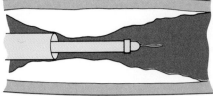 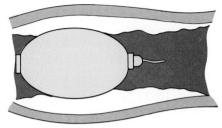

1. Guide catheter is inserted into blocked area

2. Thinner balloon-tipped tube is threaded through catheter and catheter is pulled back so that balloon is positioned at area of fatty plaque buildup

3. Balloon is inflated several times and withdrawn through catheter

Coronary Angioplasty and Lasers

Balloon angioplasty is a less dangerous approach than coronary bypass surgery to unclogging arteries. A catheter is inserted into an artery in the arm or leg, and guided to the blocked artery in the heart. A small tube with a tiny balloon at its tip is then threaded through the larger tube until it reaches the plaque-clogged area. The balloon is then inflated to squeeze the plaque against the artery walls in order to increase the area for the flow of blood (see Figure 15.6). Over 100,000 balloon angioplasties are performed annually; approximately 1–3 percent of angioplasty patients die and another 5 percent eventually need bypass surgery.[16] The technique is effective in 85 percent of all patients; however, the same artery will eventually clog again in 30–40 percent of the cases.

Laser surgery shows promise as a technique to clean out clogged arteries by burning away fatty deposits to clear the way for blood flow. Short bursts of intense laser light vaporize the plaque. Laser-heated thermal probes, hot balloons, and catheter tip turbines are also being tested as additional alternatives to bypass surgery.

Heart Transplants and Artificial Hearts

A new heart is the only cure for a variety of heart disorders. Survival rates for human heart transplant patients have greatly improved in recent years, largely due to drugs that prevent rejection of the new heart. Over 80 percent of human heart recipients are alive after one year, more than 50 percent survive for five years, and 67 percent of the survivors are in good health.

Artificial hearts may have their place as temporary replacements to keep a patient alive until a human heart can be located. All five initial recipients of artificial hearts developed serious complications, including strokes, and all died. Researchers are pursuing new approaches to artificial hearts, including those not dependent on external power sources.

Conclusion

Diseases of the cardiovascular system, particularly heart disease and stroke, represent major health problems in the United States. These chronic and degenerative diseases appear to begin in the first decade of life and slowly and silently progress until, much later, they strike. By the time first symptoms appear, such as angina pains or high blood pressure, preventive techniques have lost much of their effectiveness, although lifestyle changes may still delay the progression of the disease.

Several factors contribute to cardiovascular disease: sex, race, obesity, high blood lipid levels, hypertension, stress, sedentary living, smoking, diabetes, genetic makeup, contraceptive pills, and the aging process. Most of these factors are directly related to lifestyle. Only genetic makeup, sex, race, and the aging process are uncontrollable. Taking charge of your life can greatly reduce the risk of early coronary heart disease and stroke.

Summary

1. The most common form of cardiovascular disease and stroke is atherosclerosis, resulting from plaque buildup in the two coronary arteries and their branches, which supply blood and oxygen to the heart muscle, and the carotid arteries, which supply oxygen to the brain. It is a silent disease that begins in childhood and appears to accelerate in the third decade of life (age 20 to 30).

2. Atherosclerosis is caused by a high number of fats in the bloodstream, resulting from a high-cholesterol diet.

3. Although several drugs approved by the FDA lower LDL cholesterol and raise HDL cholesterol, diet and exercise remain the initial treatment for most people.

4. Clogging of the coronary arteries may result in a heart attack from artery closure or angina pectoris from a partial closure that limits oxygen supply to the heart and produces pain.

5. A mild stroke occurs when the brain is deprived of adequate blood supply for a short period of time. Transitory ischemic attacks are warning signs of clogging in the vessels supplying the brain. Many victims of stroke make significant progress toward a complete recovery.

6. The exact cause of many cases of sudden cardiac death, common in middle-age and older men and women, is still unknown.

7. Heart problems in children generally involve congenital defects or damage to the heart muscle following rheumatic fever or prolonged upper respiratory streptococcal infections (strep throat).

8. Heart disease and stroke can be prevented through diagnosis and sound lifestyle choices (regular exercise, absence of smoking, maintenance of normal body weight and body fat, and a careful diet that manages intake of saturated and unsaturated fat). These lifestyle choices are most beneficial when begun early in life and continued throughout adulthood.

9. Exercise contributes to a reduction in the incidence of early heart disease and stroke by controlling body weight and fat, increasing the amount of HDL in the blood, reducing blood fibrin levels, increasing the diameter of the arteries, and improving the efficiency of the heart and circulatory system.

10. Research shows that burning 1,200 calories weekly during aerobic exercise reduces the risk of heart attack by 20–25 percent, burning 2,000 calories reduces the risk by 35 percent, and burning 5,000 calories by 50 percent. These calories can be burned through a combination of different exercise programs.

11. Nonsmokers who live with a smoker have a 20–30 percent higher risk of dying from heart disease than do other nonsmokers.

12. In 90 percent of the cases, the cause of high blood pressure is unknown. While exercise and diet changes may help control mild hypertension, others may need to resort to antihypertensive medications.

13. Approximately 3 to 4 million Americans suffer from silent ischemia without pain and may have a heart attack without actually knowing it.

14. The incidence of heart disease and stroke is declining in the United States.

15. Individuals should consult with their physicians before resorting to aspirin therapy as a technique to prevent a heart attack or stroke. Evidence suggests that the risks for some individuals exceed the benefits.

16. Studies have shown evidence of plaque reversal in the coronary arteries following an aggressive therapy to lower blood cholesterol. Such a therapy consists of a healthy heart diet, regular aerobic exercise, and medication.

Questions for Personal Growth

1. Are you at risk for heart disease in the future? Identify those factors that you anticipate will play a role in the development of heart disease in ten or twenty years. Develop a five point plan to reduce your risk of future difficulty.

2. Do you have a healthy heart diet? Analyze your fat and cholesterol intake and identify the major sources of each in your diet. What changes can you make to reduce your total dietary fat intake, particularly saturated fat and cholesterol?

3. How does your current exercise program measure up? Do you engage in a regular aerobic exercise program four times weekly, at your target heart rate, for twenty to thirty continuous minutes? If not, your program is not very effective in helping you manage blood lipids or in providing protection from heart disease. Consider another exercise program and give it a try for several months.

4. Complete the game of H-E-A-L-T-H for your parents (see Exploring Your Health 15.4). Identify their overall risk of heart disease and the specific risk factors over which they have control. Discuss a complete program to reduce their risk of cardiovascular disease.

5. Sudden cardiac arrest is more common in adults who have recently experienced a single traumatic experience, such as a vicious argument, an auto accident, or an outburst of anger. Identify the high-stress situations in the life of your parents and discuss the dangers as well as ways to avoid the situations.

6. Heart disease is a pediatric problem that begins very early in life, by age 3. Do you have brothers and sisters or children of your own? If so, examine their eating and exercise behavior and devise a plan to make needed changes.

7. You can avoid problems with varicose veins in the future by making some changes now. If you are concerned about varicose veins or have a history of the problem in your family, devise a plan that you can begin to follow immediately to prevent early wear and tear on the veins in your lower extremities.

8. Now that you have had an opportunity to identify your basic personality type, analyze your typical day and identify some changes to make things less hurried, stressful, and anxiety ridden. Consider the typical things you do in a normal day and how you approach them. Record your suggestions on a 3" × 5" card and carry it with you, referring to the suggestions on a regular basis until the changes are permanent.

References

1. American Heart Association, *1990 Heart Facts* (Dallas: American Heart Association, 7320 Greenville Avenue, Zip Code 75231).

2. K. H. Cooper, *Controlling Cholesterol* (New York: Bantam Books, 1988).

3. George B. Dintiman, Robert G. Davis, Jude C. Pennington, and Stephen S. Stone, *Discovering Lifetime Fitness: Concepts of Fitness and Weight Control* (St. Paul, Minn.: West, 1989).

4. American Heart Association, *1990 Heart Facts.*

5. Ibid.

6. American Heart Association, *1990 Stroke Facts* (1990).

7. David Monagan, "Sudden Death," *Discover* (January 1986): 64–71.

8. American Heart Association, *1990 Heart Facts.*

9. Ibid.

10. Joint National Committee on Detection, Evaluation, and Treatment of High Blood Pressure, NIH Publication No. 84-10088 (Washington, D.C.: U.S. Department of Health and Human Services, 1986).

11. Meyer Friedman and Diane Ulmer, *Treating Type A Behavior and Your Heart* (New York: Knopf, 1974), pp. 193–207.

12. American Heart Association, *1990 Heart Facts.*

13. "Reversing Heart Disease," *U.S. News and World Report* (August 6, 1990): 5.

14. K. H. Cooper, *Controlling Cholesterol.*

15. Judy Ismach, "Halt That Heart Attack," *American Health* (January–February 1988).

16. Kenneth Kent, "Coronary Angioplasty: A Decade of Experience," *New England Journal of Medicine* (April 30, 1987).

CHAPTER OBJECTIVES

After reading this chapter, you should understand:

- That cancer is not a single disease, but rather a group of more than 100 diseases that involve abnormal cell growth.

- Some of the things that cause various types of cancer, including occupational and environmental agents, viruses, radiation, and hereditary factors.

- Several common cancers, such as bladder, breast, colorectal, and prostate cancer, as well as specific forms of diagnosis and treatment for each of them.

- General forms of diagnosis and treatment for cancers, including traditional technologies such as radiation therapy, chemotherapy, and surgery, as well as newer technologies such as the use of high-tech diagnostic equipment, interferon, and genetic research.

- Specific strategies for reducing your own and other peoples' risk of getting cancer.

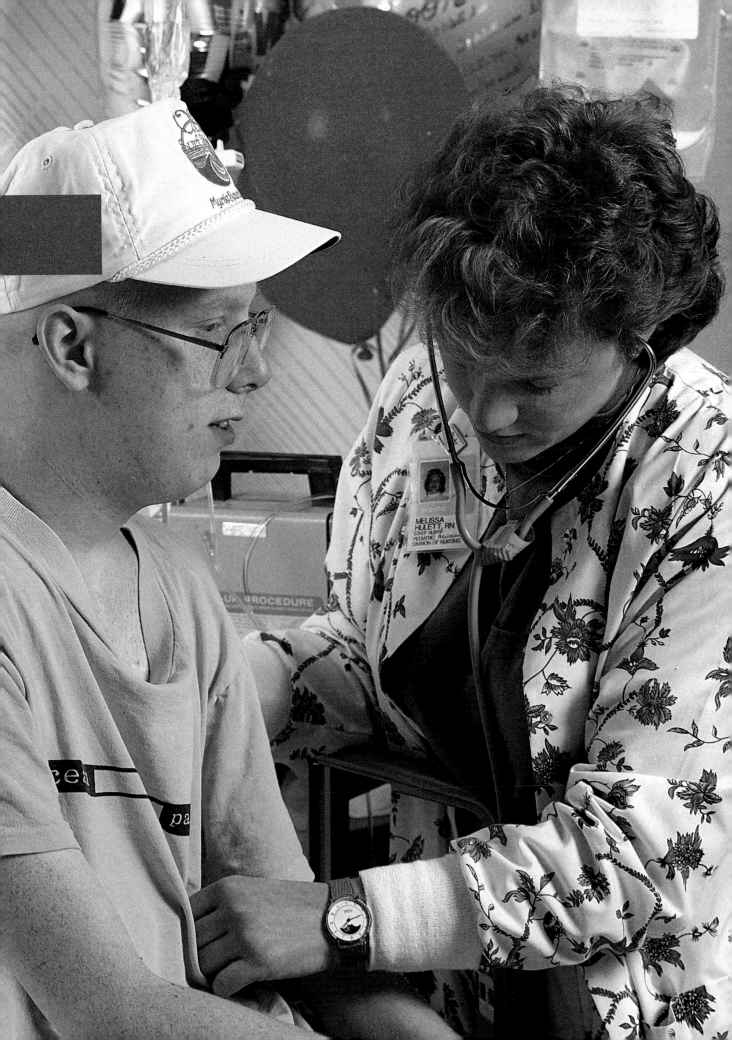

cancer Not a single disease, but a group of more than 100 diseases that are characterized by abnormal cell growth.

metastasis The spread of cancer cells through the circulatory and lymphatic systems to other parts of the body, causing cancer in new areas of the body.

remission A situation in which cancer remains asymptomatic, when it ceases to grow or to spread, or when it disappears.

carcinomas Cancers that begin in the epithelial cells (the linings) of the lungs, digestive organs, reproductive organs, mouth, and other body cavities.

sarcomas Cancers that arise in the mesodermal or middle layers of the tissues that form the bones, muscles, and connective tissues.

lymphomas Cancers that begin in the infection-fighting regions of the body—principally the lymphatic system.

Cancer is one of the leading killers in the United States, second only to heart disease. Over 510,000 people will die from cancer this year (13,977 people a day, about one every 62 seconds), and about 30 percent of the American population or 76 million people will eventually develop cancer. An estimated 1,040,000 new cases were diagnosed in 1990.[1] In spite of this data, however, the future looks encouraging. A cure has already been found for some types of cancer, and with continued public education and early detection, cure rates will continue to rise. New treatment methods and greater public awareness also offer hope in terms of both prevention and cure. Evidence suggesting that lifestyle is a significant factor in the prevention of certain types of cancer has encouraged millions of Americans to quit smoking, initiate aerobic exercise programs, alter nutritional habits, use regular self-examination techniques, avoid contact with known carcinogens, and stay informed of recent medical advances. These lifestyle changes will help to reduce the incidence of various types of cancer in the future. Researchers also continue to uncover information that brings us closer to the eradication of this dreaded disease.

What Is Cancer?

Cancer is not a single disease but rather a group of more than 100 diseases involving abnormal cell growth. In normal body cells, the rate of cell division is under precise control. Cancer cells, in contrast, grow wildly, divide rapidly, and assume irregular shapes; tumors develop and invade nearby normal tissue. These abnormal cells eventually spread to distant body areas via the blood and lymphatic system; this process of spreading is referred to as **metastasis** (see Figure 16.1). The spread of cancer to other body parts has already occurred in six of ten patients at the time of diagnosis. For those individuals, eradicating the deadly cells is much more difficult.

Cancer is capable of destroying the body in a number of ways, eventually resulting in death. Cancer cells actively divide and crowd out normal specialized cells; they rob vital nutrients from and "starve" nor-

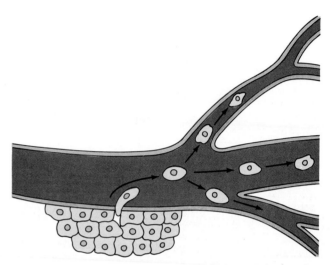

FIGURE 16.1 • Metastasis is a process in which cancerous cells entering a blood vessel spread to distant body areas.

mal cells. Eventually, normal tissues, organs, and body systems cannot perform their vital functions and death occurs. Malignant tumors may obstruct blood vessels, the digestive and urinary tracts, or other body parts, eliminating the normal function of an entire system or organ. Tumors may also decrease or eliminate the intake or absorption of nutrients causing the body literally to waste away, or they may decrease the capacity of the lungs to oxygenate blood. In addition, the body's immune system is weakened and death may occur from the inability to fight invading pathogens. Patients are considered cured if there is no evidence of cancer for five years; others may survive in **remission**, an asymptomatic state in which the spread of cancerous cells is assumed to be temporarily stopped.

Year 2000 National Health Objective

Cancer is the nation's second leading killer. To reverse the rise in overall cancer deaths, one national health objective seeks to achieve a cancer-caused fatality rate of no more than 130 people per 100,000 people. In 1987, 330 deaths occurred per 100,000 from some form of cancer.

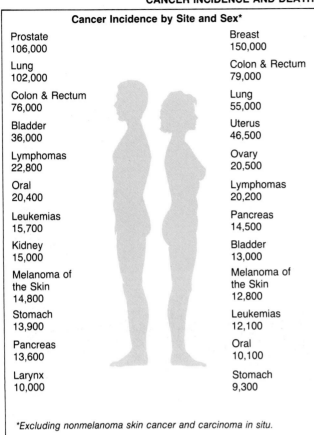

Cancer Incidence by Site and Sex*	
Prostate 106,000	Breast 150,000
Lung 102,000	Colon & Rectum 79,000
Colon & Rectum 76,000	Lung 55,000
Bladder 36,000	Uterus 46,500
Lymphomas 22,800	Ovary 20,500
Oral 20,400	Lymphomas 20,200
Leukemias 15,700	Pancreas 14,500
Kidney 15,000	Bladder 13,000
Melanoma of the Skin 14,800	Melanoma of the Skin 12,800
Stomach 13,900	Leukemias 12,100
Pancreas 13,600	Oral 10,100
Larynx 10,000	Stomach 9,300

*Excluding nonmelanoma skin cancer and carcinoma in situ.

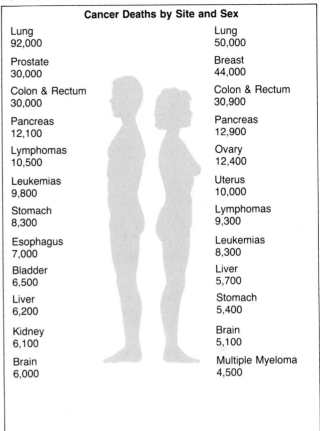

Cancer Deaths by Site and Sex	
Lung 92,000	Lung 50,000
Prostate 30,000	Breast 44,000
Colon & Rectum 30,000	Colon & Rectum 30,900
Pancreas 12,100	Pancreas 12,900
Lymphomas 10,500	Ovary 12,400
Leukemias 9,800	Uterus 10,000
Stomach 8,300	Lymphomas 9,300
Esophagus 7,000	Leukemias 8,300
Bladder 6,500	Liver 5,700
Liver 6,200	Stomach 5,400
Kidney 6,100	Brain 5,100
Brain 6,000	Multiple Myeloma 4,500

FIGURE 16.2 • Selected Cancer Sites.

Source: Data from the American Cancer Society, *Cancer Facts and Figures* (1990).

The various forms of cancer are named according to the type of tissue involved. **Carcinomas** begin in the epithelial cells, which form the lining of the lungs, digestive organs, reproductive organs, skin, mouth, and other body cavities. Carcinomas tend to spread through the circulatory or lymphatic system forming solid tumors. With early detection, treatment can be successful. A second major type of cancer arises in the mesodermal or middle layers of tissue that form the bones, muscles, and connective tissue. **Sarcomas,** as these are known, tend to spread through the blood stream forming solid tumors. Although less common, they are more difficult to treat and control. **Lymphomas** develop in the infection-fighting regions of the body and metastasize through the lymph system, forming solid tumors. Hodgkin's disease, an example of one type of lymphoma, is now being successfully treated. *Leukemia* is a cancer of the blood-forming parts of the body, such as the bone marrow and spleen. These nonsolid tumors are characterized by an abnormally high number of white blood cells. Treatment advances have greatly extended life in many patients. Sites for cancer and incidence by sex are shown in Figure 16.2.

Use Exploring Your Health 16.1 to reveal your knowledge about cancer.

Causes of Cancer

Researchers theorize that cancer is produced from a basic change in the nucleic acid chain located in the nucleus of the cell. DNA (deoxyribonucleic acid) may control the rate of cell division. RNA (ribonucleic acid) appears to assist DNA with this control. It is believed that factors inside or outside the cell may act on the DNA or RNA through a physical or chemical disturbance and result in abnormal, erratic cell division.

The World Health Organization estimates that up to 85 percent of all cancer cases are the result of exposure to environmental factors. Of the 1,400 chemicals, drugs, and pollutants suspected of causing cancer, 22 have been declared carcinogenic to humans. Uncovering cancer-causing substances is no easy task and is complicated by three problems: the twenty- to thirty-five year "latent" period between exposure and symptoms of the disease occurring, the amount of exposure that produces cancer, and the controversy over whether animal test results can be applied to humans. Regardless of these obstacles, it is evident that the environment has become a major target of cancer researchers (see Table 16.1).

Exploring Your Health 16.1

Misconceptions About Cancer

A complicated, baffling disease such as cancer is subject to considerable speculation and misinformation. To find out what you know about cancer, complete the following true-false test.

	True	False
1. Cancer is contagious.	T	F
2. Cancer may be caused by a single injury to the body.	T	F
3. Use of aluminum cooking utensils causes cancer.	T	F
4. The chances of contracting cancer are increased by even light or moderate consumption of alcohol.	T	F
5. The use of synthetic or chemical fertilizers rather than organic types causes cancer.	T	F
6. Water fluoridation causes cancer.	T	F
7. Breast tumors are always malignant.	T	F
8. Vaccination for smallpox leaves one more susceptible to cancer.	T	F
9. Birth control pills cause cancer.	T	F
10. Cancer cannot be cured once it is discovered in the body.	T	F

Scoring Give yourself one point for each correct answer. If you marked all items false, you have a perfect score. Each of the statements is incorrect.

Asbestos, a naturally occurring mineral used in insulation and fireproofing, has been shown to contribute to cancer formation. Asbestos removal for many older buildings is a necessary, dangerous, and potentially very lucrative business.

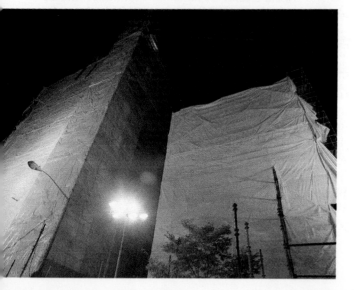

Occupational Agents

Certain physical and chemical environmental agents tend to contribute to cancer formation. In 1775, coal soot was identified as a contributor to cancer of the scrotum. One hundred years later, during the Industrial Revolution, a type of lubricating oil constantly sprinkled on men working beside cotton-spinning machines was also linked to this type of cancer. The air in mines contains a fine radioactive dust which can cause lung cancer in miners. During the 1920s, bone cancer was observed in factory workers who painted numbers on the hands of watch faces with a radium compound to make them glow in the dark. By twirling the end of a fine brush in their mouths to acquire a "tip" before dipping the brush into the compound, the workers absorbed minute quantities of radium, which eventually worked into the bones.

Among the occupational agents suspected of con-

Congenital causes, or cancer occurring during the development of the embryo during the prenatal period, involve a few special groups of tumors affecting infants, children, and young adults. Congenital tumors (most are benign) account for only a small fraction of tumors and cancer.

New findings in genetics have identified the importance of **oncogenes;** the genes found in tumor cells whose activation is associated with the transformation of normal cells into cancer cells. An analysis of the products of these oncogenes may predict which tumors are likely to recur after surgery.

Precancerous Conditions

Some precancerous conditions—but not all—tend to develop into cancer, with the cause of cancer being the same as the cause for the precancerous condition. Benign tumors, a mass or overgrowth of cells in the mouth, lip, tongue, or cheek or a patch of cells on the skin (small scab, scaly patch, brown to black warts) fall into the category of precancerous conditions. Moles are not precancerous, and the average person has about twenty-two to twenty-three of them. A mole that is constantly irritated is much more likely to become malignant. Benign tumors should be removed as soon

as possible, regardless of how low the probability of developing cancer is.

Tobacco Use

As we saw in Chapter 12, there is a strong link between tobacco use and lung cancer, cancer of the lip and mouth, and cancer of the pharynx, larynx, esophagus, pancreas, and bladder. Smoking accounts for approximately 30 percent of all cancers. The incidence of lung cancer is related to the number of cigarettes smoked, the degree of inhalation, and the number of years one has smoked. The American Cancer Society estimates that cigarette smoking is responsible for 85 percent of

Year 2000
National Health Objective

Smoking and other uses of tobacco are the most preventable causes of cancer. In recognition of this fact, one national health objective is to reduce cigarette smoking to a prevalence of no more than 15 percent among people age 20 and over, compared to 29 percent in 1987 for people in the same age group.

lung cancer cases among men and 43 percent among women—more than 75 percent overall.[3] The gap between male and female levels of lung cancer has been narrowing, due to the increased number of women who have been smoking for ten years or more. Use of smokeless tobacco also increases the risk of cancer of the mouth, larynx, throat, and esophagus.

Other Cancer Risk Factors

Estrogen Use of estrogen treatment to control menopause symptoms increases the risk of endometrial cancer. Only after individual evaluations by a physician should estrogen therapy be used.

Alcohol Excessive alcohol consumption in any form increases the risk of oral cancer and cancers of the larynx, throat, esophagus, and liver, especially when accompanied by cigarette smoking or the use of smokeless tobacco.

Nutrition The risk of colon, breast, and uterine cancer increases in obese individuals. High-fat diets may be associated with the development of cancer of the breast, colon, and prostate; and salt-cured, smoked, and nitrite-cured foods have been linked to esophageal and stomach cancer.

Obesity Available data from the first two years (1986 and 1987) of the American Cancer Society's Cancer Prevention Study II indicate that the cancer mortality rate of men who are 40 percent or more overweight is 2.25 times higher than for men of average weight. Obese women were 1.5 times as likely to die of cancer as women of average weight.

Some Common Cancers and Their Detection

A list of seven warning signals for cancer has been developed by the American Cancer Society (see Table 16.2). These symptoms may be an indication of other,

TABLE 16.2

Cancer's 7 Warning Signals

Change in bowel or bladder habits.
A sore that does not heal.
Unusual bleeding or discharge.
Thickening or lump in breast or elsewhere.
Indigestion or difficulty in swallowing.
Obvious change in wart or mole.
Nagging cough or hoarseness.
If *you* have a warning signal, see your doctor!

Source: Reprinted by permission of the American Cancer Society.

less serious ailments. Nonetheless, they should be brought to the immediate attention of a physician.

Early detection requires that you become alert to changes in your body. For people without symptoms of cancer, the American Cancer Society has developed guidelines for cancer-related checkups by age (Table 16.3).

Let's discuss some of the most common cancers and their symptoms. We'll also briefly discuss specific diagnoses and treatments for each cancer as needed, although this chapter also features a separate section on cancer treatment in general.

Bladder Cancer

An estimated 49,000 new cases of bladder cancer were diagnosed in 1990 (36,000 in men, 13,000 in women) and approximately 9,700 people died of this disease. Symptoms include blood in the urine and increased frequency of urination. The greatest single risk factor is smoking, which is estimated to be responsible for 47 percent of all bladder cancer deaths among men and for 37 percent among women.

Diagnostic techniques include the visual examination of the bladder wall with a cystoscope. Surgery or surgery in combination with other treatments is re-

Recommended Guidelines for Selected Cancer Diagnostic Tests in People Without Symptoms

Type of Cancer	Diagnostic Test	Frequency/Special Notes
Lung	Chest x-ray	Not recommended in the absence of symptoms
	Sputum Analysis	Not recommended in the absence of symptoms
Breast	Self-examination	Monthly after the age of 20
	Physician's Exam	Once every 3 years between 20–40 Once every year after age 40
	Mammography	Baseline mammogram between ages of 35–39 Mammogram every 1–2 yrs for women between ages of 40–49 Mammogram every year after 50
Uterus	Pelvic Exam	Every 3 years between ages of 20–40* Every year after age of 40
	Pap Smear	Every 3 years after two initial negative tests one year apart
	Endometrial Tissue Sample	At menopause if at risk
Colon & Rectal	Digital Exam	Every year after age of 40
	Stool Blood Test (Guaiac Slide)	Every year after age of 50
	Sigmoidoscopy	Every 3–5 years after two initial negative tests 1 year apart
Prostate	Digital Exam	Every year after the age of 40 with regular physical
Testicular	Self-examination	Monthly after age of 20

*includes women under 20 if sexually active
Source: American Cancer Society, 1987.

sponsible for a five-year survival rate of 87 percent when detected in the localized state; 43 percent and 9 percent respectively, when regional and distant disease is involved.

Bone Cancer

Cancer of the bone is most common in children and young adults between the ages of 10 and 20. It strikes approximately 2,100 people each year and causes 1,100 deaths. Malignant bone tumors develop in the skeletal system (primary tumors), develop outside the bone but metastasize into skeletal tissue (secondary tumors), or involve related benign conditions that may develop into cancer. Although injury and an increased production of a growth factor are suspect, the cause remains unknown. The most common symptom is pain in a bone or joint, generally in regions of the knee, thigh, arm, ribs, and pelvis. Unexplained swelling may also be a symptom of an expanding tumor.

Bone cancer treatment may involve surgery (removal of bone sections or amputation), chemotherapy, and radiation therapy. Survival rates have been stead-ily increasing even for osteogenic sarcoma, the most common form of bone cancer, where 30 percent of children are alive and well for three to five years after treatment.

Breast Cancer

This leading cause of cancer deaths (150,900 new cases in 1990, 44,300 deaths) involves approximately one out of every ten women at some time. Symptoms include breast changes that persist such as lumps, thickening, swelling, dimpling, skin irritation, distortion, retraction or scaliness of the nipple, and nipple pain, discharge, or tenderness, and swollen lymph nodes under the armpit. Most lumps in the breast are not cancerous; however, any lump should be carefully examined by a physician. Risk factors include age (over 50), family history, a first childbirth after age 30, or childlessness.

Early detection is critical. Breast self-examination should take place monthly for all women over 20 years of age one week after the end of their menstrual period (see Exploring Your Health 16.2). It is important to

mammography A radiological medical test to diagnose cancer of the breast.

Pap test A simple test used to diagnose precancerous and cancerous conditions of the cervix and uterus.

Exploring Your Health 16.2

Breast Self-Examination

Master the following technique and examine your breasts during your bath or shower once per month. Regular examination will soon get you used to the normal feel of your breast. Keep a record of your examination dates and the results. Indicate the type and location of any nodule, changes in the contour of each breast, swelling, dimpling of skin, changes in the nipple, or any discharge. Consult your physician immediately if you notice any of these symptoms.

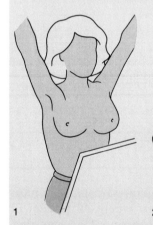

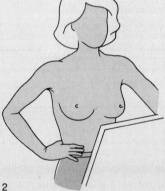

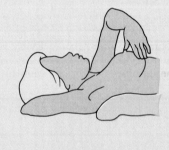

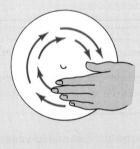

1   2   3   4

1. In the shower. Examine your breasts during your bath or shower, since hands glide more easily over wet skin. Hold your fingers flat and move them gently over every part of each breast. Use the right hand to examine the left breast and the left hand for the right breast. Check for any lump, hard knot, or thickening.

2. Before a mirror. Inspect your breasts with arms at your sides. Next, raise your arms high overhead. Look for any changes in the contour of each breast: a swelling, dimpling of skin, or changes in the nipple.

Then rest your palms on your hips and press down firmly to flex your chest muscles. Left and right breast will not exactly match—few women's breasts do. Again look for changes and irregularities. Regular inspection shows what is normal for you and will give you confidence in your examination.

3. Lying down. To examine your right breast, put a pillow or folded towel under your right shoulder. Place your right hand behind your head: this distributes tissue more evenly on the chest. With the left hand, fingers flat, press gently in small circular motions around an imaginary clockface. Begin at outermost top of your right breast for 12 o'clock, then move to 1 o'clock and so on around the circle back to 12. (A ridge of firm tissue in the lower curve of each breast is normal).

4. Then move 1 inch inward, toward the nipple and keep circling to examine every part of your breast, including the nipple. This requires at least three more circles. Now slowly repeat the procedure on your left breast with a pillow under your left shoulder and left hand behind your head. Notice how your breast structure feels.

Finally, squeeze the nipple of each breast gently between thumb and index finger. Any discharge, clear or bloody, should be reported to your doctor immediately.

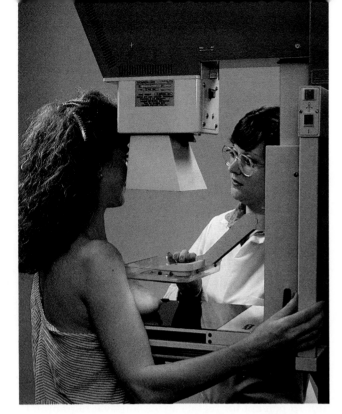

Monthly breast self-examination should be supplemented by mammography if any irregularities in breast tissue are found or if the woman is experiencing any pain or swelling of the breasts that cannot be linked to the menstrual period or other obvious causes. Mammography can detect cancers that are still too small to feel. The American Cancer Society therefore recommends that women who are not in a high-risk group should have one mammogram between the ages of 35 and 39, one every one or two years between the ages of 40 and 49, and one every year after age 50.

Year 2000 National Health Objective

One national health objective aims at the reduction of breast cancer deaths to no more than 20.6 per 100,000 women. In 1987, 22.9 per 100,000 women died from breast cancer. In addition, an attempt is being made to increase to at least 80 percent the proportion of women age 40 and older, who receive a clinical breast examination and a mammogram, and to increase to at least 60 percent the proportion of women age 50 and older who have received mammograms within the preceding one to two years. In 1987, only 36 percent of women age 40 and older, and 25 percent of women age 50 and older met this objective. The federal government will also ensure that mammograms meet quality standards by monitoring and certifying at least 80 percent of mammography facilities. In 1990, an estimated 18 to 21 percent were certified by the American College of Radiology.

complete the examination at the same time each month. **Mammography** (x-ray examination with low level radiation) is effective in revealing cancers too small to be felt by an examiner.

Treatment of breast cancer may involve *lumpectomy* (local removal of the tumor), *mastectomy* (removal of the entire breast), *radical mastectomy* (removal of the breast and the surrounding areas), radiation therapy, chemotherapy, hormone manipulation therapy, or the use of two or more methods in combination. New breast reconstruction techniques after a mastectomy have produced excellent results.[4] The five-year survival rate for localized breast cancer is 90 percent, 68 percent for cancer that has spread regionally and 18 percent for distant metastases.

Ovarian Cancer

This disease is often silent, showing no symptoms until late in its development. An enlarged abdomen is the most common sign. Women over 40, who have persistent, unexplained vague digestive disturbances, such as stomach discomfort, gas, and distention may need a thorough evaluation for ovarian cancer. There were an estimated 20,500 new cases and 12,400 deaths from ovarian cancer in 1990. Factors such as age at first live birth, age at first pregnancy, and the number of pregnancies appear to be associated with the development of ovarian cancer. Rates are also higher for Jewish women and women who have never married. Women who have breast or endometrial cancer double their chances of acquiring ovarian cancer. Periodic, regular pelvic examinations are critical to early detection. Surgery, radiation therapy, and drug therapy are available as treatment options. Modern chemotherapeutic agents have played a major role in increasing overall five-year survival rates to 38 percent, 85 percent among those who are treated early.

Uterine Cancer

An estimated 46,500 new cases of uterine cancer were reported in 1990, including 13,500 cases of cancer of the cervix and 33,000 cases of cancer of the body of the uterus (the endometrium), with an estimated 6,000 deaths from cervical cancer and 4,000 from endometrial cancer. The **Pap test,** a microscopic examination of cells scraped from the cervix and body of the uterus, and regular checkups have reduced the overall death rate by 70 percent over the past 40 years. Symptoms include unusual bleeding outside of the normal menstrual period (or after menopause), or other discharge. Risk factors for cervical cancer include early age at first intercourse, multiple sex partners, cigarette smoking, and certain sexually transmitted diseases. Risk factors for endometrial cancer include a history of infertility, failure to ovulate, prolonged estrogen therapy, and obesity. The Pap test is highly effective in detecting early uterine cancer and partially effective for detecting endometrial cancer. High-risk women should also have an endometrial tissue sample at menopause.

Treatment involves surgery or radiation or a com-

leukemia Cancers that form in the blood-forming parts of the body, the bone marrow and the spleen. These nonsolid tumors are characterized by an abnormally high number of white blood cells.

Year 2000 National Health Objective

Death from cancer of the uterus and cervix is preventable and curable in a significant number of cases. One national health objective emphasizes a reduction in the number of deaths to no more than 1.3 per 100,000 women, compared to 2.8 per 100,000 reported in 1987. An additional national health objective involves an increase to at least 95 percent the proportion of women age 18 and older who have ever received a Pap test, and to at least 85 percent those who received a Pap test within the preceding one to three years. In 1987, 88 percent "ever" were tested and 75 percent were tested within the previous one to three years. The government is also striving to ensure that Pap tests meet quality standards by monitoring and certifying all cytology.

bination of the two. The five-year survival rates for all cervical cancer patients is 67 percent, 88 percent for patients diagnosed early. If the disease is in situ (in its original place), the survival rate is 100 percent. In endometrial cancer, overall survival rates are 85 percent, 92 percent if discovered in the precancerous lesion stage.

Cancer of the Colon or Rectum

An estimated 155,000 new cases of *colorectal* cancer (110,000 of colon cancer and 45,000 of rectum cancer) occurred in 1990, with a total of 60,900 deaths (53,300 from colon cancer, 7,600 from rectum cancer). Symptoms include rectal bleeding, blood in stools (bright red or black) or changes in bowel habits (diarrhea or constipation, abdominal discomfort or pain).[5] Risk factors include a personal or family history of cancer or polyps of the colon or rectum, inflammatory bowel disease, and high-fat, low-fiber diets. Among the various diagnostic procedures available, a physician can feel for a tumor in the rectum, use a proctosigmoidoscope to see the lower ten to twelve inches of the intestine, conduct a stool blood slide test, examine x-rays of the large in-

testine following a barium enema, conduct a biopsy (examine sample tissue microscopically) of suspected tissue, examine the stools, or use a colonoscope to view the entire colon.[6]

Surgery combined with radiation is the most effective treatment for colorectal cancer. *Colostomy* (creation of an abdominal opening for the elimination of body wastes) is occasionally used for rectal cancer patients. The five year survival rate for early detected localized colorectal cancer is 87 percent for colon cancer and 79 percent for rectal cancer. Survival rates drop to 58 percent and 46 percent when cancer has spread to involve adjacent organs or lymph nodes.

Year 2000 National Health Objective

Death from colorectal cancer is far too high. One national health objective seeks to reduce these deaths to no more than 13.2 per 100,000 people. In 1987, 14.4 per 100,000 people died of colorectal cancer. An attempt is also being made to increase to at least 50 percent the proportion of people age 50 and older who have received fecal occult blood testing within the preceding one to two years, and to increase to at least 40 percent those who have ever received proctosigmoidoscopy. In 1987, 27 percent of people had received fecal occult blood testing in the previous two years, and 25 percent had received proctosigmoidoscopy.

Hodgkin's Disease

Hodgkin's disease accounts for over 50 percent of the cases of lymphatic system cancer, a disease of young adults, in individuals age 20 to 40, and less than 10 percent in individuals less than 10 or older than age 60. The median age for non-Hodgkins lymphoma (cancer of the lymph glands not associated with Hodgkins disease) is 50 years. Approximately 7,400 new cases of Hodgkin's disease and 35,600 of non-Hodgkin's lymphomas were identified in 1990, causing an estimated 600 and 8,700 deaths, respectively. Hodgkin's disease apparently begins in an area of the lymph system and spreads throughout the lymphatic network. Abnormal white blood cells multiply rapidly, leaving fewer normal cells to conduct their infection-fighting function and making patients more susceptible to numerous infections. In the advanced stages, tumors may develop in lymph node areas and in the lungs, and the abdominal organs and bones may be involved. The actual cause is unknown, although several types of bacteria and viruses and the presence of an abnormal immune state are suspected of contributing to the disease. Symptoms include swollen lymph glands in the neck, armpit, or groin that persist for more than three weeks, persistent fatigue, back or abdominal pain, weight loss, fever, itching, night sweats, nausea, and vomiting.

Treatment for Hodgkin's disease involves use of super-voltage x-rays or a combination of radiation and chemotherapy. In well-equipped centers in the United States, Hodgkin's disease is diagnosed accurately in its early stages, and cured in 90 percent of the cases. Even in the advanced stages, combinations of drugs, with radiation, cure over 50 percent of the patients, with five-year survival rates over 70 percent.

Leukemia

Leukemia remains a leading cause of death in children age 4 to 14, with 27,800 new cases of acute and chronic leukemia reported in 1990, and an estimated 18,100 deaths. Affecting the blood-manufacturing organs, bone marrow, spleen, and lymph glands, **leukemia** is characterized by large numbers of white blood cells or immature white cells. These abnormal cells crowd out normal white cells that fight infection, platelets that control hemorrhaging, and red blood cells that prevent anemia. Early symptoms include fatigue, paleness, weight loss, repeated infections, bruising, and nosebleeds or other hemorrhages. Acute leukemia in children appears suddenly, with symptoms similar to a cold, and it progresses rapidly. The lymph nodes, spleen, and liver become enlarged. The cause of most cases of leukemia is unknown. Down's syndrome and other genetic abnormalities and excessive exposure to ionizing radiation and chemicals such as benzene (a commercial product in lead-free gasoline) are suspect causes. A newly discovered retrovirus (HTLV-1) causes some forms of leukemia and lymphoma.

Although early detection is difficult, it is aided by blood tests and bone marrow biopsy. Treatment involves chemotherapy to kill the attacking abnormal cells, transfusions of blood components, antibiotics, new anticancer drugs, and bone marrow transplants for certain leukemias. The overall five-year survival rate is 34 percent. Survival rates for acute lymphocytic leukemia patients have increased from 4 percent in the early 1960s to 48 percent in the 1980s.

Liver Cancer

This is one of the most widespread, deadly forms of cancer. A preventive vaccine for hepatitis B should be taken by people preparing for surgery that may require substantial blood transfusions. Hepatitis B vaccine helps prevent both liver cancer and hepatitis B.

Liver cancer treatment involves radiation therapy, surgery, and liver transplants. Five-year survival rates are approximately 4 percent.

Lung Cancer

Lung cancer is difficult to diagnose in time for effective treatment because it can be rather advanced by the time diagnosis occurs from using the usual procedures for detection, such as x-ray and examination of a portion of lung tissue (biopsy). Persistent hoarseness, coughing, chest pain, spitting of blood, recurring pneumonia, or bronchitis are some of the overt symptoms. There were an estimated 157,000 new cases and 142,000 deaths in 1990. The incidence of lung cancer continues its slow decline for men (81.9 per 100,000) and its slow increase for women (36.4 per 100,000). In 1987, for the first time, more women died of lung cancer than breast cancer. Risk factors include tobacco smoke (the primary cause), asbestos exposure, arsenic, atmospheric pollution, radioactive ores, metals (nickel, silver, chromium, cadmium, berryllium, cobalt, selenium, and steel), and chemical products (chloromethyl ethers).[7] Residential radon may also increase the risk, especially in cigarette smokers. Sidestream cigarette smoke may increase the risk for nonsmokers.

Early detection involves chest x-rays, analysis of cell type in sputum (a mixture of saliva and mucous from the lungs and bronchial tubes, usually coughed up and ejected from the mouth) and fiberoptic examination of the bronchial passages. Treatment depends upon the type and stage of the cancer and may include surgery, radiation therapy, and chemotherapy. The treatment of choice for localized cancer is surgery. In small-cell cancer, chemotherapy alone or in combination with radiation has replaced surgery, with a high percentage of patients experiencing long remissions. Overall, the five-year survival rate for lung cancer is 14 percent, 36 percent for cases detected when the disease is localized.

Year 2000 National Health Objective

The federal government is striving to slow the rise in lung cancer deaths to achieve a rate of no more than 42 per 100,000 people, improving on the 37.9 per 100,000 identified in 1987.

Pancreatic Cancer

More than 25,000 Americans annually—double the rate of twenty years ago—now die of pancreatic cancer. Over 28,000 new cases are diagnosed each year, making this the fifth leading cancer killer. Although very little is known about its causes or its prevention, several chemical agents (cleaners, gasoline) and tobacco, coffee, alcohol, and tea have been suspected. The risk increases with age; the majority of cases occur in individuals between the ages of 65 and 79. Risk factors include smoking (twice the incidence for smokers), sex and race (more common in men, 50 percent more cases among black Americans), and high-fat diets. The fact that pancreatic cancer is a silent disease occurring without symptoms until advanced stages makes early detection difficult.

Although a biopsy provides fairly accurate diagnosis, pancreatic cancer is generally already in the advanced stages. Ultrasound imaging and computerized tomography (CT) scans are currently being studied to provide earlier detection. Surgery, radiation therapy, and anticancer drugs have little influence on the disease. In 59 percent of the cases, diagnosis occurs so late that these techniques are not used. Only 3 percent of patients live more than five years after diagnosis.

Oral Cancer

An estimated 30,500 new cases (two times more men than women) of oral cancer and 8,350 deaths were reported in 1990. Symptoms include a sore that bleeds easily and fails to heal, a lump or thickening, a red or white patch that does not go away, and difficulty in chewing, swallowing, or moving the tongue or jaws. Risk factors include tobacco use (cigarettes, cigar, pipe, or smokeless tobacco) and excessive use of alcohol. Dentists and primary care physicians have the best opportunity to detect abnormal tissue changes at the curable stage.

Treatment involves radiation therapy and surgery. Five-year survival rates depend upon the location of the cancer and range from 32 percent for cancer of the pharynx to 92 percent for lip cancer.

Prostate Cancer

The prostate gland is the leading site of cancer in men, striking over 106,000 American men annually, resulting in over 30,000 deaths. Blood in the urine or semen can be a sign, but more often such symptoms indicate a bacterial infection of the prostate or bladder. Weak or interrupted flow of urine, inability to urinate, difficulty starting or stopping the urine flow, frequent urination (especially at night), blood in the urine, pain or burning on urination, continuing pain in the lower back, pelvis, or upper thighs are nonspecific symptoms that also occur with benign conditions, such as infection or prostate enlargement. The risk increases with age, with over 80 percent of all prostate cancers diagnosed in men over the age of 65. African-Americans have the highest incidence rate in the world and some familial association, either due to genetic or environmental factors, has been found. Additional risk factors include high-fat diets and exposure to cadmium.[8]

Prostate cancer can be diagnosed during a digital rectal examination. Prostate ultrasound (sound waves with frequencies beyond the upper limit audible to human ears) examination may also reveal cancers too small to be detected by rectal examination.

Surgery, alone or in combination with radiation or hormones, and anticancer drugs can control prostate cancer for long periods of time by shrinking the tumor and relieving the pain. Even with early detection, fewer than 10 percent of newly discovered cases submit to surgery for fear of becoming impotent. In the past, nine out of ten men lost their ability to achieve an erection after the surgery. Dr. Patrick C.

**Year 2000
National Health Objective**

Another national health objective seeks to reduce deaths due to cancer of the oral cavity and pharynx to no more than 10.5 per 100,000 men age 45 to 74, and to 4.1 per 100,000 women age 45 to 74 (There were 12.1 per 100,000 men, and 4.1 per 100,000 women in 1987).

Walsh of Johns Hopkins University Hospital and others have performed a new procedure called nerve-sparing radical retropubic prostatectomy on over 400 males, with 72 percent retaining their potency. The five-year survival rate for patients diagnosed early while the tumor is localized is 84 percent with an overall survival rate of 70 percent.

Testicular Cancer

Cancer of the testes afflicts approximately 5,900 men each year. It is most often found in men age 20 to 35 and is the most common tumor in men age 20 to 25. Testicular cancer is more likely to occur in men whose testes never descend to the scrotum or descend after the age of six. Testicular cancer is more common in white males; the incidence in blacks and Asians is very low. The most common sign is a pea-sized lump, usually painless in the early stages. Other symptoms include enlargement of a testicle, accumulation of fluid, blood in the scrotum, a feeling of heaviness in the scrotum, a dull ache in the lower abdomen or the groin, pain or discomfort in a testicle or in the scrotum, and enlargement or tenderness in the chest around the nipples. Seminomas make up approximately 40 percent of the cases of testicular cancer and nonseminomas the remaining 60 percent. If any of these symptoms persist for as long as two weeks, a physician should be consulted. Regular self-examination of the testicles is the most common means of early detection (see Exploring Your Health 16.3). Diagnosis involves personal and family history, examination of the scrotum, a chest x-ray, and blood and urine tests. If these exams do not reveal an infection or other disorder, cancer may be suspected. An *inguinal orchiectomy* may be performed and the affected testicle removed through the groin to allow microscopic examination by a pathologist. Neither the scrotum nor the testicle is cut in order to avoid local metastasis should cancer be present.

Testicular cancer is almost always curable if detected early. The disease also responds well to treatment even if it has spread to other body parts. Surgery, radiation therapy, and chemotherapy are used as single treatments or in combination.

Exploring Your Health 16.3

Testicular Self-Examination

Follow the instructions in the diagram below carefully and examine your testes immediately after your next hot bath or shower. Heat causes the testicles to descend and the scrotal skin to relax, making it easier to find unusual lumps. Examine each testicle by placing the index and middle fingers of both hands on the underside of the testicle and the thumbs on the top. Gently roll the testicle between your thumb and fingers, feeling for small lumps. Changes or anything abnormal will appear at the front or side of your testicle.

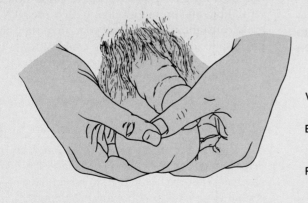

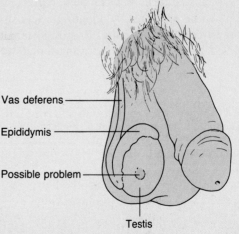

Vas deferens

Epididymis

Possible problem

Testis

Did you find any unusual lumps?

Are there any unusual signs of any kind?

Are there any markings or lumps at any site?

Keep in mind that not all lumps are a sign of testicular cancer. Unusual lumps at any location, however, should be checked by a physician. Early detection greatly increases your chances of a complete cure. Repeat the examination every month and record your findings.

Skin Cancer

In spite of the fact that more than 8,000 people die from skin cancer each year (such cancers generally are found on the face, neck, and hands) and that over 500,000 new cases are discovered annually,[9] the American people are much more concerned about smooth skin and a "bronzed, youthful" appearance than a healthy body. The quest for the fountain of youth and the perfect skin is a billion dollar industry in the United States. We spend a small fortune on cosmetic products to rejuvenate the skin, then resort to unsound tanning approaches, overexposure to the sun, and cigarette smoking in spite of the fact that the sun and tobacco are the two major causes of skin cancer, aging skin, and skin wrinkling. Unless we learn to protect our skin properly, skin cancers are certain to increase in the future as the earth's ozone layer continues to diminish, exposing us to more dangerous sun rays. The good news is that your personal behavior can prevent skin cancer and premature skin aging. Your present behavior will actually determine your risk of skin cancer in the future. Even one single blistering sunburn episode as a child may double your chance of skin cancer later in life. Early diagnosis and treatment will also greatly increase the chances of a complete cure.

The skin can be protected by adopting a few simple behaviors throughout your life. It is important to protect yourself from all ultraviolet radiation (UVR):

Often the desire to have that "healthy" bronzed look overrides good common sense when it comes to lying out in the sun. Keep in mind that it only takes one (yes, one) blistering sunburn in your youth to double your chances of developing skin cancer later in life.

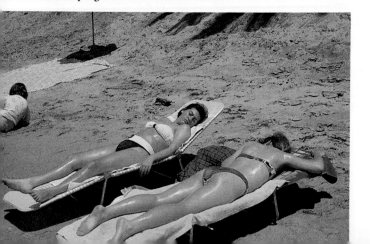

ultraviolet A (UVA), ultraviolet B (UVB), and ultraviolet C (UVC). All three waves are received from the sun, although the UVC rays are blocked by the ozone layer. As the ozone layer diminishes, some UVC rays will get through and increase the risk of skin burning and skin cancer. The shorter UVB wave lengths (blocked by glass windows) have long been associated with sunburn and skin cancer and are stronger in southern climates and most dangerous during the summer between the hours of 10 A.M. and 2 P.M. UVA waves (received through windows), once viewed as a safe tanning ray, have also been found to cause skin damage, wrinkling, and premature aging. Because UVA rays are more constant all day and all year long, they are nearly impossible to avoid. Both UVA and UVB rays work together to cause skin burning and cancer.

Follow this nine-point program to keep your skin healthy and cancer free:

1. **Identify Your Skin Type** Everyone has a different degree of natural protection from the sun. Fair-skinned people have less, dark-skinned people have more; both should use sunscreen. Young children should be provided with extra protection, greater than the "sun protection factor" (SPF) recommendations shown in Table 16.4, because they tend to stay in the sun longer. Infants should be kept out of the sun unless they wear protective clothing. Very young children should be exposed to the sun for only short periods of time and be protected with sunscreen as soon as they are 6 months of age. Identify your skin type from the information in Table 16.4.

TABLE 16.4

Identifying Skin Type

Type	Characteristics	Burn Time in Summer Sun	Recommended SPF (Sun Protection Factor)
I	Always burns, never tans. Very fair with red or blond hair, and freckles.	7 Minutes	High, such as PreSun 29–39
II	Burns easily, tans minimally. Usually fair-skinned people.	15 Minutes	High, such as PreSun 29
III	Sometimes burns, gradually tans.	21 Minutes	15 or greater
IV	Minimum burning, always tans. White with medium pigmentation.	28 Minutes	15
V	Very seldom burns, always tans. Medium to heavy pigmentation.	2–3 Hours	at least 8
VI	Never burns, but tans darkly. Blacks and others with heavy pigmentation.	3 Hours+	at least 8

2. Begin a Regular Self-Examination Program Now The American Cancer Society recommends a monthly self-exam immediately after a bath or shower, using a full-length mirror and a hand mirror. Such a procedure is one of your best weapons for early detection.[10] Complete Exploring Your Health 16.4 to begin your regular self-examination program.

3. Learn to Recognize the Warning Signs of Melanoma There are four basic warning signs of melanoma. They are referred to as the ABCDs. Most of the moles, freckles, and other blemishes on your skin are "normal." However, if you notice a blemish that exhibits **A**symmetry, **B**order irregularity, **C**olor change, or **D**iameter greater than 6 mm, you may want to consult a dermatologist. This is especially important if another member of your family has experienced numerous skin cancers or melanoma. Other warning signs include changes in the surface of a mole (scaliness, oozing, bleeding, or an increase in elevation or thickness), spread of pigment from the border into surrounding skin, change in sensation in the area (such as itchiness), and tenderness or pain.

4. Select and Use a UVB and UVA Skin Protection Product Sunscreens labeled "broad spectrum" provide protection from both UVB and UVA rays. Keep in mind that the once ignored UVA rays penetrate deeper into the dermis (the bottom skin layer), causing photoaging, a breakdown of the elastic tissue supporting the skin. This causes wrinkling, sagging, and a leathery appearance. Phototoxic reactions also occur. Itching, red blistery burns occur with sun exposure while people are taking certain medications, such as antibiotics or diuretics. Although the sun protection factor (SPF) is listed on the label, it only refers to the amount of UVB blocked. An SPF of 15 will adequately protect most skin types. If your skin begins to redden after 10 minutes of exposure, an SPF of 15 would allow the same exposure for 150 minutes $(10 \times 15 = 150)$ before burning would occur. The lighter your skin, the higher the SPF needed. To be safe, protect your skin with a minimum SPF of 15. Applying additional sunscreen after 150 minutes does not extend your time in the sun; you will still burn and damage the skin.

It is also important to use a sunscreen during high altitude activities, such as mountain climbing and skiing, because there is less atmosphere to absorb the sun's rays. The sun is also stronger near the equator. The sun's rays are also as damaging to your skin on cloudy, hazy days.

5. Apply a Generous Amount of Sunscreen to Your Face (cheeks, nose, forehead, chin, neck, arms, and hands) Sunscreen should be used even on cloudy days when you plan to be outdoors longer than fifteen to twenty minutes. Avoid any makeup for five to ten minutes, until the sunscreen is dry.

6. Limit Your Sun Exposure Even with a Sunscreen and Avoid Midday Sun (10 A.M.– 2 P.M.) Keep in mind that even sitting in the shade does not protect you from sunburn. Children should be taught to avoid sun when their shadow is shorter than they are.

7. Avoid Baby Oil or a Metal Reflector to Increase Tanning Both of these approaches can cause severe burns and skin damage. Sand, snow, con-

Exploring Your Health 16.4

Skin Self-Examination

Examine your entire body at home after bathing. Pay particular attention to the head, face, neck, shoulder, and ear areas during your self-exam, as well as the tops and bottoms of your feet and the front and back of your hands. For each mark on your body, place a corresponding mark on the drawing above at the approximate location. Describe the mark briefly (size, color, type). Refer to "3. Learn to Recognize the Warning Signs of Melanoma" in the text to evaluate various marks. See your physician immediately if any suspicious marks are found.

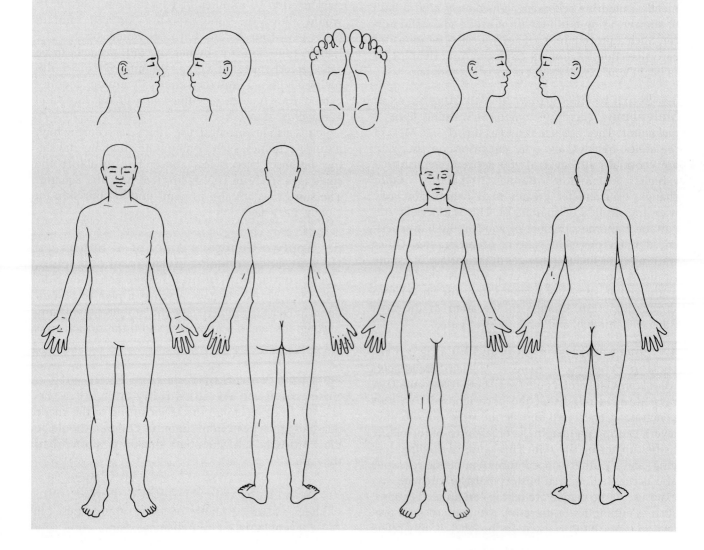

crete, and water can also reflect more than half of the sun's rays onto your skin.

8.   Wear Protective Clothing when Forced to Remain Outside for Long Periods of Time (hat with visor, shirt, long pants)   No sunscreen provides sufficient protection against lengthy periods of on-the-job exposure to the sun.

9.   Avoid Tanning Salons Regardless of the Claims Made by Owners   The UV light emitted by tanning booths causes sunburn and premature aging, and it will increase the risk of skin cancer.

Stomach and Esophageal Cancer

Cancer of the stomach now accounts for less than 3 percent of all cancers. Approximately 23,200 new cases are diagnosed each year, and 13,700 deaths occur. Cancer of the esophagus accounts for less than 1 percent of all cancer, with an estimated 10,600 new cases identified annually, and 9,500 deaths. Men are more likely to develop both types of cancers than women; 70 percent of esophageal and 60 percent of stomach cancer cases and deaths occur among men. Cancers of the stomach and esophagus often invade other organs of the digestive system and may spread by metastasis to the lungs, bones, kidneys, brain, skin, and in females, to the uterus. Esophageal cancer commonly spreads to the lungs and liver.

Risk factors for stomach cancer include diet and acid imbalance. High starch, low-fiber intake, salt-cured, pickled, and chemically preserved foods, and naturally occurring nitrates that may be converted to nitrites and nitrosamines are suspect. Stomach cancer is also linked to low stomach acid or total absence of stomach acid. The most common early symptom is indigestion, vague abdominal discomfort, a feeling of fullness after meals, unexplained gas, nausea, and heartburn that continues for weeks. Diagnosis includes x-rays and *gastroscopy* (using an instrument to see into the gastrointestinal tract) with biopsy and brushings to examine cells. Risk factors for esophagus cancer include tobacco smoking and the consumption of alcohol, gastric reflux patients (stomach acid flowing back into the esophagus), and direct contact with lye. The most common early symptom is difficulty in swallowing, first with solid foods and later with soft foods and liquids. X-rays and *esophaguscopy* (using an instrument to see into the esophagus) with biopsy and washings are effective diagnostic techniques.

The treatment of choice for stomach cancer is surgery to remove part, or all, of the stomach and the adjacent lymph nodes. Even with removal of the entire stomach, patients can adjust by eating small meals and making other dietary changes. Chemotherapy is also used to reduce the size of primary or metastatic

tumors. Five-year survival rates with early detection is over 50 percent, but with surrounding tissue or lymph node involvement, rates fall to about 15 to 20 percent. Surgery is also the treatment of choice for cancer involving the lower portion of the esophagus. The lower esophagus and upper stomach are removed and the two reconnected with a tube by pulling up part of the stomach. Radiation and chemotherapy may also be used to treat tumors in the upper esophagus and to provide symptom relief. Because early detection is difficult, five-year survival rates are low. For surgery patients with lower esophagus involvement, survival rates exceed 20 percent.

Diagnosis and Treatment of Cancer

The three main forms of treatment for cancer are radiation, surgery, and chemotherapy. The choice of treatment (or treatments) depends on the type of cancer and the extent to which it has spread. For example, surgery is most successful at treating cancers that have not spread beyond the original site, whereas chemotherapy and radiation are used to treat cancers that have spread into different areas of the body.

Radiation Therapy

Radiation treatment involves using x-rays, radium, and the betatron. Cancer cells are more vulnerable than healthy cells to x-rays and radium. The ideal dosage would destroy cancer cells, with minimal damage to normal cells. Often, however, the dose required to destroy cancer cells permanently damages surrounding normal cells. Some kinds of cancer can be entirely destroyed using radiation. High-voltage x-rays have proved successful in treating cancer, as have streams of electrical charges from the atom-smashing betatron.[11]

Interstitial implants (radioactive sources) have been inserted directly into malignancies such as inoperable brain tumors. Interstitial hyperthermia (heating cancer cells) in the head, neck, colon, and rectum is being used to make cancer cells more vulnerable to radiation. Tubes are inserted into cancer cells before using radio-frequency waves to heat malignancies to 108 to 110 degrees. Intraoperative radiotherapy involves radiation during surgery. This procedure allows 20 to 30 percent more radiation at the cancer cells and limits damage to normal tissue. Radiosensitizing and radioprotective drugs are being used to make cancer cells more vulnerable or normal cells more resistant. Particle therapy involves the bombarding of tumors with charged particles that penetrate to a specific depth and deliver their energy, with little scattering of radiation to normal tissue. This procedure permits the use of doses equivalent to over 100,000 chest x-rays without the associated damage to normal tissue.

immunotherapy A cancer treatment involving the stimulation of the body's own disease-fighting systems to combat cancer.

Surgery

Surgery is also employed in the treatment of cancer for removal of tumors. Three out of four women with breast cancer can now be saved through surgery, depending on the stage of the disease. *Radical mastectomy* (removal of the entire breast and surrounding muscles) is no longer considered necessary in the early stages of the disease. A modified mastectomy (removal of the affected part of the breast and surrounding lymph nodes) or *lumpectomy* (removal of the tumor and the surrounding tissue only) followed by radiation is just as effective as radical surgery. Regardless of the location and size of the tumor, there is no difference in survival rates.

Chemotherapy

Chemotherapy is a treatment that uses chemicals (drugs) to seek out and attack cancer cells. More than twenty-five drugs have been identified that will poison cancer cells and stop or slow their growth; all of them damage normal cells and cannot be used indefinitely. In addition, most of the drugs have serious side effects. The control of hormones in the body has been used with varying degrees of success in treating breast cancer and prostate cancer.[12]

It is clear that chemicals can alter the genetic message of cancer cells and change them into cells that can no longer grow. Although this principle of transforming cancer to benign cells, called differentiation therapy, is still in the experimental stages, it shows great promise.

Bone Marrow Transplants

Bone marrow transplants are sometimes used to treat leukemia. Unless a compatible donor is found, the "warrior cells" (T lymphocytes) attack the leukemia patient, producing a fatal condition called graft versus host disease. For the procedure to succeed, marrow must come from any identical twin or a brother or sister with closely matched blood. Less than 30 percent of leukemia patients have such a donor.

Researchers are evaluating a new technique in which a portion of the patient's own marrow is removed before treatment, saved, and later restored by transplantation. This procedure eliminates the problem of locating a suitable donor and allows the patient to tolerate larger doses of anticancer drugs or radiation therapy.

Advances in Cancer Diagnosis and Management

In recent years, dramatic advances have taken place in both the diagnosis and management of cancer. Whereas, thirty years ago, only 25 percent of cancer patients survived for five years (the criteria used to define "cure") after treatment without recurrence of the disease, the overall cure rate today is 40 percent. Early detection is now followed by a precise staging of the disease and the use of more than one type of therapy, often in combination.

A summary of the most recent diagnosis and treatment advances follows:

- *Thymosis,* a biological response modifier produced by the thymus gland and altered by researchers, has shown promise when used with chemotherapy.
- A genetic fusing of cancer cells is being used to produce disease-fighting antibodies that seek out chosen targets on cancer cells.
- Progress is being made in detecting both the presence and location of cancer.
- Intensive drug therapy is being used successfully before surgery.
- Chemical injections near the spine help relieve some cancer patients of pain.
- *Retinoids,* synthetic "cousins" of vitamin A, have prevented bladder and breast cancers in mice and rats and have promise against cancer of the lung, esophagus, and pancreas in humans.
- More than fifty drugs have been found effective against certain cancers.
- Improved diagnostic and surgical equipment such as lasers make surgery more precise.
- The surgical procedure of replacing only a section of a bone rather than amputating a leg or arm is being used effectively.
- High-frequency sound waves (*ultrasound*) are being used to locate some tumors more precisely.

- **Immunotherapy,** using the body's own disease-fighting systems to combat cancer, is an area of hope. See this chapter's "A Question of Ethics" box for a discussion of one case of immunotherapy.

- Risk profiles are being developed for most types of cancers to select the best time for detection tests.

- The transfusion of blood components is available for cancer therapy.

- Five chromosome abnormalities linked with five particular types of acute nonlymphocytic leukemia have been identified.

- DNA changes are being analyzed in a test to determine if one is susceptible to colon cancer.

- *Monoclonal antibodies,* (man-made copies of natural antibodies) are being used to track down cancer cells anywhere in the body. Similar techniques are being used to deliver radiation to cancer cells.

- New high-technology diagnostic imaging techniques are replacing exploratory surgery for some patients. Magnetic resonance imaging (MRI) employs a huge electromagnet to detect hidden tumors by mapping on a computer screen the vi-

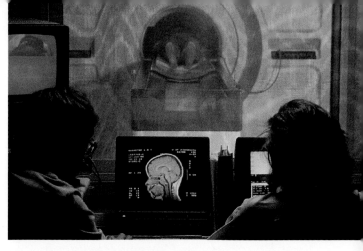

Magnetic Resonance Imaging (MRI) is a powerful, high-technology diagnostic tool. Using a giant electromagnet, the MRI machine detects tumors by sensing the vibrations of certain atoms in the body.

brations of the various atoms in the body. Computerized tomography (CT scanning) uses x-rays to examine the brain and other body parts. Both of these painless procedures more accurately show a tumor's shape and location than previously used methods.

A Question of Ethics

A Case of Immunotherapy: Benefit or Exploitation?

On May 22, 1991, National Public Radio's "All Things Considered" news broadcast featured a story about a small Massachusetts-based company that offers a type of immunotherapy for people with advanced kidney cancer. Although approximately half of the people diagnosed with kidney cancer live at least five years, most people diagnosed with advanced cases of kidney cancer die within a few months. The company mentioned above—a for-profit private company founded by a group of physicians and business people—claims that their therapy helps people with advanced kidney cancer live up to two and a half times longer than they would without this treatment. The therapy basically involves removing white cells (lymphocytes) from the patient's blood, treating these cells with proteins taken from the patient's own body in order to stimulate the white cells' cancer-fighting properties, and then placing these "recharged" white cells back into the patient's body. There are a total of a dozen treatments, offered at a cost of about $21,000.

Even though it is expensive, this sounds to many people like a very positive and hopeful form of treatment for cancer patients who face almost certain death. However, prominent members of the health care community have questioned both the ethics and the legality of this company's operations. They say that this company is actively avoiding regulation by exploiting loopholes in the policies of the U.S. Food and Drug Administration and that it is profiting from the desperate hopes of dying people. In fact, the company never received the approval of the U.S. Food and Drug Administration.

Most new medical treatments and therapies require exhaustive evidence of their effectiveness before the FDA will approve them. The law does allow some therapies to be performed without extensive study beforehand, as long as these therapies are clearly identified as being "experimental." This company opened its doors for business on the basis of one experimental study performed by its own personnel and claims that it offers a full-fledged (nonexperimental) therapy. The company also claims that it does not need FDA approval to operate because its therapy does not involve the use of drugs.

Furthermore, all of the company's operations occur within the state of Massachusetts (intrastate); the FDA has the authority to regulate only operations that cross state lines (interstate). Some medical professionals have suggested that this may be further proof that the company is trying to avoid federal regulation altogether.

Legal "grey areas" between private industry and federal regulation are nothing new and are certainly not confined to the health care industry. Questions of legality aside, do you believe it is right for private companies to offer therapies that have not undergone the rigorous testing normally associated with new drugs and medical procedures? Who should determine exactly where to draw the line between what is potentially beneficial treatment and what may be exploitation for financial gain? The federal government? The public? Private industry? What do you think?

Source: National Public Radio, "All Things Considered," broadcast May 22, 1991. Analysis prepared by David Baron. Transcript. Washington, D.C., 1991.

New Frontiers in Cancer Research

Frontiers in cancer research into the next century will involve a number of areas:

1. Interferon research. Originally discovered as an antiviral agent, interferon is now being used successfully in the treatment of a number of types of cancer, and an attempt is underway to further improve its effectiveness by combining interferon with more conventional chemotherapeutic drugs and the use of mixtures of different interferons.

2. Genetic engineering. Recombinant DNA is now used to produce interferon. The production of more powerful new drugs, correcting impaired immune systems, and modifying heredity are being explored.

3. Mechanisms of carcinogenesis. Investigation is underway to further understand how tumors arise.

4. Cell growth and regulation. New ways are being studied to check the unregulated growth of tumor cells.

Get Involved!

Furthering Cancer Risk Awareness

Although cancer is the nation's number two killer, many of the 510,000 annual deaths could be prevented. According to the American Cancer Society, over 42,000 cancer deaths could be prevented each year with early detection. Over 142,000 lives are lost from cancer caused by tobacco smoking, and over 540,000 skin cancers could be prevented by protection from the sun's rays. This unnecessary waste of precious life also brings financial disaster to millions of families, yet people continue to practice unhealthy lifestyles and to believe that "It won't happen to me." The overall medical costs for cancer accounted for 10 percent of the total cost of disease in the United States and exceeded $71.6 billion dollars in 1989 ($21.8 billion for direct costs, $8.6 billion in losses due to decreased productivity, and $41.2 billion in mortality costs). Cancer also produces considerable emotional and physical pain. One way to protect yourself from these hardships in the future is to minimize your personal risks of cancer and that of others around you. Consider these suggestions:

1. A complete ban on all tobacco products must eventually occur in the United States if a number of types of cancer are ever to be eradicated. The ban on public smoking, the elimination of certain types of advertisements, and the antismoking educational blitz underway is a start. If the momentum stops, however, the powerful tobacco industry will grease its advertising wheels and make up the lost ground. We must keep the pressure on by opposing public smoking, supporting antismoking programs and campaigns against smokeless tobacco, and by setting an example for the youth of this nation.

2. If you are a young woman and have not had sexual intercourse, consider delaying intercourse to reduce your risk of cervical cancer.

3. If you are sexually active, limit your number of partners and practice safe sex (see Chapter 5).

4. Actively encourage your friends and family to follow your example of a healthy lifestyle that involves regular aerobic exercise, a diet high in complex carbohydrates and low in fat and calories, the maintenance of normal body weight and fat, and the absence of tobacco and alcohol.

5. Talk with your health instructor about scheduling a "Self-Examination" workshop on campus to teach students the proper ways to examine oneself for breast, testicular, and skin cancer.

6. Ask your instructor about any potentially hazardous building materials in your instructional environment. Schedule a meeting with the chief of buildings and grounds to learn what is being done to make your university environment safe.

7. Volunteer your services at the local hospital and spend time with children who are terminally ill cancer patients.

5. Drug development. New cancer fighting drugs are being tested that are less toxic for normal cells and more potent against tumor cells.

6. Psychosocial, behavioral and nutritional influences. The role of nutrition, environment, and physical condition in influencing a person's general health and the chances of contracting and coping with cancer are under investigation.

7. The study of metastasis. Researchers have already discovered that genes control a tumor cell's capacity to spread, to enter the bloodstream, and to travel to distant locations in the body. One gene appears to prevent metastasis as long as it remains intact; new information in this area could prevent over 50 percent of all cancer deaths.

Reducing the Risk of Getting Cancer

Not all cancers can be prevented. However, most lung cancers, caused by cigarette smoking, and most skin cancers, caused by frequent overexposure to direct sunlight, can be prevented by avoiding the causes. Some occupationally or environmentally induced cancers can also be prevented by eliminating or reducing contact with carcinogenic agents (for example, bladder cancer among workers in the dye industry and lung cancer in asbestos workers). There is also enough scientific evidence to suggest certain precautions that should be taken throughout life to reduce risk:

Primary Prevention

Primary prevention involves steps to avoid those factors that may lead to the development of cancer:

- Abstain from using tobacco in any form, including the smokeless varieties.
- Eliminate or reduce your consumption of alcohol; drink only in moderation.

- Avoid contact with known carcinogens whenever possible. Have your house and work environment checked for radon levels and potentially hazardous materials.
- Avoid lowering your body resistance by "crash" dieting or by placing unusually heavy demands on your body for prolonged periods of time.
- Decrease your exposure to the sun, avoid sun bathing for long periods of time, and use a sunscreen with the appropriate SPF for your skin type anytime you plan to be in the sun.
- Follow a dietary plan that involves increasing your consumption of vitamins A and C, cruciferous vegetables, fiber, selenium, and omega-3 fatty acids (anchovies, herring, mackerel, sablefish, salmon, fresh tuna, whitefish, bass, bluefish, hake, halibut, mullet, ocean perch, pollack, rainbow trout, rock fish, sea trout, smelt, and oysters). Reduce your consumption of artificial sweeteners, heat-charred food, nitrite-cured or smoked foods, fat, and calories.[13]
- Maintain normal body weight and body fat.
- Consult your physician before resorting to estrogen therapy.

Secondary Prevention

Secondary prevention involves steps to be taken to diagnose a cancer or precursor of cancer as early as possible:

- Memorize the seven cancer danger signals (Table 16.2) and be alerted to these changes in your body.
- Adhere to the guidelines for early detection of cancer in people without symptoms, as shown in Table 16.3.
- Learn the breast self-examination technique (females) and the testes self-examination technique (males) and use this method monthly.
- Learn the skin self-examination and examine your skin periodically.
- Report any family history of cancer to your doctor.

Conclusion

Progress in the prevention, early detection, and treatment of various forms of cancer continues. There has been a steady rise in the age-adjusted national death rate, largely due to increases in the incidence of cancer of the lung. For many major types of cancer, age-adjusted cancer death rates have leveled off or declined over the past fifty years. The incidences of brain cancers, multiple myelomas or bone marrow cancers, breast and skin cancers have increased. Five-year survival rates continue to increase, dramatically in some areas. Although new treatment techniques are promising, complete eradication of the disease will probably not occur in this decade. Early detection and surgery still provide the highest complete cure rate for most types of cancer. A number of lifestyle changes have also been shown to reduce one's risk of acquiring cancer.

Summary

1. Cancer is responsible for more than 510,000 deaths each year. Over 6 million Americans are alive today who have had cancer; 3 million were diagnosed five or more years ago.

2. Cancer is not a single disease; it is a group of more than 100 diseases involving abnormal cell growth.

3. The four basic types of cancer are carcinoma, sarcoma, lymphoma, and leukemia.

4. Although cancer strikes at any age (it kills more children ages 3 to 14 than any other disease), it is more likely to occur with advancing age.

5. Although the exact causes of most types of cancer are unknown, cancer has been associated with carcinogens, environmental pollution, x-rays, radon, chronic irritation, viruses, radiation, the sun's rays, hereditary factors, tobacco use (including the use of smokeless tobacco and the effects of secondhand smoke), precancerous conditions, alcohol use, obesity, prolonged estrogen therapy, and diet.

6. Children living near overhead power lines are twice as likely to develop leukemia as those who live elsewhere.

7. A healthy lifestyle will provide considerable protection from various types of cancer.

8. Localized cancer is largely curable; once metastasis occurs to surrounding tissue and distant areas, survival rates decrease.

9. A complete cure for most types of cancer depends upon early detection. Early detection requires the full cooperation of the individual who must secure regular checkups as recommended by the American Cancer Society. People should recognize the cancer danger signs, and practice regular self-examination techniques.

10. Breast, skin, and testicular self-examination techniques provide an effective means of early detection. Other simple laboratory procedures, such as the Pap test and similar examinations, can be performed by a physician.

11. Treatment techniques continue to improve the five-year survival rates, and researchers are pursuing new avenues that show promise for the eradication of certain types of cancer and the control of others.

Questions for Personal Growth

1. Early detection greatly increases the cure rate for most types of cancer. Since the incidence of cancer also increases with age, your parents are much more at risk than college students. Provide your mother and father with instructions to perform breast and skin self-examinations. Encourage them to read the material and record their examination dates.

2. Lifestyle and cancer are related in a number of areas. Identify the key behaviors in your life that may actually protect you from cancer. Identify those behaviors that place you at greater risk.

3. You spend countless hours in your home and in the workplace; yet these areas may impose a health hazard. Purchase a radon testing kit at your local hardware store to determine whether the levels of radon in your house are safe. Inspect your workplace for various chemicals and materials that may impose a health hazard. Ask the building supervisor about the materials used to complete the structure.

4. Heredity is a risk factor for some types of cancers. Talk with your parents and grandparents to see if anyone in your family has had cancer in the previous generations. Are there any patterns concerning specific types of cancers in your family history?

5. Do you or any of your friends or family smoke? If so, discuss the cancer risks of cigarette, pipe, and cigar smoking and encourage individuals to join a smoking cessation group.

6. Study the seven cancer warning signals. Do you know anyone who exhibits any of these symptoms? If so, encourage them to secure a physical examination as soon as possible.

References

1. American Cancer Society, *Cancer Facts and Figures* (1990).
2. "Feeling Safer at the VDT," *U.S. News and World Report* (March 25, 1991): 17.
3. Ibid.
4. National Cancer Institute, "What You Need to Know About Breast Cancer," NIH Publication No. 89-1556 (1989).
5. Hecht, Annabel, "The Colon Goes Up, Over, Down, and Out," Department of Health and Human Services (Washington, D.C.: Public Health Service, Food and Drug Administration, U.S. Government Printing Office, 1989).
6. American Cancer Society, *Facts on Colorectal Cancer* (1988).
7. American Cancer Society, *Facts on Lung Cancer* (1987).
8. U.S. Department of Health and Human Services, Public Health Service, NIH, "What You Need to Know About Prostate Cancer" (1988).
9. *New Sun Sense: The ABC's of UVB, UVA, SPF, and PPF* (Santa Ana, Calif.: Herbert Laboratories, 1989).
10. *Skin Wellness: Self-Exam Body Man* (Dallas, Tex.: Mary Kay Cosmetics, 1989).
11. U.S. Department of Health and Human Services, Public Health Service, NIH, "Radiation Therapy and You: A Guide to Self-Help During Treatment" (1987).
12. U.S. Department of Health and Human Services, Public Health Service, NIH, "Chemotherapy & You: A Guide to Self-Help During Treatment" (1987).
13. U.S. Department of Health and Human Services, Public Health Service, NIH, "Diet, Nutrition, and Cancer Prevention: The Good News" (1987).

CHAPTER
17

Aging

CHAPTER OBJECTIVES

After reading this chapter, you should understand:

- How the American emphasis on youthfulness has led to a kind of discrimination against older people, and why this ageism is both unfair and unwise.

- Several theories that attempt to explain exactly why we age, and how our lifestyle influences how long and how well we will live.

- What changes we can anticipate as we grow older, what we can do to reduce our susceptibility to debilitating physical conditions, and how we can increase our enjoyment of certain aspects of our lives, such as sexuality, in old age.

- The possible effects of aging on some cognitive abilities such as speech, reasoning, and memory.

- Why and how aging should and can be a period of pleasure and fulfillment in a person's life.

- Why poverty and old age are closely linked in our society.

CHAPTER OUTLINE

Ageism

Aging: Theories and Lifestyle Changes

Physical Health and Aging

Cognitive Functioning and Aging

Social Adjustment and Aging

Aging and Economics

The Future

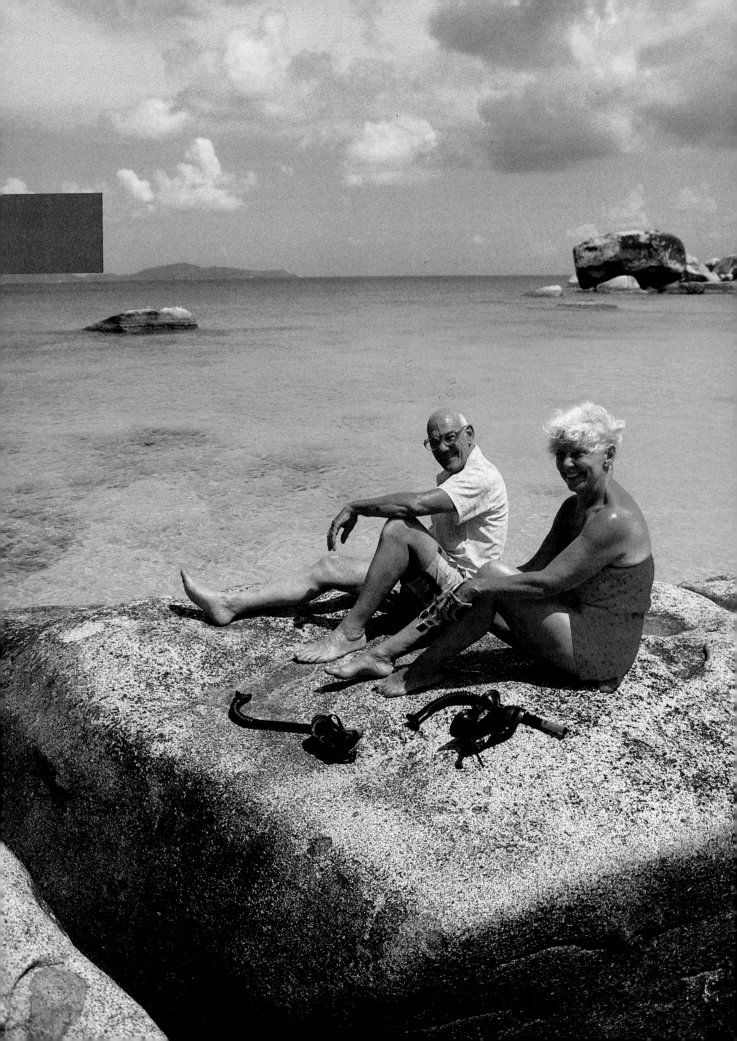

ageism A negative attitude toward growing old and toward old people; a common prejudice against older people (senior citizens), as reflected in stereotypes and derogatory language about older people.

The time to prepare for successful aging is now. Chances are extremely good that you will experience both the joy and the frustrations of old age in the future. Your concern for parents and grandparents also makes this a very important topic for you. Needless to say, the number of people over 65 years of age continues to increase (see Table 17.1). In fact, by the year 2000, older people will be the dominant population group (see Figure 17.1). By the year 2033, more than one in every five Americans will be an older person.[1] Children born in 1985 can expect to live a minimum of seventy-three years; it is projected that a baby born in the year 2000 will live eighty-five years.

Old age is a fact of life, and with it comes some real challenges, such as physical, mental, and emotional changes, reduced income, declining health, loss of loved ones, and the need to cope with new roles. Many of these problems are not the direct result of age but rather difficulties experienced by older people because of the kinds of solutions society has adopted to deal with large numbers of individuals over 65. Since 65 was arbitrarily selected by those who drafted the Social Security legislation in 1935 as the age one becomes eligible for retirement benefits, the seventh decade has been associated with old age in the United States. Many feel Americans are actually programmed to retire and die at a time when they should be at their peak of productivity. Certainly, there is nothing biologically magic about the seventh decade in terms of physical and mental deterioration. In fact, we will see as we read and study this chapter that what you do as a young adult plays a major role in determining when you are *physiologically* old and that there is a big difference in the way different people age, a difference between chronological and physiological age. How old you are physiologically at age 65 or 70 may depend on your current lifestyle.

In addition, our nation's youth need to improve their skills in communicating with and understanding our nation's senior citizens, or "seniors." This chapter attempts to provide the necessary information to help you improve those skills in the home, social networks, and the workplace, and to help you begin thinking about and preparing for your older years.

Ageism

Never before has there been so many people over the age of 65. It is no wonder that this modern phenomenon has society perplexed about its treatment of this segment of the population. Even television and movies often portray older people as feeble-minded, physically and mentally impaired, unable to cope with daily routines, and a burden to society, particularly the younger generation. Industry and institutions of higher learning are reluctant to hire older individuals; landlords often avoid them as tenants; physicians may patronize them to the point of embarrassment; and the average youngster is taught to merely tolerate rather than respect and learn from seniors.[2]

TABLE 17.1

Population Age 65 and Over in the United States, 1900–1986

Year	Number (in Thousands)	Percentage of Total Population
1900	3,099	4.1
1910	3,986	4.3
1920	4,929	4.7
1930	6,705	5.4
1940	9,031	6.8
1950	12,397	8.2
1960	16,679	9.2
1970	20,177	9.9
1980	25,551	11.3
1986 (July 1)	29,172	12.1

Source: U.S. Bureau of the Census, *Current Population Reports* (Washington, D.C.: U.S. Government Printing Office, 1982); and U.S. Bureau of the Census, Current Population Reports, Series P-25, No. 1000. *Estimates of the Population of the United States, by Age, Sex, and Race: 1980 to 1986* (Washington, D.C.: U.S. Government Printing Office, 1987).

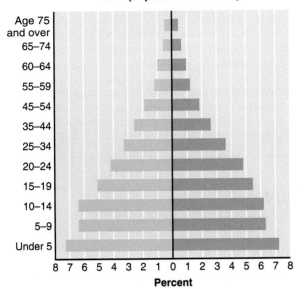

1870 (Population 40 million)

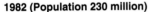

2000 (Population 260 million, projected)

Men   Women

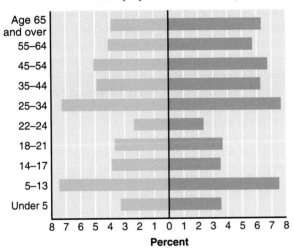

1982 (Population 230 million)

FIGURE 17.1 • Ageism and other problems of aging—physical, psychological, social, and financial—become more urgent as the population gets older. These three population pyramids show how the proportion of older people in the U.S. population is increasing. Younger people predominated in 1870, but the reverse will be true by 2000.

Sources: 1870, Judah Matras, *Populations and Societies* (Englewood Cliffs, N.J.: Prentice-Hall, 1973), p. 49. © 1973. Reprinted by permission of Prentice-Hall, Inc., Englewood Cliffs, N.J.; 1982 and 2000, adapted from U.S. Bureau of the Census, *Statistical Abstracts of the United States, 1989* (Washintgon, D.C.: U.S. Government Printing Office, 1989).

Old age is also mistakenly associated with senility, foul mood, and helplessness. Terms like "rickety," "decrepit," "codger," "geezer," "biddy," "hag," "old crank," "old miser," "cantankerous," and much worse are generally reserved for older people.[3] A little gray hair or loss of hair, a few wrinkles, and you may qualify for some of these adjectives in our society. All in fun? Perhaps not, for this type of attitude seems to be getting worse among all age groups, particularly among the nation's youth. Unfortunately, many of the solutions society has adopted to deal with older people are reflections of this negative thinking, referred to as

ageism. For many, old age is not nearly as much a problem as is the way society deals with it.

The emphasis placed on youth in the United States is clearly excessive and emotionally unhealthy. Aging is a natural process. In many cultures older individuals are respected for their experience, intelligence, and advice. In the United States, however, older people often reduce their social interaction in spite of their need and desire for it; they gradually withdraw as they lose their influence in society. Fortunately, with the increasing number of older people, groups of senior activists, such as the Gray Panthers and the American

primary aging The basic and inevitable process of aging, which is rooted in biological and genetic factors, regardless of health factors and lifestyle.

secondary aging The disabilities arising from degenerative diseases, such as arthritis and atherosclerosis; often such diseases can be delayed, prevented, or cured through medicine and good health habits.

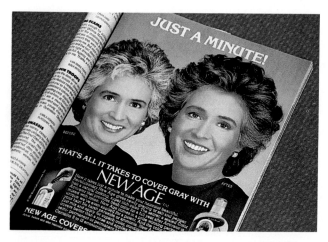

Our society persists in believing that "young" is the only good way to be. Faced with the fact that most of us will reach old age some day, do you think this is a reasonable belief?

Association of Retired Persons have emerged to work toward raising the status of seniors. As people become better informed about aging, society's view of these life passages will become more healthy.

How do you view older people? Complete Exploring Your Health 17.1 to find out.

Aging: Theories and Lifestyle Changes

Theories of Aging

Primary aging is biological, rooted in genetics and inevitable, regardless of health and daily routine. This biological process occurs at different rates for different people and may be modified or delayed through exercise, drugs, and changes in lifestyle. But the end result remains the same in time—aging and death. **Secondary aging** refers to disabilities resulting from degenerative diseases, such as arthritis, atherosclerosis, diabetes, and heart disease.

Several theories have been proposed to explain the reasons for the aging process. Let's briefly discuss some of these theories.

Free Radical Theory This popular theory has received the most support of all aging theories. Aging is said to be caused by the damaging effect of so-called *free-radicals*, chemical by-products of cell metabolism. The body does not get along well with these free-radicals produced in energy processes involving oxygen.

Exploring Your Health 17.1

How Do You View Older People?

Score each question numerically from 1 to 3 as follows: 1, untrue; 2, partially true; 3, true:

_____ 1. By the age of 65, intellectual deterioration is already noticeable.

_____ 2. People become ugly and unattractive with aging.

_____ 3. Older people rarely participate in sex due to a loss of interest.

_____ 4. Older people should be placed in special homes for the aged where they can be with individuals with similar interests and concerns.

_____ 5. Older people are "out of touch" with the real world and have very little understanding of today's youth.

_____ 6. Older people have little or no interest in current affairs.

_____ 7. The working individual loses efficiency in the sixth or seventh decade and should retire.

_____ 8. Older individuals are inflexible and uninterested in new ideas and concepts.

Interpretation 8–10 — you view the older individual as a normal, productive member of society; 11–13 — you tend to feel the older individual functions differently from other members of our society; 14 or higher — you systematically evaluate the older individual in a negative fashion.

Free radicals are suspected of accelerating the aging process and causing cancer, hypertension, senility, and immune system disorders. Reducing the number of free radicals in mice through diet manipulation has been shown to increase life span and resistance and inhibit certain cancers. Such a diet, designed to produce fewer "bad" free radicals, contains adequate nutrition, minimal amounts of saturated fats, 50–100 mg of selenium (a trace mineral); adequate vitamin E and C (suspected of reducing the adverse effects of free radicals); low protein, low fat, and low calories (reduced by 60 percent of usual consumption over five years, which is low enough to reduce total body weight), and high carbohydrate intake.

Genetic Theory
This theory suggests that we inherit cell makeup, which in turn controls aging. A "biological clock" ticks away one's life span and controls aging along the way. Some scientists feel the pituitary gland secretes a substance that controls the clock and degenerative changes. Other researchers focus on the thymus gland and feel that with the provision of replacement thymus hormones the efficiency of the body's immune system would decline more slowly with passing years and life span would increase.

Defective DNA or Genetic Material Theory
According to this theory, somehow the DNA becomes defective, thereby causing the synthesis of defective protein, until the organism is unable to function properly and deteriorates.

Errors Theory
This theory states that the body, at some point, begins to make errors in protein synthesis and produces changed proteins. As the body's immune system reacts against these changed proteins, cells are destroyed and body functions impaired, resulting in aging.

Aging Hits Theory
This theory argues that aging is a result of random events, accumulating errors that affect the body several times each year throughout life, which in turn affect cell life.

Accumulation of Deleterious Material Theory
This theory suggests that the body builds up unstable and harmful material that produces various detrimental biological changes, such as alterations in chromosomes, build-up in pigment, and alterations in macromolecules.

Stress-stimulated Response of the Adrenal Glands Theory
A relationship is proposed between aging and exercise. It is known that exercise stimulates both the adrenal cortex and the medulla, and this theory suggests that a cellular mechanism is responsible for increased life span through exercise.

Loss of Nerve Cells in the Brain Theory
Aging is suggested to be directly related to the nerve cells in the brain responsible for keeping body tissues finely tuned. Since nerve tissue neither divides nor is replaced, it is believed to be more prone to aging.

Hormone Imbalance Theory
Aging is strongly linked to the hormones.

Cross-linking of Molecules Theory
Theoretically, aging occurs when giant molecules in cells, such as DNA, link with other molecules, which then become unable to function properly. Exactly what causes this phenomenon is unknown.

Autoimmune Theory
This theory suggests that the DNA changes, thereby altering protein synthesis and creating protein the body's immune system does not recognize. The immune system's attack on these foreign proteins results in physiological aging.

Improving Longevity Through Lifestyle Changes

The theories of aging concern bodily processes that we as individuals can't control. However, several aging processes can be altered and longevity may be improved by adopting certain lifestyle changes.

Life expectancy in the United States has risen from about 54.1 years in 1920 to 73.3 years in 1986.[4] Much of the increase can be attributed to reduced infant mortality rates and control of childhood diseases. The majority of deaths in the age range of 10 to 70 years are

Regular exercise plays an important part in staying physically and mentally healthy during older years.

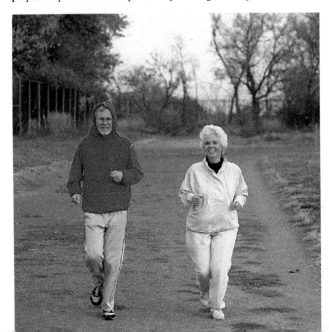

TABLE ◆ 17.2

Lifestyle Risk Factors Associated with the Leading Causes of Death in the United States

Cause of Death	Lifestyle Risk Factors
Heart disease	Smoking, high blood pressure, high serum cholesterol, diabetes, obesity, lack of exercise, stress
Cancer	Smoking, alcohol, sun exposure, radiation, worksite hazards, environmental pollution, obesity, diet
Stroke	High blood pressure, high serum cholesterol, smoking, diet, obesity, lack of exercise, stress
Accidents Motor vehicle	Alcohol, nonuse of seat belts, speed, automobile design, roadway design
Other than motor vehicle	Alcohol, smoking, product design, home hazards, handgun availability
Chronic obstructive pulmonary diseases	Smoking, environmental pollutants, worksite hazards
Influenza/ pneumonia	Vaccination status, smoking, alcohol, diet
Diabetes	Obesity, diet
Suicide	Stress, alcohol and drug misuse, handgun availability
Chronic liver disease and cirrhosis	Alcohol
Atherosclerosis	Smoking, high blood pressure, high serum cholesterol, diabetes, obesity, lack of exercise, stress

Source: From J. E. Fielding, "Health Promotion and Disease Prevention at the Worksite," p. 239. Reproduced, with permission, from the *Annual Review of Public Health*, vol. 5. © 1984 by Annual Reviews Inc.

accidental or due to degenerative diseases. Because degenerative diseases are related to lifestyle, many believe that changes in lifestyle can lead to a significant increase in longevity.

Table 17.2 lists the lifestyle factors associated with the leading causes of death in the United States. Among the most important are overweight and obesity, smoking, poor nutritional habits, excessive stress, and inactivity. Adopting the right lifestyle may even help prevent some of the more common ailments occurring in older people, as shown in Figure 17.2.

Overweight is a particularly important contributor to artery damage, and the process of clogging of the arteries can start very early in life. Fat deposits that lead to hardening of the arteries and related age-associated diseases, such as stroke, senility, and coronary heart disease, have been identified in children as young as 10 years of age.

Cigarette smoking accelerates artery clogging and greatly increases the risk of death from coronary artery disease, heart attack, and stroke in the adult years. The incidence of cancer, chronic bronchitis, and emphysema also increases.

FIGURE 17.2 ◆ The majority of older people have at least one chronic disease and many have multiple problems.
Source: National Institutes on Aging. FDA Consumer/October 1988.

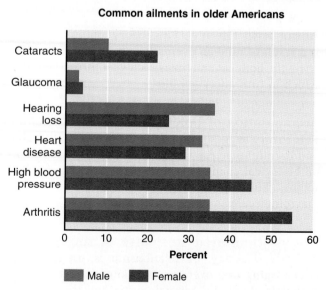

Common ailments in older Americans

■ Male ■ Female

Excessive stress has also been associated with a number of life-threatening diseases such as ulcers, mental illness, hypertension, heart disease, stroke, cancer, and diabetes mellitus. Learning to manage stress throughout one's life may be a very valuable means of increasing life expectancy.

Inactivity as a lifestyle factor in early death is especially prevalent among Americans. The average American leads a sedentary life throughout adulthood. Although aerobic exercise, such as jogging, fast walking, lap swimming, and other healthy activities are becoming increasingly popular, it is still true that fewer than 50 percent of the American people exercise at least twice per week.

Although there are no guarantees of longer life, you can improve your chances by making certain lifestyle changes. Lifestyle changes that incorporate the following healthy behaviors should increase the likelihood that an individual will be free from certain types of diseases and able to live a healthier, perhaps longer life:

- Engage in an aerobic exercise program (see Chapter 9) at least three times weekly throughout life.
- Avoid smoking cigarettes or using tobacco in any form (see Chapter 12).
- Eat a balanced diet and drink alcohol only in moderation (see Chapters 7 and 11).
- Control body weight and maintain minimal body fat (see Chapter 8).
- Control high blood pressure and diabetes (see Chapters 13 and 15).
- Reduce excessive emotional stress (see Chapter 3).
- Remain socially active throughout life, keeping mentally alert and involved as much as possible.
- Use all body systems; the cliché "use it or lose it" has implications for all systems, including sexual activity and mental functions.
- Adopt a lifestyle conducive to the prevention of chronic and degenerative diseases (see Chapters 13–16).
- Learn to live with yourself and accept your limitations (mental, physical, and economic).

Physical Health and Aging

Too much emphasis is placed on the physical changes that come with aging. These changes are natural adaptations of the human body as it ages. Being fully aware of what changes may be expected can help us adjust and accept the changes as they occur. A summary of the findings to date is shown in Table 17.3.[5] As discussed, your behavior as a young adult and throughout life has a bearing on when and how much some of these changes occur. None of the changes are as dramatic as some may anticipate and all are natural.

TABLE 17.3

Physical Changes Occurring with Age

Skin	Wrinkles occur from facial expressions as skin becomes less elastic, thins, and spreads.
Eyes	The lens hardens; the amount of light reaching the retina declines; glasses are needed to read; peripheral vision, night vision, adjustment to the dark, and the ability to distinguish between blues and greens decrease.
Head	Features become more distinguished; the head grows larger.
Hair	Hair thins out and shrinks, some men become bald; men acquire hair on other parts of the body.
Mouth	The ability to taste diminishes somewhat, the mouth becomes drier, and the voice pitch rises slightly.
Teeth	The amount of enamel decreases; tooth loss may occur if gums are not taken care of.
Ears	Hearing diminishes slightly each decade.
Kidneys	The amount of waste that kidneys filter decreases with age.
Sex	Sexual activity decreases somewhat; obtaining an erection, vaginal lubrication, reaching orgasm, and recovering all take longer.
Height	Some loss of height occurs as the bones of the spine move closer together.
Weight, fat, muscle	Additional weight and fat accumulate; the ratio of muscle mass to body fat decreases
Stamina, heart	Maximum oxygen uptake (amount of oxygen that can be taken in and used) diminishes with each decade.
Reflexes	Reflexes slow only slightly.

osteoporosis The weakening of bones as a result of decalcification; often considered a normal part of aging.

Lifestyle during the college years often carries over into old age. Young adults who exercise regularly, eat right, practice sound nutrition, manage weight and fat, avoid smoking, and use alcohol and other drugs in moderation tend to continue these health practices throughout life. More important, these behaviors will have a strong influence on future health. The twenties and thirties represent years when invisible physiological changes occur: The total number of cells in the body decreases, cells become less efficient in burning fuel for energy, and cells use that energy less efficiently. In addition, active nucleic acids, such as DNA,

are present in lower concentrations, which affects how we renew and repair tissue. Because of lowered DNA, there is a decrease in the production of a variety of chemicals, mainly those responsible for keeping the body functioning exactly as it was designed to function. The visible signs of aging, such as those listed in Table 17.3, may be far less important than these invisible changes.

Skin Aging

The condition of your skin changes considerably over time. From *age 20 to 29,* your skin will be the most healthy, smooth, and radiant. Skin is still renewing itself in the early twenties with cells rising to the outer surface layer of the skin (outside the epidermis) and shedding every three to four weeks. This process slows down in the late twenties. If you neglect to protect your skin during these "sunworshipping years," the sun could cause you to look much older or it could produce skin cancer. It is during these critical years that the skin must be protected through an absence of smoking, a proper diet, regular exercise, and the use of a good skin care routine.

From *age 30 to 39,* tiny wrinkles generally appear around the mouth and eyes where skin is thinnest and driest. Men also develop forehead lines. Years of sun abuse produce smile and frown lines, squint lines, and freckles and make the skin more taut and rough.

From *age 40 to 49,* facial expressions performed thousands of times increase lines from the bottom of the nose to the corners of the mouth (from smiling), vertical lines between the eyebrows (from scowling), and "crow's feet" around the eyes (from squinting). Under-eye puffiness, drooping eyelids, dryness, and other skin irritations may also appear. Males, with their thicker skin, hair follicles that act like supporting beams to anchor skin in place, and shaving, which speeds up new cell formation and the removal of dead surface cells, tend to keep their skin younger looking.

From *age 50 to 59,* wrinkles are deeper, lines are more pronounced, skin elasticity has decreased, and the skin is drier. Men exhibit jowls and hands begin to show wrinkles, redness, protruding veins, and tiny folds around knuckles.

From *age 60 and older,* muscle and skeletal tissue loss occurs and body mass shrinks. To accommodate this change, skin increases and sags. Muscles around the eyes weaken, bags form, and the tips of the nose and earlobes may drop. The skin feels rougher, skin color may be uneven, liver spots occur in the form of enlarged freckle-like dark areas, and itching is common. The years of sun have taken their toll as the risk of superficial skin cancer and melanoma doubles.[6]

Infectious Diseases

Infectious diseases and injuries have more serious consequences in people of advanced age.[7] With age, minor injuries such as cuts and scrapes are more likely to become infected. Along with a decrease in the body's ability to repair itself comes a less efficient immune system, making us more vulnerable to attack by *pathogens* (disease-producing organisms). Preventive inoculations against some infections such as pneumococcal pneumonia and influenza are helpful.

Noninfectious or Chronic and Degenerative Diseases

Chronic conditions that gradually worsen as the body's resistance and repair mechanisms become less efficient are the greatest cause of death and disability in older people. Cardiovascular diseases, such as heart disease and cerebrovascular accident (stroke), hypertension, and atherosclerosis, are the number-one chronic disease of the elderly, accounting for more than 60 percent of deaths in those over age 65 (see Chapter 13). Cancer (20.4 percent) ranks second among causes of death, with over one-half of all types of cancers found in those over 65 years of age, possibly due to long exposure to triggering factors and the inefficiency of the immune system (see Chapter 13). Influenza and pneumonia (3.6 percent) and diabetes mellitus (2.2 percent) are two additional diseases commonly affecting older people.[8] The incidence of autoimmune diseases (see Chapter 13), such as rheumatoid arthritis and others affecting connective tissue, also increases with age.

Osteoporosis   In people of all ages, bone is in a constant state of change referred to as *remodeling.* Small quantities of old bone are lost through resorption by the body and new bone is formed to counter the loss. In some people, the formation of new bone fails to keep pace with the resorption of old bone, which produces a condition known as **osteoporosis** (porous bones).

Calcium, phosphorus, and vitamin D are the three major building blocks of bone tissue. Approximately 80 to 90 percent of your body's phosphorus and 99 percent of its calcium are located in your skeleton. Bones act as a kind of storage space for these important minerals, giving and taking them to and from the

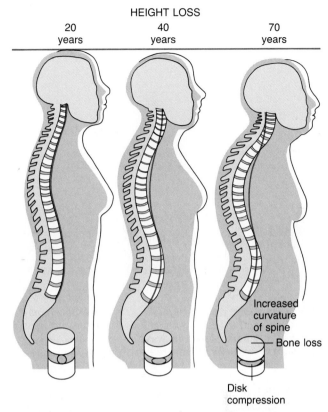

HEIGHT LOSS

| 20 years | 40 years | 70 years |

Increased curvature of spine

Bone loss

Disk compression

FIGURE 17.3   •   One of the effects of osteoporosis is compression of the spinal cord through bone mineral loss, which results in decreased height and curvature of the back with age. Proper diet, exercise, and medication can greatly reduce these effects.

blood and other body fluids to maintain proper concentrations. People who have a low dietary intake of foods rich in calcium, phosphorous, and vitamin D therefore run the risk of developing weak, brittle skeletons, especially later in life.[9] These changes are usually not obvious in your younger years. Osteoporosis develops silently and painlessly and normally goes unnoticed until a bone actually breaks or noticeable height has been lost. In its advanced stages it can cause considerable suffering, economic problems, and even death.

Osteoporosis is a major concern among older people. Although a reduction in some bone mass occurs "naturally" and may not affect normal functioning, a high percentage of postmenopausal women and some older men experience loss of enough skeletal mass to greatly increase the risk of fractures in the hip, wrists, spine, and other bones (see Figure 17.3). Approximately 200,000 people suffer from broken hips each year; 12 to 20 percent of these people die from complications of their fractures and many others are permanently incapacitated. A condition referred to as *crush* (spinal fractures) occurs when one or more vertebrae collapse from the weight of the upright body on bones that have become brittle and weak due to mineral loss. Another condition, called *dowager's hump,* results in loss of height and severe back pain. Bone loss in the

Exploring Your Health 17.2

How Healthy Will You Be in Your Old Age?

Research shows that lifestyle is highly related to health and well-being. Although there is no way to accurately predict your future health, it is clear that how you live the first three decades of your life will affect your health in old age. Some of the more important habits you practice today that may affect your future health are included in this activity. Place the number of the item best describing your current behavior in the space provided at the left of the category. Total your score and consult the scoring chart below to estimate your chances of having an active, healthy late adulthood:

_____ **Cigarette Smoking Habits**
(daily consumption)
0. Nonsmoker who never smoked
1. Nonsmoker who quit
3. One-half to one pack cigarettes; pipe or cigar smoker
5. Smokeless tobacco user
7. One to one and one-half packs cigarettes
9. One and one-half to two packs cigarettes
10. More than two packs per day

_____ **Exercise Habits**
1. Regular aerobic exercise 20 minutes or more at the target heart rate level, a minimum of three times weekly
2. Tennis, racquetball, handball, squash, full-court basketball, or equivalent sport, a minimum of four times weekly
3. Aerobic exercise two to three times weekly

4. Sports participation exercise two to three times weekly
5. Occasional exercise one to two times weekly
6. Sedentary—never exercise

_____ **Eating Habits**
1. Regular, balanced meals from the basic food groups with moderate consumption of saturated fats, salt, and sugar, and adequate fiber intake
2. Follow most of the factors listed above
3. Skip breakfast or noon meal regularly
4. Snack between meals and before bedtime on high-calorie foods
5. Consume four or more drinks of alcohol daily
6. High fat content in the diet

_____ **Weight Control**
1. Body weight (according to weight charts) and body fat are within the recommended ranges (less than 15 percent for men and 20 percent for women) and stable
2. Slightly overweight: approximately 20 percent above recommended weight on charts and between 16 and 20 percent (for men) or 21 and 25 percent (for women) body fat as determined by skinfold measures or underwater weighing
3. Underweight: approximately 20 percent below recommended weight on charts and less than 7 percent body fat (unless you are a highly conditioned athlete)
4. "Seesaw" up and down through use of two to three diets annually to

remain close to standard described in item two
5. More than 30 percent above recommended ranges on weight charts or in excess of 25 percent (for men) or 30 percent (for women) body fat
7. More than 40 percent above recommended ranges on weight charts or in excess of 40 percent body fat

_____ **Health Care**
1. Regular medical and dental check-ups, including examinations in high cancer risk areas (colon, breast, testicles, lungs, and so forth)
3. Regular medical and dental check-ups without examinations in high cancer risk areas
5. Occasional physical examinations for special occasions, such as company check-ups, obtaining new insurance policies, and so forth
7. Rarely secure medical or dental check-ups

_____ **Stress Management**
1. Type B behavior pattern
2. Type A behavior pattern that is under control, motivating your work habits but not adding constant stress; presence of pleasurable relaxation in daily routine
3. Some signs of Type A behavior and some signs of Type B behavior
4. Type A behavior pattern

Scoring Probability of having an active, healthy late adulthood: excellent: 6–9; fair: 10–14; poor: 15 or more.

jaw may also cause oral health problems and tooth loss.

Who is at risk for osteoporosis? In addition to people who do not consume enough calcium, phosphorus, and vitamin D in their diets, connections between osteoporosis and smoking, alcohol use, and sedentary living have also been established. In addition, some cases point to the possibility of certain physical, hormonal, and genetic factors in developing osteoporosis.

The primary mode of preventing osteoporosis is to reach middle and old age with as much bone mass as possible. This goal is especially important for females, who in the current older population are eight times more likely than males to develop osteoporosis because of less bone and muscle mass, less frequent exercise, and less consumption of calcium-rich foods. There are four areas of your lifestyle and your body's functioning that you should pay attention to in order to reduce your risk of developing osteoporosis:

1. **Nutrition** (men and women). Sufficient calcium, phosphorus, and vitamin D are critical. Too much protein, alcohol, caffeine, fiber, and vitamin A may harm your body's bone production. See Chapter 7 on Nutrition for further information on forming proper dietary habits.

2. **Exercise** (men and women). Inactive individuals lose bone mass at a rapid rate. Although it is important to develop good exercise habits early in life, older people should not think that it's too late to fight the effects of osteoporosis. Walking, jogging, racquetball, squash, tennis, handball, golf, and aerobic dance are all forms of exercise that provide excellent work for the long bones, bring dietary calcium to the bones, and generally stimulate bone formation.[10]

3. **Smoking** (especially women). Women who smoke have been found to possess less bone mass than nonsmokers.

4. **Estrogen** (women only). If your body is not producing enough estrogen to cause menstruation, it is probably not producing enough to avoid bone mineral loss. As estrogen production decreases, the bones contribute more calcium to meet the body's needs. You should consult your physician about this. *Hormone replacement therapy,* which involves the use of drugs that produce hormonal changes, is one possible way of dealing with this problem.

Sexuality and Older Age

One of the most notable signs of aging for women is the cessation of menstruation and ovulation. These events, referred to as *menopause* or "change of life," may cause emotional and physical problems in some women. Skin may become dry and less elastic. Lubrication secretions in the vagina may be reduced. Some women experience sudden sensation of heat (hot flashes). But only about 25 percent of women experi-

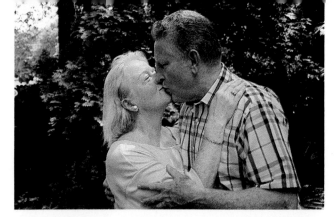

Sexual feelings last throughout life. Your present attitude about sexuality may indicate how sexually active you will be in older years.

ence disturbing symptoms that require a physician's care. The loss of fertility may place considerable stress on some women. However, research suggests that for most, middle age may bring a sense of freedom from worry about unwanted pregnancy and a heightened interest in sexual activity.

While some men experience reduced sexual drive during middle age, reproductive changes similar to those in women do not occur. The average man remains fertile and capable of sexual relations throughout life. However, men do require more time to achieve erections as they grow older, and they ejaculate with less force.

Sexuality in old age is more problematic. While some older individuals continue to be sexually active, others who are still healthy and have a healthy partner fail to do so because of societal attitudes. The myths that old people are not supposed to have sexual feelings and that to continue sexual activity in old age is shameful are still prevalent. These attitudes arise long before people reach old age. Your present attitude and your own sexual adjustment are probably the best indicators of whether you'll continue to be sexually active in your later years. It is a choice you can make.

Cognitive Functioning and Aging

For the healthy individual, verbal skills, reasoning ability, and IQ should improve during middle adulthood (ages 40 to 60). After the age of 60, some cognitive skills diminish, although this decline is small in many healthy individuals. Other cognitive skills may not decline at all. Studies have shown that when older people are motivated, improvements occur in short-term memory, alertness, and mental activity.[11] In an atmosphere of challenge, usefulness, and love, rather than boredom, mental abilities should decline only slightly with age. Long-term memory does decline in many, but not all, older people, although this decline is moderate and not nearly as great as people imagine. Both genetics and environment play a part in determining the amount of intellectual decline in later life. Studies

Alzheimer's disease A brain disorder, affecting 6 to 8 percent of the older population over 65; it is characterized by memory loss, and gradually leads to a generalized inability to function independently.

dementia A term used to describe both Alzheimer's disease and a nonspecific progressive mental impairment found in some older people.

successful aging A life characterized by satisfaction and high morale in old age, usually the result of high activity and engagement of the older person in his or her society and environment.

A Question of Ethics

Is It Ethical for Manufacturers to Bombard the American Public with Antiaging Products?

Although getting old is a natural, unavoidable part of life, our society continues to send out thousands of inaccurate messages that it doesn't have to happen, at least not so fast. To slow down the aging process or at least to look decades younger, one only has to undergo cosmetic surgery (face lifts, tummy, thigh, and buttocks tucks, fat removal from anywhere and everywhere), have a hair transplant, or purchase a special product to rejuvenate one's aging skin or body. Unfortunately, the cost of trying to stay young is steep—thousands of dollars for special operations and monthly costs as high as $100 for special products, at a time in life when retired Americans are living with reduced incomes. In 1986, the famous Dr. Christian Barnard was censured by dermatologists for endorsing Alfin Fragrances, Inc.'s Glycel antiaging cream in ads imply-

ing he had made a major discovery about the aging process. Others who have advertised products indicating that their use will take up to ten years off your looks without expensive plastic surgery have been criticized openly by the Better Business Bureau and medical experts. One of the few products that appears to be capable of really making a difference in rejuvenating aging skin is Retin A, an expensive item that shows considerable promise in eliminating some, but not all, wrinkles and making skin smoother.

As we age skin becomes thinner and more fragile. Retin A has been shown to thicken forearm skin by 40 percent. Its use turns over epidermal cells, selectively encourages damaged cells to come to the surface and slough off, and encourages new cell growth. Old cells are peeled away and the number of fine blood vessels

near the skin surface increases and causes some smoothing of the skin.

Should such a trend be permitted to continue? Although products can make some improvement in the appearance of the skin, there are no fountains of youth. The chances of any product serving to slow the aging process are quite slim. Doesn't our senior population have enough to worry about dealing with economic and health concerns? Should they be subjected to constant reminders of their passing years? Should they be given continuous false hopes of an eternal youth? One has to wonder how this trend affects the mental health of our senior population and whether something should be done to stop this practice.

What do you think?

of identical twins indicate that they are much more alike in their cognitive functioning in the older years than fraternal twins or unrelated individuals. Negative surroundings, expectations of intellectual decline, and the absence of stimulation in one's environment are also critical factors that influence cognitive performance in older people.

Older individuals who stay involved in interesting and challenging intellectual activities are less likely to decline in cognitive performance. In fact, such an environment may actually reverse cognitive declines that have already occurred. So-called crystalized intelligence, the accumulation of abilities gained through instruction such as vocabulary, general information, and mathematical rules, should continue into old age.

"Fluid" intelligence, the general ability to detect relationships and transform information which is resistant to education and instruction, declines somewhat by late adulthood in most individuals.[12]

Alzheimer's Disease and Dementia

The idea that most older people become senile is nothing more than a myth. There is a brain disorder known as **Alzheimer's disease,** which affects approximately 6 to 8 percent of older people (about one in forty people over the age of 65, causing about 120,000 deaths per year).[13] Figure 17.4 depicts the estimated increase in the incidence of Alzheimer's disease from 1980 to 2030.

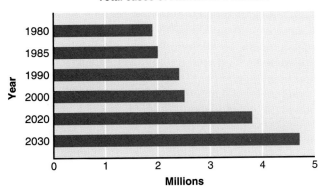

Total cases of Alzheimer's disease

FIGURE 17.4 • Alzheimer's Outlook, 1980 to 2030.
Source: Estimates by the National Institute on Aging.

Symptoms of Alzheimer's may be evident as early as age 40, or not until after age 80, although it is much more common in older people. After diagnosis, patients generally pass through three stages over a five to fifteen year period. In the *early stage* of Alzheimer's disease, patients develop persistent forgetfulness, are unable to recall names and experience difficulty in making lists, reading maps, and performing other simple chores. In the *middle stage,* it becomes more clear that the condition is something other than occasional absentmindedness, as patients experience considerable difficulty in talking, making simple explanations, and following directions. Mood changes, such as feelings of anger, paranoia, and clinical depression arise. In the later more *severe stage* patients may be unable to recognize family members, lose bodily functions and speech, and need constant care.

Several genetic links to Alzheimer's disease have been uncovered. In some families, five or six people in generation after generation develop the disease. Another recent genetic link is the connection between Alzheimer's and Down's syndrome, a birth defect associated with a duplication of chromosome 21, which causes mental retardation and a shortened life span. As Down's patients reach age 30 to 40, memory problems and dementia are common. Examination of brain tissue has revealed numerous similarities between Down's syndrome and Alzheimer's. The Down's-Alzheimer's link provides hope that chromosomal studies, an active area of research, will eventually lead to a process that alters the mutation to prevent the disease from occurring.

Treatment for Alzheimer's is steadily improving, although it is still in the experimental stages. Some new drugs show promise of slowing the disease and improving the quality of life by making patients more comfortable. Since Alzheimer's is more likely to affect new memories, patients relate to old tunes and respond to music. Pets are also helpful in renewing memories and providing comfort.

The term **dementia** is used to describe two conditions: (1) specific chronic, progressive, and irreversible conditions such as Alzheimer's disease, and (2) nonspecific progressive mental impairment, sometimes reversible, in at least three of the following areas: language, memory, visual-spatial skills, emotion or personality, and cognition. Drugs (the most common cause), systemic illnesses, conditions affecting nerves in the brain, exogenous toxins (heavy metals, solvents and industrial agents, pollution), and aging are the main causes of dementia.[14] The AIDS virus has also been found in the brain cells of people diagnosed as dementia patients. Success in the treatment of both reversible and irreversible dementia is increasing, and the tendency to treat dementia in older people as an irreversible condition is changing.

Social Adjustment and Aging

The last years of life should be a time of pleasure and fulfillment, a time to reflect on life with satisfaction. Unfortunately, the self-esteem, self-confidence, and satisfaction of the aged are threatened by cultural attitudes associated with physical appearance, abilities, and social roles. A reduction in both abilities and responsibilities can produce feelings of inadequacy and low self-worth. How then do older people adjust psychologically and socially?

Successful Aging

Consider two theories of **successful aging,** which we define as satisfaction and high morale in old age.

The *activity theory* suggests that increasing regular,

Successful aging involves pursuing old and new physical, social, intelluctual, and emotional activities. Many activities combine all of these elements.

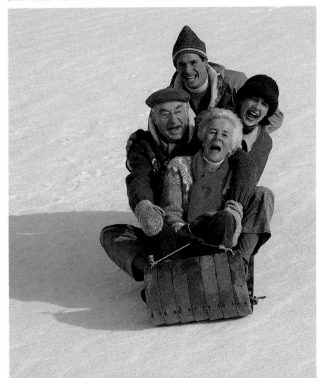

mid-life crisis A period of confusion, doubt, depression, and anxiety experienced by many middle-aged men and women; it is related to growing older and to the psychological and physical changes inherent in that process.

meaningful activity in one's profession and social organizations or beginning new pursuits is one way older people cope more successfully and live more meaningful lives. Most experts agree that what older people need to retain their function is physical activity, social contacts, and intellectual and emotional stimulation.

The *disengagement theory* is the opposite side of the coin and suggests that aging individuals and society mutually disengage from one another. Modern American society clearly has lesser expectations of older persons and socially "excuses" them from many tasks and responsibilities. Older people consequently become preoccupied with themselves, are content to relax, withdraw, and let others take their former roles in society. The two theories are not entirely mutually exclusive. The time eventually comes when activity is no longer meaningful or possible, and the individual and society must disengage from one another.

Studies indicate that successful aging is associated with good health, job satisfaction, an emotionally stable marital relationship, physical activity, and secondary group activity (activity with friends). This and other research tends to support the activity theory of aging.[15]

Mid-Life Crisis

Although some experts feel **mid-life crisis** is just another developmental stage we all pass through, not everyone goes through the experience. Opponents of the developmental stage theory argue that mid-life crisis is triggered by too much stress in a short time period. Such stress may be a divorce, the death of a family member, financial loss, or other factors all occurring within a period of six to twelve months or so. Although menopause and hormonal changes have been associated with mid-life crisis in women, men also experience mid-life crisis. What hits a man when he hits 40? No one seems to know, yet some men vigorously try to recapture their youth with sports cars, young women, athletics, and other behaviors common to young males. In some families, it is a stressful period of time that eventually passes. The realization that many of these feelings are natural and common to most people of similar ages helps to shorten the adjustment period.

Widowhood

Of the more than 12 million widowed men and women in the United States, approximately 11 million are widows. Women outlive men by ten or more years. Assuming that the ten-year difference in life span between men and women will continue, approximately 75 percent of wives will be widowed at some time in their lives. The average age of widows is 56 and the probability of remarriage is quite low. The first year after death of a mate is the most difficult; there is a high death rate for the surviving spouse and an increased likelihood of suicide. Both widows and widowers find adjustment difficult. Widows are more likely to suffer from chronic disabling physical ailments and face financial difficulties resulting from reduced income. In addition, widows find that they are often excluded from social gatherings, have no one to escort them to social functions, are viewed with suspicion by some married women, and often can find friends only among other widows. Widowers are particularly susceptible to coronary heart disease, and they suffer a number of simultaneous role changes, such as loss of job, reduced income, loss of spouse, loss of health, and inability to assume the domestic responsibilities shouldered by the wife during the marriage. Widows, on the other hand, generally established more independent mid-life roles when children left home.

Remarriage

In general, older widows tend not to remarry and seek other widows as friends, whereas older widowers remarry within one year of the death of their spouses. Widows who remarry do so an average of seven years after the death of their husbands. Widowers have many more women to choose from in their age group but are more apt to marry younger women. The widow is less likely to marry a younger man because this is not as accepted in our society.

Most widows and widowers marry old friends, childhood lovers, or former neighbors. The majority of marriages that occur late in life are successful; few end in divorce.

It is becoming more common for older couples to seek alternatives to marriage. Living together provides love, security, comfort, and companionship; it also prevents a reduction in Social Security benefits or in a widow's pension.

Retirement

Retirement means different things to different people. In our youth-oriented society, many people look on retirement as a signpost of old age. It is often assumed that retired people have difficulty adjusting to the loss of their primary role in life—that of productive worker. How true this is depends on several factors. People who have been forced to retire before they wanted to may indeed feel a sense of rejection and loss. However, there are many others who look forward to retirement at 65 or even earlier as a chance to experience new challenges or simply to enjoy a more relaxing lifestyle.

One important factor in how people feel about retirement is income. Many people retire voluntarily before the age of 65 if they are financially solvent. Concern about their financial future is often what keeps people on the job until the age of 65. Another factor in how people view retirement is whether they have planned for it. The adjustment is much easier for individuals who have planned for their retirement in terms of finances, activities, and the like.

What can be done to help people prepare for retirement? Our society as a whole needs to change its attitude. We believe that people should not be forced to retire before they are ready. It is time for Americans to begin to value older individuals, use their talents, and treat them with respect and dignity. Similarly, older persons should stop viewing themselves as useless and should perform useful activities throughout life. This means developing a healthy involvement and positive attitudes from childhood on. What does retirement mean to you? What can you do to prepare yourself for this life passage? Do you want to retire early or work as long as you can? Why? How will you handle it if you are forced to retire before you want to? Use Exploring Your Health 17.3 to answer these questions.

Programs Available to Older People

Your chances of needing custodial care (sheltered living arrangements for older people, such as nursing homes or homes for the aged) during the retirement years are approximately one in twenty-four. Many people are placed in custodial care because they lack family ties or are a burden to their relatives. In some countries, institutionalizing a family member is unheard of, since it is assumed to be the responsibility of the offspring. In the United States, the cost of securing adequate care in institutions is becoming prohibitive. Perhaps it is time to adopt a similar custom and assume responsibility for our own seniors. Home care is more personal and less traumatic for seniors, and less expensive to all concerned. Alternatives are available for older people who are not in need of constant medical

---

Exploring Your Health 17.3

Planning Your Future, Today!

It is never too early to plan for retirement and old age. Even young college students like yourself will be old someday, and some of the decisions you make now and immediately after graduation will affect your future physical health, mental health, and economic security. Make a list of the things you can do *now* and *within the next few years* in each of the areas listed below to help secure your future:

Retirement (IRA and other retirement policies):

_____

_____

_____

Health insurance (short- and long-term plans):

_____

_____

_____

Health care:

_____

_____

_____

Preventive health care and your health behaviors:

_____

_____

_____

Special interests and hobbies:

_____

_____

_____

gerontology The study of aging as a scientific discipline; *geriatrics* is the medical treatment of older people.

Issues in Health

Are Retirement Communities Helpful?

Pro Over 25 million Americans are over 65, and this population of older people is expected to increase as the birth rate falls and better medical care and preventive medicine increase life expectancy beyond the age of 73. Society still has not learned to use the skills and knowledge of senior citizens, and adjustment to the retirement years is traumatic for approximately 30 percent of Americans who decide to leave their working days behind them. The decision to remain in the community or enter a retirement community presents a unique set of problems.

Retirement can make people feel useless. Work identity is of major importance to most men and women. In addition, friendships may center around work. Retirement often results in a loss of identity and contact with work friends. The one or two close relationships that an individual has had through work may disappear. Retirement communities provide the opportunity to establish new close relationships, particularly a close friendship which psychiatrists feel is important to adjustment in the later years. Proponents of retirement communities argue that new friendships are easily developed among peers who are experiencing similar changes in their lives. These communities also provide ideal settings for widows and widowers to meet individuals of their own age and increase the opportunity for courtship, marriage, and alternatives to marriage.

Con Opponents of the retirement community concept argue that such communities are often located far from one's residence, forcing a move that takes the individual away from close friends and relatives. This separation and new environment can be traumatic. Retirement communities also separate older people from the rest of society and perpetuate the myth that the old are misfits and have no significant contribution to make. Suddenly, retired individuals are faced with a totally new environment, new friends, and new roles, and they are completely isolated from the society in which they worked and played for sixty years or more. So many drastic changes, it is argued, may be too much for some individuals to handle. In addition, many of these communities are too expensive for individuals who rely on Social Security benefits for their financial support.

What do you think?

---

attention, such as retirement communities and "networking" organizations that allow older people to secure support or help.

A wide variety of programs are now available to assist older people in practically every phase of their lives. In addition, these programs are expanding to better meet the needs of seniors:

- **The Older Americans Act.** Passed in 1965, this act established the Administration of Aging within the federal government, which requires states to establish units on aging and authorizes state and community social service programs. Homemaker services, transportation, congregate meals, nutrition education counseling, and a foster grandparent program were funded.

- **Senior centers.** These centers have developed a variety of programs to aid healthy older people remain active in community life.

- **The Foster Grandparents program.** This is a project designed to provide employment for older workers. Foster Grandparents work twenty hours weekly at minimum wage in child-care institutions. Budget reductions under the Reagan administration forced a decrease in the number of these programs. Unfortunately, state and local governments have not been able to pick up the costs of funding them as originally planned.

- **The National Institute on Aging (NIA).** The NIA deals with scientific inquiry into issues and concerns of seniors and research on aging. Located within the National Institute of Health, the NIA supports research on health-related topics, such as nutrition, Alzheimer's disease, and biological indicators of aging, as well as sociological topics. The development of **gerontology** (the study of aging) as a scientific discipline is credited to the NIA.

Findings benefit the older population and improve society's treatment of them.

- **Social Security.** This is by far the most important government program assisting the economic needs of the older people. Unfortunately, it has become very expensive for those still in the workforce and inadequate for those forced to live on its benefits alone.
- **National health insurance.** Medicare and Medicaid (not solely for the aged) help defray some of the health-care costs of the older people.
- **Homemaker services.** These services help seniors with laundering, shopping, and preparing meals; however, services are not paid by Medicare.
- **Meal programs.** These programs evolved from the Comprehensive Services Amendment to the Older Americans Act in 1972 and help improve the nutrition of older people by providing one hot meal a day, five days per week.
- **Geriatric day care centers.** Centers are developing for older people with mental and physical impairments who can remain in the community if support services are available.

You, the reader, are probably between the ages of 18 and 21, so most of these programs are not going to mean anything to you personally right now. However, you probably have older friends or relatives who might be interested in—or who might even need—these programs. But ask yourself: Is that it? Do these programs represent all that can be done for and with the older people in my life? Is there anything I can and should do?

Older People and You

Many young people are uncomfortable or impatient with the older people in their lives. Part of the reason for this, as we have mentioned, is that our society places a premium on youthfulness. Other reasons include a fear of growing older, a fear of the mortality (dying and death) that aging points to, and the hectic lifestyles that society often tells young people they should be leading—lifestyles that don't allow time for spending with people who can't help us get that promotion, close that deal, or improve ourselves in some other obvious (preferably material) way.

On a broad, societal level, it is becoming increasingly clearer that young Americans—whether they like it or not—are going to have to get over these fears and attitudes and develop new ways of thinking about and coping with the needs, lifestyles, and social and political goals of older people. It is hoped that you will be able to think positively about these necessary changes. Certainly, if you cannot think about them in terms of other people, perhaps you should keep in mind that you, too, are aging. How would you like to be viewed by younger people when you are old enough to be called a senior?

On the level of individuals and families, many young Americans are facing the prospect of seeing their parents and grandparents live to increasingly older ages. This may be a mixed blessing, for while some older Americans remain healthy and self-sufficient right up to the day they die, the vast majority of seniors will eventually arrive at a time when they will no longer be able to live independently. Have you experienced a situation like this? What was your response to this situation?

Giving and Receiving Care There are many ways to spend time with older people in your own family and in your local community. Besides occasional visits for companionship and conversation, you can make a real contribution to the lives of older people in fairly simple, everyday ways. Doing household chores, providing the grocery shopping, doing personal finances, paying bills, and providing transportation are all potential problems for older people who are trying to live independently.

If the older person needs more attention than you or other people can give, then it may be time to consider getting the help of a care-giving facility such as a day care center or nursing home. Helping an older person choose such facilities can be a very difficult—and often an emotionally painful—task. Sometimes, the older person has little choice because of finances or specific health problems. Nursing homes in particular represent a significant financial commitment. In 1990, the average cost of a nursing home was over $3000 *per month,* plus other medical expenses. Medicaid will pay for nursing home care only after an individual's savings have been used up. In effect, many older people are forced to become "paupers" in order to receive adequate health care. It is to be hoped that a solution will be found to this rather cruel situation in our present health-care system.

Aging and Economics

In our society, poverty and old age are closely linked. Those who have individual retirement accounts, adequate pensions, and sufficient finances are in the minority. In fact, inadequate Social Security checks are the sole support of many older people.[16] More than 25 percent of the seniors live on incomes below the poverty level. Women and other minorities are forced to function on even less income during their retirement years. In addition, government health programs such as Medicare (see Chapter 20) do not fully cover medical costs (physician, drugs, hospital, nursing). Age discrimination in employment and forced retirement make it difficult for older people to supplement their Social Security income. Initiating private retirement plans if you are self-employed, and using IRAs, tax sheltered annuities, and other investments early in your career can eliminate these problems. Unfortunately, financial planning for the future must be done at a time when people most need the dollars that should be set aside for older years. A financial adviser can help you begin looking ahead during your first job. Small payments become large investments after thirty or more years and can make the difference in the quality of your retirement years.

The Future

"Grow old along with me! The best is yet to be." Some experts predict that these words of Robert Browning will come true in future decades as a larger, more vigorous older population transforms America from a youth-oriented society to a mature society. By sheer

A larger, longer-lived, and more vigorous population of seniors is already changing the fabric of American social and political life. Do you think this is a good trend? Why? Why not?

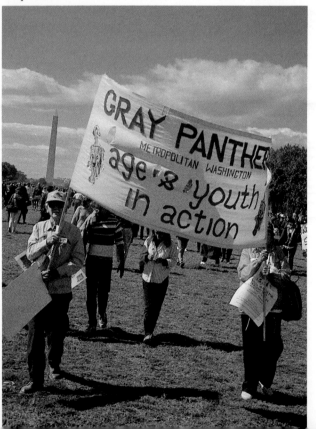

Get Involved!

Discouraging Ageism

Aging is a normal, unavoidable part of life. Even those who lead the "perfect" life will eventually exhibit the changes of passing time. Successful aging encourages people to take care of their minds and bodies and to enjoy each decade. Your preparation for successful aging should begin now as college students. During this critical time, there is much you can do to prepare for your later years and to change the way older people are viewed in the United States.

1.   Seek the knowledge of older people in your family and learn to profit from their years of experience.
2.   Encourage seniors to keep physically and mentally active, to practice sound nutrition, and to engage in valuable leisure and work pursuits.
3.   Treat older people with respect and kindness and learn to be tolerant of the varying behaviors of individuals of all ages. Discourage "ageism" and avoid evaluating human beings by their outward appearances.
4.   Encourage the use of older people as a valuable work resource in your community.
5.   Volunteer your services whenever possible to programs for seniors, such as Meals on Wheels. Visit nursing homes and include the elderly as important members of your social group.
6.   Adopt a healthy lifestyle now that includes regular aerobic exercise, proper nutrition, limited use of alcohol and other drugs, no smoking, relaxation, and worthwhile leisure pursuits.
7.   Learn to enjoy each decade of life, accepting the physical changes that occur as normal stages of development. Continue to live a physically and mentally active life.

numbers, seniors will have considerable political and economic leverage. The Census Bureau estimates that the number of Americans 65 and over will more than double from 26.8 million in 1983 to 65.8 million in 2033.[17] Should senior citizens unite their voting efforts, a clash with the young for a bigger piece of the pie is certain to occur. Programs for senior citizens could jump from the current 28 percent of the federal budget to as much as 65 percent. Some futurists indicate that the projected increase in life span to nearly 75 for men and 83 for women is far too low and predict a life expectancy of nearly 120 years, with some people living to 150.

It is also predicted that discoveries in genetics and immunology will make it possible to slow the aging process so that people who are 70 will look 35. Future generations of older people may also be more active physically, intellectually, politically, and economically; better educated; and productive much longer than present-day seniors. At this point, the wisdom, judgment, and experience of older people will be valuable in the workplace, and people's attitudes toward seniors should change from one of mere tolerance to one of respect.

Projected low birth rates, which will reduce the workforce, may keep senior citizens working much longer, well into their seventies. Some segments of the economy will also experience a labor shortage. This will bring about a more flexible definition of retirement and permit individuals to stay on after the mandatory retirement age. It is already clear that the Social Security retirement age will be increased before the baby-boom generation reaches 65 in approximately 2010.

Not everyone is so optimistic about longevity and health in the years to come. With medical costs continuing to rise (see Chapter 20), the number of older people needing medical care at a reasonable price will also increase. It is therefore theoretically possible to have a large population of dependent individuals who are chronically ill. On the other side of the coin, some social scientists predict that seniors of the future will be in good health and have much more disposable income, enabling them to live independently in housing that is not segregated by age.

Conclusion

Aging is a topic that needs to be studied and discussed by college-age students. Successful aging requires a thorough understanding of the physical (visible and invisible), mental, and emotional changes that occur through the years. The real challenge of aging lies in adapting to these changes. With proper planning that also involves a healthy lifestyle during the college and later years, you are much more likely to reach old age in better health, and in a better mental, emotional, and economic state. It is important to remember that wide variations exist from individual to individual in the manner and speed of aging. Chronological and physiological age can differ by twenty-five years or more. To a degree, this difference is determined by the way you take care of your body and mind throughout life.

Summary

1. Aging is a natural process; many cultures respect the aged for their experience, wisdom, and advice. Senior activists such as the Gray Panthers are working toward improving the status of seniors in the United States.

2. Systematic negative views toward older people, referred to as ageism, are common in the United States. As the number of healthy, productive people over 65 continues to increase and older people become more influential both politically and economically, this attitude may change.

3. Futurists predict a tremendous gain in life span in the future, with an expected life of over 100 years.

4. Several theories attempt to explain the aging process: free radical theory, the genetic theory, the defective DNA theory, the errors theory, the theory of aging hits, the theory of accumulation of deleterious material, the stress-stimulated response theory, the theory of loss of brain nerve cells, the hormone imbalance theory, the cross-linking of molecules theory, and the autoimmune theory.

5. Tremendous differences between individuals exist in the manner and rate of aging.

6. Too much emphasis is placed on the physical side of aging. People must learn to accept these changes in their bodies as natural occurrences. In general, changes in personal appearance and health are not nearly as dramatic as individuals anticipate.

7. The aging process can be influenced and even slowed by exercise, absence of smoking, proper nutrition and moderate alcohol and drug use, maintenance of proper body weight and body fat, preventive medical and dental care, removal of excess stress, maintenance of social activity, use of all body systems, and learning to accept oneself.

8. Your present lifestyle is certain to affect your future health as a senior citizen.

9. You can delay the rate and type of skin changes that occur with age by taking proper care of your skin through the use of sunscreens, limiting your exposure to the sun, eliminating the use of tobacco, eating wisely, and engaging in regular exercise.

10. A less efficient immune system makes the older person more vulnerable to attack by disease-producing organisms.

11. Chronic conditions that gradually worsen with age are the greatest cause of death and disability in older people.

12. Age-related bone loss (osteoporosis) can be kept to a minimum through proper nutrition, absence of tobacco and alcohol, regular exercise, and hormone replacement therapy.

13. In most cases, older individuals with the proper attitude can remain sexually active throughout life.

14. There are both physical and mental advantages that accompany aging, and these need to be viewed positively and emphasized.

15. Just how much mental decline occurs in later life is determined by both genetics and environment. In individuals who remain challenged and interested in intellectual activities only a slight decline is likely. For the 6 to 8 percent of older people affected by Alzheimer's disease, progressive deterioration of memory and other mental functions occurs over a period of three to ten years. Although the total number of reported cases is expected to increase steadily, treatment procedures are also improving and research funding increasing each year.

16. In the fourth or fifth decades of life, some women and men experience symptoms of midlife crisis, possibly triggered by excess stress, hormonal changes, or the sudden realization that one is growing older. Some experts feel that various degrees of these changes are natural and merely part of another period of growth and development.

17. Approximately 75 percent of wives will be widowed at some time in their lives. Older widows tend not to remarry, whereas older widowers tend to remarry within one year of the death of their spouses.

18. By planning during the early years and throughout life, one can arrange to meet retirement with adequate finances for an enjoyable life.

19. Retirement is viewed differently by different people. Some consider it the end of their productivity, whereas others look forward to it as an opportunity for new experiences.

20. Only a small percentage of seniors are in need of institutional care during their retirement years; the majority are economically and physically self-sufficient. Less expensive alternatives to institutional care are becoming available in the United States for those who cannot take care of themselves. In addition, the number and type of formal services for older people continue to increase.

21. More creative approaches are needed to harness the energy of those older people who want and need to work into productive and financially beneficial jobs that will make them more economically self-sufficient and improve our economy.

22. As the number of people over 65 increases to a projected 65.8 million in the year 2033, programs for older people will also increase. It is also projected that seniors of the future will be more active physically, intellectually, politically, and economically.

Questions for Personal Growth

1. Prepare a ten-point program that you can begin to follow now that will keep you physically and mentally healthy through the years.

2. List six to ten key suggestions that will improve the physical and mental health of your grandparents. Talk to your grandparents about your stud-

ies on aging and discuss these items openly. Can you bring about one or two important changes in their lives?

3. List your five biggest fears of growing old. Describe a plan to cope with these concerns.

4. To help eliminate some of your fears of aging, identify and interview two older male and female faculty members (one over 60 and one over the age of 70) who are physically active in sports, such as jogging, cycling, tennis, racquetball, squash, handball, aerobic dance, or another exercise program. Compare their activity level to those of the students in your class.

5. As the decades pass, values change. What is extremely important to you now will be replaced by other factors as time passes. List the five most important things in your life today. What do you think are the five most important factors in the life of a 40, 50, 60, and 70 year old? Compare your lists.

6. Prepare a financial plan leading to independence at age 65 to 70. Ask one of your parents to review the plan and make suggestions.

7. The too frequent use of drugs is a common problem among older people. In some cases, the "pill" box or home pharmacy begins to occupy most waking hours. What types of medication are your parents or grandparents using? Can you provide alternatives to any of these drugs?

8. Genetics obviously plays a role in the aging process. Research your family tree and record the cause of death of your grandparents and great grandparents and their families. List the diseases affecting each individual. Are any of these diseases linked to lifestyle? What can you do to avoid some of these disorders in your old age?

9. Mid-life crisis seems to occur in at least one family member. Identify someone in your family who has experienced this problem. What do you feel were the contributing factors? What could have been done to prevent the crisis?

References

1. "If You Live to Be 100—It Won't Be Unusual," *U.S. News and World Report* (May 9, 1983).

2. James J. Strain, "Ageism in the Medical Profession," *Geriatrics* 36, 4 (April 1981): 158–165.

3. Judith Rodin and Ellen Langer, "Aging Labels: The Decline of Control and the Fall of Self-Esteem," *Journal of Social Issues* 36, 2 (1980): 12–29.

4. U.S. Bureau of the Census, Current Population Reports, Series P-25, No. 1000, *Estimates of the Population of the United States by Age, Sex, and Race 1980–1986* (U.S. Government Printing Office, Washington, D.C.: 1987).

5. Strain, "Ageism in the Medical Profession."

6. *How Your Skin Ages and What You Can Do About It* (Kenilworth, N.J.: Schering Corp., 1990).

7. Martin S. Finkelstein, "Unusual Features of Infections in the Aging," *Geriatrics* 37, 4 (April 1982): 65–78.

8. Metropolitan Life Foundation, *Statistical Bulletin* 63, 1 (January–March 1982): 2.

9. R. P. Hershey, "The Role of Diet and Activity in the Treatment of Osteoporosis," in *Diet and Exercise Synergism in Health Maintenance*, eds., P. L. W. White and T. M. Mondeika (Chicago: American Medical Association, 1982), pp. 153–159.

10. C. J. Lee, G. S. Lawler, and G. H. Johnson, "Effects of Supplementation of the Diets with Calcium and Calcium-Rich Foods on Bone Density of Elderly Females with Osteoporosis," *American Journal of Clinical Nutrition* 34 (1981): 819–823.

11. Rodin and Langer, "Aging Labels."

12. Wortman and Loftus, *Psychology*, 3e (New York: Random House, 1988), pp. 232–233.

13. Rachael Filinson, "Chronic Illness and Care Provision: A Study of Alzheimer's Disease," in *Social Bonds in Later Life*, eds., Warren Peterson and Jill Quadagno (Beverly Hills, Calif.: Sage, 1985).

14. "Behind Spreading Fear of Two Modern Plagues," *U.S. News and World Report* (August 12, 1985), in *Health 87/88*, ed., Richard Yarian (Guilford, Conn.: Duskin, 1987).

15. Dan Leviton and Linda Campanelli Santoro, eds., *Health, Physical Education, Recreation and Dance for the Older Adult: A Modular Approach* (Reston, Va.: American Alliance for Health, Physical Education, Recreation, and Dance, 1980).

16. Jill Quadagno, *Aging*. Unpublished document, University of Kansas (1985).

17. U.S. Bureau of the Census, Current Population Reports, Series P-25, No. 1000, *Estimates of the Population of the United States by Age, Sex, and Race*.

CHAPTER 18

Dying and Death

CHAPTER OBJECTIVES

After reading this chapter, you should understand:

- The struggle to arrive at a meaningful and comprehensive definition of death and how we form our attitudes toward death.

- What dying is, how people who are dying may be cared for, and how dying may be understood in terms of a dying "process" with several stages.

- Why planning for death is important and what legal papers should be placed in order in preparation for one's own death. These papers may include a Living Will, instructions about Durable Power of Attorney, Organ Donor Cards, and instructions concerning euthanasia.

- Why we grieve and mourn, the difference between grief and mourning, the importance of grief work, and the special problems associated with the death of a child.

- The different kinds of funeral and burial arrangements that are available and the decisions that need to be made about them —preferably before the death occurs.

CHAPTER OUTLINE

Death: Definitions and Attitudes

Dying

Planning for Death

Grief and Mourning

Funerals and Burial Arrangements

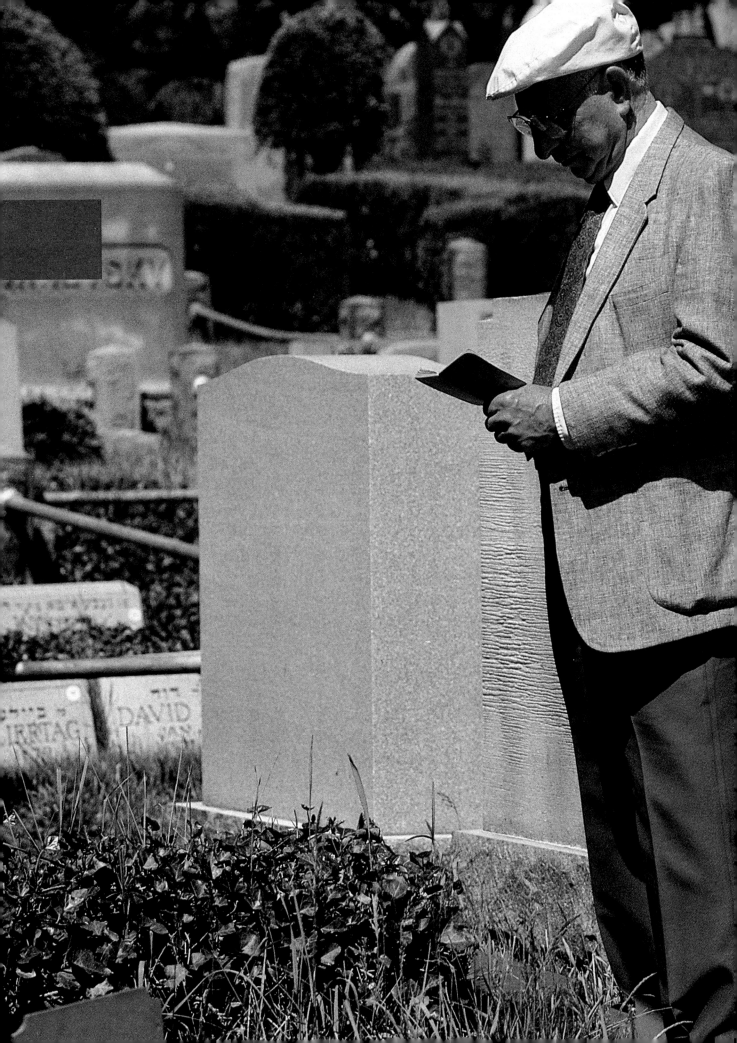

brain death A medical definition of death that includes the criteria of unresponsiveness, unreceptiveness, lack of movement, lack of breathing, lack of reflex, and a total lack of brain wave (EEG) activity.

electroencephalogram (EEG) A medical measure of the electrical impulses within the brain (brain wave activity).

Death is for all of us both a public and private experience. When we were transfixed to our television sets during the launching of the Challenger space shuttle, as were millions of school children, in 1987, and when we observed its explosion and the death of its crew, we grieved publicly. But when a pet or a loved one dies, we grieve privately. Try as we may, these experiences are unavoidable; they are a part of life. If you are unscarred by the death of someone you loved, you are indeed fortunate. You are also in the minority and should realize that this privileged state is temporary. No one lives forever.

Death is a part of life. It is such a vital part of life that without it the quality of our existence would be seriously diminished. Imagine what kind of motivation you would have if you knew you would live forever. Would you study hard? Work hard? Would you treat people well? Would you enjoy the risks you take (riding a roller coaster, white-water rafting, skydiving)? Would you enjoy getting older and older, with increasing disability? You see, death contributes much to our lives.

Furthermore, death allows for the cyclical nature of life. Depending on how we wish our dead bodies—or remains—to be handled, we may be able to contribute to other people's lives (for example, through organ donations for transplants) as well as to the nutrition and growth of other environmentally important forms of life (for example, grass, trees, and small organisms). Because of other living things we are alive, and because of us others will live. If we did not die, the crowded earth would not be able to house new lives.

In this chapter, we confront our mortality by considering death and the dying process. As a part of that discussion, we also study grieving, funerals, and organ transplants.

Death: Definitions and Attitudes

Definitions of Death(s)

Although it would seem reasonable to assume we all know what is meant by death, there are actually several different forms of death and conceptions of them. Most dictionaries define death as "the ending of life in a person, animal, or plant, in which all vital functions cease permanently." However, recent additions to medical technology tend to challenge such straightforward definitions. Has the life of a person whose heart is kept pumping by a machine "ended"? And what if doctors can keep most, but not all, of a person's vital functions working?

Many people think of the signs of death as obvious. They imagine a pale, bluish complexion, lack of breathing or heartbeat, and sensory unresponsiveness. These are indeed all indications of death. Nevertheless, for medical specialists to determine that death has occurred is often not so easy. Is someone who is in a coma, only being maintained by medical technology, alive or dead? If that person's heartbeat can be maintained by machinery and his or her lungs filled regularly by a respirator, is he or she alive or dead? When should medical personnel cease providing care for the patient? In other words, when has he or she died?

The need for a reliable definition of death becomes even more urgent when we recognize that someone might be waiting for a donor's organ—the heart, for instance. Do we let a donor in a deathlike state die so that the waiting patient can receive the donor's heart, or do we use modern technology to keep the donor breathing and the heart beating? Clearly, a definition of death that goes beyond maintaining people in a vegetablelike state is needed.

Brain Death   A Harvard Medical School committee developed a definition that is referred to as **brain death**. The four criteria of brain death are:[1]

- **Unreceptiveness and unresponsiveness.** A total unawareness of externally applied stimuli and inner need, accompanied by complete unresponsiveness. Even the most intensely painful stimuli evoke no vocal or other response, not even a groan, withdrawal of a limb, or quickening of respiration.

- **No movements or breathing.** Observation covering a period of at least one hour by physicians is adequate to satisfy the criteria of no spontaneous muscular movements or spontaneous respiration.

- **No reflexes.** No swallowing, yawning, and so forth. Pupils are fixed and dilated and do not respond to a direct source of bright light.

- **Flat electroencephalogram (EEG).** An **electro-encephalogram (EEG)** measures a person's brain wave activity. Different brain wave patterns occur when you are awake and thinking and when you are asleep and dreaming. When an electroencephalogram cannot detect *any* brain wave activity for a period of at least ten to twenty minutes—a flat EEG—you may legally be declared to have suffered *brain death*.

The committee recommends that all of these tests be repeated at least twenty-four hours later. If no change has occurred, the physician may pronounce the patient dead.

We should emphasize that a flat EEG reading by itself is not necessarily a good indicator of death. A recent popular movie takes its title from the flat EEG reading we typically associate with death. The movie, *Flatliners*, describes the attempts of several medical student friends to experience "death"—a flat EEG reading—and be resuscitated before their deaths become permanent. These students realized that because EEGs only pick up electrical activity from the outer layers of the brain, leaving the physical parts "alive," they would "return" to life if their brains could begin functioning again. In fact, however, a flat EEG reading can indicate the death of the outer layer of the brain while failing to register such vital functions as breathing, beating of the heart, and reflex activity. Again, we are confronted with the question: What is death?

Uniform Determination of Death Act Another group of medical professionals, The President's Commission for the Study of Ethical Problems in Medicine and Biomedical and Behavioral Research, developed the Uniform Determination of Death Act of 1981, which states that a person is dead when he or she has sustained either (1) irreversible cessation of circulatory and respiratory functions, or (2) irreversible cessation of all functions of the entire brain, including the brainstem. In light of new medical technologies, however, it is difficult to say who should determine when either cessation of functioning is "irreversible."

Other Significant Deaths Yet we can also speak of other forms of death. For example, the loss of a limb could be considered the death of a body part. The loss of a significant relationship could be considered the death of that relationship. We all should be aware that the grief that accompanies these forms of death is often no less intense than the grief that accompanies a person's death.

Thus, when you really think about it, "brain death," "cessation of functioning," or other forms of "loss" cannot individually or collectively define death comprehensively. Although there are moral and ethical imperatives—prompted by issues like organ transplants and euthanasia—for a solid, lasting definition of

death in terms of society, defining death seems to want to remain a very individual matter. People are seldom "prepared" for a death, especially when it is the death of a loved one, even after the loved one has suffered a long illness or disease inevitably resulting in death. We still take our definitions of death more or less on faith, each of us really deciding for himself or herself when death has actually occurred—even after a medical professional has pronounced and "finalized" its occurrence. Should we strive toward a comprehensive definition of death for the good of society? How would you define death for other people? How would you define your own death?

While we struggle to find a definition of death, we must also reconcile ourselves with it. Let's examine how people try to reconcile themselves with death through their attitudes toward death and dying.

American Attitudes toward Death

Only a few decades ago, sex was a taboo topic not discussed in mixed company. Today, in much the same way, death is not considered an appropriate topic for conversation. The denial of death is implicit in the way we treat dying people. Since few people die at home, we seldom come in contact with the dead. We idolize youth and vilify old age. Face lifts are in, wrinkles out. Many adults dress in as youthful a style as possible. Children are seldom taken to funerals and seldom visit a graveyard. Richard Dumont and Dennis Foss describe this attitude of denial when they write, "When I am, death is not. . . . When death is, I am not. Therefore we can never have anything to do with the dead."[2]

Even our terminology for death is indicative of this attitude. We refer to the dead as "passed away," "departed," "gone to heaven," and "laid to rest." In the end, they all mean the same. We will all be confronted by death at some time in our lives; therefore to deny it or never to consider its significance in a rational manner seems unhealthy.

> *Our attitudes toward our individual deaths . . . affect not only the way we view death, but also the way in which we live our lives. If one views his death with horror, he may have considerable difficulty in mustering the courage necessary to cross a street in heavy traffic. If, on the other hand, death is conceived as a pleasurable and exciting experience, one may not hesitate to walk a tightrope or go over Niagara Falls in a barrel. Furthermore, as at least one writer in the area of death research has suggested, the type of immortality we seek affects our behavior. If we seek biological immortality (through our children) or social immortality (through works or deeds that testify to our existence and live on in the minds of others), our philosophy toward life may be carpe diem . . . seize the day (live it up). On the other hand, if we seek a transcendental immortality (life hereafter), we may try to live a life of good deeds, so that we will be judged favorably after death by the supernatural forces.[3]*

Death educators believe that the study of death and dying may provide clues to our behavior. The

dying The process by which living matter arrives at death.

hospice A special facility or service that provides for the care of dying patients at their home or in a homelike setting.

amount of risk we are willing to take may be a function of our conception of death. And, as we noted previously, during the later years of our lives we strive for a feeling of continuity; that is, we try to achieve a sense of identification with all of humanity.

How do you conceptualize death? How does this conceptualization affect your behavior? Complete Exploring Your Health 18.1 to find out.

Dying

Dying is the process by which living matter arrives at death. One view is that you begin to die as soon as you are born. In a sense this is true because in our bodies cells are constantly dying and being replaced. However, we will consider dying as an event that is closely associated with death, either in time or in some disease state. For example, if you get into an automobile accident and emerge in such hopeless condition that attending physicians consider it a matter of time before you die, then you are dying. Or, if you have AIDS and, on the average, have only a couple of years to live, we can say you are in the process of dying. Most people do not fear death as much as the process of dying—particularly if dying is accompanied by pain. Over 70 percent of the people who die in the United States have chronic degenerative diseases which usually include a prolonged period of dying.[4] Consequently, more and more attention is being directed at ways to ease the fear and pain of dying people. Drugs such as LSD and marijuana have been used in research settings to control the pain (both physical and psychological) experienced by dying patients. Yet, some dying patients would rather not be "drugged." In these cases, understanding family members and hospital personnel can go a long way in relieving unnecessary suffering. For example, if a member of your family is dying you could acquire the help of a social worker so financial concerns are attended to, arrange for a psychologist to respond to the fear and anxiety, and request a member of your religion's clergy to counsel your dying loved one. Most hospitals and nursing homes offer assistance in arranging for these services. Consistent with the theme of this book, it is not only your death to which attention should be directed. You are a member of a larger soci-

ety and, therefore, you have responsibilities related to the death of other people with whom you share that society. We encourage you not to shirk those responsibilities. Many hospitals now offer counseling services for dying patients and their families.

In addition to these and other practices, a whole new environment in which to die has evolved. Over 90 percent of all people die in institutions, where care is often expensive and dehumanizing. A study to determine where people would want to die found that 75 percent of the respondents did not want to die in a hospital and 82 percent did not want to die in a nursing home; 63 percent preferred to die at home. A different system of care for terminally ill patients of all ages attempts to meet the needs that people have expressed of being able to die in a loving environment, close to their family.

Hospice centers are uniquely organized to be responsive to the needs of dying patients and their families. Have you ever considered volunteering some time to work at a hospice center?

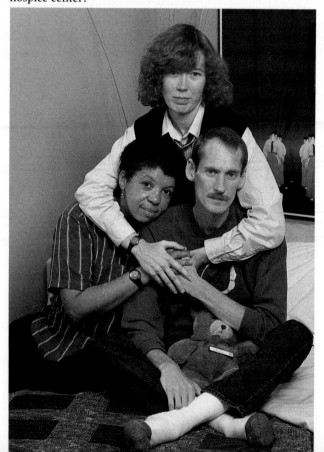

Exploring Your Health 18.1

Attitudes toward Death

What are your attitudes regarding death? Circle the number to the left of each item below with which you agree:

249 The thought of death is a glorious thought.
247 When I think of death I am most satisfied.
245 Thoughts of death are wonderful thoughts.
243 The thought of death is very pleasant.
241 The thought of death is comforting.
239 I find it fairly easy to think of death.
237 The thought of death isn't so bad.
235 I do not mind thinking of death.
233 I can accept the thought of death.
231 To think of death is common.

229 I don't fear thoughts of death, but I don't like them either.
227 Thinking about death is overvalued by many.
225 Thinking of death is not fundamental to me.
223 I find it difficult to think of death.
221 I regret the thought of death.
219 The thought of death is an awful thought.
217 The thought of death is dreadful.
215 The thought of death is traumatic.
213 I hate the sound of the word death.
211 The thought of death is outrageous.

If you discuss the results of this exercise with your classmates, you will find that attitudes toward death vary greatly.

Interpretation To determine your attitude toward death, disregard the first digit of the numbers (2), place a decimal point between the remaining two digits, and average all the circled responses. The average will correspond to an attitude statement or will fall between two attitude statements. This represents your attitude toward death. For example, if you circled numbers 241, 235, and 215, the computation would look like this:
$4.1 + 3.5 + 1.5 = 9.1$
$9.1 \div 3 = 3.0$ (to the nearest tenth)
Your attitude would fall between the attitude statements 231 and 229 on the above scale, because there is no item numbered 230.

Source: Dale V. Hardt, "Development of an Investigatory Instrument to Measure Attitudes Toward Death," *Journal of School Health* 45 (February 1976): 96–99. Copyright, 1976, American School Health Association, Kent, Ohio 44240. Reprinted by permission.

The Hospice System

A **hospice,** which means "care to travelers" (in this case, on the way to death), is a special facility that cares for dying patients in a homelike setting. Hospices are intended to perform the following functions:

- Provide medical care for the continuing control of symptoms such as pain and nausea.
- Concentrate on bedside nursing to provide comfort, close attention to easing physical distress, interpersonal interactions, attention to feeding, emotional support, and so forth.
- Focus on the family unit and allow the patient and family to cope with the situation.
- Include both the patient and the family by developing open communications.
- Involve community volunteers, many of whom are widows or widowers, in such varied activities as assisting with patient care, gardening, working in a day-care center, and helping in the business office.
- Provide spiritual care through ecumenical services, discussion groups, and an atmosphere of love and concern.

- Provide a comprehensive program of outpatient and inpatient care to meet a variety of patient and family needs.
- Foster a spirit of friendliness and encourage individuals to participate in a facility that is more homelike than a hospital.
- Establish built-in supports for staff and volunteers so that they can carry on their demanding work.

Hospices take various forms:

- **Freestanding.** A separate facility with beds, staff, and economic independence.
- **Extended care facility.** Part of a nursing home set aside for a hospice.
- **Home care.** Sometimes called a hospice without walls. Care is provided at one's home by trained hospice staff available twenty-four hours a day.
- **Hospital-affiliated but free-standing.** A separate facility but located near and owned by a hospital.
- **Hospital-based.** Either part of a hospital set aside for a hospice or home care provided by the hospital and its specially trained staff.

Hospices and conventional care facilities (hospi-

thanatologist Someone who studies or who is an expert on death and dying.

TABLE 18.1	

Hospice versus Conventional Care

Hospice Care	Conventional Care
Program under medical direction.	Physician-directed.
Care delivered by interdisciplinary team.	Occasional "team" care.
Focus on relief of symptoms.	Focus on cure and rehabilitation.
Emphasis on care in the home.	Emphasis on institutional care.
Patient/family is the unit of care.	Patient is the unit of care.
Services available 24 hours, 7 days a week.	Limited services in home, with full institutional care.
Bereavement support for survivors, pre- and postdeath.	Usually no bereavement support.
Integrated and coordinated attention to spiritual, social, psychological needs of patient/family.	Usually limited attention to spiritual, social, psychological needs of patient/family.

tals, nursing homes) differ in some respects and are similar in others. The characteristics of each are presented in Table 18.1.

Understanding the Stages of Dying

Another means of meeting the needs of dying people is to recognize and respond to the stages of the dying process. The work of psychiatrist and **thanatologist** (someone who studies and is an expert on death and dying) Elisabeth Kübler-Ross is often used as a guide in recognizing the stages of dying. Dr. Kübler-Ross identified five phases that dying people usually experience: *denial* of impending death; *anger* at having to die; *bargaining* (for example, "If I could have one more month

I'd spend it doing only good"); *depression;* and, finally, *acceptance* of death.[5] These five stages are depicted in Figure 18.1.

At the denial stage, the family can help the patient by discussing the medical evidence at hand. Perhaps a second opinion will verify the patient's condition. Family members can acknowledge the value of denial as a protective device: "It must be difficult to accept that you're going to die."

At the anger stage, families can let patients know that they have a right to be angry and that their anger will have an outlet; it will not be suppressed but rather encouraged. After all, wouldn't you be angry if you learned that your life would soon end?

Bargaining is a way of staving off the inevitable. Death is imminent, regardless of the deals one makes, and the family needs to help the patient realize that: "I, too, wish I could give one month of my life so you could live that much longer, but unfortunately neither of us can make such a deal." Such statements will help the patient recognize the futility of bargaining.

Depression, too, is understandable. As with anger, the patient should be encouraged to discuss feelings of depression with family members, and the family should accept these emotions. Too often, the family attempts to make the patient feel better by denying expressions of depression: "Come on, you don't really feel like that." It would be more valuable to acknowledge these feelings: "What a heavy burden you must bear. I can understand you're feeling depressed. I'm sure I would too. Do you want to talk about it?"

Acceptance of death is the goal of the terminally ill; not all such patients reach this stage. For those who do, the family should be ready to help them organize their affairs so that they feel everything is in order. The will should be updated if necessary, a list of bank accounts drawn up, health and life insurance policies at hand, and funeral and burial arrangements made.

People move through these stages at different rates and may move back and forth between stages or not go through all of them, but they do describe a process that the terminally ill commonly experience. The obvious implication is that dying people need different types of communications and relationships at different stages. In any case, it may do the dying person a disservice to avoid discussing his or her condition. Family,

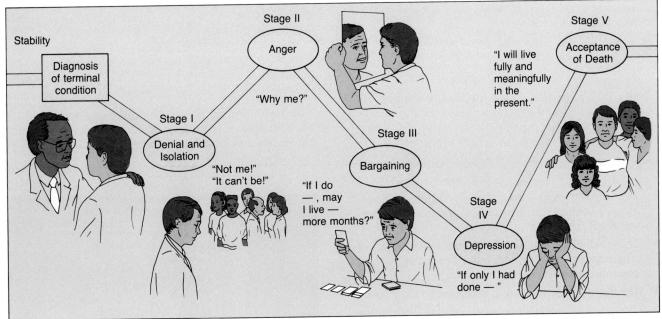

FIGURE 18.1 • Kübler-Ross's stages of dying as experienced by the dying person.

friends, and caregivers should help the dying person through these stages by listening to and encouraging the individual and by respecting his or her special needs, several of which include:

- The need to participate in one's own death, to know one is dying. Even though terminally ill patients may act as though they do not know or do not want to know that they are dying, loved ones

and the medical staff should undeniably state the fact and address their feelings. Denial is generally unhealthy and interferes with meaningful communication with loved ones—the best medicine available at this point.

- The need to live to the end with dignity.
- The need for hope—not necessarily hope for the preservation of life, but the hope that accompanies faith and meaningful living.

Issues in Health

Bill of Rights for Terminal Patients

Ten prominent doctors developed the following lists of rights they believe are due to terminal patients:

- Doctors should decrease or halt aggressive treatment if it would only prolong an uncomfortable process of dying.
  —But the patient or the family should decide, if possible.
- Doctors and hospitals should respect a patient's right to refuse treatment.
  —And doctors should take the time to tell the patients their choices, rather than leave them adrift in a mass of medical facts and opinion.
- A patient's refusal of treatment should not be called a sign of incompetency.

- A doctor who isn't sure about a patient's chances of recovery should consult specialists.
- The rare report of a similar patient who survived should not become an overriding reason to continue treatment.
- Appropriate and compassionate care should have priority over undue fears of criminal or civil liability, or advice of lawyers "whose primary objective is to minimize liability."
- Patients should seldom, if ever, be denied the truth, since the anxiety of the unknown can be more upsetting.
- In patients who are not brain-dead but are in a "persistent vegetative state," or in a hopelessly ill pa-

tient who is also "severely and irreversibly demented [and] merely passively accepting" food and care, it is justifiable to withhold antibiotics and artificial nutrition if the patient, by prior wishes, would have agreed and the family agrees.
- Even in "elderly patients with permanent mild impairment of competence," the "pleasantly senile," emergency resuscitation and intensive care may be applied "sparingly," guided again by the patient's and family's wishes and the patient's prospects.

Do you agree with each of these rights? Which do you believe are more important?

Living Will A written statement, legally binding, that instructs doctors and others on the medical procedures to be used in case of catastrophic illness or accident because of which the writer of the will is incapable of making or communicating decisions. The will applies in situations in which the writer cannot regain a normal life or is terminally ill.

- The need to work through and ventilate feelings of guilt, denial, jealousy, anguish, and other coping emotions.
- The need to be listened to without censure or anger and to be accepted, regardless of the defense mechanisms used.
- The need to feel valued as a person.
- The need to give and be given to long after he or she is able to give.
- The need to be remembered.
- The need to function at some level, even if it's only deciding what to have for dinner.
- The need for meaningful communication (not necessarily verbal).
- The need for family and friends to resolve their own defense mechanisms and not to inflict unrealistic expectations on the dying person. Those who cannot face their own deaths can hardly help a dying person accept it calmly.
- The need to maintain self-confidence, security, and self-esteem.
- The need of some terminally ill people to receive permission from their loved ones to die.

Planning for Death

Recognizing that we are merely mortal, that we will die one day, and that we can't know with any assuredness just when that day will be, it is important that each of us plan for our deaths. Exploring Your Health 18.2 will help with this planning. Long before death is anticipated it is advisable to have certain legal papers in order. These include a living will, a power of attorney (particularly for health matters), an organ donor card if you choose to donate organs, and instructions regarding funeral and burial arrangements.

The Living Will

Medical science has developed numerous technologies to keep people alive. There are respirators that maintain breathing, heart-lung machines that keep the heart beating and the blood circulating, and tubes in-

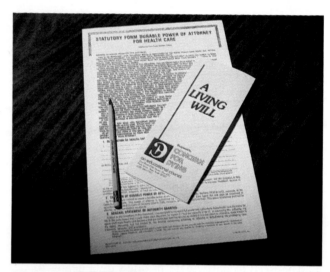

Preparing for your death is best done well in advance of knowing when you are going to die. Although you may be perfectly healthy (you think), it is recommended that you have a will and, if you wish, a Living Will or Durable Power of Attorney. Do you have these? When will you take steps to obtain these?

serted through the nose into the alimentary canal by which to feed patients unable to be fed in any other manner. Some people argue that to be kept barely alive in this fashion is not to be "alive" at all. They would prefer being allowed to die as painlessly and in as dignified a manner as possible rather than having their physicians resort to last minute "heroic" medical procedures. Everyone has a right to make this decision for herself or himself. However, if you become incapacitated—for instance, in a coma—and that decision needs to be made for you (usually by a family member), then a problem may arise. Because the medical professions are obligated by law and ethical codes of conduct to work to keep patients alive, they may hesitate to perform any actions that would not prolong life —even a comatose life. In addition, they may hesitate to perform any actions that might actually shorten life (such as taking a patient off a respirator when the prognosis is that the patient will not be able to breathe on his or her own).

Such was the case with Nancy Cruzan. Nancy lay in a comatose state in a Missouri hospital as a result of an auto accident. The part of her brain that controlled

Exploring Your Health 18.2

Death Questions and Decisions

If you were to die today, what would you want people to say about you? Imagine you are a reporter for your local newspaper and write your obituary:

_____

_____

_____

_____

_____

Who would you want to read this obituary?

_____

_____

_____

List below your most valued material possessions. Beside each possession listed, write the name of the person you would like to see receive this possession upon your death:

1. _____

2. _____

3. _____

4. _____

5. _____

Who will miss you most when you die? Why?

_____

_____

_____

What do you want done with your body when you die? Why?

_____

_____

_____

Would you like to donate your organs for research? Why or why not?

_____

_____

_____

Do you want your life sustained regardless of your condition? Why or why not?

_____

_____

_____

thought and voluntary movement had been destroyed. However, the part of her brain that controlled breathing was still functional. It was predicted that Nancy could live in this way for years. Because she could not swallow, Nancy needed to be fed through a feeding tube. After seven years, when she was 32 years old, her parents requested that the feeding tube be removed and that Nancy Cruzan be allowed to die physically (they argued that the "real" Nancy had died years earlier). The hospital refused and the case eventually had to be decided by the United States Supreme Court. On June 25, 1990, the Court sided with the hospital and against Nancy's parents. They ruled that in order for life-sustaining measures to be withheld, there had to be "clear and convincing" proof that the person would not have wanted these measures employed. As a result, experts are even more adamant regarding the need to have such instructions in writing than they were before.

It should be noted that Nancy Cruzan's parents eventually went back to court and were able to demonstrate—clearly and convincingly—that Nancy would not have wanted to be kept alive given her condition. This was no easy task, requiring testimony regarding conversations that Nancy had had and documents she had written. The feeding tube was then removed and soon thereafter, in the latter part of 1990, Nancy died.

Nancy Cruzan's case was not the first to receive such widespread publicity. In 1975, Karen Ann Quinlan of New Jersey became comatose after ingesting alcohol and tranquilizers. Karen became the center of a national debate over the "right to die" when her doctors refused her parents' request that she be taken off the respirator that was breathing for her. In 1976, the United States Supreme Court ruled Karen could be removed from life support systems at her parents' request, as long as there was no reasonable chance of recovery. The irony was that after being removed from the respirator, Karen lived without any life support for almost nine years until she died of pneumonia on June 11, 1985.

If you wish not to prolong life with heroic medical procedures—some of which might be painful, embarrassing, and costly—you should consider filing a **Living Will**. A Living Will is a written statement, witnessed by someone else, that instructs doctors not to use life-prolonging medical procedures when your condition is hopeless and when there is no chance of regaining a meaningful life. A sample Living Will is presented in Figure 18.2.

Modifications to this will can be made as one wishes. For example, you might want to cross out some life-sustaining procedures because those are the ones you would like the doctors to try. "Comfort measures" referred to in the sample Living Will are medication, nursing care, and other treatment administered for the purpose of keeping one as comfortable and free from pain as possible. One section of the Living Will ("Other personal instructions") allows it to be personalized with additional instructions. The Living Will should be signed and dated, witnessed by two people who are not blood relatives or beneficiaries identified in your property will, and renewed each year to keep it current.

You might also want to include a Proxy Designation Clause as part of your Living Will. This clause identifies someone entrusted to make medical decisions in accordance with your wishes at a time when you are unable to make those decisions for yourself.

Once the Living Will is completed, several copies should be made: one for your files, one for your medical file housed in your doctor's office, and one for relatives whom you have asked to maintain a file of your personal papers. In addition, a reduced copy should be kept in your wallet in case it needs to be used immediately. Keeping the Living Will in a Safety Deposit Box

A Question of Ethics

Is It Ethical to Withhold Treatment from Ill People?

Scientific and medical breakthroughs have occurred so quickly and been so effective that our society is often in a quandary about their value. Consider the cases of heart transplant recipients Barney Clark and William Shroeder. They were dying because their hearts could no longer support their bodies. Both agreed to have artificial hearts surgically implanted in their chests. Barney Clark, a 61-year-old retired dentist, was the first recipient of an artificial heart. Clark was operated on December 2, 1982, and lived with his new artificial heart until his death on March 23, 1983. Aside from repeated physical problems and being tethered to the pump that operated his new heart, his family described him as different after the surgery. He never was the same old Barney. His personality—his essence?—was lost and interactions he had after the transplants were unlike those before. And yet to withhold treatment would certainly have meant the end of Clark's life.

William Shroeder was the second artificial heart transplant patient. He received his transplanted heart on November 25, 1984 and lived until August 6, 1986. Throughout those 620 days, Shroeder lived only a short time outside the hospital and suffered from repeated strokes that left him physically debilitated. After Schroeder died, mechanical hearts became considered as merely stopgap, temporary measures while people waited for real hearts that could be transplanted.

But these are only two cases, and they both received more than their share of media coverage and hype. There are countless stories of people in comas who miraculously and inexplicably recover to live relatively normal lives. And there are countless stories of comatose people who remain that way for years—never coming out of these comas but rather diminishing the quality of their families' lives by the continuous financial and emotional trauma.

Should we keep these people alive by regular feedings or by maintaining them on respirators? Or should we stop all care so they can finally die?

If we can keep a baby with a severe birth defect alive, even though we know death will be inevitable in a few months or years, should we do so? What if the baby would be experiencing pain during his or her life? What if, as occurred not too long ago, the baby could be kept alive by transplanting a baboon's heart?

These are not easy questions to answer. Often, all we can do is select the best of terrible choices. What's more, we can expect these dilemmas to increase rather than decrease in frequency, since scientific and medical advances are being made rapidly and repeatedly.

How would you answer these questions? How would you advise that our society control scientific and medical advances so that they are used ethically?

To My Family, Doctors, and All Those Concerned with My Care

I, _____ , being of sound mind, make this statement as a directive to be followed if for any reason I become unable to participate in decisions regarding my medical care.

I direct that life-sustaining procedures should be withheld or withdrawn if I have an illness, disease or injury, or experience extreme mental deterioration, such that there is no reasonable expectation of recovering or regaining a meaningful quality of life.

These life-sustaining procedures that may be withheld or withdrawn include, but are not limited to:

SURGERY   ANTIBIOTICS   CARDIAC RESUSCITATION
RESPIRATORY SUPPORT   ARTIFICIALLY ADMINISTERED FEEDING AND FLUIDS

I further direct that treatment be limited to comfort measures only, even if they shorten my life.
You may delete any provision above by drawing a line through it and adding your initials.

Other personal instructions:

These directions express my legal right to refuse treatment. Therefore, I expect my family, doctors, and all those concerned with my care to regard themselves as legally and morally bound to act in accord with my wishes, and in so doing to be free from any liability for having followed my directions.

Signed _____   Date _____

Witness _____   Witness _____

PROXY DESIGNATION CLAUSE

If you wish, you may use this section to designate someone to make treatment decisions if you are unable to do so.
Your Living Will Declaration will be in effect even if you have not designated a proxy

I authorize the following person to implement my Living Will Declaration by accepting, refusing and/or making decisions about treatment and hospitalization:

Name _____

Address _____

If the person I have named above is unable to act on my behalf, I authorize the following person to do so:

Name _____

Address _____

I have discussed my wishes with these persons and trust their judgment on my behalf.

Signed _____   Date _____

Witness _____   Witness _____

FIGURE 18.2   •   Living Will Declaration
Source: Courtesy of Society for the Right to Die, 250 West 57 Street, New York, NY 10107.

is not recommended because it may not be readily available when needed.

Living Wills are recognized by most states as representative of a person's wishes and are, therefore, legally binding. However, the specific form appearing in Figure 18.2 may not be binding in your state. You can obtain your state's legally binding form by requesting one from the Society for the Right to Die, 250 West 57 Street, New York, NY 10107.

Durable Power of Attorney

Living Wills have several drawbacks: (1) They are not uniform; as stated previously, you need to obtain your

Durable Power of Attorney Often written in conjunction with a Living Will, a Durable Power of Attorney is legally binding and instructs a person to act as agent or attorney for another person who is incapacitated by illness or accident.

state's particular Living Will form. (2) They refer to the withholding of treatment exclusively, rather than speak to the right to have treatment when that is appropriate. (3) Some state laws require Living Wills to be reaffirmed periodically, which people may forget to do; other states require that the person be told the condition is terminal before the Living Will can apply; and in still other states (five states at last count) the Living Will must be filed with the court. Finally, (5) Living Wills cannot be written for a child or an incompetent adult except in a few states.

These drawbacks have led experts to recommend the filing of a **Durable Power of Attorney** instead of or in conjunction with a Living Will. The Durable Power of Attorney can apply when a person is not terminally ill but temporarily incapacitated, protects a person's right to have treatment as well as to have it withheld, and avoids the need to anticipate all possible

FIGURE 18.3 • Durable Power of Attorney for Health-Care Decisions

---

Durable Power of Attorney for Health-Care Decisions

I, **(your name)**, hereby appoint: **(name, address and phone numbers)** as my attorney in fact to make health care decisions for me if I become unable to make my own health care decisions. This gives my attorney in fact the power to grant, refuse or withdraw consent on my behalf for any health care service, treatment or procedure. My attorney in fact has the authority to talk to health care personnel, get information and sign forms necessary to carry out these decisions.

If the person named as my attorney in fact is not available or is unable to act as my attorney in fact, I appoint the following persons to serve in the order listed below:

(Names, addresses, phone numbers of two persons)

With this document, I intend to create a power of attorney for health care, which shall take effect if I become incapable of making my own health care decisions and shall continue during that incapacity.

My attorney in fact shall make health care decisions as I direct below or as I make known to my attorney in fact in some other way.

(a) Statement of directives concerning life-prolonging care, treatment, services and procedures.

(b) Special provisions and limitations:

By my signature I indicate that I understand the purpose and effect of this document. I sign my name to this form on **(date)**, at **(address)**.

(Your signature)

WITNESSES

I declare that the person who signed or acknowledged this document is personally known to me, that the person signed or acknowledged this durable power of attorney for health care in my presence, and that the person appears to be of sound mind and under no duress, fraud or undue influence. I am not the person appointed as the attorney in fact by this document, nor am I the health care provider to the principal or an employee of the health care provider of the principal.

(Date, and print names, signatures and addresses of two witnesses)

At least one of the witnesses listed above shall sign the following declaration:

I further declare that I am not related to the principal by blood, marriage or adoption, and, to the best of my knowledge, I am not entitled to any part of the estate of the principal under a currently existing will or by operation of law.

(Signatures)

situations in which decisions might have to be made. A Power of Attorney is a written instrument of agreement authorizing a person to act as the agent or attorney for another person. By adding the words, ''This power of attorney shall not be affected by my subsequent disability or incapacity,'' a Durable Power of Attorney is created.

Another option is the Durable Power of Attorney for Health-Care Decisions, which limits a person's ability to make decisions for another person in health-related matters. An example of a Durable Power of Attorney for Health-Care Decisions appears in Figure 18.3. An attorney should be consulted to assure the Durable Power of Attorney is valid in your state.

Organ Donor Cards

In 1987 there were approximately 11,000 organ transplants done in the United States. However, there were 13,000 people on waiting lists to receive organs. The shortage of organs to transplant is reflected in the following figures for 1987:

1. Hearts—1,512 transplanted; 900 persons on waiting list
2. Liver—1,182 transplanted; 500 on waiting list
3. Pancreas—127 transplanted; 100 on waiting list
4. Heart-Lung—43 transplanted; 200 on waiting list

There may be religious or other reasons why you may

There are many people on waiting lists to receive organs they need to live because there aren't enough organs being donated. Have you thought about donating organs upon your death? If so, have you filled out an organ donor card?

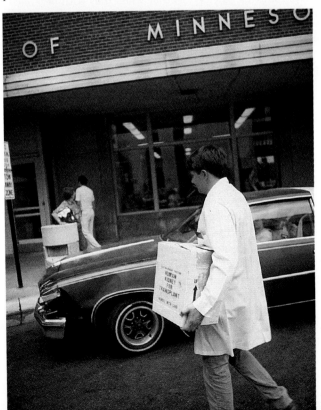

FIGURE 18.4 • Sample Uniform Donor Card for an Anatomical Gift

not want to donate organs (for example, Orthodox Jewish law prohibits mutilation of the body, which means no organ donations or autopsies). However, if you do choose to donate certain organs, an Organ Donor Card should be completed and your family notified. An example of a Uniform Donor Card appears in Figure 18.4 and can be obtained from the National Kidney Foundation or your local motor vehicle bureau. This card should be copied, with one copy kept in your wallet and another copy kept with your personal papers. For many people, knowing that their death will mean that others may live is very comforting.

Euthanasia

Part of the need of some terminally ill people is to be able to end their lives when they wish, usually short of extensive pain or disability. As you can imagine, this is a controversial area. Most of us would have great difficulty seeing a loved one end his or her life, even when they are in a good deal of pain. Death is so permanent!

passive euthanasia The withholding of life-supporting treatment or other measures that would prolong the life of a person who would certainly die otherwise.

dyathanasia A term that is synonymous with passive euthanasia.

active euthanasia Actions that hasten or cause the death of someone who is terminally ill and without hope of recovery; also called "mercy killing."

grief The emotions of anger and sadness and the sense of loss that follow after the death of a loved one.

mourning The manner in which grief is manifested.

bereavement The time period during which one mourns the death of a loved one.

Euthanasia: An "Unnatural" Form of Dying?

It was 1990 and Janet Adkins was becoming progressively incapacitated by Alzheimer's disease. She couldn't bear the thought of losing control of her life, and the emotional and financial burden her family would experience in having to care for her as her disease got worse weighed heavily on her mind. Then she heard of Dr. Jack Kevorkian. Dr. Kevorkian had developed a "suicide machine" that intravenously dripped life-taking chemicals into one's body, ending life in a "controlled" manner. After assessing Janet's condition, Dr. Kevorkian agreed to insert an intravenous needle into Janet's arm—a needle connected to containers of the life-taking chemicals—and

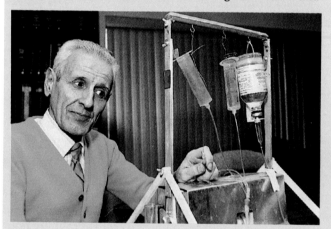

allow her to decide when to push a specially placed button that would release the chemicals into her body. Soon Janet had pushed the button and was dead, and a controversy regarding the ethics of physicians who assist patients to end their lives ensued.

People who are terminally ill, who know they will soon die, sometimes decide to end their lives before experiencing pain or disability. This form of suicide is called *euthanasia*. When others withhold life supporting treatment—such as not reviving a person who suffers a fourth and massive heart attack—it is termed *passive euthanasia*, also called *dyathanasia*. When an action is actually taken to cause someone's death—such as that taken by Dr. Kevorkian—it is termed *active euthanasia*.

Some argue that euthanasia gives families excuses for avoiding the financial and emotional responsibilities associated with chronic and expensive illnesses, and it gives doctors a reason for ending lives prematurely in order to acquire organs for transplant operations. Others take the view of Norman Cousins, former editor of the *Saturday Review*. When Cousins heard of an elderly couple committing suicide together when they both became terminally ill, he wrote, "Why are so many people more readily appalled by an unnatural form of dying than by an unnatural form of living?"

Are you in favor of euthanasia? If so, which form? Passive? Active? Both? Under what conditions?

And yet, when someone you love is in great discomfort, in a coma, or in some other state of existence you have difficulty defining as "living," and this condition is judged to be irreversible, you, too, might consider a swift, merciful death to be in that person's best interest. Such an action is termed *euthanasia*.

Euthanasia is the putting to death, painlessly, of someone suffering from an incurable life-taking condition. **Passive euthanasia**—sometimes called **dyathanasia**—is the withholding of life-supporting treatment or measures that would prolong life. The withholding of this treatment accelerates dying (some would say, naturally). Examples of passive euthanasia are to not put someone on a respirator to maintain his

or her breathing or to not insert a feeding tube to provide nutrients for that person's body. **Active euthanasia** is when an action is taken to actually cause someone's death: for example, injecting a lethal dose of medication or placing a deadly amount of sleeping pills in someone's drink. This is sometimes referred to as "mercy killing."

Although many Americans oppose the taking of a life, even under the conditions previously described, most support some form of euthanasia when appropriate.

If you decide that some form of euthanasia is acceptable for you under selected circumstances, you need to clarify what those circumstances are and include those instructions in your Living Will. In addition, you need to make sure that your physician will abide by these wishes.

Grief and Mourning

Grief is the combination of distressing emotions felt as a result of the death of a loved one. Anger, sadness, and a profound sense of loss are examples of feelings experienced when people grieve. When experiencing the death of a loved one, people also mourn. **Mourning** is the manner in which grief is manifested during the period of **bereavement** (the time during which someone is grieving). The way in which people mourn varies from religion to religion and from culture to culture. Your religion's instructions or culture's standards for mourning may include burial, cremation (burning the body at extremely high temperatures until all that remains are ashes), refraining from certain behaviors (drinking, dancing, eating certain foods) for some specified period of time, or a wake or period of shiva during which other people visit to express their sympathy.

The grieving process runs a predictable course, as described in Table 18.2. Each of the stages of ordinary grief is necessary, and together they serve to return the bereaved person to a normal life. The first stage is shock and disbelief. The grieving person may feel numb and weep for several days after the death. The second stage is a sense of profound sadness and longing for the deceased. The grieving person may be preoccupied with thoughts of the deceased and may even sense the presence of the dead person. Sadness, crying, loss of appetite, an apathetic attitude, and difficulty in sleeping all characterize the second stage of grief. In the third stage, the grieving person becomes more accustomed to the reality of the death and fewer episodes of sadness occur. This stage marks a return to normal activities, and the bereaved person learns to live with the fact of the death.

Grief Work

When a loved one dies, the survivor's grief can be so intense for a time that nothing else seems to matter. Grief is hard work—*grief work*. Psychologists recommend three steps for working out one's grief:

- Facing up to the death and not denying it.
- Breaking bonds with the deceased (for example, disposing of his or her clothes).
- Finding new interests in activities and relationships.

It is not easy to follow these steps, and grief needs to run its course before the bereaved can resume a normal life.

Grief has been found to have the potential for

TABLE	18.2

Stages of Ordinary Grief

Timetable	Manifestations
Stage 1 Begins immediately after death; lasts one to three days.	Shock Disbelief, denial Numbness Weeping Wailing Agitation
Stage 2 Peaks between two to four weeks after death; begins to subside after three months; lasts up to one year.	Painful longing Preoccupation Memories Mental images of the deceased Sense of the deceased being present Sadness Tearfulness Insomnia Loss of appetite Loss of interest Irritability Restlessness
Stage 3 Should occur within a year after death.	Resolution Decreasing episodes of sadness Ability to recall the past with pleasure Resumption of ordinary activities

Source: Robert B. White and Leroy T. Gathman, "The Syndrome of Ordinary Grief," *American Family Physician* 8 (1973): 98. Reprinted with permission of the American Academy of Family Physicians.

causing serious health problems, in particular, in the elderly. For example, it is well established that widowed persons have a greater chance of dying than nonwidowed persons, and that the risk is greatest immediately after bereavement.

Contrary to the belief of many college students with whom we've spoken, you can do a lot to help someone who is grieving. Even without training in counseling (something you might want to consider and to which we refer in the "Get Involved!" box at the conclusion of this chapter), your expressions of concern, your willingness to listen, and your physical presence can be "just what the doctor ordered" (or in this case, what was ordered instead of needing a doctor). Don't devalue the love you can give just when it is needed the most. This love may be the most powerful healing "drug" available at the time.

Sometimes the grieving person needs professional assistance in getting through the stages of grief, in which case, a physician, a psychologist or psychiatrist, a member of the clergy, or a close relative may be able to help. Psychiatrists may prescribe sleeping pills for the bereaved, but they caution that daytime sedatives or tranquilizers may interfere with the natural course that grief must run. Extended psychotherapy may be required for the bereaved person who remains fixated at the first or second stage of grief. Since grief can result in physical illness as well, care should be taken to prevent or respond quickly to such conditions. The bereaved should be encouraged to maintain a nutritionally balanced diet, get enough sleep, and so forth —in other words, to take care of their own health in spite of how depressed they feel.

When a Child Dies

As one of the authors of this textbook (JSG), I had a very emotional experience during a workshop I was presenting on stress management. From the back of the room, a woman who appeared to be in her early thirties, raised her hand to ask a question: "What can you do to manage the stress from the death of your child?" How could anyone not feel sad for this woman? The answer she received couldn't possibly make a dent in the grief she was feeling, but I attempted to help her by responding, "There really is no way to manage such stress. It must be terrible to have to experience the death of a child. Time usually helps in the healing, as does a lot of crying, praying, and sharing your grief with other loved ones and friends." In addition, I made sure to spend some time speaking with her after the workshop.

1. I spoke with her about using resources in her community, for example, counseling services of-

fered privately or through the health department or mental health association.

2. I spoke with her about making sure to care for her own health by attempting to get enough sleep, eating well, exercising regularly, and employing some means of relaxation daily.

3. I cautioned her to refrain from "quick cures"— such as alcohol or other drugs—that would only provide temporary relief at the expense of greater damage. Besides, I continued, when the effects of the drugs wore off, the problem would still be there.

4. I beseeched her to focus her attention, as best she could, on the good times she shared with her child rather than on the loss. (Remember our discussion of "Selective Awareness" in Chapter 3 on Stress.)

5. I alerted her to attempts some people make to replace their lost child. They may become pregnant or adopt another child, and then place unrealistic and unhealthy expectations on that child to be like the deceased. Realize, I told her, that your loss is irreplaceable, but that it doesn't mean you can't enjoy still another child in a new but just as fulfilling way.

Although the loss of any loved one is traumatic, the loss of a child is especially so. After all, the expected order of death is reversed: the *parent* is supposed to die *first*! Well, in death there is no "supposed to." What occurs, occurs. If you know someone whose child recently died, or if this should occur sometime in the future, be particularly sensitive. Realize that there is much you can do to help. Although there is no magic that will make the pain disappear, your caring and concern will be greatly appreciated. A wordless hug, a few tears, and a "seemingly" ineffective, "I'm so sorry," may be all you can offer, but offering all you can will help the bereaved cope with his or her loss.

Other Losses

There are other losses in life that can affect people almost as profoundly as the death of a loved one. For example, as you grow older and more independent, your parents lose you; that is, they lose your dependence on them, your actual presence in the home, or part of

Issues in Health

Should Dead Bodies Be Used for Medical Research?

Medical researchers and doctors have suggested that bodies of recently dead people be hooked up to life-support systems so they can be used for research.

Pro "Neomorts"—as these dead bodies have come to be known—could serve several purposes: They could be used to keep organs viable until they can be transplanted. They could be used to experiment with new surgical techniques and medications. In the case of a pregnant woman, her body could be kept alive until the baby is viable and can be removed.

Since these are dead bodies, advocates argue there is no problem using them in this way; there is no chance of revival. In addition, these bodies would only be used if either the person before death or the family after death agreed. Arguing for neomort usage, advocates have lobbied for the development of a "neomortorium"—a facility to house neomorts and to organize research on them.

Con Opponents of the use of recently dead bodies for research and other purposes argue that they are reminded of Frankenstein. They be-

lieve the human body is inviolable; it is not to be experimented on. Furthermore, if doctors knew the body would be used after death, they might not work as diligently to keep that person alive. The fact that there are no national or state regulations concerning neomorts, nor any medical group (for example, the American Medical Association) policies, also worries opponents.

Do you think neomortoriums should be established? Under what circumstances and for what purposes, if any, do you think it appropriate to use dead bodies as neomorts?

your time and love when you meet someone with whom you fall in love. Though it is perhaps not readily obvious, they mourn this loss; and if they don't have something in which they can take an active interest (work, hobby, and so forth), they may dwell on this loss so that it affects their health. Develop ways to help your parents, or the parents of someone close to you, deal with this loss.

Funerals and Burial Arrangements

Every society memorializes the death of a person with some sort of ceremony. The ritual seems to satisfy deeply felt human needs. Family closeness and the support of friends and clergy aid the living in dealing with their grief. Be it a wake or sitting "shiva" or a memorial service, the family and group support those in mourning receive at this time is an important component of the healing process.

By the time a death has occurred, funeral and burial arrangements should have long ago been decided upon so that all that needs to be done is to put them into place. In the United States, most people choose burial as the means of disposing of the body. Although a growing number of people are selecting cremation, for most there is a desire to preserve the remains and mark the spot of burial for surviving family members.

Funerals and the Consumer

The typical funeral in our society costs over $4,000 (see Table 18.3). It isn't surprising, then, that there is now a trend toward more simple funerals. Regardless

TABLE 18.3

What Funerals Cost

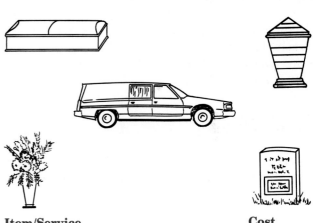

Item/Service	Cost
Casket	$300 to $12,000
Hearse	$90 to $190
Limousines	$50 to $190/hour
Funeral home staff	$500 to $1,000
Embalming	$150 to $250
Other preparations of the remains	$50 to $90
Use of funeral home for a service	$125 to $250
Use of funeral home for visitation	$150 to $275
Cremation	$600 to $1,100

Source: Federated Funeral Directors cited in "Getting the Best Value for a Funeral," *USA Today* (February 20, 1989): 3B.

embalming The replacement of the blood in a corpse with various fluids to make the body more presentable for a funeral, to prepare the body for transport, or to preserve the body if refrigeration is not available.

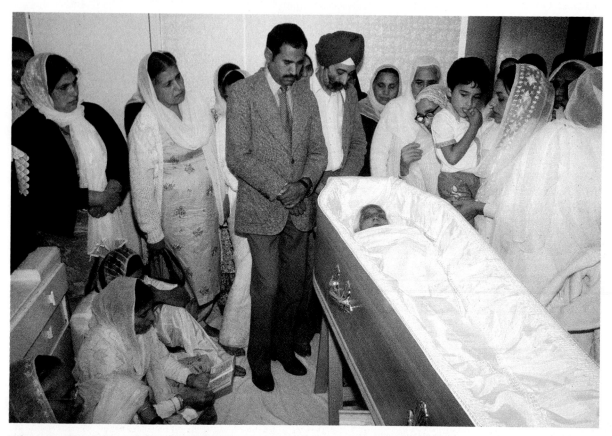

When you die, there are several options. You can be cremated, buried after a funeral, or merely have a memorial service without a funeral. Which would you prefer? Have you notified anyone of your preference? Perhaps you should.

of the type of funeral chosen, certain services are provided. The funeral home will transport the body, provide facilities for the eulogy or viewing of the body, use their equipment to embalm or cremate it, acquire the death certificate, place the body in a casket for burial, and assist the family in filing the necessary papers to receive whatever death benefits they are entitled to (for example, Social Security or Veterans Administration benefits).

Should a funeral and burial be chosen, several associated decisions are required. For example:

1. Which funeral home will be used?

2. In which cemetery will the deceased be buried?

3. Will a casket be used? If so, what kind (wood, metal)? At what cost? Will you use a grave liner (a concrete container that lines the grave to prevent the earth from caving in when the casket deteriorates) or a vault?

4. Who will the grave marker be purchased from? Some cemeteries require that you purchase it from them; others do not, but may have an exorbitant charge for installing it if purchased elsewhere. How much are you willing to spend on a grave marker? What should it say?

5. Should the deceased be embalmed? Some states require **embalming**—replacing the blood with various embalming fluids to make the body appear more presentable. Under certain circum-

stances embalming is required (for example, if the body is transported over state lines, if the person died of a communicable disease, or if the body is to be held for over twenty-four hours before burial or cremation and adequate refrigeration facilities are not available).

Other costs associated with funerals are the cost of clergy, the cost of the cemetery plot, and the cost of opening and closing the grave.

Because several decisions need to be made—embalm or not, type of casket or urn to purchase, where to bury, where to get the grave marker, burial or cremation, which funeral home to use—it is wise to make funeral arrangements before the death, if possible. These decisions can then be given careful consideration rather than being made hastily and at a time of great emotion.

A common consumer complaint is that funeral home directors deceive family members about funeral and burial arrangements. Complaints have been made that they charge excessive fees and encourage unnecessary services and that they use clients' feelings of guilt, or that they incorrectly describe state regulations to influence the mourners to pay for these unnecessary services. In 1984, in response to these complaints, the Federal Trade Commission required funeral directors to:

1. Give customers an itemized list of prices at the beginning of any discussion of funeral goods or services.

2. Disclose prices over the telephone when asked to do so.

3. Tell customers that embalming is not legally required in most cases.

4. Disclose in writing the existence of any mark-ups imposed on "cash advance items" such as flowers or death notices.

Get Involved!

Helping Other People in Dying and Death

What did you think when you first looked at the title of this chapter? You probably felt at least a little uncomfortable with the subject of dying and death, right? Admittedly, it is not a happy or pleasant subject. After all, life is so much more, well, "alive" than death! Now that you've come to the end of the chapter, however, we hope that you understand how death is a natural part of life; that it is as necessary and, in a way, as "good" for all life as birth.

Each of us must work out our own feelings regarding dying and death. This can be a lonely process, but it doesn't have to be. By helping other people confront and cope with their own deaths or the deaths of loved ones, and by helping others after your own death (for example, through organ donations), you may be able to touch a deep, powerful part of your own humanity, a part of you that you want to share with other people.

Here are some specific ways you can contribute to the health of your community, nation, and world in terms of dying and death:

1. If consistent with your religious beliefs, instruct family members that you should be cremated rather than buried in the ground. If you believe that land is scarce and should be used for the living, you will be helping to create a "demand" for cremation that will set an example for others to forego burial.

2. If consistent with your religious beliefs, complete an organ donor card so others will actually benefit from your death. You can help others see by donating your cornea, and help others live by donating other vital organs. Since there is a shortage of organs for trans-

planting, donating your organs will be of tremendous help.

3. Complete a property will that provides resources (money or other assets) for charitable purposes. There are many people living in poverty conditions that can benefit from financial contributions or the use of your clothing or other possessions.

4. Devote your time to assist the functioning of a local hospice or hospital that treats the terminally ill. Either provide services consistent with any expertise you possess, or offer to conduct other chores that will save the hospice money that can be better used in direct services for its patients.

5. Lobby legislators to vote for regulations regarding the terminally ill about which you hold strong beliefs. That might mean advocating active euthanasia if you believe that is appropriate, or advocating laws prohibiting any form of euthanasia if you believe that view is correct.

6. Conduct a survey of funeral parlors and print a listing of the services they offer and the prices they charge. Perhaps local groups such as the Health Department or the American Association of Retired Persons will distribute this listing for you.

7. Enroll in a counseling course offered at your school or through a local mental health association so you can be prepared to help friends and relatives cope at times of grief. During this course, make especially sure to develop such skills as listening and expressing empathy effectively. Learn to know when to refer someone in mourning to professional services when necessary.

cremation The incineration of a corpse in a special oven at a very high temperature.

memorial service A ceremonial gathering of the family and friends of a deceased person to remember that person; often done in lieu of a funeral or when there is no corpse.

In addition, funeral directors were forbidden to do the following:

1. Tell customers they need to buy a casket if they want a "direct" cremation.
2. Tell customers there is a legal requirement to buy an outside burial container for a casket, unless state or local law or a cemetery requires it.
3. Tell customers that any law, cemetery, or crematorium requires them to buy a certain item or service if such a requirement is not true.
4. Claim that any funeral goods (such as sealed caskets) or services (such as embalming) will delay a body's decomposition for a long, or indefinite, time after burial. Customers cannot be told that a

casket or vault will protect a body from water, insects, and so forth if that is not true.

The penalty for violating any section of the FTC regulations was to be a $10,000 fine.

Cremation and Memorial Service

Another option becoming increasingly popular is cremation with a memorial service following, or a memorial service by itself. **Cremation** is the burning of the body in a special oven at very high temperatures until all that remains are ashes. **Memorial services** are gatherings of people to recall the life of the deceased.

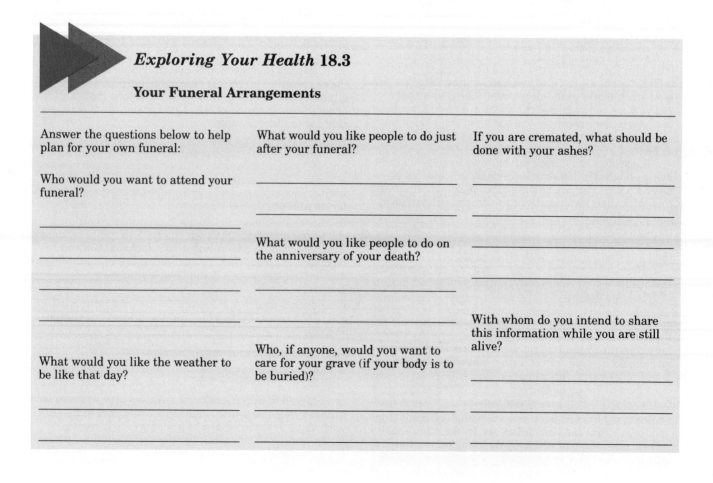

Exploring Your Health 18.3

Your Funeral Arrangements

Answer the questions below to help plan for your own funeral:

Who would you want to attend your funeral?

_____

_____

_____

What would you like the weather to be like that day?

_____

_____

What would you like people to do just after your funeral?

_____

_____

What would you like people to do on the anniversary of your death?

_____

_____

Who, if anyone, would you want to care for your grave (if your body is to be buried)?

If you are cremated, what should be done with your ashes?

_____

_____

_____

With whom do you intend to share this information while you are still alive?

_____

_____

When a body may not be available for burial or cremation—for example, when a soldier is declared Missing in Action—a memorial service may be the only option. Memorial services can take any number of forms. Some involve objects from the deceased's life. For example, at one memorial service a father stood in front of a painting by his deceased daughter and spoke of her love of art. Another alternative is for the service to present a biography of the deceased. In this case the family might be responsible for researching phases of the deceased's life and making brief presentations at the service. Often this approach results in the family learning things about their loved one's life they would have never learned otherwise. Other forms of memorial services include the Jewish practice of saying kad-dish and lighting a yahrzeit candle one year after the death, or the Catholic practice of offering an anniversary mass for the repose of the soul.

Any form of memorial service that meets the needs of both the deceased and the bereaved family members can be organized given sufficient time for planning. If friends from across the country are expected to participate, for instance, time for them to be able to travel to the service would have to be provided. If a history of the deceased is to be presented, time must be available to research his or her life. Even within these limitations, however, much is possible. Exploring Your Health 18.3 will help you plan for your funeral.

Conclusion

Dying and death are topics that need to be discussed and studied. We need to improve both the way people die and the way they live their lives. A study of dying and death can help to serve both these needs. Your conception of death influences your decisions and behavior in life. To come to grips with your death, your mortality, is to make better sense of your life and make you better able to help those who are dying. To appreciate the role of grief is to be better able to help the bereaved.

Completing Exploring Your Health 18.4 will help identify your feelings about dying and death.

Exploring Your Health 18.4

Identifying Your Feelings About Dying and Death

To identify some of your thoughts and feelings about dying and death, complete the following sentences:

1. Death is _____

_____

2. I would like to die at _____

_____

3. I don't want to live past _____

_____

4. I would like to have at my bedside when I die

_____

5. When I die, I will be proud that when I was living I

_____

6. My greatest fear about death is

_____

_____

7. When I die, I'll be glad that when I was living I didn't

_____

_____

8. If I were to die today, my biggest regret would be

_____

_____

9. When I die, I will be glad to get away from

_____

_____

10. When I die, I want people to say

_____

_____

What can you learn about your life from the sentences you have just completed?

_____

_____

_____

Summary

1. Most people know when they are dying, and most wish to die at home, yet over 90 percent of Americans die in institutions, and over 70 percent die of degenerative diseases, sometimes in pain.

2. The hospice—meaning care to travelers—is a special facility that cares for dying persons in a homelike setting.

3. The five stages of the dying process described by Elisabeth Kübler-Ross are denial, anger, bargaining, depression, and acceptance. Thanatologists tell us that not everyone passes through all of these stages in the exact order suggested by Kübler-Ross.

4. Our view of death affects how we live our lives. If we think death is the end of everything, we might try to experience as much of life as possible; if we think there is an afterlife whose quality depends on how we live this life, we might be especially kind and charitable.

5. Brain death consists of four components: unreceptiveness and unresponsiveness, no movements or breathing, no reflexes, and a flat electroencephalogram.

6. Preparing for dying and death requires completing a Living Will, a Durable Power of Attorney, Organ Donor Cards if you plan to donate any organs, and making explicit funeral plans and arrangements. Without these documents it is possible that your wishes may be disregarded regarding how you will be treated if severely ill or how your funeral will be conducted.

7. Grief is the combination of distressing emotions felt as a result of the death of a loved one. Mourning is the manner that grief is manifested during the period of bereavement (the time during which someone is grieving). The way in which people mourn varies depending upon the religion and culture of the bereaved.

8. Grief has been described as occurring in three stages. The first stage is one of shock and disbelief, the second stage consists of painful longing for the deceased, and the third stage is marked by a return to normal activities and acceptance of the loss.

9. Funerals can take many different forms and vary greatly in cost, depending on which services are included.

Questions for Personal Growth

1. The realization that you are mortal can provide you with a sense of urgency about doing things you might otherwise have put off. What are the things you want to make sure you do soon? What are the things you want to avoid doing?

2. What is it that you can leave on this earth as a heritage? Who will benefit from your being alive? What will you leave behind that will be valued? How can you organize your life to maximize this heritage?

3. Even if you are young, you never know exactly when you will die. Considering this fact, what plans have you made for your death? Have you completed a Living Will? A Durable Power of Attorney? An Organ Donor Card if you want to donate organs upon your death? Does your family know what you desire regarding a funeral, burial, or memorial service? When will you make these arrangements?

4. Do you know what members of your family want done when they die? With their possessions? With their bodies? With their organs? Have you specifically discussed these matters with your family?

5. What can you do for people for whom you care when they experience grief? How can you help them during their time of bereavement? What can you do for grieving people whom you know only as acquaintances?

6. How can our society make adjustments to be more sympathetic to people in mourning? For example, what changes in the tax laws ought to be made? What should legislation regarding inheritances allow and not allow?

References

1. Report of the Ad Hoc Committee of the Harvard Medical School to Examine the Definition of Brain Death, "A Definition of Irreversible Coma," *Journal of the American Medical Association* 205 (1968): 337–340.

2. Richard Dumont and Dennis Foss, *The American View of Death: Acceptance or Denial?* (Cambridge, Mass.: Schenkman, 1972), p. 104.

3. Edgar N. Jackson, "Grief," in Earl A. Grollman, ed., *Concerning Death: A Practical Guide for the Living* (Boston: Beacon Press, 1974), p. 9.

4. P. Ebersole and P. Hess, *Toward Healthy Aging: Human Needs and Nursing Response* (St. Louis, Mo.: C. V. Mosby, 1985).

5. Elisabeth Kübler-Ross, *On Death and Dying* (New York: Macmillan, 1969).

CHAPTER
19

Preventive Health Care and the Consumer

CHAPTER OBJECTIVES

After reading this chapter, you should understand:

- The concept of self-care.

- How quacks use false advertising and other methods to lure consumers to spend their money on medications, foods, and devices that ostensibly promote health but may actually damage health.

- How to be a smarter consumer when it comes to generic versus brand-name drugs.

- Why consumers spend millions of dollars each year on cosmetic products.

- Basic strategies for reducing your risk of food poisoning, as well as basic information about food-product labeling.

- How various government and private bureaus and agencies work to protect consumers from unsafe food and health-care products.

- How you can judge health-care advertising and when you should be skeptical or seek the advice of your physician.

CHAPTER OUTLINE

Preventive Health Care

Quackery

Drugs and the Consumer

Cosmetic Products: Myths and Facts

Nutrition and the Consumer

Protecting the Consumer: Your Advocates

Learning to Judge Advertising

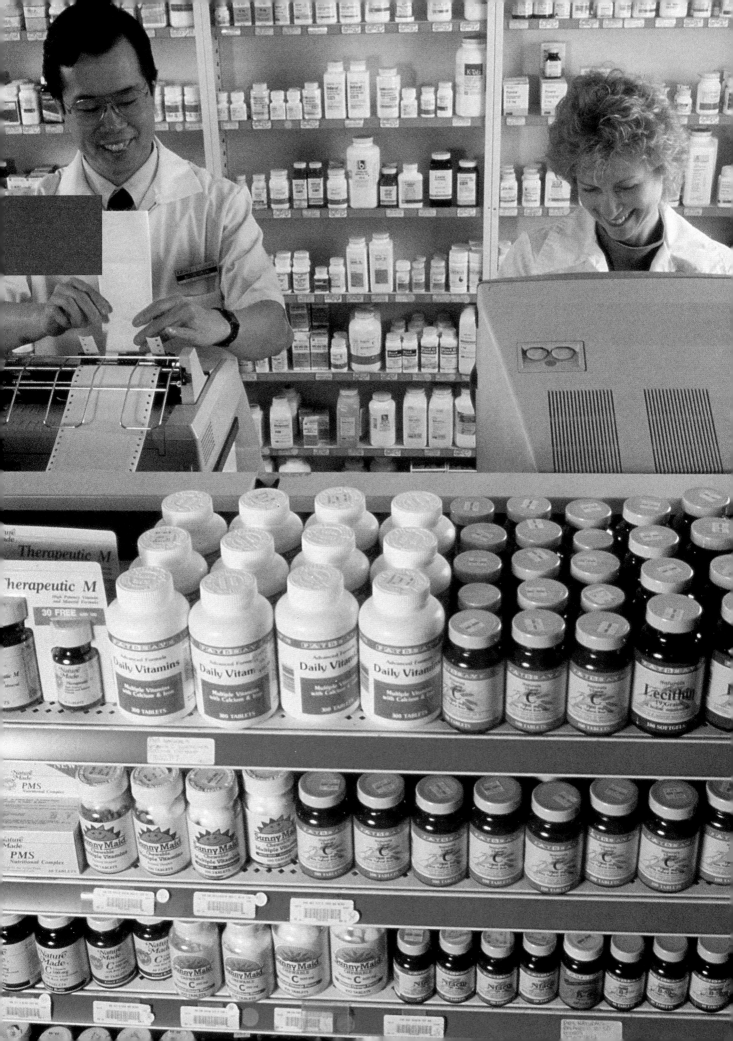

self-care When an individual takes responsibility for the monitoring of his or her own health, determining when to use self-treatment and when to seek the help of health-care specialists.

radial pulse The pulse as taken by placing the index and middle fingers in the hollow of the wrist at the

base of the thumb in order to palpate the wrist artery.

carotid pulse The pulse as taken by placing the index and middle fingers in the hollow of the neck under the jaw bone in order to palpate the carotid artery.

Everyone in our society is the guardian of his or her own health, and we are all responsible for our own preventive health care. In addition, a good member of society is concerned about, and actively involved in, the health and well-being of others. This chapter deals with self-care techniques; self-medication for common, uncomplicated injuries and illnesses; home treatment of minor injuries and illnesses, knowing when a physician's care is or is not needed; and helping others with their self-care problems. It is important to become a "healthy skeptic" as you evaluate the many "scientific" claims and counterclaims about these products.

Your voice and the voice of other consumers can make a difference. In fact, most investigations of health-related products are initiated by consumer complaints. Because it is impossible for the various government and private agencies to monitor the influx of all new products, each individual must assume this responsibility by asking hard questions about advertising claims and costs.

This chapter, therefore, also provides information about the preventive health care movement and health-related products, and it suggests ways for you to evaluate advertising claims, take action through federal, state, or private agencies, and help others benefit from your knowledge.

Preventive Health Care

The Self-Care Movement

Self-care requires that individuals learn about their bodies, monitor their bodily functions, and determine when and how to use medical resources (doctors, hospitals, clinics, and the like). In addition, self-care carries with it the responsibility of establishing a healthy lifestyle. This involves regular exercise, proper nutrition, maintenance of normal body weight, minimal stress, avoidance of tobacco smoking, and moderate use of alcohol, over-the-counter drugs, and prescription drugs. In recent years, self-care has gained widespread acceptance. Many people believe that requiring each individual to take more responsibility for his or her own health is the most effective form of preventive medicine.

Year 2000 National Health Objective

In order to encourage self-care, one Year 2000 National Health Objective seeks to increase to at least 40 percent the proportion of people with chronic and disabling conditions who receive formal patient education, including information about community and self-help resources, as an integral part of the management of their condition.

An important part of self-care includes learning about the symptoms of common complaints and knowing when to treat yourself and when to seek help from medical practitioners. Several self-care books provide health information in terms that any consumer can understand. Here's a brief bibliography of self-care books. Check with your university or community library for further sources of information in this area.

Fries, James, *Take Care of Yourself* (Reading, Mass.: Addison-Wesley, 1990).

Pantell, R. H., et al., *Taking Care of Your Child*, rev. ed. (Reading, Mass.: Addison-Wesley, 1984).

Hashim, A. S., *How to Be Your Child's Doctor Sometimes* (A. S. Hashim, 1984).

Graedon, Joe, *People's Pharmacy*, rev. ed. (New York: St. Martin's Press: 1989).

Self-medication, which is a part of self-care, involves using over-the-counter drugs to relieve symptoms of headaches and the common cold. However, self-medication can be abused, particularly if people rely on it too much, do not inform themselves about the effects of drugs, misdiagnose their ailment, or are unaware of their own reactions to particular medications (see Chapter 10).

When to Seek Help

To take care of your health, you need to know when to seek help. In general, a visit to your doctor is indicated when any of the following occurs:

- Oral temperature above 101°F.
- Severe pain that is persistent or recurrent.
- Abdominal pain persisting for more than three hours or accompanied by nausea.
- Repeated digestive upset.
- Fatigue over a long period with no apparent cause.
- Unanticipated weight loss or gain.
- Dizziness or fainting.
- Bleeding without apparent injury.
- Personality changes without any apparent explanation.
- Any of the seven warning signals of cancer (see Table 16.2 in Chapter 16).
- Headache persisting for more than one day.
- Joint pain persisting for more than a few days.
- Shortness of breath.
- Unusual discharge from some body part.

Self-Care Skills

With minimum practice and time, you can learn to identify changes in your health and determine when you should report these findings to your physician and when you can safely treat yourself. Careful observation of your body will help you decide whether to see a physician for diagnosis. Refer to Figure 19.1 while you read through these suggestions.

Temperature   Buy a thermometer and master the proper technique of taking accurate temperature readings. Report the exact temperature to the physician rather than relying on "feel." Several types of forehead thermometers that provide "ballpark" readings are available for use with young children. It is recommended, however, that a rectal or oral thermometer also be used and exact readings reported to the physician.

Pulse   Learn to count your heart rate accurately using the carotid or radial pulse. It is important to remain quiet in a sitting or lying position for five minutes before counting your pulse. The **radial pulse** is taken by placing the index and middle fingers of the left hand in the hollow of the wrist at the base of the thumb. Move the fingers around until you find a strong pulse. The **carotid pulse** is taken by placing these same two fingers in the hollow of the neck on the left side (under the jaw bone). Only gentle pressure should be applied. The number of beats should be

FIGURE 19.1   •   Basic Self-Care Skills: More Than an Apple a Day

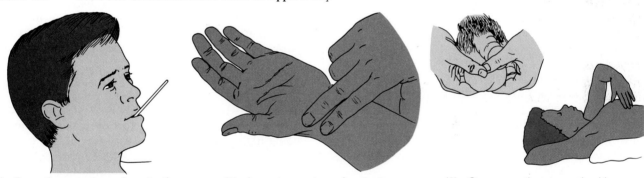

(1) Buy a thermometer and master the proper technique of taking accurate temperature readings.

(2) Learn to count your heart rate accurately by using the carotid (neck) or radial (wrist) pulse.

(3) Once a month, women should perform a breast self-exam and men should perform a testicular self-exam.

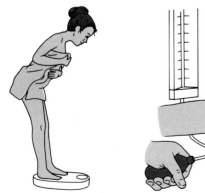

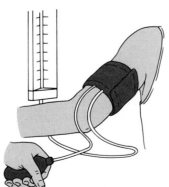

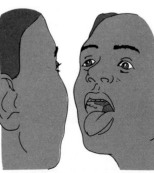

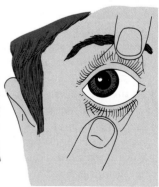

(4) Weigh yourself periodically at the same time of day and under the same conditions.

(5) Have your blood pressure checked regularly.

(6) Learn to recognize a healthy throat so that you can catch a small problem before it becomes a big one.

(7) Learn to recognize the symptoms of various eye problems.

blood pressure The pressure of the blood as it flows through and presses against the arterial walls of the body; an important measure of cardiovascular and general health.

glaucoma An eye disorder characterized by increased pressure within the eye; a serious disease causing blindness if not treated, but easily controlled with medication.

conjunctivitis An infection of the mucous membranes (conjunctiva) lining the inner surface of the eyelids and covering the surface of the whites of the eyes; also called "pinkeye."

counted for thirty seconds, then multiplied by two. Learn to recognize regular and irregular beats, such as skipping or palpitating, and describe the problem accurately to your physician. Record your normal resting pulse to provide some basis for comparison.

Breast and Testicular Cancer

Women should learn the breast self-exam, and men should learn to perform the testicular self-exam. Both should be done monthly (see Chapter 16).

Body Weight and Fat

Weigh yourself periodically at the same time of day and under the same conditions. In addition, it is helpful to pinch yourself in the abdominal area, thighs, and back of arms as a crude measure of body fat (see Chapter 8 for skinfold measures). Be able to provide accurate data on weight loss or gain over a specific period of time.

Blood Pressure

Blood pressure refers to the pressure of the blood against arterial walls during the beating or systolic stage and during the resting or diastolic stage. Recent findings of the association of hypertension and cardiovascular disease place the cutoff for "minimal" risk (high normal blood pressure) at a diastolic reading of 85–89 mm Hg and a systolic reading of more than 140 (see Chapter 15).[1]

Coin-operated blood pressure machines can be used for a rough indication of blood pressure but not as the basis for self-medication, altering therapy, or ignoring the instructions of a doctor. It is important to realize that machines may be inaccurate and that your blood pressure can vary from day to day as a result of emotions, bladder distention, climate changes, exertion, pain, and medication. Therefore, a single reading may not accurately characterize your blood pressure. If you do not have a *stethoscope* (to listen to your heartbeat) and *sphygmomanometer* (to measure your arterial blood pressure) or do not know someone who can use this equipment properly, use the coin-operated machine to estimate your pressure, and consult a physician if your pressure falls outside the suggested ranges. The reading will be more accurate if you first rest in a sitting position for five to ten minutes. Also, it is very difficult to take your own blood pressure unless you are extremely adept at the procedure.

Throat

Learn what a healthy throat looks like so that you can recognize the symptoms of a problem. Inflammation, swelling, and white or yellow patches at the back of the throat are all indicators of infection. Examining the throat yourself is useful, but it may not reveal whether the infection is bacterial (strep throat) or viral. If someone in your family has a persistent sore throat, you should call your doctor to determine whether an office examination is indicated. The doctor can take a throat culture to determine if bacterial infection is present. You can also have a throat culture taken at a medical laboratory, if this is more convenient. If the culture is positive, your physician will start antibiotic therapy. If the culture is negative, you can treat the problem at home with throat lozenges, aspirin, and salt water gargle. Using a humidifier or vaporizer is also helpful because the humid air will keep your throat from drying out.

Eyes

Eye pain may be caused by injury, infection, or disease, such as **glaucoma** (pressure within the eye being higher than normal). Tired eyes after a long period of close work are normal. Severe pain behind the eye may be a symptom of a migraine headache. Pain below the eye may be caused by sinus problems. Pain in both eyes on exposure to bright light is a common symptom of some viral infections and will disappear as the infection improves. A physician should be consulted if pain is severe and persists for more than forty-eight hours. If pain is associated with tiredness or flu, home treatment can be used (resting the eyes, taking aspirin, and avoiding bright light).

For vision problems, such as temporary blindness (partial or complete), blurred vision, blocked vision, or changes in vision, an ophthalmologist should be consulted.

Eye burning, itching, and discharge are generally symptoms of **conjunctivitis,** or "pinkeye," an infection of the mucous membranes (*conjunctiva*) lining the inner surface of the eyelids. Wearing dark glasses or goggles at work to avoid a particular allergic exposure may help. If the condition remains, the discharge gets thicker, eye pain develops, or vision is impaired, see an ophthalmologist.

Contact Lenses An association has recently been established between *Acanthamoeba keratitis*, a corneal infection, and soft contact lens use. The infection produces severe pain and irritation and often mimics other infections such as herpes. Although only 75 cases have been reported to the Centers for Disease Control since the infection was first identified in 1973, the seriousness of the infection and the fact that the number of cases has doubled in five years have alarmed many of the more than 21 million American contact users. Antimicrobal drugs are generally ineffective, and corneal transplants are necessary. Other contact lens-related problems such as irritation, swelling and scratching, infection, and ulcers are more common. Perhaps, attention to *Acanthamoeba keratitis* will improve the impact of the message that contact users need to exercise very special care: (1) lenses should be rinsed regularly in a commercial saline solution (homemade solutions are more likely to become contaminated), (2) lenses should be removed when swimming, (3) lenses should fit perfectly and cause no irritation, and (4) extended-wear lenses should be kept in the eyes no longer than six days before overnight removal and sterilization. Bacteria must be killed by use of a multistep process. Lenses are removed and a commercial cleanser is rubbed in before the soap is rinsed away in a saline solution. Next, lenses are disinfected either in an electrical heating unit (heat disinfection) or overnight rinsing in a commercially prepared chemical disinfectant (cold disinfection). The next morning, lenses are rinsed with saline or wetting solution and placed back into the eyes. Daily-wear soft lenses should be disinfected every day; extended-wear lenses approximately every six days.[2]

Home Medical Tests

Use of home medical tests can help reduce your medical costs, help you keep a closer watch on chronic conditions, and assist you with the early detection of a number of health problems. Home medical testing has also been a financial boon to manufacturers, with sales expected to reach $2.2 billion by 1995. People are now testing their eyesight, stool, urine, blood, and blood pressure in search of clues to various health concerns such as pregnancy, gastrointestinal disease, infection, ovulation, diabetes, hypertension, and other conditions. These tests are inexpensive, simple to use, and fairly reliable.

Self-testing products fall into three categories: (1) those that help diagnose a specific condition or disease in people with symptoms, (2) screening tests that identify indications of disease in people without symptoms,

and (3) doctor-recommended monitoring devices for on-going checkups on an existing condition. When these tests are performed in conjunction with medical guidance, they can be extremely helpful.

In addition to self-testing for blood pressure, which was discussed above, some of the more common specific tests available to the consumer include:

Blood Glucose Monitoring This is a one- to two-minute test to measure the level of glucose in the blood and should be used in conjunction with a physician. The user pricks a finger or earlobe to obtain a drop of blood and then places it on a chemically treated test strip. After a period of time the blood is blotted or wiped off the strip and eventually matched to a color guide for diagnosis.

Ovulation Monitoring This test measures the amount of luteinizing hormone (LH) in the urine. Once daily for one week in the middle of the menstrual cycle, a chemically treated strip is dipped in a urine specimen. The strip is compared to a color guide to indicate the time of the LH surge and the start of ovulation. The test takes twenty minutes to one hour to complete.

Pregnancy Testing In this test, the HCG (human chorionic gonadotropin) hormone produced by a developing placenta is detected by mixing chemicals with a urine specimen. A positive result is signaled (in some brands) by the presence or absence of a ring formation, as you look down the tube. Accuracy is increased when women delay testing until at least seven to nine days after the missed period should have occurred. The test takes from twenty minutes to two hours.

Urinary Tract Infections In this test, a chemically treated strip is dipped in a urine specimen on three consecutive mornings. The test detects *nitrite* in urine. Although urine contains small amounts of nitrite, the bacteria that cause most urinary tract infections change nitrate in urine into nitrite.

Hidden Fecal Blood A stool specimen is brought into contact with hydrogen peroxide and guaiac (a kind of wood resin). If hidden blood is present, a color change will appear. Samples should be taken from three separate bowel movements. Results are produced in thirty seconds to sixteen minutes.

One disadvantage of home medical tests is the risk of misinterpreting or overrelying on test results. There is the danger that some people will take a single abnormal reading as a diagnosis of illness or a normal reading as a cure. The Department of Health and Human Services offers these precautions to promote self-testing safety and effectiveness:[3]

rebound congestion The tendency of nasal passages to become more inflamed and swollen after a topical decongestant, which has been applied to relieve nasal stuffiness, has ceased to work.

irritable bowel syndrome Constipation or diarrhea caused by intestinal spasms, usually related to worry, fear, and anxiety.

1. For test kits containing chemicals, note the expiration date and avoid purchasing products if the date is past.
2. Consider whether the product needs protection from heat or cold and follow storage directions.
3. Study the package insert carefully, reading it first for a general view, then meticulously to master the specific steps.
4. Consult a pharmacist or other health professional to clarify something you don't understand.
5. Learn what the test is intended to do and its limitations.
6. Elicit help for tests involving color if you are colorblind.
7. Note and follow special precautions.
8. Follow instructions exactly and in exactly the same sequence.
9. Before collecting a urine sample, wash the container thoroughly and rinse out all soap, unless a container is present in the kit.
10. When a step is timed, be precise and use a watch with a second hand.
11. Note and follow what you should do if results are positive, negative, or unclear.
12. Keep accurate records of results.
13. Keep test kits containing chemicals out of the reach of children and discard used test materials as directed.

Self-Medication

Many common health problems can be taken care of at home with a few basic supplies used wisely (see Table 19.1).

Colds and Coughs

As we saw briefly in Chapter 13, a cold is an infection of the membrane lining the upper respiratory tract, including the nose, the sinuses, and the throat. The average American contracts between four and eight colds a year. Although it is known how colds are caused by viruses and how these viruses are transmitted from one individual to another, little is known about how to prevent or cure them. All that can be done is relieve the symptoms. Left un-

TABLE 19.1

Your Home Pharmacy

Items in bold print are basic requirements. Other preparations may find use in some households. Keep all medicines out of the reach of children.

Ailment	Medication
Allergy	Antihistamines Nose drops and sprays
Cold and coughs	Cold tablets/cough syrups
Constipation	Milk of magnesia, bulk laxatives
Dental problems (preventive)	Sodium fluoride
Diarrhea	**Kaopectate,** paregoric
Eye irritations	Eye drops and artificial tears
Hemorrhoids	Hemorrhoid preparations
Pain and fever (in children)	**Aspirin, acetaminophen** Liquid acetaminophen,* aspirin rectal suppositories
Poisoning (to induce vomiting)	Syrup of ipecac*
Fungus	Antifungal preparations
Sunburn (preventive)	Sunscreen agents
Sprains	**Elastic bandages**
Stomach, upset	**Antacid, nonabsorbable**
Wounds (minor) (antiseptic) (soaking agent)	**Adhesive tape, bandages** Hydrogen peroxide **Sodium bicarbonate** (baking soda)

* Items are for homes with small children.
Source: Donald M. Vickery and James F. Fries, *Take Care of Yourself: A Consumer's Guide to Medical Care,* rev. ed. (Reading, Mass.: Addison-Wesley, 1986), p. 44. Reprinted with permission.

treated, a common cold will last approximately seven days, with treatment it will last a week. Aspirin or acetaminophen relieves fever and aching, and decongestants shrink swollen nasal membranes. Topical decongestants work faster and are more effective than the oral type. Overuse can lead to **rebound congestion,** resulting in stuffiness that is worse than the original problem. With each application, some irritation and inflammation occurs. Eventually, the more the product is used, the more irritated, inflamed, and blocked up the nasal passages become. Steroid drugs may be needed to break the cycle.

About one-half of individuals with colds develop a cough. Review the section in Chapter 10 titled "Cough Medicine" for information about self-medication for coughs.

Diarrhea and Constipation Bowel dysfunction often reflects emotional stresses. Stress may cause opposing responses in different people or in the same individual, speeding up bowel transit time to produce diarrhea, slowing bowel transit time to cause constipation, or stress may lead to intestinal spasms with alternating periods of diarrhea and constipation. When these conditions persist or recur and are accompanied by worry, fear, and anxiety, they are generally diagnosed as **irritable bowel syndrome.** This complex disorder is triggered by a number of factors, including emotional upset.

Refer to the section in Chapter 10 titled "Laxatives" for information about dealing with diarrhea and constipation.

Hemorrhoids Americans spend more than $75 million on hemorrhoid suppositories, cleansers, creams, and ointments each year. Most products sell on the same claim—temporary relief of pain and itching. No product has been shown to shrink swollen hemorrhoids. To minimize the symptoms and also help to prevent the condition from developing: (1) Add fiber to your diet; because straining due to constipation is a main cause, avoiding constipation is important. (2) Practice good anal care to control irritation and itching; keep skin around the anus dry and clean and use toilet paper moistened with warm water rather than vigorous wiping with dry toilet paper. Premoistened wipes are also helpful. (3) Use a light sprinkling of talcum powder and avoid tight undergarments and pantyhose, opting for loose cotton underwear to control perspiration. (4) Use a sitz bath (sitting in warm water for ten to fifteen minutes) as needed. The best hemorrhoid products, such as Preparation H, cleansing pads, and Tucks Pads, help keep the anus clean. Suppositories are of questionable value. Creams are preferable to ointments and may help soothe irritation. For persistent irritation, itching, pain, or bleeding, consult your physician.

Pain and Fever As we saw in Chapter 10, aspirin is available generically as acetylsalicylate. Aspirin does relieve pain, common headaches, fever, and inflamma-

tion; however, aspirin also irritates the stomach lining and causes slight bleeding which is more pronounced in combination with alcohol, heparin, warfarin, and other anticoagulants. Acetaminophen (Anacin-3, Tylenol, Tempra, Excedrin) also relieves pain, fever, and common headaches, although it is not antiinflammatory like aspirin. Large doses increase the drug effect of warfarin and other oral anticoagulants, causing bleeding. Liver damage may also occur with overdoses of acetaminophen or use with barbiturates.[4] Both aspirin and acetaminophen should be used cautiously. Take aspirin with a full glass of water to reduce the chances of irritating the stomach lining. For infants and small children with fever, it is a good practice to give acetaminophen, because some children have a reaction to aspirin. *Reye's syndrome*, a potentially fatal disease in children, is suspected of being related to the use of aspirin. If fever or pain persists, consult your doctor.

Poisoning For the ingestion of certain poisonous materials, the recommended emergency treatment is to induce vomiting with syrup of ipecac (prepared from the dried roots of a certain plant). However, vomiting should not be induced for poisons that are highly acidic or alkaline. If a household produced has been ingested, read the label to find out what the antidote is, and call your local poison control center. Appendix B provides more information on first aid for poisoning.

Stomach Upset Heartburn, sour stomach, and acid indigestion refer to the same basic symptom that indicates an upset stomach. Heartburn generally begins low in the front of the chest and rises toward the throat, and acid indigestion and sour stomach means that stomach juice has entered the mouth. Most lay people refer to the term "upset stomach" for all three complaints, which explains why manufacturers claim their product relieves upset stomach. Self-medication with antacids should be limited to no more than once per week for the treatment of occasional heartburn. Misuse of antacids can aggravate certain gastrointestinal problems and mask others. For occasional problems, consider the following suggestions: (1) avoid the use of any antacid for longer than two weeks; (2) restrict sodium bicarbonate antacids to occasional use; (3) avoid calcium carbonate antacids for prolonged periods; (4) choose products with magnesium and aluminum ingredients and those low in sodium, but avoid taking antacids that contain aluminum, calcium, or magnesium at the same time you are taking prescription antibiotics containing tetracycline; (5) chew tablet-form antacids thoroughly; and (6) consult your physician if symptoms persist.

Use Exploring Your Health 19.1 to determine the cost, purpose, and effectiveness of the items in your medicine cabinet.

quacks People who used false advertising and other inducements to entice consumers to purchase and use bogus medical procedures, medicines, and health-care products.

generic drug A pharmaceutical drug that is produced after the patent has expired on the original brand-name drug; generic drugs have the same formulation, safety, and effectiveness as brand-name drugs, but they are indicated by their chemical names and usually cost less than their brand-name counterparts.

Exploring Your Health 19.1

The Home Medicine Cabinet

Other than first-aid equipment, only a small number of safe supplies are needed in your home medicine cabinet to treat common ailments not requiring a physician (refer to Table 19.1).

Prepare a list of the items in your home medicine cabinet, and complete the information at left: Circle the unnecessary, unsafe, or ineffective items. Are you spending your health dollars wisely or being influenced by advertising?

Item	Cost	Purpose	Effectiveness

Home Treatment of Common Injuries

For most household emergencies, home first aid can be applied and a visit to a physician eliminated. The key is to recognize symptoms that merit a physician's care. Appendix B summarizes common illnesses and injuries and lists cues that suggest physician care versus home care.

Quackery

Misrepresentation of health products and services is a profitable con game that drains the American public of billions of dollars each year. **Quacks** are people who use false advertising and a variety of other lures to entice consumers to spend their money on drugs, mechanical devices, foods, and other products that do no good and can be harmful.

Quacks have existed for millennia and continue to thrive for several reasons. People fear pain, illness, aging, and death. Those who have a serious disease that modern medicine cannot cure may be especially vulnerable to quacks. And, unfortunately, every new legitimate achievement of modern medical research makes it easier for quacks to convince people that they too have developed a cure. Also, many people suffer from conditions that will eventually improve without any treatment. Ailments of this sort disappear by themselves during the course of a quack's expensive treatment, and the quack gets the credit and the publicity. Finally, a quack can diagnose any condition as "cancer," prescribe some special cure, and win over a host of new patients—who may actually have cancer.

Mail-Order Quacks

Mail-order quacks promote drugs, food fads, and devices to energize, revitalize, develop, or cure just about anything imaginable. Mail-order quackery is typified by advertisements promoting a copper bracelet as a cure for arthritis. Such quack advertisements make their way into the home through all types of media, both print and visual. The days of the traveling medicine show may be gone; however, the huckster is still very much with us in quack advertisements.

One of the most extensive investigations of mail-order health advertising was conducted by the Pennsylvania Medical Society in 1977. Five hundred nationally circulated magazines were surveyed, one-fourth of which were found to carry mail-order ads for

Exploring Your Health 19.2

How Common Is Health Quackery?

health products. Typical products included bust developers, weight reducers, hair-loss remedies, blemish removers, longevity formulas, aphrodisiacs, sexual pleasure devices, penis enlargers, and impotency cures. Practically all the ads shared one characteristic, according to the Pennsylvania Medical Society: They were misleading.[5]

Recognizing Quackery

How can you tell if you're dealing with a quack? Some tip-offs include:

- Promise or guarantee of a quick cure.
- Use of a "secret remedy" or unorthodox treatment.
- Use of advertising to gain patients, especially ads in sensational magazines, such as those related to faith healing.
- Testimonials by patients who have been cured.
- Claims that a product will cure a wide variety of ailments.
- Request for payments in advance.
- Use of scare tactics, such as warnings of harmful consequences if a product being promoted isn't used.
- Claims from the sponsor of the product that the medical profession is against them.

Quacks have been around for millenia, thriving on people's fears about pain, aging, disease, and death.

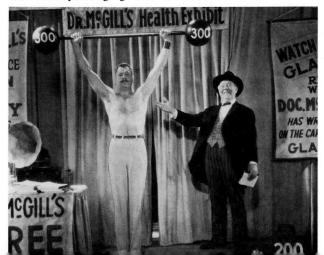

Quackery endangers both your pocketbook and your health. Fake treatments may delay early and accurate diagnosis and appropriate treatment until the problem is very serious. Your best protection is to analyze carefully all products or treatment methods you are considering. In most cases, using good sense is enough. Sometimes it may be necessary to contact your doctor or a reputable agency or nonprofit organization for advice. One good resource for information on drugs is a publication called *The Medicine Show,* an unbiased report on numerous products by the editors of *Consumer Reports.*[6] Other sources of health-related consumer information are the National Health Council; the World Health Organization; the Food and Drug Administration; the Department of Health and Human Services; and various nonprofit associations, such as the American Heart Association, the American Lung Association, the American Cancer Society, and the American Medical Association.

Drugs and the Consumer

The High Cost of Drugs

Many drugs have both a trademarked brand name and a generic name. A **generic drug** is the term for a prescription or nonprescription drug that is the same as a brand-name drug. Most brand name drugs are developed under a patent designed to protect a drug firm's investment by giving them the sole right to sell the drug. Generic versions of a drug may be sold by competing companies only after the patent expires—approximately seventeen years after the discovery of the drug. When a patent on a particular drug has expired, marketplace competition enters the picture, and generic versions are usually sold for less than the brand name product.

The following information will help you decide between generic and brand name drugs:

1. A generic drug contains exactly the same active ingredients as the brand-name drug and is required to be just as safe and effective. Generics

acne Skin blemishes, such as pimples and blackheads, caused by excessively oily skin; a common complaint of the adolescent and young adult years.

Issues in Health

Should the Sale of Over-the-Counter Stimulants Be Eliminated?

Nodoz Tablets, Amostat Tablets, Pep-Back, Tirend Tablets, and *Vivaran* are some of the common products advertised and sold over-the-counter to keep people alert and awake. Manufacturers emphasize the need for over-the-counter stimulants to handle monotonous activity, such as highway driving, fatigue, and boredom, and merely to stay awake while studying or working.

Pro Proponents of over-the-counter stimulants argue that these products are no different or more dangerous than foods and beverages containing caffeine, such as coffee, tea, hot cocoa, and some soft drinks. An over-the-counter stimulant may actually save lives by keeping one awake while driving or performing some delicate task. In addition, small doses of caffeine (50 to 200 milligrams)

stimulate brain functions and encourage creative thoughts. Such doses eliminate feelings of fatigue and drowsiness. Caffeine use is widespread and helpful to students, truck drivers, executives, physicians and other professionals, and people who merely need to stay awake to perform some task. These products perform a valuable function and should be readily available to the public.

Con Opponents of over-the-counter stimulants point out that any stimulant is dangerous and must be used with caution. For fatigue, it is argued, rest is the best remedy, and resorting to drugs may become psychologically addicting and eventually lead to the use of more powerful and dangerous stimulants. Although it is debatable whether stimulants are addicting, serious symptoms are pro-

duced upon withdrawal. Evidence indicates that a number of weight loss products, such as Dexatrim, are being abused as stimulants, and that they are taken in much higher doses than recommended. In low doses, stimulants do heighten the body's sensitivity and improve mental performance, but high doses also produce states of hyperactivity and hyperexcitement, behavioral fixations, and severe health consequences. Food drugs provide enough stimulation, it is argued, and over-the-counter pills that make it easy to increase the dose tenfold or more is asking for trouble.

What do you think? Should over-the-counter stimulants be eliminated?

must be identical in strength, dosage, form, and route of administration, and they must release the same amount of the drug into the body as the brand-name drug.

2. The 1984 Drug Price Competition and Patent Restoration Act does not lower any of the standards for generic drugs. Since the ingredients of generic drugs have already undergone the elaborate testing required for the production of the brand name drug, duplicate testing is not required. It must be shown, however, that the generic version is just as effective.

3. A generic drug must have the same therapeutic effect as its brand-name counterpart and deliver to the bloodstream or other site the same amount of active ingredient.

4. A generic drug must act on the body in exactly the same way as the brand-name version.

5. Generic drugs are produced in the same type of modern facilities as the brand-name drugs that meet FDA standards.

6. There is no evidence that generic drugs produce a higher incidence or a greater number of side effects than brand-name drugs.

Any physician can prescribe drugs by the generic name; however, drug companies try hard to persuade doctors to prescribe their more expensive brand name. A drug containing the same active ingredient often is put out in many forms, combinations, and brand names. Keeping up with this endless drug market is nearly impossible for the physician, who therefore tends to rely on medical advertisements supplied by the drug industry. Expensive advertising—not research as claimed by the drug industry—have pushed up the cost of all drugs.

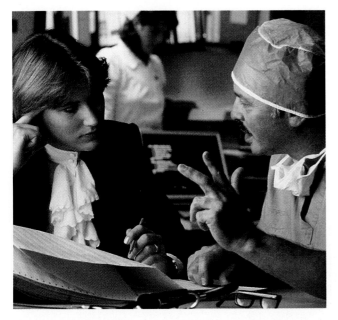

Drug companies work hard to make sure doctors prescribe brand name drugs rather than their less expensive generic counterparts. Pharmaceutical salespeople regularly visit doctors to inform them about new drug products—and to encourage them to prescribe only brand name products.

Industry-Related Problems

In general, the American public has a great deal of faith in the drug industry. Unfortunately, there are several problems with this industry, including inadequate testing of new drugs, withholding of clinical testing data, biased studies, and publications that promote the sale of a product. To complicate the picture, new drugs enter the market at a fantastic rate; many of them contain the same basic ingredient but carry a new brand name. At the center of all these problems is the physician, who is the target of practically all market strategy in drug advertising.

Protect Yourself: Read Labels

Federal law requires that labeling of over-the-counter drugs provide all necessary directions for use by the consumer, including conditions under which the drug should *not* be taken (special instructions for infants,

children, the elderly, pregnant women, or people with certain medical conditions). These labeling standards are very thorough and cover several points that will help ensure better protection for the user, such as directions for use, warnings, drug interaction precautions, and active ingredients (see Figure 19.2).

Cosmetic Products: Myths and Facts

Skin Products

Acne Preparations Hormonal changes in adolescents increase the size of skin oil glands and change the amounts of oil produced. In many teenagers, pores become blocked causing some form of **acne** or skin blemishes on the face, back, and chest. Some form of acne occurs in 80 to 90 percent of all teenagers. Inadequate washing, eating certain foods, and the use of moisturizers have little to do with causing acne, although certain foods may aggravate the condition. Acne is caused by skin oils, not dirt or moisturizers. Flare-ups may be reduced by washing the face with a mild soap several times daily; avoiding chocolate, nuts, dairy foods, salt, colas, shellfish, and other foods (if these foods encourage flare-ups); using an over-the-counter product or soap and water instead of facial creams for cleaning (creams close the pores); keeping the skin as clean as possible; removing blackheads with a blackhead extractor after applying hot, wet compresses for ten minutes (avoid squeezing blackheads); and protecting the skin with a skin protection factor (SPF) of at least 15 in the sun. If flare-ups still persist, a dermatologist may be consulted.

Skin Rejuvenation Americans spend millions of dollars each year on skin products that claim to restore a youthful appearance to aging skin. Unfortunately, these products don't work. Studies of products containing hormones, turtle oil, shark oil, buttermilk, and so forth, reveal the same thing—no change in skin prop-

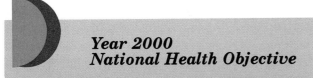

Acne is a common problem in many teenagers and young adults. Most acne can be controlled by general skin cleanliness and over-the-counter preparations.

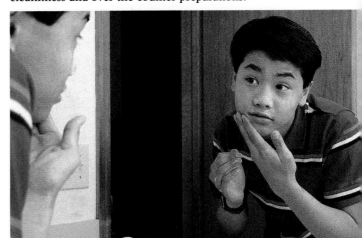

hyperpigmentation An excessive darkening of the skin, usually in certain areas, caused by too much exposure to the sun, disease, oral contraceptives, and pregnancy.

cryosurgery Freezing the skin or other tissue with liquid nitrogen; sometimes used as a treatment for age spots.

electrolysis The permanent removal of unwanted body hair through the use of an electrical current administered by the injection of a needle into the hair follicle.

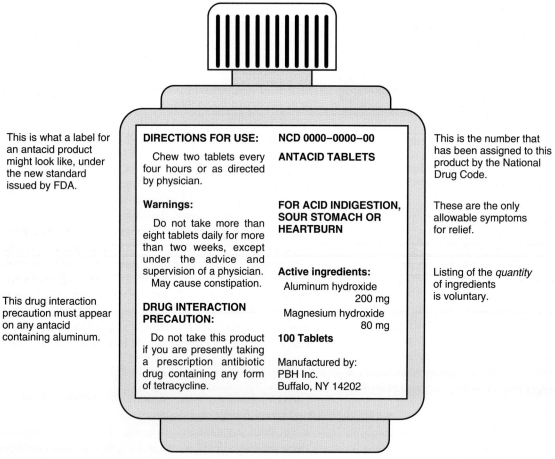

This is what a label for an antacid product might look like, under the new standard issued by FDA.

This drug interaction precaution must appear on any antacid containing aluminum.

DIRECTIONS FOR USE:

Chew two tablets every four hours or as directed by physician.

Warnings:

Do not take more than eight tablets daily for more than two weeks, except under the advice and supervision of a physician. May cause constipation.

DRUG INTERACTION PRECAUTION:

Do not take this product if you are presently taking a prescription antibiotic drug containing any form of tetracycline.

NCD 0000–0000–00

ANTACID TABLETS

FOR ACID INDIGESTION, SOUR STOMACH OR HEARTBURN

Active ingredients:
Aluminum hydroxide
200 mg
Magnesium hydroxide
80 mg
100 Tablets

Manufactured by:
PBH Inc.
Buffalo, NY 14202

This is the number that has been assigned to this product by the National Drug Code.

These are the only allowable symptoms for relief.

Listing of the *quantity* of ingredients is voluntary.

FIGURE 19.2 • Sample Drug Label under the FDA Standard.

erties. Because hormones can be absorbed through the skin, they are unsafe and particularly dangerous to individuals with a family history of breast disorders or cancer of the genital organs. Such products are no more effective than old-fashioned emollient cream. After the age of 30, it may be helpful to apply a moisturizer and to avoid heated rooms, hot showers, sun, dry air, and chlorine, which dry the skin and increase the need for a moisturizer. The moisturizer should be applied all over the body while the skin is still wet after bathing. Women who have previously used water-based makeup as teenagers should change to oil-based products after the age of 30 because extra moisture is needed as time passes.[7] Studies indicate that *Retin A* has some promise in delaying skin aging and restoring skin

to a more youthful appearance. As we age, skin becomes thinner and more fragile. Retin A tends to thicken the skin by turning over epidermal cells, by selectively encouraging damaged cells to come to the surface and slough off, and by encouraging new cell growth. Old cells are peeled away and the number of small blood vessels near the skin surface increase and cause some smoothing of the skin. The milder forms of Retin A now available produce fewer side effects than the earlier topical products.

Age Spots   Chronic exposure to the sun, skin disease, other diseases, use of oral contraceptives, and pregnancy are some of the causes of **hyperpigmen-**

tation, or excess darkening of the skin. Fade creams attempt to lighten the blemishes. Fade cream commercials promise a rapid disappearance of brown spots or freckles. But according to the FDA,[8] fade creams do not always work (they are more effective against flat brown blemishes such as freckles and age spots), and when they do, it may take several months to see results. One must rub in the cream twice daily to achieve and maintain fading. If the treatment is stopped, a faded spot will redarken. Also, faded areas must be kept out of the sun or protected by clothing. Some fade creams now contain a sunscreen. Alternative approaches include the use of foundation creams to cover up skin blemishes or the use of **cryosurgery** (freezing the skin with liquid nitrogen) and laser surgery by a dermatologist to remove the spot permanently.

Suntan Products   See the section in Chapter 16 titled "Skin Cancer" for a discussion of skin cancer, skin care, and suntan products.

Deodorants and Antiperspirants   Body odor occurs through the action of bacteria on secretions from the skin's glands. The best natural protection against odor is bathing with an ordinary bath soap. Following the bath, a *deodorant* (to mask body odors) or *antiperspirant* (to reduce perspiration) may be applied. No product prevents profuse sweating during vigorous exercise or in hot, humid weather. Sweating is a natural process that is important to body functions and should not be totally prevented. If you have an odor problem, bathe regularly and use a deodorant or antiperspirant.

Hair Products

Hair Removers   In our country, it is considered unattractive for women to have body or facial hair. There are basically two approaches to the removal of such hair: temporary treatments that must be repeated and a permanent, "one treatment" method.

The following methods are temporary. Because they remove hair above the root level, the hair will grow back.

- Chemicals soften and dissolve the hair shaft without disturbing the root. Skin reactions to these chemicals are common.
- A wax stick composed of resin and turpentine, warmed and applied to hairy areas, tears the hair away from the roots when the wax hardens.
- Tweezers pluck out hair; however, this method is painful and runs the risk of infection from unclean skin and tweezers.
- A fine pumice stone, if used daily and rubbed against soap-lathered hair, prevents hair from appearing above the skin.
- Shaving underarms and legs removes hair above the skin. Shaving will *not* coarsen hair or increase its growth.

Some women prefer to remove facial and body hair permanently. **Electrolysis** is the only method that can permanently remove unwanted hair. The hair follicle is completely destroyed by injecting a fine electric needle down the root of the follicle and providing low electric current. A dermatologist can recommend a trained electrolysist. The procedure requires patience, good eyesight, coordination, time, and—money! To re-

---

Exploring Your Health 19.3

Are You a Big Health Products Consumer?

To determine whether you are a big consumer of health products, write down what you would do in the following situations:

You have indigestion or stomach upset. _____

You have had trouble sleeping for several nights. _____

You have a cold with stuffiness. _____

You have dandruff. _____

You have a headache. _____

You have recently noticed that your breath seems bad. _____

You have a mild cough. _____

You have an outbreak of blemishes. _____

You want a quick suntan. _____

Your eyes are bloodshot from lack of sleep. _____

Did most of your answers involve using a health product? If so, are you satisfied that you're making wise choices? Given what you've learned, will you change your purchasing habits when it comes to health-related products?

duce chances of infection, only a few hairs on the upper lip are removed at one visit.

Hair-Coloring Products Products that change the color of the hair either penetrate the hair shaft and remain until the hair grows out or remain only until the hair is washed. The majority of these products can produce skin irritations and require some caution. Before you use one, try this test: Put a small amount of the product behind one ear or on the inside of an elbow. Allow to dry and do not wash this area for twenty-four hours. If itching, burning, swelling, or any other irritation occurs, avoid this product. If you should happen to use a product on the hair and get an irritation, shampoo again with soap and water, follow with hydrogen peroxide, and follow once again with a soap shampoo. All hair color products should be kept away from the eyes.

Hair-Restoring Products Baldness is apparently genetic and, as men grow older, the hair-growing follicles on top of the head become more sensitive to dihydrotestosterone, a hormone produced by the skin. Experts believe that it is a person's hormones that cause baldness rather than excessive shampooing, use of inexpensive shampoos, wearing a hat, or not letting the scalp breathe. Some hair loss is natural, with the average person losing about 50 to 100 hairs per day.

The American public has been bombarded with mail-order and television promotion of special ointments, drugs, and other treatments to cure baldness. Before-and-after testimony attempts to convince the American male that any bald spot can be restored with "new growth" hair in a short period of time. Antihormone drugs used in the past feminized men, stimulating breast growth, raising the pitch of the voice, and eliminating facial hair. A drug developed by Upjohn called minoxidil (a compound developed to relieve high blood pressure that is applied topically in 2–3 percent solutions) has shown considerable promise, without interfering with the hormone system. Even modest hair-growth results reported by Upjohn in 1986 sent company stock skyrocketing and other pharmaceutical firms to their laboratories. The evidence is now available to show that new scalp hair growth does occur for

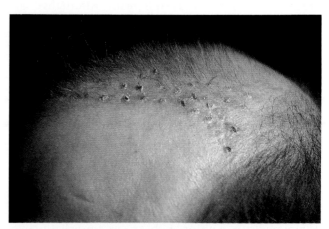

Most hair-restoring medications yield modest results. Surgery is available, but it is expensive and the results may not be any better in the long run. Could you learn to live with baldness?

one-third of its users; fuzz for a third; and no hair at all for the other one-third.[9]

Acquiring a new head of hair is expensive. Approximately $1,000 per year is the charge for topically applied solutions and scalp patch transplants may cost as much as $15,000 and take a year or two to complete. **Scalp reduction** is a technique that reduces the amount of new hair a patient needs by cutting out a strip of skin from the bald area and sewing the edges of the scalp together to move the hair on the sides of the head closer to the top. The technique costs from $1,500 to $2,000. Transplants and scalp reduction carry some risks of infection and produce pain, swelling, inflammation, and temporary numbness. Finding a surgeon who is capable of producing adequate results in a safe manner is not easy. Some surgeons use questionable techniques and the results are often disappointing.

Dandruff Even in its healthiest condition, the scalp exhibits a mild degree of scaling. The sebaceous glands add oil secretions *(sebum)* to the dead skin scales to form **dandruff.** Dandruff is a scalp problem, not a hair problem, and is not nearly as widespread or serious as advertisements portray. Now that most people wash their hair almost daily, flakes are washed away before they fall. There is nothing wrong with washing one's hair daily, or as often as you want. Most inexpensive shampoos contain adequate cleaning and conditioning ingredients.

Antidandruff shampoos are considered a drug, rather than a cosmetic, by the Food and Drug Administration. The exact cause of excessive flaking is unknown and it is doubtful that germs are the cause as indicated by some advertisers. Severe dandruff can be controlled, not cured, through use of one of the five ingredients in the over-the-counter dandruff shampoos deemed safe and effective by the FDA: coal-tar preparations (Denorex and Tegrin), salicylic acid (P & S, S-Seb), selenium sulfide (Selsun), zinc pyrithione (Head and Shoulders, Sebulin, Zincon), and sulfur preparations (Sebulex, Vanseb). Dandruff imposes no medical consequence although severe flaking can be a sign of a disease, such as seborrheic, dermatitis, and psoriasis, which may require special treatment by a physician.

Products for Teeth and Eyes

Mouthwashes and Gargles Although mouthwashes may taste good, there is no evidence that they are any more effective in treating a sore throat or eliminating bad breath than pure water. In fact, continuous use of mouthwash can actually cause excessive drying of the mucous membranes of the oral cavity.

Unpleasant mouth odor, produced from eating garlic or onions or from smoking, does not originate in the mouth. The aroma is carried from the intestines to the lungs and expired into the air. Very little odor exists in particles that remain in the mouth and teeth. Therefore, gargling has little effect other than to mask the unpleasant odor with a pleasant smell, such as mint. It is not possible to absorb the odor, in spite of what the ads for some products claim.

To limit the bad morning taste and reduce mouth odor by 75 percent, brush your teeth thoroughly before going to bed and upon waking, and brush both your teeth and your tongue after each meal.

Toothpastes and Tooth Decay Although about one-third of all tooth decay has been eliminated, it is still a serious problem in the United States. Bacteria are present in the mouth and on the teeth at all times waiting to grab onto fermentable carbohydrate (practically all the food we eat, not just sugar). When this happens the pH in the mouth is lowered and the tooth enamel may dissolve, causing cavities (bacteria + fermentable carbohydrate over time = cavities). Even Aspartame, present in NutraSweet, is unsafe for the teeth. Since Aspartame is 250 times sweeter than one teaspoon of sugar and since it is difficult to market an item as small as 1/250 of a teaspoon, fermentable carbohydrates are added to each pack of Aspartame.

Upon rising in the morning the pH in the mouth is neutral (7). After eating, pH drops below 4 or 3 for thirty to ninety minutes, creating the right climate for a "plaque" or acid attack on the enamel, particularly in the secluded areas between the teeth. These acid attacks occur a number of times daily depending upon how often one snacks. Some experts feel that raising the pH in the mouth is one way to help prevent tooth decay. Flossing the teeth after eating, brushing the teeth with toothpaste containing baking soda, chewing Trident chewing gum, and eating certain foods, such as cheddar, gouda, brie, blue, and swiss cheese, will raise the pH in the mouth. If you live in an area with fluoridated water, brushing your teeth with water or baking soda will give the same or better results as other toothpastes, providing you brush properly and use dental floss. Otherwise, choose a fluoride toothpaste or ask your dentist for a fluoride treatment. Do not spend money on toothpaste products that guarantee "whiteness." These have abrasives that can cause excessive wear on the teeth.

Eye Washes The most effective way to remove irritating material from the eye is through natural tears. Frequent use of eye drops may delay early diagnosis of a serious disorder, such as glaucoma, which causes 15 percent of all blindness.

Eye discomfort can result from visual problems, eye fatigue, bacteria and viruses, or allergic sensitivity to dust or pollens. If symptoms persist for more than two or three days, consult a physician. For relief of simple eye irritation, apply iced, wet compresses for fifteen minutes or place several drops of cold water in the lower lid with an eye dropper. If eye irritation continues, consult your physician or ophthalmologist.

Nutrition and the Consumer

We have emphasized throughout this book that proper nutrition plays an extremely important role in good health. Chapter 7 was devoted to nutrition exclusively, but we believe it is important to discuss several consumer-related nutrition topics here. These include food poisoning, product labeling, and seals of approval.

Minimizing the Risks of Food Poisoning

Practically any food, perishable or nonperishable, carries the potential for food poisoning. For food to transmit disease, it must contain a disease-producing agent (bacteria, toxin-forming mold, virus) or be contaminated through handling, and it must be consumed in sufficient quantity to cause symptoms.

Highly vulnerable food items, such as poultry, require special care. Some studies indicate that approximately 35 to 50 percent, or as high as one in two uncooked chickens and turkeys, contain salmonella. Even if inspectors could identify bacteria-laden meat, the problem could not be solved. Almost half of all chickens in the United States, for example, would have to be destroyed. Unpasteurized milk, cracked eggs, and undercooked fish are additional sources of salmonella. Although 56,500 cases of salmonella and campylobacter infection are reported annually, the Centers for Disease Control in Atlanta, Georgia, estimate that over 4 million people are affected by these bacteria each year. In addition, the number of reported cases is increasing dramatically. During Thanksgiving and Christmas, the risk increases considerably. Unfortunately, meat, poultry, or fish contaminated with these bacteria do not look or smell bad. It also takes about 12 hours after eating contaminated food to develop the symptoms of diarrhea, nausea, stomach cramps, and fever. Most people think they are developing influenza. Critics indicate that the federal government and the meat and poultry industries have done very little to prevent the spread of salmonella and campylobacter bacteria. High-speed assembly lines spread microorganisms by bringing clean carcasses into contact with contaminated surfaces; animals are raised in such close quarters that bacteria pass freely from one to another; little testing takes place for harmful hormones, pesticides or chemical residues of any kind; no inspection exists for domestically harvested fish; little funding is available to improve tests for bacterial contamination; and the government does not require meat labels that could tell consumers how to avoid getting sick from the bacteria.[10]

Fortunately, there is much the consumer can do to reduce the risk of contamination and even eliminate the problem. Wise shopping, proper cooking, and proper storage offers the best protection. Consider these suggestions:

Shopping

- Examine each shopping item to detect signs of spoilage, such as a torn package, an imperfect seal, or a bulging can. Avoid any package that is not tightly wrapped or contains tears.

- Be certain to examine the expiration date, the "sell by" or "best-if-used-by" date, and avoid outdated items.
- Avoid buying food stored above the "frost line" of supermarket freezer or refrigerator display cases.
- Avoid purchasing perishable products, such as milk, meat, or desserts, that are not adequately refrigerated. Purchase perishable foods in small quantities.
- Transport food immediately from the store to your home; never leave groceries in a hot car, where disease-producing bacteria can multiply. Make the grocery store your last stop before returning home.

Storing

- Read labels at home for special storing instructions.
- Avoid storing food in a cabinet with a drainpipe, such as under the kitchen sink.
- Avoid leaving leftover food on the table after a meal while you socialize; store it in the refrigerator immediately.
- Keep poultry and other meat frozen or refrigerated.
- Thaw meat only in the refrigerator.
- Never refreeze items unless the ice crystals are present in the meat; otherwise, cook immediately.
- Store meat in the coldest part of the refrigerator; never keep uncooked meat at room temperature for more than two hours.
- Devise a system to identify the time of storage, and use older items first.
- Learn the approximate amount of time the food can be safely stored, such as the following times for turkey and other poultry:

In Freezer—Frozen

Frozen turkey parts	6 months
Whole turkey	12 months
Turkey deli products	1–2 months
Leftover cooked turkey	4 months

In Refrigerator—40°F

Fresh turkey in original wrapping	1–2 days
Large turkey parts	3–4 days
Leftover cooked turkey	1–2 days

Preparation and Cooking

- Examine foods carefully before cooking. Avoid tasting any food that appears spoiled; use odor or appearance as your guide, discarding anything that is suspect.
- Keep hot foods hot (140°F or above) and cold foods cold (40°F or below); avoid partially cooking meat; always finish the cooking once it is started.
- Discard any perishable food that was not refrigerated.
- Avoid using the same knife to cut uncooked meats and other foods; contamination can be transmitted from one food to the other.
- Wash all items thoroughly that were used for thawing, storage, preparation, and serving, including dishcloths, sponges, cutting surfaces, knives, pans, and thermometers.
- Wash your hands before and after serving food, and after diapering a baby or using the bathroom.
- Use hard plastic or acrylic cutting boards instead of wooden surfaces.
- Use a clean plate for serving items once they are cooked.
- Cook pork, stuffed turkey, and other meats until the inner part reaches a temperature of 165°F to kill infectious microorganisms; use a thermometer to determine when this temperature is reached.
- Stuff turkey immediately before cooking, or cook stuffing in a separate dish.
- Remove stuffing from turkey immediately after cooking. Place uneaten portions in a separate container before storing in the refrigerator.
- Reheat leftovers thoroughly to at least 165°F; boil leftover gravy for at least one minute before serving.
- Serve cooked foods as soon as possible.

Product Labeling

The information on food products is your guide to wise food purchasing. It helps you choose foods low in sodium, saturated fat, and sugar; high in fiber; and with the proper vitamins, minerals, and number of calories. In addition, the U.S. Recommended Daily Allowances (RDAs) allow you to compare the nutritive value and relative costs of different foods.

Any food label providing nutrition information must include:

- Net contents—number and size of servings per container (weight, fluid measure, or numerical count).
- Ingredients—listed by common name in order of the largest percentage; for example, if sugar is listed first, the primary ingredient is sugar; number of calories, amount of protein, carbohydrates, fat, and sodium (in grams) per serving, amounts of eight nutrients (protein, vitamin A, thiamin, riboflavin, niacin, vitamin C, calcium, and iron) in one serving expressed as a percentage of U.S. RDAs.

For a thorough discussion on food labeling, see Chapter 7.

Seals of Approval

Approximately ten new seals of approval that are bestowed by nonprofit or trade groups have appeared on the market recently, joining old mainstays such as the Good Housekeeping seal and Underwriters Laboratories seal. Although a product with a seal of approval is in general deserving of it, it is difficult for consumers to know the underlying ground rules for "approval" in the first place. Products without a seal may not be inferior, only indicative of a manufacturer who did not want to pay a five-figure fee. Examples of the new breed of seals include Green Cross (identifies recycling or biodegradability of products), American College of Nutrition (identifies cooking oils low in saturated fat), and NutriClean (certifies the absence of detected pesticide residues on fruits and vegetables). The use of seals of approval in combination with careful reading of product labels offers additional guidance to consumers in a wide variety of areas.

Protecting the Consumer: Your Advocates

Federal Agencies

The Food and Drug Administration Approximately 4,500 employees of the Food and Drug Administration (FDA) are faced with the nearly impossible task of surveying thousands of food, drug, and cosmetic companies in the United States. This organization operates in four main areas.

1. The Bureau of Drugs verifies the safety and effectiveness of all drugs. Companies must submit information on new drugs for investigation before they can be used in human tests.
2. The Bureau of Foods and Pesticides attempts to assure safe, pure, and wholesome foods. Food

plants are inspected, ingredients of food products are examined, and packaging and labeling are checked. Safe levels for chemical food additives, such as preservatives, flavoring, and coloring, are established.

3. The Bureau of Veterinary Medicine enforces similar requirements for veterinary drugs and devices for optimum animal health and safety.

4. The Office of Product Safety enforces the Federal Hazardous Substances Act to protect the public from accidents involving chemicals.

The Federal Trade Commission The Federal Trade Commission (FTC) is required by law to keep competition free and fair. Key areas of concern for the

Get Involved!

Preventive Health Care and the Consumer

There is much you can do to keep yourself healthy and to save on medical costs. The first step involves accepting full responsibility for your own health. Such a responsibility requires some understanding of the human body and a basic knowledge about and a few skills in determining normal and abnormal symptoms. In addition, consumer awareness is necessary to help you work through the often inaccurate claims of numerous manufacturers about their products.

1. An effective self-care program requires some organization and planning. Unless you take the time to identify the recommended time periods for regular physical examinations and specific checkups and record these dates on a calendar, it is unlikely that you will secure proper preventive care. An annual schedule that includes appointments with your physician and a reminder of periodic self-examination dates, and the results of previous visits and examinations, is a valuable self-care tool.

2. It is also important to form the habit of questioning all claims of manufacturers about their products and to evaluate these claims against your basic understanding of the human body and against the independent research on the product. One must avoid "jumping on the bandwagon" with new products until independent testing indicates effectiveness and safety.

3. You can also protect your health and that of your family by maintaining a safe, practical home medicine cabinet, purchasing appropriate home medical tests, and following sound nutritional principles in relation to food purchasing, storage, preparation, and cooking.

4. Another effective technique of self-care involves practice. It is helpful to review and study the literature on first aid and CPR procedures, for example, and to safely practice on friends and family members the various rescue techniques for choking and stopped breathing. Practice is also necessary in the areas of blood pressure measurement, pulse rate measurement, throat examination, eye examination, and in the monitoring of other body functions if these techniques are to be performed accurately.

5. You can also use a number of approaches to get actively involved in the preventive health care of others. For example, constructively confront your classmates, friends, and relatives about their use of questionable products. Explain the limitations and dangers of these products and suggest a more sound approach. Letter writing to complain about the false advertisement of a health product is another effective method for consumers. You can voice your concern to the appropriate government or private agency. These groups rely on consumers to help them identify problem areas in health care.

6. Seniors are particularly vulnerable to misinformation designed to entice spending on unneeded and often dangerous health products. Plan to visit and speak with older people in an attempt to identify questionable products and practices. Pay close attention to unsound advertisements that target seniors. Identify three or four problem products or practices and initiate a letter-writing campaign with your classmates.

A Question of Ethics

Should Food Labeling Be Completely Standardized and Strictly Controlled?

Food manufacturers have learned to play the health game. Clever packaging and careful labeling can fool many customers into believing that they are purchasing a health product. Sugar, for example, is listed under many aliases such as corn syrup, corn sweeteners, maple syrup, fructose, dextrose, sucrose, and honey. Some products list three or more different types of sugars. Although no sugar is listed first, the combined total may be greater than any single ingredient. Fat and oil can also be disguised with terms such as salad, vegetable, safflower, corn, coconut, peanut, olive, shortening, and butter, to hide from the consumer the fact that these products are almost pure fat and contain 9 calories per gram or 45 calories per teaspoon. Portions of foods are often redefined to increase the apparent nutrition of a product. The phrase "no preservatives" may be highlighted when other chemical additives are present that the consumer may wish to avoid. Deceptive phrasing is used to imply nutritional benefits when the product contains only slight amounts of the touted ingredient.

There is some evidence to indicate that food manufacturers may be taking advantage of America's preoccupation with diets to avoid heart disease. Since cholesterol isn't a food ingredient, regulations regarding labels are loose, and only food products claiming to be low cholesterol are required to list it on the nutrition part of the label. Some products indicating "no cholesterol" may still be poor choices since saturated fats such as coconut and palm oils, hydrogenated fats, or shortening may have no cholesterol but can raise cholesterol levels in the blood. Even the use of the word "lite" is deceiving. A lite corn chip, for example, is only one single calorie per chip less than the regular chip. These and other examples of deception argue strongly for more regulation and control of food products by the FDA. Only the very informed consumer, it is argued, can decode the label to avoid these pitfalls, and then, only if they have the time to do so. Also, labels are almost meaningless to anyone who has trouble with numbers.

Opponents of strict control point out that the consumer will always have to worry about deception from advertisers, regardless of the product. In fact, it is consumer's responsibility to become well informed and to make wise nutrition decisions for themselves and their family. Even if stricter regulation were necessary, it is argued, the task is not feasible, and it may actually be impossible to impose and enforce strict regulations in the United States.

What do you think?

---

consumer are the Fair Packaging and Labeling Act, The Trademark Act, the Truth in Lending Act, and the Fair Credit Report Act. The majority of violations are *misrepresentation* and *mislabeling* of products. The FTC will initiate action against a violator if the product is not what the label states or implies. You can file a confidential complaint with the FTC by explaining the facts in a letter and enclosing as much supporting evidence as possible. The FTC will initiate an investigation and take action, forcing the violator to discontinue the practice through an informal settlement or a formal complaint in court. Fines, imprisonment, or seizure of the product may follow.

Consumer Product Safety Commission   The Consumer Product Safety Act of 1972 led to the formation of the Consumer Product Safety Commission. This act was designed to protect the public against unreasonable risks of injury associated with consumer products, help consumers evaluate the safety of products, develop uniform safety standards for consumer products, and promote research on the causes and prevention of product-related deaths. The main goal of the commission is to reduce the more than 20 million annual injuries associated with consumer products by is-

suing and enforcing safety standards for more than ten thousand products. The Flammable Fabrics Act, the Federal Hazardous Substances Act, the Poison Prevention Packaging Act, and the Refrigerator Door Safety Act are also the responsibility of the commission.

U.S. Postal Service   The U.S. Postal Service is responsible for protecting the health and well-being of the nation by investigating mail fraud and attempts to sell harmful or worthless merchandise or medicines through the mail and by protecting the consumer from harassment, pornography, and some types of junk mail. Responsibility for initiating a complaint rests with the consumer. The Postal Service can only take a case to court with the evidence and witnesses you supply.

Private Agencies

Better Business Bureau   The Better Business Bureau in your community is a private, nonprofit corporation supported by private business. It assists you by mediating misunderstandings between consumers and businesses, investigating advertising misinformation and questionable activity, and supplying factual information on thousands of businesses in the United States. You can call your local office for the leaflet entitled "What Is a Better Business Bureau?" which describes the services provided.

Chamber of Commerce

Your local Chamber of Commerce also acts as a liaison between the business community and the consumer and is supported by businesses within your community. The Chamber of Commerce functions similarly to the Better Business Bureau and performs most of its work at the local level.

Medical, Dental, and Other Agencies

Other independent agencies that serve as watchdogs for the consumer include the State Medical Association and the State Dental Association (dental and medical ethics), the Legal Aid Society and the Legal Services Organization (advice on consumer problems and legal representation for those with limited income), the State Bar Association (advice and literature on common legal problems), the State Nursing Home Association (standards of care and services), the State Pharmaceutical Association (druggists, drugs, and prescriptions), the State Department of Mental Health (care and services), and the State Retail Council (liaison between retailers and consumers).

FIGURE 19.3 • Judging Health Care Products Advertising

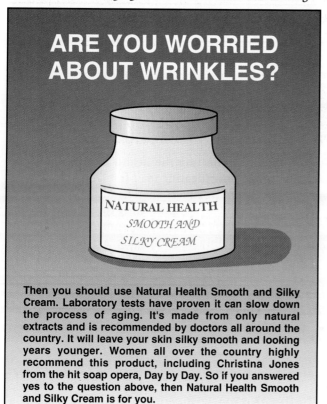

ARE YOU WORRIED ABOUT WRINKLES?

NATURAL HEALTH
SMOOTH AND
SILKY CREAM

Then you should use Natural Health Smooth and Silky Cream. Laboratory tests have proven it can slow down the process of aging. It's made from only natural extracts and is recommended by doctors all around the country. It will leave your skin silky smooth and looking years younger. Women all over the country highly recommend this product, including Christina Jones from the hit soap opera, Day by Day. So if you answered yes to the question above, then Natural Health Smooth and Silky Cream is for you.

• Is the product objectively presented without appealing to basic human needs, such as fear, love, and security? If not, you should be skeptical.

• If research findings are cited, was the research done by health scientists (not independent laboratories, which may need to show favorable results to stay in business) and published in a recognized medical journal?

• Does the commercial make unsupported claims?

• Does the advertiser use endorsements from individuals who are not scientists? Such endorsements indicate only that the company has enough money to hire a celebrity to read a script.

• Are the findings consistent? Have other investigators in other areas found the same thing?

• Is unclear information used, such as "Hospital tests showed . . . ," "Doctors recommend . . . ," or "A major study revealed . . . ," without the hospital, doctors, or study being identified?

Learning to Judge Advertising

Advertisers spend a great deal of time and money analyzing the American people. They know what motivates different people to try different products. They know what words and pictures will sell a product. You are at the mercy of the advertisers unless you learn to judge commercials and advertisements. Here are some questions to keep in mind:

- Is the product objectively presented without appealing to basic human needs, such as fear, love, and security? If not, you should be skeptical.
- If research findings are cited, was the research done by health scientists (not independent testing laboratories, which may need to show favorable results to stay in business) and published in a recognized medical journal?
- Does the commercial make unsupported claims?
- Does the advertiser use endorsements from individuals who are not scientists? Such endorsements indicate only that the company has enough money to hire a celebrity to read a script.
- Are the findings consistent? Have other investigators in other areas found the same thing?
- Is unclear information used, such as "Hospital tests showed . . . ," "Doctors recommend . . . ," or "A major study revealed . . . ," without the hospital, doctors, or study being identified?

Probably your best protection is not to buy health-related products you see advertised in magazines or on television unless you first check with your doctor or pharmacist. They can tell you whether the product has any benefit.

Conclusion

Quackery is ever-present in the United States in the treatment of illnesses and the sale of consumer products. A rather gullible public willing to spend billions of dollars on quick, easy approaches to practically anything guarantees its existence. False advertising in all forms of media remains a strong obstacle to the elimination of quackery. Fortunately, the public is slowly becoming wiser. Consumers are beginning to ask for hard evidence and to question the value of products and claims by advertisers. The FDA and other government agencies are also increasing their scrutiny of consumer products and advertising claims. The fact remains, however, that many over-the-counter medicines, cosmetics, special foods, and gadgets are a worthless waste of hard-earned money. Some are even hazardous to health. When in doubt about any product capable of affecting your health, it is wise to consult a physician before initiating any home treatment.

Summary

1. Each individual is responsible for maintaining his or her good health and for detecting and treating minor illnesses and injuries. To provide proper self-care, people need to learn more about their bodies, monitor bodily functions regularly, and use regular physician- and self-screening techniques.

2. Contact lens users must follow recommended habits of use and hygiene very carefully to avoid infections and eye damage.

3. Self-medication is an important part of self-care. Over-the-counter drugs must be carefully selected and used to treat minor illnesses and injuries, not to cure serious disease. If the symptoms of an illness persist, a physician should be consulted.

4. The proper use of reliable home medical tests can help reduce medical costs and improve both the diagnosis and the management of various health conditions.

5. There are two basic approaches to the control of quackery: legal and educational. Both approaches are the responsibility of the consumer.

6. The quack has existed for millennia and will continue to prey on the unwise consumer. Mail-order quackery relies on unfounded claims, indirect suggestion of cures, remedies, and rejuvenation, and the consumer's attraction to fast, easy solutions to complicated health problems.

7. Nonprescription medicines are not meant to—and do not—cure disease. They should be used only for temporary relief of minor symptoms. Improper use of over-the-counter drugs may aggravate symptoms or mask a condition needing physician attention.

8. To save money, ask your physician and druggist to provide you with the least expensive generic-name drug (refers to the chemical ingredient in the drug) or brand-name product.

9. Your best protection against false claims and improper use of all over-the-counter drugs is a careful study of labels.

10. Several products are on the market that result in new scalp hair growth for some, but not all, users.

11. The possibility exists for considerable deception in food labeling. Study the label carefully before making your decision.

12. The risk of food poisoning can be greatly reduced by wise purchasing, storing, and cooking practices. Your best guide to wise purchasing (cost and nutritive value) is the food label. Choose foods low in sodium, fat, and sugar; high in fiber; and with the proper vitamins, minerals, and calories.

13. More than 20 million injuries each year are associated with consumer products. Federal agencies, such as the Food and Drug Administration, the Federal Trade Commission, the Consumer Product Safety Commission, and the U.S. Postal Service, rely on the consumer to provide valuable testimony on the dangers of such products and to work with them to prosecute or remove the product from the market. Other agencies, such as the Better Business Bureau, Chamber of Commerce, and State Medical and Dental Associations, advise consumers on health-related goods and services.

14. Wise consumerism also carries the responsibility of learning to evaluate and judge advertising claims before making the decision to purchase a health-related product.

Questions for Personal Growth

1. As one of the first steps in developing a sound self-care program, it is necessary to develop a reliable record-keeping system. Secure a calendar you can use specifically for health records. Record the health examinations you have had in the past twelve months. Now, refer to the guidelines on medical checkups provided in this chapter and schedule yourself for the appropriate month three years in advance. What type of system can you establish to record all self-examination results, including the date, the findings, and the dates of needed checkups? Can you identify any hereditary tendencies that may merit more frequent checkups than is usually recommended?

2. What key medical tests should you administer on a regular basis? After you identify these tests, establish a schedule for regular self-testing and plan to record your results in the calendar established with the previous guidelines.

3. What products does your home medicine cabinet contain? Are these products safe? Outdated? Reorganize your medicine cabinet according to the recommendations provided in this chapter, discarding outdated items safely.

4. Try to recall the last time you or a member of your family was ill. How did you assess the situation? Did you administer the appropriate self-tests that helped communicate the problem to the physician? What could you have done differently?

5. Study the labels on home products dealing with the hair (hair removal, hair coloring, and hair restoration). Study the labels on deodorants and antiperspirants, eye washes, toothpastes, and other products. Evaluate the claims. Are you a victim of shrewd advertising? Do these products really do what they say they do? Which products should be eliminated or replaced?

6. Observe carefully the next time someone prepares a meal in your presence. Pay close attention to storage, food preparation, and cooking techniques. What practices were used that impose a potential health risk? What assistance could you provide to reduce the risk of food poisoning?

7. The presence of some form of quackery is evident in most households. What signs do you see in your dormitory or house in areas such as nutrition, cosmetic products, over-the-counter medications, hair care, sleep disorders, and so forth? What advice can you provide to the users of these products that may elicit a change in purchasing behavior?

References

1. "Joint Committee on Detection, Evaluation, and Treatment of High Blood Pressure" NIH Publication No. 84–1088, U.S. Department of Health and Human Services (1984).

2. Robin M. Henig, "Vision and Vanity," *Washington Post* (July 21, 1987).

3. Department of Health and Human Services, Public Health Service, Food and Drug Administration, FDA *Consumer* (1989).

4. David Zimmerman, "Drug Interactions You Should Know About," *Ladies Home Journal* (August 1985): 47–48.

5. James M. Corry, *Consumer Health: Facts, Skills, and Decisions* (Belmont, Calif: Wadsworth, 1983).

6. Consumers Union, *The New Medicine Show: Con-sumers Union's Practical Guide to Some Everyday Health Problems and Health Products* (Mount Vernon, N.Y.: Consumers Union, 1989), pp. 167–174.

7. *Skin Wellness: A Program for a Lifetime of Healthy Skin* (Dallas, Tex.: Mary Kay Cosmetics, 1989).

8. "Fade Creams," *Consumer Reports* (January 1985): 12.

9. Consumers Union, *The New Medicine Show: Consumers Union's Practical Guide to Some Everyday Health Problems and Health Products.*

10. U.S. Department of Agriculture, Food Safety and Inspection Services, "A Margin of Safety: The HACCP Approach to Food Safety Education" (March 1990).

CHAPTER

20

Choosing Medical Service and Health Insurance

CHAPTER OBJECTIVES

After reading this chapter, you should understand:

- How to select your physician and dentist, what types of physicians are available, how to talk to your physician, and how to select a hospital.

- Several alternative approaches to various aspects of health care, including acupuncture and chiropractic.

- Why it is so important to have health insurance, the various kinds of insurance providers and insurance plans that are available, and how to evaluate health insurance policies before you buy.

- How the spiraling cost of health care and increasing numbers of malpractice suits against health care providers have created a very difficult situation in the United States.

CHAPTER OUTLINE

Making Medical Care Work for You

Alternative Approaches to Health Care

Health Insurance

Problems with the Health Care System

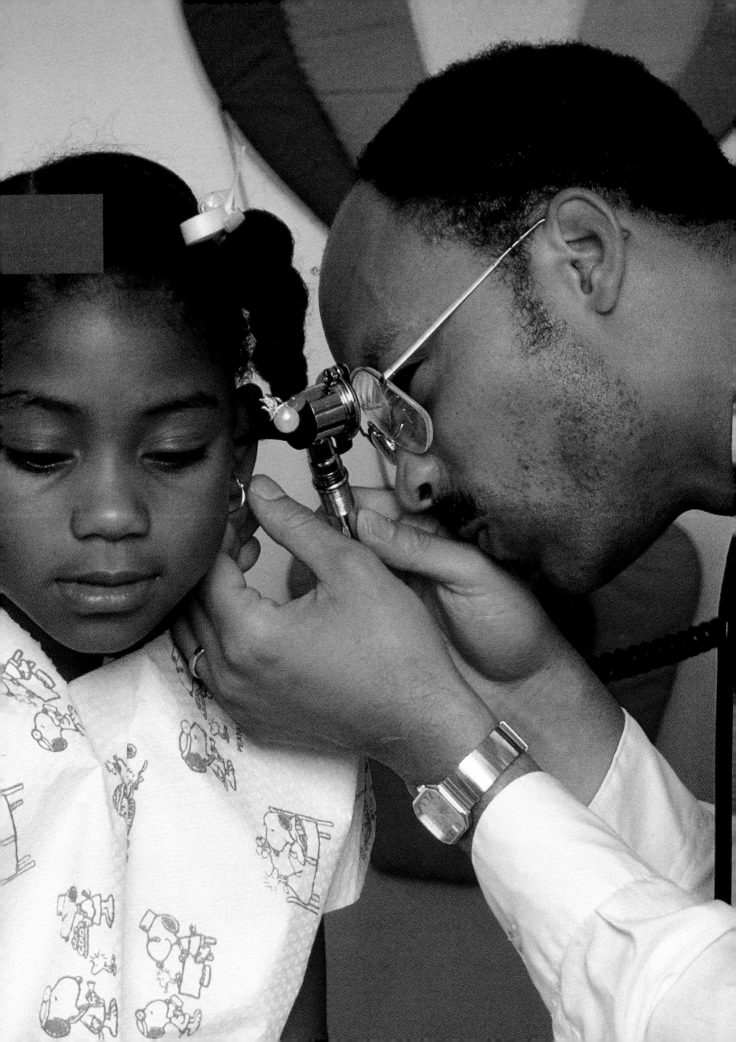

primary care physician A physician who serves as the patient's first and regular contact with medical treatment; these doctors are usually specialists in family medicine or in internal medicine.

teaching hospitals Hospitals that are associated with medical schools and serve as on-the-job training centers for doctors and nurses; the hospital staff serves as the faculty, the students are medical students, interns, residents, and student nurses.

group practice Three or more physicians working together in their various specialties.

America is currently experiencing a health care crisis. Although the United States is among the most modern, technically advanced countries in the world in medical science, the health services available to some Americans are inadequate. In addition, for a substantial portion of the population, medical care is a tremendous burden on the family budget. Medical care costs continue to rise at a much faster rate than the cost of living and at a greater rate than the average take-home pay increases of blue- and white-collar workers. We are also facing a health care crisis in terms of personnel. At present, approximately 98 percent of physicians specialize, and only 2 percent have a general practice with initial patient contact and diagnosis.

In view of this situation, securing and paying for high-quality medical care require careful planning. Each individual or family needs to know how to choose a health plan and a physician and how to monitor his or her health or the health of family members. This chapter offers some guidelines for choosing appropriate medical services.

Making Medical Care Work for You

Selecting a Physician and Dentist

Practically everyone needs a **primary care physician,** or family medicine physician, as the specialty is called, and a family dentist. Your family physician will refer you to the appropriate specialist, should the need arise. If you belong to a health maintenance organization (HMO), you must choose a doctor in that program. One method of locating a physician is to ask local relatives and friends about their physician's expertise and commitment to the patient.

Another method is to locate a medical school and its hospital affiliates in your area. Call the school and ask for a list of staff physicians. You may also secure valuable suggestions by phoning the resident on call at the local emergency room. First-year residents have had an opportunity to evaluate doctors in various situations and will generally be happy to suggest names. Keep in mind that **teaching hospitals** (those associated with a medical school) generally have the most advanced care and facilities; patients of doctors at these hospitals tend to receive considerable attention from the medical personnel.

The county medical society will also provide you with a list of physicians and information on medical schools, residency programs, and physicians' board certifications. Similar procedures can be used to locate a dentist.

After making your choice, call the doctor's office to ascertain that new patients are being accepted and to check on office hours, fees, and other information. It is also helpful to inquire about the physician's approach to preventive medicine (regular examinations, consultations, and vaccinations). Avoid making your final decision until after your first or second visit. If you sense a communication problem or notice questionable practices, continue your search.

A wise choice for family care is often a well-established **group practice,** in which three or more physicians work together in their various specialties. Records on patients are available to each physician, on-the-spot consultation is provided, and a physician who knows your health history is always available or on call nights and weekends. In addition, physicians pool their economic resources to purchase expensive equipment and hire auxiliary health staff, and can therefore offer reduced fees.

Types of Physicians

The five clinical specialties are internal medicine, surgery, pediatrics, obstetrics and gynecology, and psychiatry. There are other specialties; however, the patient rarely goes directly to physicians in such fields without a recommendation from the family doctor. Table 20.1 lists common specialists and their treatment areas.

You need to decide whether the family physician should handle the health of the entire family. A pediatrician may be desirable for children of both sexes, a gynecologist for girls over the age of twelve or thirteen. Most people need a primary care (family) physician who handles the majority of the family health problems, including referral to an appropriate specialist when necessary.

TABLE 20.1

Specialists and Areas of Treatment

Medical Specialist	Area of Specialty Treatment	Medical Specialist	Area of Specialty Treatment
Allergist	Body reactions and hypersensitivity to drugs, pollens, food, and animals.	Otolaryngologist	Diseases of the ear and larynx
		Otologist	Diseases of the ear
Anesthesiologist	Anesthesia, maintenance of vital functions during surgery and trauma	Pediatrician	Diseases in children
		Plastic surgeon	Correction of deformed or damaged external body parts
Cardiologist	Heart disease	Proctologist	Diseases of the colon, rectum, and anus
Dermatologist	Skin disease		
Endocrinologist	Internal secretions of the ductless glands	Psychiatrist	Mental and personality disorders
Family physician	Preventive medicine for the family	Radiologist	Diagnostic and therapeutic use of radiant energy
Gastroenterologist	Diseases of the digestive system	Rhinologist	Disorders of the nose
Gerontologist	Diseases and changes in old age	Urologist	Diseases of the genitourinary tract
Hematologist	Diseases of the blood and blood-forming tissues	Endodontist	Diseases of the nerve of a tooth
Internist	Illnesses of a nonsurgical nature in adults	Orthodontist	Correction and prevention of teeth irregularities and malocclusion of the jaw
Neurologist	Diseases of the nervous system		
Obstetrician	Care during pregnancy and childbirth	Pedodontist	Dental ailments in children
Ophthalmologist	Refractive errors of the eye	Periodontist	Gums and supporting tissue of the teeth
Orthopedist	Diseases of joints, bones, and spine	Prosthodontist	Construction of dentures, bridges, and crowns

Nonmedical Specialistc	Area of Specialty Treatment	Nonmedical Specialist	Area of Specialty Treatment
Optician	Grinds and sets lenses to the prescription of an oculist	Podiatrist	Treats diseases, defects, injuries of the foot
		Psychologist	Applies scientific methods to the study of human behavior
Optometrist	Measures visual acuity, prescribes glasses		
Orthoptist	Corrects defects through eye exercises		

How to Talk to Your Doctor

Your doctor will first want to know the main reason you scheduled your visit—your primary complaint, specific symptoms (temperature, blood pressure, heart rate, swelling, redness, type of pain, and so forth), medications taken, and the kinds of physical activity you are still participating in. Your doctor will also need information about previous illnesses, surgery, and treatment, as well as allergies and reactions to medication. During the physical examination, you should help the doctor by pointing out pains, lumps, growths, or previous injuries that occasionally cause pain, discomfort, or concern. During the initial examination, your doctor is trying to learn as much about your body as possible to aid diagnosis and treatment.

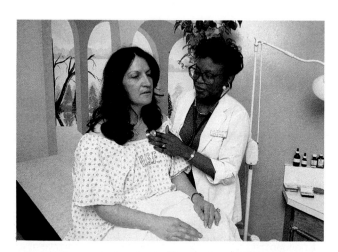
For some individuals, the family physician is the only medical contact.

specific conditions or diseases, generally for long periods.

Hospitals are also classified according to financing: voluntary, government, and private. Voluntary hospitals are public, nonprofit hospitals managed by philanthropic institutions or individuals. Financial assistance is often provided by local groups and the federal government. Government hospitals are supported by federal, state, county, or city government and are generally equipped to handle long-term illnesses. Care is provided for military and Public Health Service personnel and families and for American Indians, veterans, and merchant seamen. Private hospitals are owned by individuals or corporations with the intention of making a profit. Consequently, these hospitals are often smaller, less well equipped, understaffed,

It is up to you, the patient, to be direct and assertive, asking any question that occurs to you, no matter how trivial it may seem. Will this drug have side effects? What are they? When should I check back? How soon can I expect these symptoms to disappear? Should I go to work or school? Unless you ask, the doctor may not volunteer this information. To avoid forgetting important concerns, write them down before your visit and bring the list with you. Anything that concerns you is a fair question. Don't be hurried or permit the doctor to brush you off to rush to the next patient. Do not leave the office until you are satisfied that the doctor has answered your questions. If you are hurried, treated like a child, or cannot secure direct answers about your condition, change doctors.

Selecting a Hospital

Those who are fortunate enough to live in an area with more than one hospital have an opportunity to select the one best suited to their needs. Hospitals vary tremendously in terms of available equipment, competency of physicians and other personnel, ability to administer sophisticated tests, treatment, and surgery. General medical and surgical hospitals diagnose and treat a wide variety of health conditions, generally for short periods. Specialty hospitals admit patients with

Year 2000 National Health Objective

Several national health objectives have been established in recognition of the critical role of the primary care provider: (1) to increase to at least 50 percent the proportion of primary care providers who routinely assess and counsel their patients regarding the frequency, duration, type, and intensity of each patient's physical activity practices; (2) to increase to at least 75 percent the proportion of primary care providers who routinely counsel patients about tobacco use cessation, diet modification, and cancer-screening recommendations (approximately 52 percent of internists counseled over 75 percent of their smoking patients in 1986); (3) to increase to at least 40 percent the proportion of people age 50 and older who receive oral, skin, and digital rectal examinations during an office visit (in 1987, only 27 percent had received a digital rectal exam within the preceding year); (4) to increase to at least 75 percent the proportion of primary care providers who initiate a diet, and, if necessary, drug therapy at levels of blood cholesterol consistent with management guidelines for patients with high cholesterol; (5) to increase to at least 75 percent the proportion of primary care providers who provide nutrition assessment, counseling, and referral to a qualified nutritionist or dietitian (an estimated 50 percent met this objective in 1988).

Exploring Your Health 20.1

Your Last Physical Exam

Think about your last physical examination. How long ago was it? The areas listed below represent the major aspects recommended for a complete examination. What key areas were neglected? Do you have any symptoms that suggest a need for consultation in any area? How thorough was your physician? Did your consultation include suggestions for changes in lifestyle (exercise, smoking, eating, sleeping habits)?

_____ 1. Complete medical history, including chief complaints and present illnesses.

_____ 2. Review of health habits (eating, sleeping, exercise, smoking, anxieties).

_____ 3. Exercise EKG or stress test.

_____ 4. Exercise evaluation—body fat (skinfold measures), abdominal strength, aerobic capacity (from known 1.5-mile run, 2-mile time, Cooper's 12-minute test, or Master's Step Test administered in the office).

_____ 5. Heart disease risk profile.

_____ 6. Pulse, respiration, and blood pressure.

_____ 7. Blood work—including cholesterol and triglycerides.

_____ 8. Rectal examination.

_____ 9. Skin inspection.

_____ 10. Ear, nose, and throat.

_____ 11. Lymph nodes.

_____ 12. Chest x-ray or skin test for tuberculosis.

_____ 13. For women, Pap smear, breast and reproductive system examination.

_____ 14. For men, examination of genitalia.

_____ 15. Test for glaucoma (after age 40).

_____ 16. Urinalysis, urine cultures, and tests for blood in the stool after age 30.

---

lacking in facilities, and weak in handling emergencies. Emphasis is placed on patients with short-term illnesses who are unlikely to develop complications and are capable of paying their bills. The larger private hospitals maintain generally high standards and avoid most of the difficulties of the smaller hospitals.

Before choosing a hospital, consider the following six factors:

1. **Accreditation status.** Hospitals accredited by the Joint Commission on Accreditation have met certain standards in all phases of hospital care: selection and training of staff, equipment, facilities, food service, pharmacy, record keeping, and medical staff. Accreditation does not guarantee a

perfect hospital, nor can one be assured that broad certification of staff is required. In general, however, a voluntary hospital is superior to a private or government-funded hospital and adheres more strictly to accreditation standards.

2. **Affiliation with a medical school.** Teaching hospitals are generally equipped to provide excellent medical care for practically any illness or ailment. Only hospitals with extremely high standards are associated with medical schools.

The location and quality of emergency room care are important criteria in choosing a hospital.

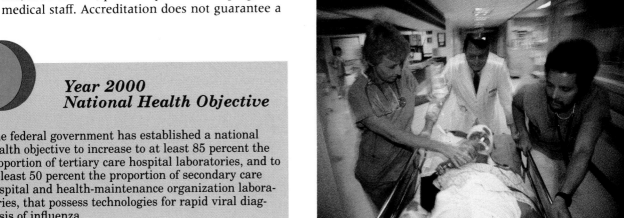

Year 2000 National Health Objective

The federal government has established a national health objective to increase to at least 85 percent the proportion of tertiary care hospital laboratories, and to at least 50 percent the proportion of secondary care hospital and health-maintenance organization laboratories, that possess technologies for rapid viral diagnosis of influenza.

acupuncture A method of medical treatment that uses needles inserted at specific points on the body to relieve pain and to bring about a treatment or cure for disease.

chiropractic A method of medical treatment originated in 1895 by David Palmer, chiropractic medicine relies on manipulation of the vertebrae and other body parts to bring about efficacious medical treatment.

You can be relatively sure that these hospitals will have a well-trained staff of experienced physicians and modern equipment.

3. **Size.** Small hospitals (two hundred beds or less) offer a narrow range of services, have few specialists, and may not be equipped to handle serious illnesses. In general, larger hospitals offer the best and most comprehensive health care.

4. **Location.** Depending on the illness, it is desirable to choose a hospital within a reasonable distance from your home. Emergency room treatment varies considerably from one hospital to another, suggesting the need to investigate this area of health care.

5. **Cost.** Cost of private and semiprivate rooms and medical services varies from hospital to hospital. It is helpful to consult your health insurance plan and discuss cost with the hospital of your choice.

6. **Ownership.** According to Consumers Union medical consultants, a voluntary hospital is your best choice.

A hospital should be used only when absolutely necessary. Many services can be provided outside the hospital for much less cost. The hospital should not be used for rest or for convenience: It is a noisy, unfamiliar environment with continuous interruptions. It is often not the best place to conduct screening tests. In addition, treatment for some ailments is more effective in a home environment.

Patient's Bill of Rights

The American Hospital Association has devised a document listing the rights of hospital patients. You should receive your copy of this *patient's bill of rights* when you are admitted to a hospital that belongs to the association. Although the patient's bill of rights is not a legal document, it does set forth standards that member hospitals are expected to follow.

The patient's bill of rights contains the following provisions:

- Considerate and respectful care.
- The right to obtain complete information concerning your diagnosis, treatment, and prognosis, in terms you can understand.

- The right to all the information you need to give informed consent (risks, benefits, alternative treatments) before treatment.
- The right to refuse treatment, once you are aware of the facts, to the extent permitted by law.
- Privacy and confidentiality (refusal to be examined in front of people who are not involved in your case, confidentiality of records).
- A reasonable response when you ask for help, including evaluation, service, and referral, as indicated by the urgency of the case.
- Information about any possible conflicts of interest (hospital ownership of labs evaluating your tests, professional relationships among doctors who are treating you).
- The right to be told if the hospital plans to make your treatment part of a research project or experiment.
- The right to an explanation of your hospital bill.
- The right to know what hospital rules apply to your conduct as a patient.
- The right to expect good follow-up care.

Awareness of your rights as a patient is a first step toward getting the quality of care you need. It is your personal responsibility to look out for yourself, insisting on good care and expressing your needs and concerns freely.

Community Health Care

Community health resources are available to all. State health departments and county or city health units exist to help residents with specific health problems. Although the most important function of city and county health departments is the education of the public, direct medical services are provided to members of the community. Immunization centers for disease control, special clinics for sexually transmitted diseases, and maternal and child health services are generally available.

In most cities, "free clinics" have evolved to treat or counsel people for undesired pregnancies, sexually transmitted diseases, and drug use. Many of these clinics treat all ailments for those who cannot afford regular medical care. Minimum funding and a shortage of personnel restrict medical services to a small number of patients and reduce services considerably; however, sympathetic care and sincere interest are provided. With more community support, free clinics could provide a real contribution to the modern medical care system.

Alternative Approaches to Health Care

Acupuncture

Acupuncture is a method of eliminating pain using needles inserted at specific points on the body. This technique has been practiced in China for thousands of years and began to attract the attention of medical practitioners in the West in the 1970s. Using acupuncture, Chinese surgeons have been able to perform operations of the head, chest, and abdomen without anesthesia. The advantages of acupuncture anesthesia are numerous: The patient is able to remain conscious during surgery, there is no risk of side effects or possible death from general anesthetics, the danger of blood clotting after surgery is reduced, and the patient does not have to spend time in a recovery room while anesthesia wears off.

The use of acupuncture as an alternative treatment for pain and other disorders is becoming more common in the United States.

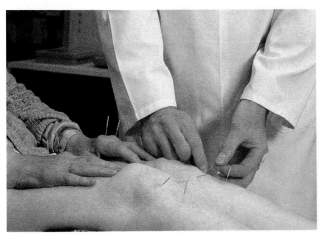

Considerable scientific investigation is under way to determine the therapeutic value of acupuncture as a treatment for nerve deafness, narcotics withdrawal, and pain. Acupuncture has been used successfully as a surgical anesthetic for root canal therapy, skin grafts, tumor biopsies, and minor surgical procedures, and it appears to be useful in abortions and childbirth as well. To date, the reasons acupuncture seems to work are unclear. The major danger with the treatment is its use by quacks who have no training. If you plan to look into the technique, seek out a licensed physician performing acupuncture under the auspices of a hospital or medical school.

Chiropractic

Chiropractic was originated in 1895 by David Palmer, who called himself a "magnetic healer." Palmer performed manual adjustments of the vertebrae in order to cure deafness and heart trouble. From his experiences evolved the theory that partly dislocated *(subluxated)* vertebrae emit heat from pressure on the nerves, and these pressures cause practically all diseases. The R. J. Chiropractic Clinic was developed by Palmer's son and became a model for future facilities. The modern-day chiropractic profession operates on the following four principles:

1. Anatomical "disrelation" (misalignment) can create functional disturbances in the body.
2. Disturbances of the nervous system are primary factors in the development of many diseases.
3. Spinal subluxations are a specific cause of nerve irritation or interference.
4. Nerve irritation at the spine may lead to a disturbance in the function of internal organs of the body (the viscerospinal principle).[1]

The controversy over and criticism of the effectiveness of chiropractic lie in the lack of support for the theoretical basis of these clinics, inadequate education and training of some chiropractors, and unsupported claims of cures for various diseases and ailments. According to the chiropractic profession, the American Medical Association and most physicians have unjustly condemned their mode of treatment. The fact that more and more insurance companies now include coverage of chiropractic services in their health plans demonstrates a new faith in the profession.[2] In addition, many people believe the approach has helped them.

Other Alternative Health-Care Approaches

There are a number of additional nontraditional approaches to standard medical care. *Naturopathy* is a method of healing that relies solely on nature, employ-

premium The amount of money paid for an insurance policy.

deductible The initial portion of an insurance claim that is paid by the insured; the higher the deductible, the lower the premium.

coinsurance clause A statement indicating that a specified percentage of insurance-covered cost must be paid by the insured after the deductible amount is subtracted.

disability insurance Private health insurance designed to provide income during periods of sickness or injury.

ing massage, physical exercise, diets based on natural foods, vitamins, fasting, vegetarianism, and combinations of air, light, water, sun, vibration, heat, rest, and electricity as treatment methods. Medicine is used sparingly; surgery and x-ray or radiation are used for diagnostic purposes only; the bacterial theory of disease is rejected; diseases are believed to be caused by the violation of nature's laws and by moral, social, and sexual conduct. *Homeopathy* follows the premise that diseases or symptoms can be cured with small doses of the same substance that causes the problem. *Faith healing* preceded the medical profession by many centuries and relies on healers who emphasize curing illnesses by the faith the individual has in God. *Hypnotherapy* (the use of hypnosis in a therapeutic setting) has been used effectively for pain alleviation in childbirth and dentistry and for the treatment of emotional problems, migraine, and vascular headaches. Exactly how the procedure works, when it should be used, and with whom is under study. The *occult* deals with what is mysterious, hidden, or obscure. Some of its practitioners include gurus, swamis, astrologers, palmists, and tea readers who turn to phrenology, numerology, astrology, and other nonscientific methods for cures.

Health Insurance

Health insurance is an absolute necessity in the United States today. Given the extremely high cost of medical care, the alternative—direct out-of-pocket payment by the patient—can pose a tremendous financial burden. Unfortunately, many individuals do not receive adequate medical coverage due to a lack of money for insurance. Approximately 15 percent of the American population has no health insurance. These individuals often delay care until there is a serious emergency. Preventive health care is also nonexistent for these people. Funding for uninsured cases who do not have the financial means to pay occurs through charitable means or through increased rates to the insured. Most Americans have some form of health insurance as part of their employment compensation, a government program, or a private health plan. Over 75 percent of the insured population is covered through group plans provided by a family member's employer. The employer may pay all or part of the premium. The rising cost of health care has brought about a dramatic increase in premiums, and many private companies can

Exploring Your Health 20.2

Are You Getting the Most from Your Doctor Visits?

Consider the last time you went to the doctor for help with a health problem. Then answer the following questions:

1. Did you think about the reasons for your visit so that you could convey them to the doctor clearly?

2. Did you tell the doctor all your symptoms, or did you try to underplay some of them?

3. Assuming that the doctor was able to diagnose your ailment, did he or she give you an understandable and satisfactory explanation of it?

4. Did the doctor answer all your questions fully and clearly? If unable to answer a question, did he or she say so?

5. Did the doctor treat you like a responsible adult, or did you feel intimidated?

6. Did you report to the doctor any medications you take or allergies and other reactions you may have to medications?

7. If the doctor prescribed a medication, did you ask about how to take it and possible side effects?

8. If you left with a prescription, did you have it filled and take it as directed for the full time period directed?

9. If the doctor told you to check back within a certain time period, did you do so?

If your response to any of these questions was negative, you may not be getting the most out of your doctor visits. What steps could you take to improve your doctor-patient relationship?

no longer afford to pay them. Small firms have a difficult time purchasing cost-effective insurance and they do not have the buying clout or cash to be self-insured. As a result, companies are reducing benefits, increasing deductibles and copayments, and seeking different approaches to coverage, such as self-insurance and multiple employer trusts, which pool many small companies and operate as one large, self-insured medical plan. If costs continue to spiral and the poor economic climate of the early 1990s continues, more and more employers will be forced to eliminate health insurance as a benefit. Insurance costs are already increasing so quickly that many people will not be able to afford to run their own businesses.

The increased cost of medical insurance has brought about a renewed interest in preventive health care. In the 1970s, approximately 30 companies offered some sort of fitness program; today, that figure exceeds 20,000. Some companies operate their own full-fledged health clubs, while others subsidize membership at local clubs or conduct clinics to stop smoking, reduce stress, lose body weight and fat, change eating habits, and reduce alcohol and drug use. Employers have discovered that preventive health care can significantly reduce insurance costs.

Several kinds of group and individual health insurance plans are available. The major components of the ideal policy are:

- Hospital insurance to cover hospital bills.
- Surgical insurance to cover doctors' operating fees.
- Regular medical insurance to pay for nonsurgical doctors' fees in and out of the hospital.
- Major medical insurance to cover a percentage of expenses incurred above a certain cost in case of major illness or injury.
- Disability or lost-income insurance to pay for living expenses if the family breadwinner is incapacitated.

Most health insurance companies are expected to follow the trend to reduce **premiums** (the amount of money paid for an insurance policy) for insurees with healthy lifestyles that include regular aerobic exercise, absence of tobacco and alcohol use, absence of other drug abuse, and maintenance of normal weight and body fat.

Few purchases that you make require such serious consideration and review on your part.

Insurance Providers

Independent Insurance Plans
More than 500 independent insurance plans are available in the United States. Some are joint ventures between union and management; others provide benefits through prepaid group practice plans. Several of these plans are nonprofit service corporations that allow a free choice of medical personnel and provide service benefits.

Commercial Insurance Plans
Profit-making insurers write both group and individual health insurance policies. Life insurance, disability insurance, and major medical insurance can also be acquired as part of a complete package. Major medical policies are designed to handle expensive medical costs not ordinarily covered by typical insurance. Maximum benefits range from $2,000 to $40,000 or more, with a **deductible** and a **coinsurance clause.** The patient pays the deductible amount out of his or her own pocket before any costs are paid by the company. The higher the deductible, the lower the premium. A coinsurance clause states that a specified percentage of the cost must be borne by the patient after the deductible amount is subtracted. A policy, for example, may pay a maximum benefit of $10,000, with a deductible clause of $500 and a coinsurance clause of 20 percent. If a portion of a total bill of $10,000 ($1,200, for example) is paid by a basic plan, the patient presents a bill of $8,800 less $500 (deductible), or $8,300. This $8,300 is subject to coinsurance (20 percent), with the patient responsible for paying $1,660. Actual reimbursement from the major medical plan amounts to $6,640 ($8,300 − $1,660). In the case of prolonged hospital care and serious illness, a coinsurance clause can mean substantial cost to the patient.

Disability Insurance
During hospitalization and convalescence, loss of income due to unemployment and expiration of accumulated sick leave threatens family security. Such a dangerous risk makes **disability insurance** a must for most families. Premiums are paid to insurance companies that, in cases of disability, pay 75 percent or more of the patient's regular monthly income. Policies are also designed to provide lump-sum benefits for loss of a limb or part of a limb or to survivors in case of accidental death.

Blue Cross and Blue Shield
Blue Cross was founded by hospital officials during the Depression to keep hospitals from going bankrupt. A small premium (about $1.00 per month) was paid in return for a specified number of days of hospital care. Every member paid the same premium, regardless of age, sex, or health status. Blue Cross gave no cash to policyholders; instead, hospitals were paid for services rendered and generally kept their charges within the ranges provided by the Blue Cross plan. As hospital workers began to demand higher wages, expensive diagnostic and treatment equipment was invented, and hospital and physician costs soared, Blue Cross premiums increased tremendously. The plan was no longer an inexpensive, simplified answer to health insurance. Industry soon discovered that it was possible to purchase policies from private companies at lower rates,

health maintenance organization (HMO) A comprehensive medical insurance plan that covers both treatment and prevention for a fixed, prepaid monthly fee.

preferred provider organization (PPO) A comprehensive medical insurance plan, similar to an HMO except that consumers may choose to select a health care facility that is not "preferred" by the plan.

particularly when their work force consisted predominantly of young male (no pregnancy risk) workers. Faced with the threat of losing its healthiest members, Blue Cross began setting premium rates by classes and selling policies based on actual risks.

Today, about seventy-five Blue Cross plans offer service benefits and provide compensation for a specified number of days in a hospital, generally covering the majority of costs (from the first dollar) of an average stay. Blue Cross and Blue Shield is a plan that primarily serves major medical needs, such as hospitalization and major surgery. Lesser medical expenses, such as physician office visits and prescription medications, are covered in part and only after payment of a deductible (usually paid quarterly). No emphasis is placed on preventive care; routine physical examinations and periodic screening (Pap smears and the like) are not covered. All Blue Cross plans must meet the approval of the American Hospital Association's Blue Cross Commission and must exist as a non-profit organization: profits must be used to improve the plan. Surgical and medical benefits are obtained through Blue Shield, which covers bills in full only for patients up to certain income levels. Many hospitals accept Blue Shield allotments for different surgical and medical procedures and do not make added charges. Rates are increased to reflect increases in hospital, surgical, and medical costs.

Managed Care Programs: HMOs and PPOs

The rising costs of health care have brought about a growth in *managed care* programs, such as those provided by health maintenance and preferred provider organizations. Such programs offer a comprehensive range of services, which include general and specialty physicians, preventive care, and the assignment of a primary physician for general care and referral.

The health care system in the United States has traditionally focused on treatment of the sick. When a patient suffers some symptoms, a physician provides treatment, and a health plan reimburses the patient for all or part of the costs for most illnesses. Little emphasis has been placed on preventive measures because

the typical health plan does not cover regular checkups, screening, and the like. **Health maintenance organizations (HMOs)** are different in that they provide comprehensive medical coverage, from a routine checkup to major surgery, from a physician visit to hospitalization, in exchange for advance payment of a fixed monthly fee. HMOs are designed to encourage subscribers to cut their costs by preventing illness. Both the physician and the patient share the financial risk of ill health. Unlike conventional health plans, HMOs guarantee that services will be made available to the consumer.

HMOs are group practices that also give doctors some incentive to keep people well; to treat illnesses before hospitalization becomes necessary; and to practice preventive medicine. Although physicians associated with HMOs are salaried, their annual bonus is based on a percentage of the profits. The cost of office staff, equipment, buildings, and malpractice and other insurance is borne by the health maintenance organization. An administrative staff also handles much of the paperwork, which can consume 15 to 25 percent of a private physician's time. This frees the doctor to spend more time with individual patients. Doctors can order lab tests or admit patients to a hospital without worrying about whether an insurance plan will cover the expense. HMO physicians also enjoy all the advantages of a typical group practice.

For the patient, HMOs offer a less expensive approach to medical care. A patient is also encouraged to seek early treatment because the prepaid monthly fee covers all services. In addition, physicians, labs, and pharmacies are sometimes organized under one roof, saving the patient valuable time. A physician is usually on call twenty-four hours a day. One disadvantage for patients belonging to most HMOs is the lack of choice in selecting a physician. A patient must see one of the physicians employed by the HMO. Figure 20.1 shows the tremendous growth of HMOs since the trend began in 1981.

In 1987, there were 626 HMOs nationally, with a total enrollment of 25,777,130 patients—a 22 percent increase from 1986. Large plans are now dominating HMO enrollment. Federally qualified plans are also a dominant force, with 81 percent of the total December

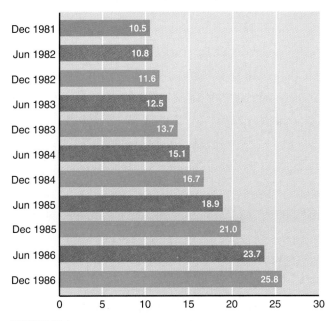

Enrollment in millions

Dec 1981	10.5
Jun 1982	10.8
Dec 1982	11.6
Jun 1983	12.5
Dec 1983	13.7
Jun 1984	15.1
Dec 1984	16.7
Jun 1985	18.9
Dec 1985	21.0
Jun 1986	23.7
Dec 1986	25.8

0   5   10   15   20   25   30

FIGURE 20.1 • HMO growth 1981–1986.

Source: The Robert Wood Johnson Foundation, *Special Report Number 2* (May 1987).

31, 1986 enrollment.[3] More competition among HMOs should bring more innovative approaches to health care delivery and financing in the future. Table 20.2 makes some comparisons between traditional health insurers, such as Blue Cross, and HMOs.

The **preferred provider organization (PPO)** is a more recent development in managed care. Insurance companies and employers contract with "preferred" physicians or hospitals for medical services, and discounted fees are provided in return for the guaranteed payment of claims. Unlike an HMO plan, a PPO plan does allow individual consumers to select a physician or medical facilities unassociated with the PPO; however, only visits to preferred physicians or facilities are likely to be paid in full. As of 1987, there were approximately 500 PPOs covering 25 to 30 million Americans.

Flexible Spending Accounts

In 1990, more than 900 companies offered *Flexible Spending Accounts* to employees to deal with rising health costs. Employees place money into the plan to pay for medical expenses that their normal health insurance doesn't cover. Employees decide at the beginning of the year how much money will be entered into the plan through payroll deductions. As medical or day-care bills are due, employees utilize the money. Money in these accounts is not taxed, even when it is spent. Beginning January 1, 1991, the IRS allowed employees to borrow against the amount earmarked for their account for the year. The main disadvantage of flexible spending accounts is that the money must be used by the end of the year or it reverts to the company.

Medicare and Medicaid   Congress amended the Social Security Act in 1965 to include Title 18 *(Medicare)* and provide a program of health insurance to individuals 65 years of age and older. Two programs were established: (1) compulsory hospital insurance financed by Social Security taxes to cover hospital care, extended-care facilities (nursing homes), and outpatient diagnostic services; and (2) voluntary medical insurance financed by individual premiums and matching funds from the government to pay medical bills not covered by hospital insurance.

The Social Security Act was also amended to include Title 19 *(Medicaid),* providing federal grants to the states to operate a medical assistance program for those already receiving public assistance from the federal government (including the elderly, blind, disabled, and families with dependent children); to assist those who have enough income to live on but not enough to cover medical expenses; and to provide help for all young people under age 21 whose parents cannot afford medical expenses.

Medicare, with its unique feature of combining compulsory and voluntary methods of payment, has resulted in improved and extended health care to millions of Americans who previously could not afford to pay for medical services. The plan removes older people, a high-risk group, from the health insurance market. It is estimated that the government now has taken over approximately 90 percent of medical costs for persons over the age of 65.

Evaluating Before You Buy

Examine your policy carefully to secure accurate answers to the following key questions:

- Is there "first dollar" coverage?
- How does a deductible of $100, $500, or more affect premiums? What amount is suited to your income?
- Is disability or lost-income protection provided?

If medical costs continue to rise, many of our nation's older people will not be able to afford proper medical care.

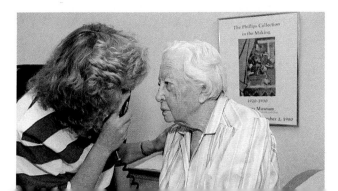

TABLE 20.2

Traditional Health Insurers and HMOs: Some Comparisons

Fee-For-Service Plans (Blue Cross/Blue Shield Standard Plan)	Typical Prepaid Plans (HMOs)
Provide health care services for a *major part* of medical expenses on a fee-for-service basis.	Provide *comprehensive* health care services in return for a prepaid monthly fee.
Typically require a quarterly deductible for small medical expenses, such as doctor's visits or prescription drugs. Some plans also require clients to pay approximately 20 percent of expenses above the deductible.	No deductible for smaller medical expenses.
Provide 100 percent coverage for major medical expenses (hospital and surgical).	Provide 100 percent coverage for major medical expenses (hospital and surgical).
Do not encourage preventive care because routine and preventive services are not covered.	Encourage preventive care because routine and preventive services are covered (e.g., physical exams, Pap smears, well baby care).
Client may select *any* participating physician or medical facility.	Client must select a *specific* HMO primary care physician and use hospitals associated with the HMO.
Client must submit claim forms to be reimbursed for some smaller services, such as physician's office visits.	Virtually no claim forms or bills are incurred by the client.
Client must secure the medical services and submit the costs for reimbursement.	Client is guaranteed that services will be made available.
May need to use a number of different physicians.	Provides all needed care under one roof.
Services generally available during regular business hours.	Services available 24 hours daily.
Waiting time is minimal.	Waiting time is generally longer.
Chance to evaluate your physician before you choose.	System may attract unqualified physicians.
Flexibility of care depends on you and your physician.	System is less flexible.
Care is personal to the degree that your choice of physicians emphasizes this aspect.	Care tends to be more impersonal.
Can choose a physician and hospital nearby.	Location may be unsuitable, requiring considerable driving time.
Prescription drugs and insulin covered at 80 percent after deductible.	$3 copayment per prescription.
Preventive care not covered.	$3 copayment per visit to primary care physician.
Skilled nursing home care in semiprivate room covered for 120 days at $65 per day.	100 percent covered up to 180 days per calendar year.

Exploring Your Health 20.3

Evaluating Your Health Insurance Plan

Now that you are familiar with the provisions of HMOs and private health plans, study the benefits of your university or family health plan. In the column to the left, list the benefits of your plan. In the right-hand column, record the problem areas (items not covered, deductible, handling of a long-term illness, first-dollar coverage, freedom to select a physician or hospital, and so forth). Is your policy adequate for you at this time? Are you assured of high-quality physician and hospital care? Would a long-term hospital illness place undue financial burden on you and your family? Would an HMO provide better and less expensive coverage?

Benefits

1. _____
2. _____
3. _____
4. _____
5. _____

Problem Areas

1. _____
2. _____
3. _____
4. _____
5. _____

What portion of your monthly salary is involved? For how long? Is there provision for permanent disability?

- Is there a lump-sum payment to dependents in case of your death?

- Is full coverage provided for hospital, medical, and surgical costs? What dollar restrictions are placed on length of stay, costs for various surgical and medical procedures, cost of drugs, and special treatments? Are physicians' costs covered both in and out of the hospital?

- Is major medical insurance available for serious illnesses or accidents?

- Are expenses for care during pregnancy and delivery covered?

- Are reduced rates available for policyholders not in need of coverage for pregnancy? Are reduced rates available to nonsmokers? Nondrinkers? Individuals in good health?

- Is this a "commercial" policy (one that can be canceled if the holder becomes a bad risk after the claim for the current illness is paid); a "guaranteed-renewable" policy (the holder has the right to continue until age 65, as long as premiums are paid on time; and premiums cannot be raised unless they are increased for everyone in the insured's classification); or a "noncancelable guaranteed-renewable" policy (the insured can keep the policy until age 65 or, in some cases, for life, without any change in provision, including

rates). Premiums rise with both the noncancelable guaranteed-renewable and the guaranteed-renewable policies.

- Is a group policy available? Group rates are generally lower, and health risks are accepted in the plan that ordinarily are not handled on an individual basis.

- Is coverage provided for mental and emotional disorders?

- Does your policy use the term "accidental bodily injury" if it covers expense sustained as a result of accident (this wording tends to guarantee coverage for injuries by a willful attempt to cause you bodily harm)?

- Is coverage provided for dental care?

- What provisions are available for coverage of dependents?

- What is the grace period for late premiums before cancellation occurs?

- Do any restrictive clauses eliminate payment for previously existing illnesses or require a waiting period before such illnesses are covered?

Your state insurance department can also be of assistance. It will provide an analysis of any policy, explain its terms, provide information on the ease or difficulty of securing payment on claims, and clarify any feature of the policy you don't understand.

Problems with the Health Care System

Cost

The cost of hospital, physician, and dental care continues to rise. Experts now predict that the cost of indigent care to hospitals will increase 80 percent by 1995 and that, during that same period, 10 percent of the nation's hospitals will close. The number of community hospital closures across the nation increased 45 percent in 1986, with a total of 83 hospitals (71 community and 12 speciality hospitals) closing in 1986.[4]

From 1965 to 1987, health-care expenses increased 1000 percent: from an average of approximately $176 to $1758 annually for every person in the United States, as shown in Figure 20.2. As of 1989, Americans spent $1.3 billion dollars daily for health care.

Access to adequate care in the future is expected to be strongly influenced by age, severity of illness, and ability to pay. The cost of technology, hidden costs (increase in the number of small tests and procedures such as mass screening for AIDS), artificial organ transplants, the AIDS pandemic, increases in the cost of medical professional liability, and the ability to prolong life (not necessarily at a high-quality level) will drive costs even higher. Government changes offer little hope of relief for the average consumer since high costs of health care will continue to dictate policy in the next five to ten years.

Results of health care studies in the United States such as those summarized in Figure 20.3 demonstrate a deterioration in access to medical care among the nation's poor, minority, and uninsured citizens. Some improvements in access noted in 1982 have also been reversed. These segments of the population are also least able to take advantage of new forms of health care delivery.[5]

The medical profession remains a self-regulating body, with the American Medical Association (AMA) controlling the supply of physicians through state licensing laws and limited admissions to medical school. In addition, the medical profession continues to evaluate performance through peer review. This type of autonomy is blamed by some for the resistance of the profession to lowering its prices. Defenders of higher prices note that the cost of initiating a private dental or

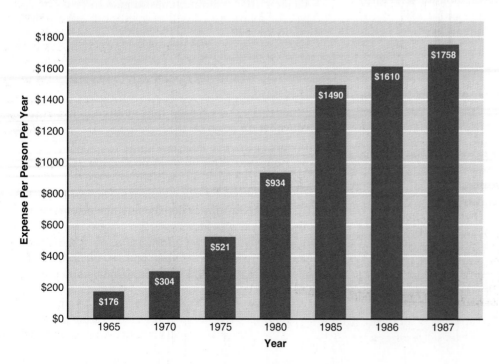

FIGURE 20.2 • Health Care Expenses Per Person, 1965 to 1987

Source: Health Insurance Association, *1989 Source Book of Health Insurance Data* (Washington, D.C.: Health Insurance Association of America, 1989).

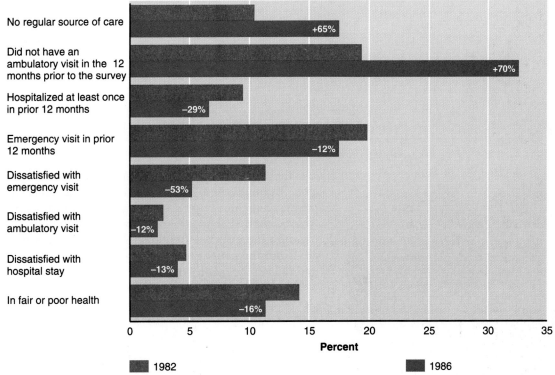

Enrollment in millions

Category	
No regular source of care	+65%
Did not have an ambulatory visit in the 12 months prior to the survey	+70%
Hospitalized at least once in prior 12 months	−29%
Emergency visit in prior 12 months	−12%
Dissatisfied with emergency visit	−53%
Dissatisfied with ambulatory visit	−12%
Dissatisfied with hospital stay	−13%
In fair or poor health	−16%

Percent

■ 1982   ■ 1986

FIGURE 20.3 • Changes in access to medical care.
Source: Medical Economic Digest (May 30, 1987). Used by permission.

medical practice is high, and overhead for private offices, including high malpractice protection premiums, is also high. To avoid some of these expenses, group practices have become popular as a means of sharing costs and providing physicians with more free time. Unfortunately, this approach has not yet translated into lower costs for patients. New technology and the cost of developing and producing modern diagnostic and treatment equipment continues to push hospital costs up. Fortunately, there is some relief in sight for the consumer.

Year 2000 National Health Objective

Recognizing the need for improved medical care for all Americans, especially Hispanics, blacks, and low-income people, the federal government is striving to increase to at least 95 percent the proportion of people who have a specific source of on-going primary care for coordination of their preventive and episodic health care. In 1986, less than 82 percent met this objective and 18 percent reported having no physician, clinic, or hospital as a regular source of care. In addition, the government is striving to improve financing and delivery of clinical preventive services so that virtually no American has a financial barrier to receiving, at a minimum, the screening, counseling, and immunization services recommended by the U.S. government.

The trend toward using paraprofessionals (nonphysicians) such as nurse practitioners and physician's assistants to perform some routine medical care has some potential. In some cases, individuals such as university exercise physiologists and physical educators are part of a team that includes physicians. Such teams can provide key preventive service through prescription exercise, nutrition, and weight-control guidance. These professionals are becoming more and more important in the health care system, since it is now recognized that the key to better health and lower cost of health care for the individual lies in prevention of disease through a lifestyle that includes proper nutrition, regular aerobic exercise, weight management, wise use of drugs, home care of the teeth and body, and regular checkups.

Competition among physicians and hospitals who are now advertising, trimming fees, posting prices, making special deals for large groups, and offering new services should drive prices down. The growing number of physicians (247,000 in 1963, 425,000 in 1983, 500,000 in 1990) will also reduce prices as competition for patients increases.[6] Whoever can control the flow of patients will make the most money. Physicians in the future will try to reduce the number of patients they send to the hospital to maintain their income, while hospitals will be interested in admitting more patients. Some feel hospitals will branch out to provide primary care in the community through group practices in out-patient departments and emergency

Year 2000 National Health Objective

Recognizing the importance of regular checkups and preventive health care, one national health objective seeks to increase to at least 50 percent the proportion of people who have received, as a minimum within the appropriate interval, all of the screening and immunization services and at least one of the counseling services appropriate for their age and gender.

rooms. The competition among physicians and hospitals and between physicians and hospitals could translate into lower costs for the patient. The focus will be on reducing costs while improving care.

The traditional fee-for-service system of reimbursing physicians may not survive in the United States. Patient revenue growth continues to diminish, averaging only 6.6 percent between 1984 and 1987, less than

half the 15.2 percent average annual growth rate from 1977 through 1983.[7] As competition for patients increases, a greater number of physicians will be forced to seek salaried employment with health maintenance organizations. Such a trend could shift physician loyalty from the patient to the employment organization and reduce the quality of patient care.

Checkups and Screening: Too Many Unnecessary Expenses?

The annual physical examination was once a major feature of preventive medicine in the United States. In recent years, however, the annual physical examination has been criticized as an unnecessary expense, particularly when a person is in good health. It is estimated that at least 25 percent of all medical tests are unnecessary. Although there are good reasons for some medical tests, too many tests are useless and drive up costs while contributing little to patient care (see Issues in Health: "Is Defensive Medicine Really Ef-

Issues in Health

Is Defensive Medicine Really Effective?

To reduce the risk of malpractice claims and improve patient care, physicians have initiated what is called "defensive medicine": extra precautions to cover all avenues for potential suit should something go wrong. Failure to diagnose, failure to follow up abnormal test results, and communication errors such as failure to inform patients of material risks and to document informed consent are some of the more common grounds for actions against physicians.[8]

Pro Proponents of defensive medicine argue that both the patient and the physician profit. The patient benefits from a number of additional

routine tests that provide important data for both diagnosis and treatment. At the very least, the patient has more confidence in the diagnosis. Eventually, it is argued, liability insurance premiums will decrease and the savings will be passed along to the patient. Defensive medicine also forces the physician to maintain better record keeping (estimated at over $31,000 annually per physician), spend more time with each patient, and diagnose and treat patients more carefully.

Con Opponents point out that defensive medicine has been around for several years and there is no sign of reduction in either the frequency or

severity of malpractice claims. In fact, claims continue to rise. In addition, defensive medicine may cost the patient more out-of-pocket money in the long run because of the extra diagnostic tests. Patients also suffer the physical discomfort of numerous unnecessary tests, some of which carry medical risks. To date, there is no evidence to show that physicians' fear of liability results in improved diagnosis or treatment; taking steps to reduce the chances of a malpractice suit does not necessarily translate into reducing the risk of disease.

What do you think? Should the practice be continued?

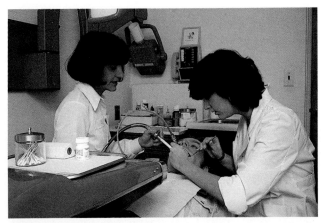

Regular dental checkups and cleaning can prevent tooth and gum problems later in life.

condition prior to symptoms, whether early diagnosis and treatment alters the progress of the disease, and whether the test is accurate, relatively risk-free, and inexpensive.

Regular dental checkups are important at all ages and are critical during adolescence and the late teens, when a high rate of dental decay and periodontal disease is common. A minimum of one visit every six months is recommended for college-age students, as well as for all adults. Preventive dentistry is a very effective means of protecting against tooth and gum diseases later in life.

Medicine Meets the Law: Malpractice

The malpractice crisis appears to be getting worse. According to the American Medical Association, the number of malpractice suits against doctors, the size of the jury awards for damages, and the cost of malpractice insurance are all soaring. Twenty of every hundred physicians face a lawsuit today, compared to twelve per hundred in 1979.

fective?''). Healthy individuals need to select screening tests that are useful to them. It is important to analyze whether a diagnostic test will reveal a significant health problem, whether you are at risk for the disease or disorder, whether the test can detect the disease or

A Question of Ethics

Securing Adequate Medical Care—A Privilege or a Right?

Soaring medical costs may eventually make private health care a privilege only the upper-middle and upper classes can afford. The less economically fortunate would then be forced to use the services of public health agencies and free clinics. Expenditures for medical care in the United States have mounted rapidly. The figure was $139 billion in 1976, more than $180 billion in 1978, $200 billion in 1980, $350 billion in 1983, and over 460 billion in 1989. Increases in private physician, hospital, and insurance fees for the individual are staggering. If the trend continues, only a small percentage of the American people will be capable of financing health care for their families.

The view that every citizen has a right to adequate medical care is gaining support. More than a dozen national health insurance bills have been proposed by congressional representatives and interested groups. The Kennedy-Corman plan proposes shifting the financing of health care to the government and doing away with private health insurance firms. The plan is based on the idea that significant changes must be made,

not only in the financing of health care, but in the way medicine is practiced, hospitals are run, and costs are controlled. A 1 percent income tax, an employer's tax, and money from the general revenues would be used to finance the plan.

Some experts sense a move toward medical rationing and the allocation of health care to certain people while depriving others. Some countries, including the United States, already use a similar approach. The state of Oregon, for example, plans to ration Medicaid benefits sometime in 1992. Priorities for over 1,600 medical treatments are being established. Rationing health care in the future will probably be based on the skills of people, their remaining productive life, and their intelligence. Under such a system, some people could not get certain treatment even if they had the money. Programs prepared by politicians that put procedures before people are being severely criticized. Regardless of the specifics, rationing presumes discrimination and wholesale plans for rationing will not be incorporated without long legal battles.

The most radical plan is a bill proposed by Representative Ronald Dellums (D-Calif.) to create a national health service similar to the one in Great Britain. By nationalizing the health care industry, this plan would eliminate fees for services; pay the salaries of doctors, who would work for the government; and provide government control of all hospitals.

Many medical personnel are skeptical about such a plan. They point out that, in other countries with government health services, efficiency has declined, costs have risen, and taxpayers have had to support an ever-growing bureaucracy.

In spite of these concerns, the demand for change is spreading to the grassroots. Most advocates of reform agree that health insurance should be mandatory and should protect every citizen and cover the costs of all forms of illness. A broad health care program will be expensive and out of the reach of most citizens unless some form of government plan is initiated.

What do you think?

Get Involved!

Choosing Medical Service and Health Insurance

The United States is experiencing a health care crisis. Rising health-care costs threaten not only the economic but also the physical well-being of all Americans. New technology, malpractice lawsuits, the spread of AIDS among people who simply cannot afford to pay for health care, and social and economic factors continue to drive the cost of health care upward. This means that in order for most families to maintain even a minimum level of professional health care, they will have to divert an increasingly larger proportion of income to health care from necessities such as food, transportation, housing, and savings as well as from luxuries and leisure items and activities.

The American people and federal and state governments are fast approaching a time when some very painful and far-reaching decisions will have to be made about health care in this country. Some of these decisions may involve the creation, for example, of some form of "nationalized" health care. Many people are upset with this particular idea because they believe it would ultimately limit the individual's choices (even more than in the case of an HMO or PPO) and possibly reduce the overall quality of medical treatment. Other people claim that a highly unfair, two-tiered health "system" is emerging in the United States, with younger, wealthier, and healthier people enjoying substantially better health care than older, less wealthy, and less healthy people.

We urge you to educate yourself about the causes and some of the possible solutions to the current health care crisis. Some of your self-education will probably involve moral and political decisions on your part. Hopefully, the information you gather and think about will also provide you with a solid basis for getting involved in some of the decisions that federal and state governments and health care organizations will have to make about health care in this country.

In the meantime, there are some things you can do for yourself and for the other people in your life to keep the cost of health care down:

1. Take charge of your own medical care and encourage family and friends to do so as well. Consult the interns at a local hospital to identify physicians and dentists who emphasize *preventive* health care. Medical and dental care that focus on prevention rather than treatment after the fact will be much less expensive in the long run and provide a healthier life.

2. Review the health insurance policies of several insurance companies or organizations and see if reduced premiums are offered for a healthy lifestyle that includes the limited use of alcohol, absence of smoking, regular exercise, and the maintenance of normal body weight and fat. Do you or people you know already have policies that do not offer reduced premiums for a healthy lifestyle? If so, why not?

3. Visit your student health care office and discuss the possibility of including self-care sessions at the annual university health fair or health awareness day.

4. Get directly involved in the health care systems of your community by volunteering to work a few hours each week with a local ambulance service or a free clinic.

Insurance carriers have raised malpractice premiums 400 to 600 percent in the past ten years. It is not unusual for physicians in high-risk specialties such as neurosurgery, anesthesiology, obstetrics, and orthopedics to pay an annual premium in excess of $100,000. These increased premiums result in billions of dollars that are added to the nation's health care bill.

Obviously, the patient is paying the bill through higher costs in all aspects of health care. Some alarmed physicians respond to the threat of malpractice suits by ordering expensive tests, that ordinarily would not be used, to rule out all possibilities of misdiagnosis and improper treatment. This also increases the cost to the patient and insurance carriers.

The American Medical Association is urging tougher screening of potential physicians in medical schools and tougher peer-review procedures as a means of eliminating incompetent physicians. Hospitals are using computers to analyze treatment trends of physicians to identify potentially risky practices early. Solving the problem of the many capricious lawsuits against competent physicians seems to be the larger issue, however, as awards for unrealistic claims seem to be increasing.

For the patient, concern with the quality of health care in the United States is rising. While no hard evidence exists of a trend toward low-quality care, examples of poor services, lack of individual attention, and dangerous and even fatal treatment can be found. Old-fashioned faith in the physician is dwindling in spite of modern medical advances.

In fairness to the medical profession, it appears that the increase in the number of malpractice suits is due largely to rising consumerism rather than to poor medical practice. Individuals are demanding better value for their money and greater accountability for all products, including medical care. But if the trend continues, the patient will become an even bigger financial loser, for the physician is also a businessperson who must make a profit. Higher costs will certainly be passed along via higher cost of health care and insurance.

Conclusion

The United States is facing a health care crisis. Rising medical costs are already so high that some families avoid or delay treatment. The introduction of Medicaid and Medicare has been of some help; however, Social Security costs have soared as a result. Moreover, disease may increase if the widespread physical abuse (smoking, overeating, and so on) and sedentary lifestyles of the American public continue. Any significant change in longevity and quality of life will come from two areas: the improved physical fitness of the nation and the improved health care of individuals through early detection of disease. The first area is completely free of cost; the second has the potential to drain family finances. A comprehensive health insurance plan is imperative for individuals of all ages to avoid bankruptcy due to illness. Such a plan, coupled with a careful monitoring of body changes and certain lifestyle practices (sound nutrition, regular exercise, abstention from smoking) can result in a life relatively free from disease.

Summary

1. Each individual should carefully select a primary care (family) physician to provide family health care and make referrals to specialists when needed. A physician should be chosen only after you have consulted your friends or neighbors, the local medical school, or the county medical society.

2. It is the patient's responsibility to be direct and assertive when communicating with the doctor. It is also the patient's right to receive direct, honest answers about his or her condition.

3. Patients should select a hospital carefully, considering such factors as accreditation status and affiliation with a medical school.

4. Acupuncture, an alternative approach to medical care, eliminates pain by inserting needles at specific points on the body. The practice remains controversial. If you want to explore this treatment method, seek out a licensed physician performing under the auspices of a hospital or medical school.

5. Chiropractic, another controversial alternative approach to medical care, uses manual adjustments of the vertebrae to cure various conditions and ailments. More and more insurance companies are including coverage of chiropractic services.

6. Fee-for-service health plans, such as Blue Cross, provide health care services for a major part of medical expenses by reimbursing all or part of the expenses associated with hospitalization and major surgery. Coverage is not provided for routine physical exams or screening. Health maintenance organizations offer comprehensive health care in return for a fixed monthly fee. There is no deductible for small medical expenses. HMOs encourage preventive care.

7. Preferred provider organizations, a popular form of managed care, involves insurance companies and employers who jointly contract with physicians and hospitals. In return for guaranteed payment of claims, discounted fees are provided to the employees of the companies.

8. To offset the rising cost of health care, some companies have introduced Flexible Spending Accounts in which employees place untaxed money into a plan to pay for expenses that are uncovered by their health plan.

9. An annual physical examination may not be necessary for healthy individuals, and it is important for those individuals to analyze carefully the various screening tests performed as part of their physical exam to determine which tests are appropriate.

10. It is important to evaluate the services of a health plan carefully before choosing one—to determine if your anticipated needs and those of your family will be met with limited additional cost to you.

11. An alarming number of Americans do not have access to adequate health care. Age, the severity of the illness, and the ability to pay will continue to dominate medical care in the future and further discriminate against the nation's poor.

12. The number of malpractice cases and the size of monetary awards for damages is increasing dramatically. The American Medical Association is urging stricter screening of medical students as one method of combating malpractice. It is not yet clear what portion of the increase is due to consumerism and the trend to sue and what is attributable to the incompetence of physicians and other health care personnel. The debate continues over whether defensive medicine reduces health costs or improves health care for the patient.

Questions for Personal Growth

1. In modern medicine, there are specially trained physicians for most types of ailments as well as alternatives to traditional health care. Evaluate the professional training of the chiropractic physician and describe the type of ailments you feel are adequately treated by this specialty. If you encounter a problem in any of these areas in the future, would you seek the services of a chiropractor? Why? Why not?

2. Prepare a list of all the medical services you have used in the past twelve months (for example, specialists, hospitals, outpatient surgery centers, community clinics, or home care programs). Rate each experience and list one positive and one negative feature.

3. List the name and specialty area of each health-care provider used by you and your family. What procedures did you use to select your primary care physician and the specialists? How do you know you selected the best possible physician for your family? Describe a plan to evaluate these doctors now.

4. The next time you visit your physician, make a list of all your medical concerns, related or unre-lated to your visit. After your examination, go over each question with your physician, making sure you understand the responses. Did your physician willingly take the time to respond to your concerns? Were the responses adequate and easy to understand? If your physician is not willing to discuss health-related information with you, what steps can you take?

5. Identify your most serious medical concern. By using the criteria discussed in this chapter, evaluate the effectiveness of hospitals in your area in treating this medical problem in emergency situations. Which hospital would provide you with the best care?

6. Health insurance plans vary considerably throughout the United States in terms of cost and coverage. Before you select a private plan, it is important to compare a number of policies. Evaluate your current policy based on the criteria provided in this chapter. Now compare your policy to at least two other plans available in your area.

7. The increased number of malpractice suits is a major factor in the rising costs of medical care in the United States. What do you think could be

done to minimize the size and number of lawsuits in the future?

8. Another factor responsible for rising health-care costs for some individuals is the overuse and unnecessary use of health-care services. What guidelines should be followed to determine if physician care is needed? What steps can safely be taken prior to a visit with a physician? What changes could you make in your lifestyle that may reduce medical costs in the future?

9. Compare your current medical insurance plan to the best HMO in your area. List the characteristics of your current plan that you dislike. Does an HMO meet your needs better than your current plan? Why? Why not?

References

1. John A. Conley, "Another Look at the Chiropractor," *Health Education* 7 (January–February 1976): 22.

2. "Executive Board Debates Chiropractic," *The Nation's Health* (May 1983): 10.

3. The Robert Wood Johnson Foundation, *Special Report Number 2* (May 1987).

4. Ron Mullner, et al., Hospitals (May 5, 1987).

5. The Robert Wood Johnson Foundation.

6. Victor Cohen, "Mastering the Medical Maze, *Washington Post* (October 10, 1984): D7.

7. *The Medical Economic Digest* (June 15, 1987).

8. Jeffrey E. Harris, "Defensive Medicine: It Costs, But Does It Work?" *Journal of the American Medical Association* (May 22, 1987).

CHAPTER 21

Our Environment

CHAPTER OBJECTIVES

After reading this chapter, you should understand:

- How air pollution affects the health of all living creatures.

- Why harmful loud sound, or "noise," produces both auditory and nonauditory ill effects on human health.

- The threat modern industrial society has posed to public water sources and aquatic habitats, and ways to deal with this threat.

- Some of the solid and chemical wastes that pollute our environment.

- What you should know about several sources of radiation that are potentially harmful to human health.

- Specific strategies you can employ to help reduce environmental pollution.

- General information about how human population growth affects our world's environment.

CHAPTER OUTLINE

Air Pollution

Noise Pollution

Water Pollution

Solid and Chemical Waste Pollution

Radiation

A Plan to Reduce Pollution

Population and Health

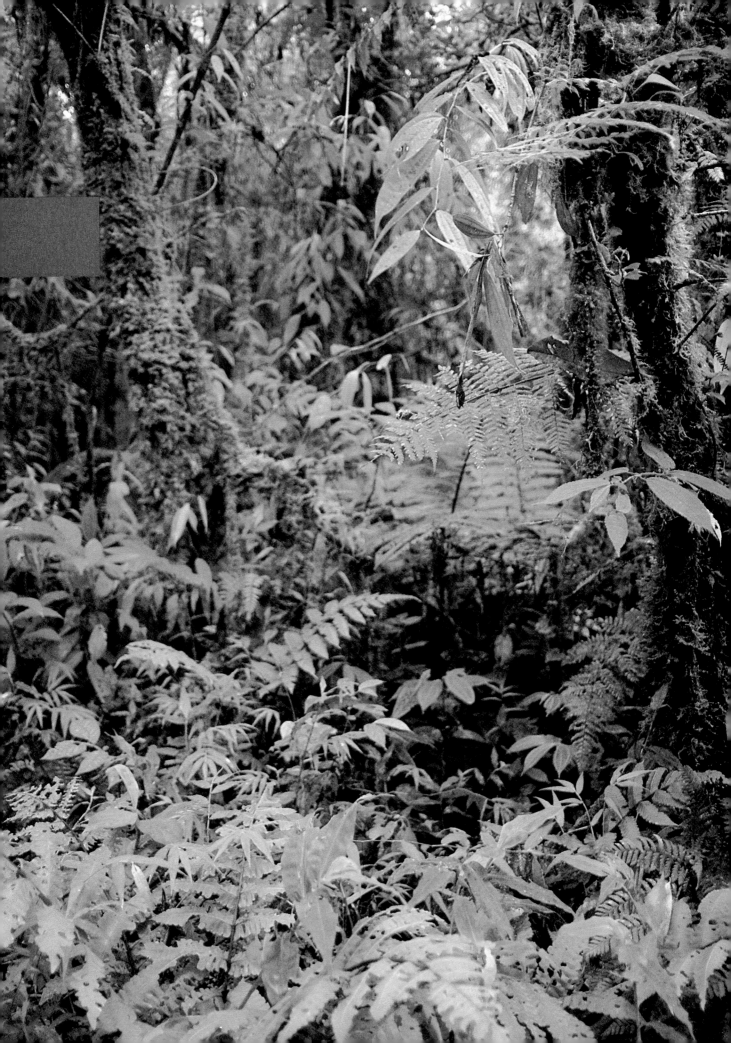

global warming The long-term warming of the earth's climate due to excessive amounts of carbon dioxide, a by-product of fossil fuel use.

greenhouse effect Warming of the earth's atmosphere and surface produced when the sun's heat is trapped by layers of carbon dioxide and other gases.

ozone layer The ozone gas in the atmosphere of the earth that protects the earth from the ultraviolet radiation of the sun; the ozone layer is damaged by air pollution.

Throughout this book we have tried to emphasize the exploration of connections between your health and the health of other people. Through most of this exploration of good health, we have made one big assumption: We will be able to achieve and maintain good health in the earth's present environment. The purpose of this chapter is to question this assumption, for in the last two decades it has become clear that we will really only be able live healthful lives *for as long as the earth's environment allows us to do so.* The fact is, we are experiencing an environmental crisis whose primary cause is—all of us. The human population has thrived, especially in the last several hundred years, and its progress has been marked by the increasing use and pollution of air, water, land, and even space.

The world has always experienced a certain level of natural environmental degradation. Erupting volcanoes, burning forests, floods, and other natural "disasters" over the centuries have caused changes in human, animal, and plant lives, changing the face of the environment and sometimes helping to cause the destruction of certain species. However, human population increases and industrial activities in only the last hundred years have caused such a manifold increase in pollution that there is now the danger that the earth will soon no longer be able to absorb the damage and, ultimately, restore the delicate balances that are necessary for a reasonably healthy environment.

Fortunately, the late 1980s witnessed a tremendous surge of public interest in environmental issues in the United States and in other countries. You are probably already aware of many of these issues, such as the incredible growth in human population, global warming and the greenhouse effect, thinning of the ozone layer in the earth's atmosphere, noise pollution, acid rain, and solid and chemical waste pollution. You may be wondering what you, as a lone individual, can possibly do about these huge problems. Believe it or not, if you are already pursuing a healthful lifestyle, you are already doing a great deal to slow environmental degradation. For example, by *not* smoking or consuming alcohol irresponsibly, you are *not* (1) polluting the air with tobacco smoke, (2) littering the ground with cigarette butts, (3) encouraging farmers to grow tobacco (and use pesticides to do so that degrade the land), (4) throwing beer cans, liquor bottles, and other packaging materials out of your car windows, (5) getting drunk, driving, and leaving your shattered car and your own shattered body by the side of the road for someone else to clean up.

Of course, there is much more that you can do to help slow the environmental degradation that threatens all of us. As we move into the next century, it is up to you to keep interest in environmental issues alive. You can and should take responsibility for your own interactions with the environment, and you should help other people realize that they, too, can do much to help. We can only give you limited information about these issues here, but we encourage you to make learning about the earth's environment a life-long pursuit.

Air Pollution

Polluted air affects the health of all living creatures, including human beings, and is responsible for a significant number of human deaths and illnesses (see Table 21.1)[1]. About 800 million tons of pollutants enter the atmosphere each year, consisting of approximately 38 percent carbon monoxide, 22 percent sulfur oxide, 17 percent particulate matter, 14 percent hydrocarbons, and 9 percent nitrogen oxides. Automobiles, factories, and power-generating plants, in that order, are the major sources of air pollution. Pollutants also produce chemical reactions from contact with sunlight, heat, and air. In addition, trash and garbage disposal, energy

Year 2000 National Health Objective

In recognition of the health advantages of clean air, one national health objective seeks to reduce human exposure to criteria air pollutants to a minimum of 85 percent of the people who live in counties that have not exceeded any EPA standard for air quality in the previous 12 months. Approximately 49.7 percent met this objective in 1988.

TABLE 21.1

Health Effects of Regulated Air Pollutants

Criteria Pollutants	Health Concerns
Ozone	Respiratory tract problems such as difficult breathing and reduced lung function. Asthma, eye irritation, nasal congestion, reduced resistance to infection, and possibly premature aging of lung tissue.
Particulate Matter	Eye and throat irritation, bronchitis, lung damage, and impaired visibility.
Carbon Monoxide	Ability of blood to carry oxygen impaired. Cardiovascular, nervous, and pulmonary systems affected.
Sulfur Dioxide	Respiratory tract problems, permanent harm to lung tissue.
Lead	Retardation and brain damage, especially in children.
Nitrogen Dioxide	Respiratory illness and lung damage.

Hazardous Air Pollutants

Asbestos	A variety of lung diseases, particularly lung cancer.
Beryllium	Primary lung disease, although also affects liver, spleen, kidneys, and lymph glands.
Mercury	Several areas of the brain as well as the kidneys and bowels affected.
Vinyl Chloride	Lung and liver cancer.
Arsenic	Causes cancer.
Radionoclides	Causes cancer.
Benzene	Leukemia.
Coke Oven Emissions	Respiratory cancer.

Source: Environmental Protection Agency, "Environmental Progress and Challenges: EPA's Update" (Washington, D.C.: EPA, Office of Policy Planning and Evaluation, August 1988), p. 13.

sources (coal and oil), and industrial chemical by-products compound the problem.

Global Warming and the Greenhouse Effect

At the 1990 global climate conclave in Geneva, scientists from around the world officially warned government officials of an environmental disaster that had been discussed in academic circles, in the media, and by the general population of the world for several years: that the atmospheric buildup of carbon dioxide, through the burning of fossil fuels (such as coal, oil, and natural gas) and the destruction of rain forests, is producing a long-term irreversible change in the earth's atmosphere. This change, referred to as **global warming,** is a gradual heating up of the earth's atmosphere. The mechanics of this warming are commonly referred to as the **greenhouse effect,** because the buildup of carbon dioxide acts like the glass of a greenhouse, letting in and trapping the sun's warmth (see Figure 21.1).

Compounding the problems of global warming and the greenhouse effect is the gradual destruction of the earth's atmospheric **ozone layer.** Ozone is a gas formed when nitrogen dioxide interacts with hydrogen. At ground level, ozone is actually a harmful pollutant that irritates the respiratory system, injures or kills people with chronic diseases, and destroys crops and vegetation. In the upper atmosphere, however, the ozone layer protects the earth's living creatures and vegetation from the intense ultraviolet radiation given off by the sun (see Figure 21.2). Chlorofluorocarbons or CFCs (chlorine, fluorine, and carbon, which are used as coolants for refrigerators and air conditioners and as propellants for aerosol spray cans and in electrical cleansers) and halon (industrial chemicals containing bromine) break down the ozone layer. A huge and growing hole in the ozone layer has been detected over the Antarctica.

What does global warming mean? Global warm-

FIGURE 21.1 • The Greenhouse Effect Traps Solar Heat.

Source: Environmental Protection Agency, "Environmental Progress and Challenges: EPA's Update" (Washington, D.C.: EPA, Office of Policy Planning and Evaluation, August 1988), p. 38.

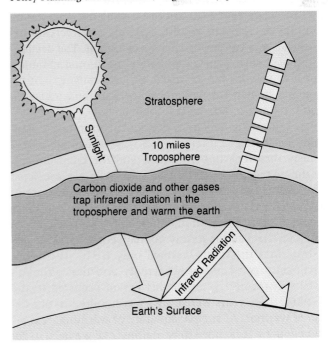

acid rain Rain that is more acidic than rain usually is or should be; a health hazard in all areas of the industrialized world.

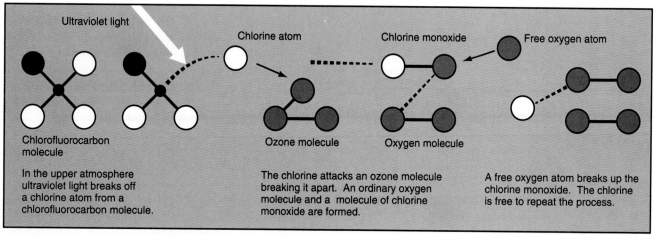

FIGURE 21.2 • How Ozone Is Destroyed.
Source: Environmental Protection Agency, ''Environmental Progress and Challenges: EPA's Update'' (Washington, D.C.: EPA, Office of Policy Planning and Evaluation, August 1988), p. 39.

ing is already believed to be partly responsible for rising sea levels and the erosion of many coastal areas. In the near future, the melting of alpine glaciers and polar ice sheets and the expansion of the ocean due to heating are expected to raise sea levels two to seven feet by the year 2100. A seven foot rise would inundate 50 to 80 percent of U.S. coastal wetlands, destroying untold numbers of wildlife habitats and recreational beaches and ruining coastal development. The destruction of the ozone layer will allow additional radiation to flow unimpeded to earth's surface, causing vast increases in skin cancers and rendering important agricultural areas arid and less productive.

Not everyone agrees that global warming is actually occurring or that, even if it is occurring, it seriously threatens human health and the environment. Climate models from the 1980s, for example, predicted an average warming of 4.2 degrees Celsius because of doubled carbon dioxide emissions. According to these models, the earth should now have warmed about 2.5°C. This has apparently not happened. Some studies show that the earth warmed only 0.3°C in the last half-century of industrial activity and that although the six warmest years of this period occurred in the 1980s, these years were only a few hundredths of a degree warmer. At such a slow rate of warming, it is argued, there is no need to be alarmed. All we need to do,

some advocates say, is wait until we have developed new technologies to replace older, polluting technologies and to clean up the mess we seem to be making now. Everything will work itself out in the end.

Although you must make up your own mind about these issues, we urge you to use a little common sense. Even if global warming is only a theoretical reality, we can all experience the direct effects of air pollution every day. We also know for certain the causes and effects of acid rain, radon, and indoor air pollution.

Acid Rain

A health hazard in all areas of the industrialized world, **acid rain** begins with emissions of sulfur dioxide (from coal-burning power plants) and nitrogen oxides (from motor vehicles and coal-burning power plants) that interact with sunlight and water vapor in the upper atmosphere to form acid compounds. During a storm, these compounds fall as acid rain or snow, or they join dust or other dry airborne particles and fall as dry deposition. Scientists blame hydrogen peroxide in the summer months for 70 to 80 percent of the transformation of sulfur dioxide from power plant and industrial smokestacks into sulfuric acid. Ozone is believed to be responsible for the remaining acid rain.

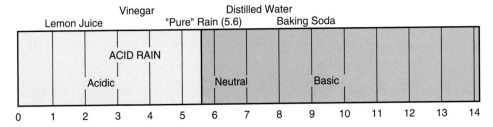

The pH scale ranges from 0 to 14. A value of 7.0 is neutral. Readings below 7.0 are acidic; readings above 7.0 are alkaline. The more pH decreases below 7.0, the more acidity increases.

Because the pH scale is logarithmic, there is a tenfold difference between one number and the one next to it. Therefore, a drop in pH from 6.0 to 5.0 represents a tenfold increase in acidity, while a drop from 6.0 to 4.0 represents a hundredfold increase.

All rain is slightly acidic. Only rain with a pH below 5.6 is considered "acid rain."

FIGURE 21.3 ◆ How "Acid" Is Acid Rain?

Source: Environmental Protection Agency, "Environmental Progress and Challenges: EPA's Update" (Washington, D.C.: EPA, Office of Policy Planning and Evaluation, August 1988), p. 28.

The majority of sulfur dioxide emissions (80 percent or more) originate in the thirty-one states east of or bordering the Mississippi River. Winds carry emissions to the Northeast. Depending on the "acidity" of the rainwater (see Figure 21.3), acid rain can damage soil, surface water, aquatic life, forests, and agricultural products.

Radon

Occurring naturally from the radioactive decay of radium-226 found in many types of rocks and soils, the major portion of indoor radon comes from the rocks and soil around buildings. Radon enters through cracks or openings in the foundation or basement. Well water and building materials account for additional sources. Radon levels vary throughout the United States and often within the same community depending upon soil concentrations, construction techniques, and ventilation. Figure 21.4 identifies the areas with potentially high radon levels in the United States. Inhaled radon particles have been shown to release ionizing radiation that damages lung tissue and leads to cancer. Some experts feel that radon is the leading cause of lung cancer among nonsmokers, responsible for 5,000 to 20,000 deaths each year. According to the EPA, over 8 million homes have radon levels exceeding four picocuries per liter of air.[2]

Indoor Air Pollution

Besides radon, other forms of indoor air pollution are becoming a major health issue. In tightly constructed, energy efficient structures, indoor pollutants may be higher than outdoor pollutants. Ventilation and the type, mixture, and amount of pollutants all play a role in adding airborne pathogens (such as viruses, bacteria, and fungi) and inorganic compounds (such as formaldehyde, chloroform, and perchlorethylene) to the air. Tobacco smoke, asbestos, biological pollutants bred in heating, ventilation, and air conditioning and humidifying systems, and pesticides cause most of the problems.

The Effects of Air Pollution

Polluted air makes the eyes water, burns the throat, and irritates the respiratory system, causing coughing, chest discomfort, and impaired breathing. Carbon monoxide interferes with the ability of blood cells to carry oxygen and impairs the function of the central nervous system. Air pollution also causes serious problems for those with preexisting conditions, such as asthma, heart disease, chronic bronchitis, and emphysema. Asbestos fibers in the air have been associated with bronchogenic cancer, mesothelioma, and other forms of malignancy. Airborne mercury, used in batteries, mildew proofing, and the production of paint, pulp, and paper, affects the central nervous system.

Year 2000 National Health Objective

Because of the relationship of home pollutants to health, one national health objective seeks to increase to at least 40 percent the proportion of homes in which occupants have tested for radon concentrations. The goal is to have these homes pose a minimal risk or to have these homes modified to reduce risk to health. In 1989, less than 5 percent of homes had been tested. In addition, a national health objective has been identified to expand to a minimum of thirty-five the number of states in which 75 percent of local jurisdictions have adopted construction standards and techniques to minimize elevated radon levels in new building areas that are determined to have elevated levels.

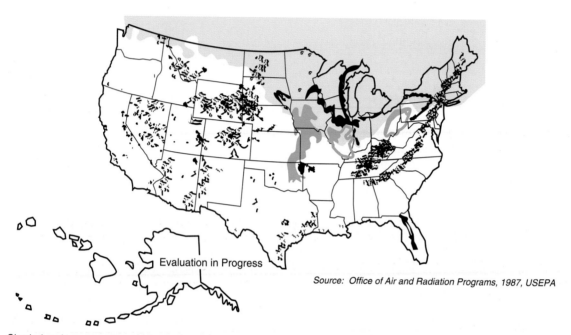

Evaluation in Progress

Source: Office of Air and Radiation Programs, 1987, USEPA

Shaded regions are areas which may have the greatest chance of producing high radon levels and the largest number of high radon levels

This map should not be used as the sole source for any radon predictions. This map cannot be used to predict locations of high radon in specific localities or to identify individual homes with high radon levels.

Local variations, including soil permeability and housing characteristics, will strongly affect indoor radon levels and any regional radon prediction.

This map is only preliminary and will be modified as research progresses.

Areas outside of shaded regions are not free of risk from elevated indoor radon levels.

Extent of continental glaciation

Geologic areas with known or expected indoor radon levels; granitic rocks, black shales, phosphatic rocks, near surface distribution of potential uranium sources.

Areas with scattered occurences of uranium bearing coals and shale

FIGURE 21.4 • Areas with Potentially High Radon Levels.

Source: Environmental Protection Agency, Environmental Progress and Challenges: EPA's Update''
(Washington, D.C.: EPA, Office of Policy Planning and Evaluation, August 1988), p. 35.

Air Pollution Legislation and Research

Because automobiles and industrial plants have been major sources of air pollution in the United States, environmentalists pressed Congress to pass a series of Clean Air Acts in 1963, 1965, and 1970. These laws required car manufacturers to cut auto emissions drasti-cally and encouraged states and cities to set up programs to reduce pollution from stationary sources. Emission control devices on automobiles have had a beneficial effect. According to the Environmental Protection Agency (EPA), from 1972 to 1977, even though more people were driving, smog levels remained stable. Ground level ozone or ''smog'' has been diffi-cult to control. The greatest success has been the reduction of lead in the air, an 87 percent decrease from 1977 to 1988. Nationwide levels of ozone, carbon monoxide, airborne particulates, sulfur dioxide, and nitrogen oxides have also declined.

The new Clean Air Act signed by President George Bush in November 1990 tightened restrictions on toxic air pollution, urban smog, and emissions causing acid rain. The bill's acid-rain provisions also placed a nationwide cap on sulfur-dioxide emissions from electric utilities. Companies that meet the new standards are given financial incentives to sell their "right" to emit a certain number of tons of sulfur dioxide annually. Those that become cleaner than the bill requires may either sell untapped credits or "bank" them for future use. This phase of the bill provides financial incentives for industry to go beyond federal standards. Competent engineers can now be assigned to the problem without undue expense to industry. It is estimated that this approach could reduce the overall cost of acid rain cleanup by $2 to $3 billion annually. Questions as to whether the incentive program can be properly policed and if it is wise to create a system of entitlements to pollute are being raised by skeptics. To date, however, experiments with tradable permits have shown promising results.

Global warming and the greenhouse effect require a carefully planned, long-range approach. Because CFCs and halon remain in the atmosphere for 175 to 200 years, correcting the problem requires a long-term commitment. To date, the only ballot proposition to cut CO_2 emissions drastically, the "Big Green" proposition in the state of California, was defeated by 26 percentage points, a margin of defeat worse than the Democratic presidential defeats of 1972 and 1984. At the Geneva conference, twenty governments did pledge to reduce their carbon dioxide emissions. Japan and Germany, for example, are vigorously working on energy-saving technologies to slash fossil-fuel use, the main source of troublesome emissions, and to secure a large piece of the technological future. Since 1974, the use of aerosols has declined. Industry has also shifted to substitute low-cost chemicals and to eliminate the nonessential use of CFCs as propellants, as mandated in 1978 by the EPA. Unfortunately, other uses of CFCs are growing. Only the United States, Canada, and a small number of European nations have banned CFC use in aerosols.

It is likely that mandated action will be required if we are ever to have really clean air. Nevertheless, individuals do have an important role to play. Exploring Your Health 21.1 asks you to consider your role in this effort.

Clean Air: Our Responsibility

Although it might seem that the problem of air pollution is insurmountable, we as individuals and as groups of individuals working together can make a difference. Consider the following possibilities, which are under our control:

- **Bicycling, walking, and using other nonpolluting transportation.** Evidence linking exercise and health is additional encouragement to walk, jog, run, or bicycle to work, if you live only a few miles away.

- **Using public transportation (buses, subways).** This approach would reduce the number of autos on the highway.

- **Purchasing a smaller car or one with a four-cylinder engine.** Small autos burn less fuel and produce less pollution than large cars.

- **Tuning your automobile engine frequently.** A well-tuned engine using lead-free gasoline emits fewer harmful by-products.

- **Owning one car instead of two.**

- **Avoiding open trash and incinerator burning.**

- **Abstaining from smoking tobacco.**

- **Reducing the use of volatile chemicals and cleaners in the home.** Household dust should be carefully emptied into a receptacle to avoid dispersion in the air.

Exploring Your Health 21.1

How Can You Help Clean Up the Air?

Before reading the suggestions in the section titled "Clean Air: Our Responsibility," write down as many ways as you can think of to contribute to cleaner air. You might consider your driving and car care habits, whether or not you smoke, and what role you could play in keeping the pressure on politicians.

decibel A measure of sound based on the pressure of sound on the human ear; 1 decibel is the faintest sound a person can hear; 120 decibels will produce physical pain in the ears.

- **Using the fireplace sparingly; burning dry wood instead of cannel coal.**
- **Driving your car less.** Avoiding unnecessary trips, combining shopping with other errands, riding a bike, walking, carpooling, and using public transportation will significantly reduce car use and exhaust emissions.
- **Planting a tree for the future and protecting the trees on your property.** Trees help cool cities, buffer noise, provide shelter and food for wildlife, and convert atmospheric carbon dioxide into oxygen. Organize a community tree planting day or join the "Global ReLeaf" campaign (dial 1-800-368-5748), a national program to reduce the greenhouse effect. Trunks and roots need protection from lawnmowers and weed eaters, mulch should be used under trees, and excavation should be avoided around the roots.
- **Testing your house and business site for radon.** Use one of the EPA approved standard methods for measuring radon levels, such as the carbon canister, to collect radon samples. Visit your local hardware store for home testing kits. To date, only a small percentage of houses and public and commercial buildings have been tested. States must step up their activity in communicating the risks and encouraging the testing of all public buildings.
- **Avoiding the purchase of aerosol spray cans and questionable cleaning products.**
- **Avoiding the burning of refuse, leaves, or trash.**

Noise Pollution

The American public is exposed to numerous sources of harmful loud sounds that produce both auditory effects (hearing loss) and nonauditory effects (stress, psychological problems, and loss of the ability to function in everyday life). Urban dwellers live with the sounds of jackhammers, garbage trucks, and automobiles. Many suburbanites have to endure the sound of freeway traffic, airplanes taking off and landing, and power mowers. In addition, the average person is also a victim of recreational noise from personal stereos, crowds, concerts, and other entertainment in close

Year 2000 National Health Objective

Because of increasing levels of noise in the workplace, the federal government is striving to reduce to no more than 15 percent the proportion of workers exposed to average daily noise levels that exceed 85 decibels.

quarters. Nonauditory problems seem to occur more from "uncontrolled" sounds such as traffic, trucks, automobiles, jets, emergency vehicles, crowd noises, and so forth. At what point is noise so loud as to be dangerous? The pressure of sound on the ear is measured in **decibels** (dB), an arbitrary unit based on the faintest sound that a person can hear. The scale is logarithmic,

Urban environments are dangerous places for the ears. Noise pollution is responsible not only for auditory problems, but also for nonauditory problems such as increased stress.

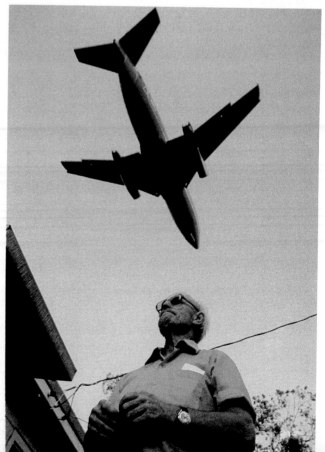

Decibels. A decibel is an arbitrary unit based on the faintest sound that a person can hear. The scale is logarithmic, so that an increase of 10 db means a tenfold increase in sound intensity, a 20 db rise a hundredfold increase, and a 30 db rise a thousandfold increase.

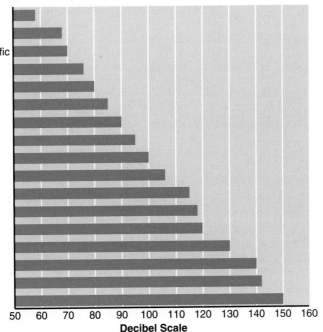

FIGURE 21.5 ♦ Common Sounds and Their Decibel Rating.

so that an increase of 10 dB means a tenfold increase in sound intensity, an increase of 20 dB means a hundredfold increase, and an increase of 30 dB means a thousandfold increase. Prolonged exposure to sounds above 70 dB is quite annoying, eight hours of exposure to 90 or more decibels produces hearing damage, and eight hours of exposure to 100 decibels produces serious damage. The hearing pain threshold is reached at about 120 decibels; eardrums may rupture at 150 decibels or more. Damage may occur with or without apparent symptoms.

Figure 21.5 lists decibel ratings for some common sounds. Gunfire (140 + decibels) is the greatest cause of recreational hearing loss, followed by rock concerts (110 to 120 decibels at a distance of four to six feet). One bullet fired is equivalent to one week's exposure to hazardous job noise; 50 bullets fired are equivalent to one year of exposure. There are also reported cases of up to 30 percent hearing loss after exposure to one rock concert. Hearing loss is common among both performers and audiences. Personal stereos played at the 100 decibel level have produced permanent hearing loss in 5 to 10 percent of users. Over 50 percent of incoming college freshmen have been shown to suffer hearing loss in the high frequency range, and their hearing capability is equivalent to that of individuals in the seventh decade of life. Hearing damage among employees in industry is also common, costing millions of dollars each year in industrial compensation.

Budget cutbacks, including the near elimination of the EPA's noise pollution control budget, has hampered the control of noise pollution in the United

Exploring Your Health 21.2

Has Exposure to Noise Decreased Your Hearing?

Surprising as it may seem, it is not unusual to find college students with impaired hearing. In some cases, these problems are related to social habits. Answer the following questions about your social environment. If you respond with "yes" to two or more questions, have your hearing checked through the health education department or nurse in your institution.

_____ Do you attend rock concerts?

_____ Do you frequent establishments that play loud music?

_____ Do you listen to your stereo with the volume turned very high?

_____ Do you live or work around loud noises, such as construction or major industry?

_____ Do you sit up front when you go to the movies?

silt The soil that is eroded and washed away from the earth's surface by the runoff of precipitation.

States. Although noises on newer models of jet plane engines, motorcycles and other motorized vehicles, and vacuum cleaners have been reduced, legislation to enforce control in factories and other buildings is lacking. Fortunately, individuals can reduce noise levels and protect their hearing by taking a few precautions:

- If you're at a rock concert, sit as far away as possible from the band.
- Learn to enjoy listening to music at home at moderate volume.
- Put drapes over windows to reduce street noises.
- Choose acoustical tile for ceilings and walls when building a house or adding a room.
- Use floor carpeting or select an apartment with carpeting in all rooms adjacent to other units.
- Locate noise-making appliances away from bedrooms, den, and living room.
- Select home sites or apartments away from truck routes, airports, industry, and business areas.
- Use special ear plugs on the job, in crowds, at rock concerts, and so forth that remove excessive sound and can actually improve hearing.

Water Pollution

Public water supplies come from rivers, lakes, underground waters, and various upland sources. The quality of water from remote upland sources tends to be excellent because it often travels hundreds of miles through unpopulated areas. Unfortunately, this is not true of our rivers and lakes, into which modern industrial society has discharged domestic sewage, industrial wastes (toxic chemicals), and agricultural wastes (animal excrement, fertilizers, insecticides, and liquid wastes from slaughterhouses and canning and packing plants). In addition, the soil erosion caused by the runoff of precipitation from the land, referred to as **silt,** provides a naturally occurring discharge into stream beds. Silt can keep needed sunlight out of water and smother the bottom-dwelling organisms. Oil spillage from the more than 1 billion tons of oil shipped by sea each year is also a major source of water pollution. Oil spillage causes damage to marine and bird life, and some clean-up methods cause even greater damage to plants and animals.

Efforts to provide safe drinking water for humans and safe surface water for fish, vegetation, and wildlife involves minimizing the contamination of ground water and surface water and monitoring and treating drinking water prior to consumption.

Drinking Water

Ground Water *Ground water* is merely precipitation that seeps into the ground. It is used for drinking by 50 percent of all Americans (120 million people; 95 percent of rural Americans). Since 1970, every state in the nation has found contaminated ground water. The current contamination and vast potential for contamination of ground water is shown in Figure 21.6. Potential contamination may come from 29,000 hazardous waste sites, millions of septic systems (one-fourth of all homes in the United States), over 180,000 surface impoundments (pits, ponds, and lagoons), approximately 500 hazardous waste land disposal facilities, 16,000 municipal and other landfills, 5 to 6 million underground storage tanks (hundreds of thousands of which are estimated to be leaking), thousands of underground injection wells, and millions of tons of ground pesticides and fertilizers.[3] Many of these sources po-

Year 2000 National Health Objective

To improve the quality of the nation's drinking water, one national health objective seeks to increase to at least 85 percent the proportion of people who receive a supply of drinking water that meets the safe drinking water standards established by the EPA. In 1988, 74 percent of the 58,099 community water systems serving about 80 percent of the population met these standards. Another objective seeks to reduce outbreaks of waterborne diseases from infectious agents and chemical poisons to no more than eleven per year. Thirty-one outbreaks per year occurred during the 1981 to 1988 period.

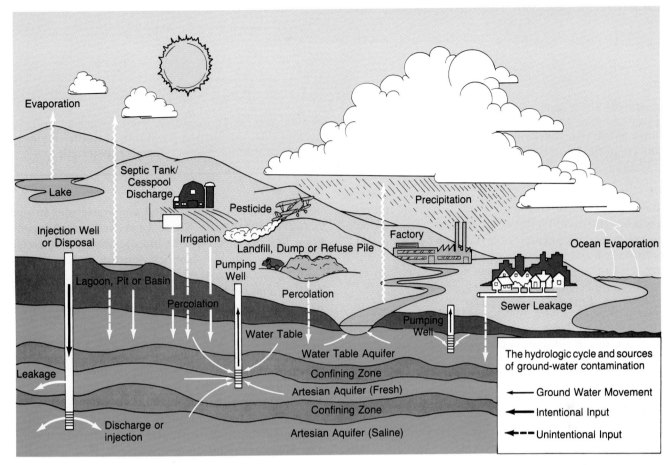

FIGURE 21.6 • Sources of Ground Water Contamination

tentially contain hundreds of chemicals that could reach ground water and contaminate drinking water wells. The EPA is primarily concerned with man-made toxic chemicals, such as synthetic organic chemicals, that contaminate some of the 40,000 community public water systems and 13 million private wells. EPA findings to date have been alarming. As many as 3,000 public water supplies using ground water exceeded EPA standards for inorganic substances, particularly fluoride and nitrates; 20 percent of all public water supply wells and 29 percent of those in urban areas had detectable levels of at least one volatile organic chemical. Sixty pesticides have been detected at various levels of contamination in 30 states, and 13 organic chemicals confirmed as carcinogens have been detected in drinking water wells.

Surface Waters   *Surface water* refers to precipitation that runs into streams, rivers, or lakes rather than filtered into the ground or evaporated. Surface water is contaminated by sewage treatment plants and factory discharges of wastes. While there have been improvements, high levels of toxic chemicals are still found in many lakes and streams. Fish living in these areas have been found with cancerous growths. Pollutants in our nation's waterways impair human health, destroy

aquatic life, and devalue recreational and aesthetic potentials. The major sources of such pollution are shown in Figure 21.7. Due to EPA efforts, conventional pollutant contamination is being fairly well controlled. Unfortunately, efforts are not keeping pace with population growth, and many lakes, rivers, and streams remain threatened.

Drinking Water at the Tap   Ground water and surface water are the main sources of tap water in the United States. Although cholera and typhoid have been eliminated in the United States, a number of contam-

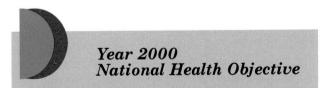

Year 2000 National Health Objective

In recognition of on-going surface water damage, one national health objective seeks to reduce potential risks to human health with a decrease to no more than 15 percent the proportion of assessed rivers, lakes, and estuaries that fail to support beneficial uses, such as fishing and swimming. In 1988, an estimated 25 percent did not support designated beneficial use.

wetlands Those lands that are adjacent to bodies of water and which are covered with water at certain times of the year; wetlands are very important resources of food and habitat for many organisms.

coastal waters Those waters from the coast to the head of tide, the farthest point inland where the influence of the tide on water levels is detected.

inants in our drinking water, such as lead, radionuclides, micro-biological contaminants, disinfection by-products, and underground injections of solid and hazardous waste, still impose health risks.

Critical Aquatic Habitats

The nation's wetlands, near coastal waters, oceans, and lakes are still in need of special protection.

Wetlands

Once regarded as wastelands, **wetlands** are now recognized as a valuable resource in our environment. In fact, wetlands are the most productive of all ecosystems. Wetland plants convert sunlight into material that serves as food for aquatic and terrestrial animals, and their land provides habitats for many forms of fish and wildlife. Wetlands improve and maintain water quality in adjacent water bodies by removing nutrients such as nitrogen and phosphorus to prevent the over-enrichment of waters. They filter harmful chemicals such as pesticides and heavy metals, and trap suspended sediments that would produce cloudiness in water. Wetlands have also been found to aid flood control by absorbing peak flows and releasing water slowly. Wetland vegetation reduces shoreline erosion. Wetlands also contribute $20 to $40 billion annually to the nation's economy through recreational and commercial fishing, hunting of waterfowl, and the production of cash crops such as rice and cranberries. In spite of their importance, our wetlands are diminishing at an alarming rate. Over 200 million acres to less than 100 million acres have been lost to agricultural development that involves drainage (responsible for 87 percent of the loss) and urban and other development. Wetlands are also threatened by chemical contamination and other forms of pollution.[4] Although government efforts have slowed wetland loss and contamination, our nation's wetlands are still threatened by loss of habitat.

Coastal Waters

Coastal waters encompass inland waters from the coast to the head of tide (the farthest point inland where the influence of tides on water level is detected). Such waters include bays, estuaries, coastal wetlands, and the coastal ocean to the point it is not affected by land and water uses in the coastal drainage basin. These waters and wetlands generate billions of dollars in income from commercial fishing, recreational fisheries, tourism, urban waterfront and private real estate development, recreational boating, and harbors. These areas also represent home to valuable fish, birds, and other wildlife. Destruction of coastal habitat has accelerated in recent years and coastal fishery, wildlife, and bird populations have been declining. Unfortunately these areas are highly vulnerable to contamination because they act as sinks for pollution from municipal sewage treatment plants, industrial plants, hazardous waste disposal areas, and they collect runoff from agricultural lands, suburban developments, city streets, and sewer and stormwater overflows. In addition, modifications from dredging channels, draining and filling wetlands, dam construction, diverting freshwater for irrigation and drinking, and shorefront construction further damage coastal environments.

Oceans and Lakes

Many countries and industries around the globe continue to dump dredged material, sewage sludge, industrial waste, and oil into oceans and lakes. Although ocean dumping of industrial waste has declined from 3 million tons in 1973 to 0.3 million tons in 1986, sewage sludge dumping increased from 5 million tons to 7.9 million tons during that same period. According to oceanographer Jacques Cousteau, we will see the death of the world's oceans in fewer than fifty years unless a cooperative effort is launched by all industrialized countries. Cousteau pointed out to the Senate Subcommittee on Oceans and the Atmosphere that ocean floors, which were free of chemicals little more than twenty years ago, are now almost devoid of living organisms. A long-term waste management strategy is needed that eventually eliminates the ocean as a dumping ground alternative.

Dealing with Water Pollution

Drinking water standards (taste, odor, color, turbidity, chemical, radiological, and bacteriological) have been established by the United States Public Health Service. Water treatment plants provide clean water relatively free from health hazards.

Common Pollutant Categories

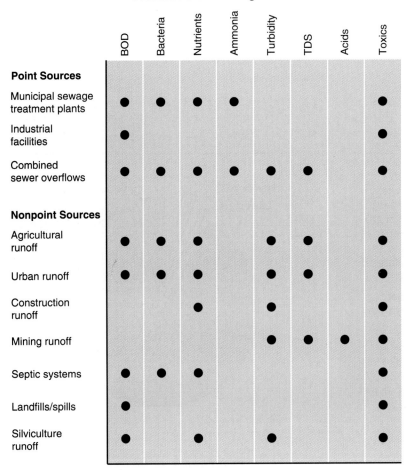

	BOD	Bacteria	Nutrients	Ammonia	Turbidity	TDS	Acids	Toxics
Point Sources								
Municipal sewage treatment plants	●	●	●	●				●
Industrial facilities	●							●
Combined sewer overflows	●	●	●	●	●	●		●
Nonpoint Sources								
Agricultural runoff	●	●	●		●	●		●
Urban runoff	●	●	●		●	●		●
Construction runoff			●		●			●
Mining runoff					●	●	●	●
Septic systems	●	●	●					●
Landfills/spills	●							●
Silviculture runoff	●		●		●			●

Source: Modified from 1986 305(b) National Report
Abbreviations: Biological Oxygen Demand, BOD; Total Dissolved Solids, TDS.

FIGURE 21.7 ◆ Pollutants and Their Sources.

Protection from waterborne infection is achieved either through purification of water supplies or treatment of waste before it enters water bodies. Purification has received the most emphasis to date, and improvement of waste treatment facilities is anticipated in the next decade. Strict enforcement of existing legislation and heavy fines could reduce contamination from industrial waste, agricultural waste, and oil spillage. There should also be increased emphasis on reuse of water, use of upstream land, restoration of land, land treatment, forest replenishment, topsoil conservation, and conversion of seawater to drinking water.

Individuals can significantly improve the safety and cleanliness of our water. Consider the following suggestions:[5]

- **Save water.** The overall demand for water can be reduced by fixing faucet leaks and leaking toilets, and by using water sparingly.
- **Maintain your septic system.** Untreated waste from failing septic systems can pollute waterways. If drains and toilets drain slowly or effluent seeps upward from the ground, your system needs attention.

- **Fertilize your lawn sparingly.** Excess fertilizer can run off into streams, rivers, and bays.
- **Reduce soil erosion on your property.** Plant trees and shrubs to reduce erosion and to soak up nutrients that pollute waterways. Install gravel ditches along driveways or patios to collect water, allowing it to filter into the soil. Resod bare patches as soon as possible, and grade all areas away from your house at a 1 percent slope or more.
- **Protect marine animals from plastic trash dangers.** Six-pack rings, fishing lines, plastic containers, balloons released into the air, and other items pose hazards to marine life who mistake these items for food or become entrapped in them.
- **Be a responsible boater.** Keep trash aboard in a closed container and avoid discharging boat sewage into waterways. Use pump-out stations at your marina and empty portable toilets at home. Avoid throwing any trash into lakes, streams, or oceans.
- **Use biodegradable detergents.**
- **Dispose of all household chemical products safely, according to the directions.** It is also

important to read the label before you purchase. Choose alternative, less harmful products whenever possible, and use the least toxic product. Dispose of chemicals in a landfill only after pouring the chemicals into a plastic container filled with kitty litter or stuffed with newspaper, allowing the chemicals to dry completely before disposal.

- **Have your drinking water tested.** If unsafe, purchase an effective filtering system or resort to bottled water for drinking.
- **Clean faucet openings on a regular basis.** Washing dishes, hands, and so forth splashes bacteria on the nozzle that can then enter the water.
- **Protect the environment at all times in your recreational use of water, land, and air.**

Solid and Chemical Waste Pollution

Household and Industrial Trash

Solid wastes produced by U.S. households and industries amount to approximately four to five pounds per person each day. More than 6 billion tons of agricultural, commercial, industrial, and domestic waste are produced each year in the United States (see Figure 21.8).[6] Most agricultural waste is plowed back into the land. Waste from industrial, municipal, utility, mining, and milling sources can pose a danger to public health and the environment. In our cities, the majority of this material is burned in large incinerators, while water-

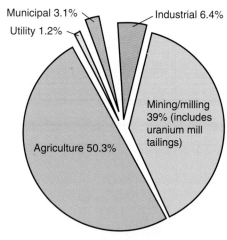

FIGURE 21.8 • 6 Billion Tons of Waste Are Generated in the United States Each Year (excludes high-level radioactive waste)
Source: Office of Solid Waste, EPA

front and harbor debris is carried out to sea or burned by private contractors. In some cities, as much as 40 percent of the municipal solid wastes are transported to dumps and landfill sites without passing through any incinerators. Another approach used has been to dump demolition materials into marshlands. As a result, it is estimated that cities use up land for solid wastes at a rate of one to two square miles per year.

In some cities, as much as 40 percent of municipal solid wastes are transported directly to dumps and landfill sites. Some cities use up land for the disposing of solid wastes at a rate of one to two square miles per year.

Year 2000 National Health Objective

In recognition of the relationship between solid waste and the water, air, and soil contamination problem in the United States, the federal government is striving to reduce human exposure to toxic agents from solid waste with a reduction in average pounds of municipal solid waste produced per person each day to no more than 3.6 pounds. A total of 4.0 pounds per person daily was produced in 1988.

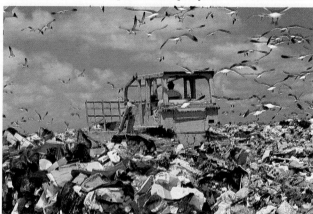

General Classification of Solid Waste Materials

Category	Description	Source
Garbage	Wastes from the preparation, cooking, and serving of food. Market refuse, waste from the handling, storage, and sale of produce and meats.	Households, institutions, and commercial concerns (hotels, stores, restaurants, markets, etc.).
Rubbish	Combustible (primarily organic): paper, cardboard, cartons, wood, boxes, excelsior, plastics, rags, cloth, bedding, leather, rubber, grass, leaves, yard trimmings. Noncombustible (primarily inorganic): metals, tin cans, metal foils, dirt, stones, bricks, ceramics, crockery, glass, bottles, other mineral refuse.	
Ashes	Residue from fires used for cooking and for heating buildings, cinders.	
Bulky wastes	Large auto parts, tires, stoves, refrigerators, other large appliances, furniture, large crates, trees, branches, palm fronds, stumps, flotage.	
Street refuse	Street sweepings, dirt, leaves, catch basin dirt, contents of litter receptacles.	Streets, sidewalks, alleys, vacant lots, etc.
Dead animals	Small animals: cats, dogs, poultry. Large animals: horses, cows.	
Abandoned vehicles	Automobiles, trucks.	
Construction and demolition wastes	Lumber, roofing, and sheathing scraps, rubble, broken concrete, plaster, conduit, pipe, wire, insulation.	
Industrial refuse	Solid wastes resulting from industrial processes and manufacturing operations (food-processing wastes; boiler house cinders; wood, plastic, and metal scraps and shavings, etc.).	Factories, power plants, etc.
Special wastes	Hazardous wastes: pathological wastes, explosives, radioactive materials. Security wastes: confidential documents, negotiable papers.	Households, hospitals, institutions, stores, industry, etc.
Animal and agricultural wastes	Manures, crop residues.	Farms, feed lots.
Sewage treatment residues	Coarse screenings, grit, septic tank sludge, dewatered sludge.	Sewage treatment plants, septic tanks.

Source: U.S. Environmental Protection Agency, Publication No. 2084, *Guidelines for Local Government on Solid-Waste Management* (Washington, D.C.: Government Printing Office, 1971), p. 42.

The general classification of solid waste materials, shown in Table 21.2, demonstrates the magnitude of the problem. These sources of solid waste pollution have led to the serious pollution problems in the United States.

Mercury

Although the human body can adapt to the trace concentrations of inorganic mercury found in the natural environment, it is unable to cope with the large amounts of organic mercury introduced into the environment by human technology. Mercury is a metal that has thousands of uses in agriculture and industry, such as protection of seeds against fungus growth, control of microorganisms that cause machinery damage, and control of mildew and bacteria growth. It is also used in paints, plastics, fluorescent lamps, tooth fillings, and many other products. According to the National Institute of Occupational Safety and Health, approximately 150,000 people in the United States are routinely exposed to mercury on the job.

lead poisoning (plumbism) A serious disease resulting from the ingestion or inhalation of lead; findings include weakness, anemia, brain damage, and mental retardation. Lead has been a serious pollutant of water, soil, and air.

Inorganic mercury causes damage to the liver, kidneys, and small intestine and creates difficulties in reabsorption and secretion. Organic mercury affects the parts of the brain that control vision, hearing, and balance. Symptoms of mercury poisoning are muscle weakness, loss of coordination, paralysis, blindness, deafness, and mental retardation. Children and developing embryos are most affected because of rapid cell growth.

Lead

It is estimated that over a million tons of lead per year are used in the manufacture of metal products, batteries, pesticides, solder for sealing food cans, and gasoline. **Lead poisoning (plumbism)** occurs as lead accumulates in the human body from the air, food, and water. The chief victims are children who live in older dwellings where the walls have been coated with lead paint. Small children have been poisoned from eating the lead-based paint flakes.

The high lead content in the environment is a problem that was created by and can also be solved by humans. Mandatory use of lead-free gasoline in newer-model autos, removal of lead paint in old buildings, and stricter control of industrial wastes are already helping to alleviate the problem. Individuals can also reduce the risk of lead poisoning by washing all fruits and vegetables carefully to remove traces of airborne lead dust, not purchasing food in cans sealed with lead soldering, not storing food in the original can (air deteriorates the soldered seam), preventing children from playing near heavily traveled roads where lead-loaded dust may be present, and covering walls that may contain lead-based paint with wallpaper.

Chemical Wastes

More than 1,500 new chemicals are produced each year, bringing the current total to more than 65,000 chemical substances on the market. Many of these products have been a boon to humanity, increasing longevity, decreasing suffering, and preventing and treating disease. Unfortunately, however, some 35,000 chemicals are classified by the Environmental Protec-

Year 2000 National Health Objective

Hazardous waste sites have been identified throughout the United States. A key national health objective seeks to eliminate significant health risks by using a national priority list hazardous sites as a measure of clean-up performance. In 1990, 1,082 sites were on the list, with health assessments conducted for approximately 1,000 of these.

tion Agency as either definitely or potentially hazardous to human health (see Table 21.3).[7]

A misconception by most Americans is that chemicals commonly used in houses, offices, and factories are safe because the government permits them to be manufactured and sold. The assumption is that someone is carefully testing the chemicals. The truth is that only ten to fifteen of the 1,500 chemicals introduced each year are studied for possible toxic effects on the brain and nervous system.[8] Chemicals may be effective, but they may also impose a significant health risk to users. More than 65,000 man-made chemicals are used in the workplace and home as cleaning fluids, solvents, paints, pesticides, and inks. Although the Toxic Substances Control Act requires chemical companies to notify the government when a new product is being manufactured and sold, the EPA does not require tests to be run on these and other chemicals unless there is some preexisting evidence of danger. Because new chemicals have no history, few are tested for toxicity. This loophole, combined with lack of funding, make the Toxic Substance Control Act inadequate to protect the public. According to a report of the National Academy of Sciences, poor toxicity data exists for 90 percent of all new chemicals used in industry and commerce. The effects of many chemicals on the market today will remain unknown due to the absence of toxicity data.

Of particular concern is the disposal of toxic wastes from mining and manufacturing. It is estimated that only 10 percent of hazardous chemical waste is being disposed of in a safe manner. The remaining 90

TABLE 21.3

Common Hazardous Wastes

Chemical	Use	Hazard
C-56	Bug and insect killer	Acutely toxic, suspected carcinogen
Trichloroethylene (TCE)	Degreaser	Suspected carcinogen
Benzidene	Dye industry	Known human carcinogen
Curene 442	Plastics industry	Suspected carcinogen
Polychlorinated biphenyls (PCBs)	Insulators, paints, and electrical circuitry	Acutely toxic, suspected carcinogen
Benzene	Solvent	Suspected carcinogen
Tris	Fire retardant	Suspected carcinogen
DDT	Bug and insect killer	Acutely toxic
Vinyl chloride	Plastics industry	Known human carcinogen
Mercury	Multiple uses	Acutely toxic
Lead	Multiple uses	Acutely toxic, suspected carcinogen
Carbon tetrachloride	Solvent	Acutely toxic, suspected carcinogen
Polybrominated biphenyls (PBBs)	Fire retardant	Effects unknown

Source: Council on Environmental Quality.

percent is being dumped indiscriminately and is certain to pose serious health problems in the future.

There is no way to determine just how many illegal toxic waste dumps exist. It is estimated that there are approximately 50,000 dump sites in the United States, about 2,000 of them posing serious health problems. Many are revealed only after flash floods, soil erosion that exposes rusting drums, or excavation.

In recent history, strong media coverage of environmental disasters such as those that happened at Love Canal, near Buffalo, New York, at Times Beach, Missouri, and at Bhopal, India, provide powerful, disturbing portraits of the suffering toxic environmental disasters can cause to entire communities.

At Love Canal, toxic industrial waste had been released into a waterway during the 1960s and 1970s until a pattern of cancers and birth defects in nearby residents was established. The entire town was evacuated and sat empty until 1991, when authorities deemed it "safe" for properties in Love Canal to be sold.

At Times Beach, dioxin, a highly toxic chemical waste, had been mixed with waste oils and spread on dirt roads to control dust. The dioxin worked its way

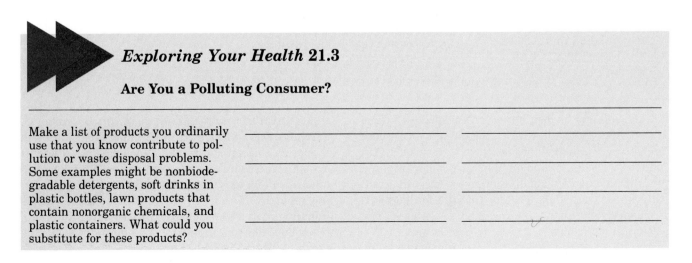

Exploring Your Health 21.3

Are You a Polluting Consumer?

Make a list of products you ordinarily use that you know contribute to pollution or waste disposal problems. Some examples might be nonbiodegradable detergents, soft drinks in plastic bottles, lawn products that contain nonorganic chemicals, and plastic containers. What could you substitute for these products?

Issues in Health

Who Are the NIMBYs, Anyway?

The unmarked garbage truck lumbered up the darkened street, past the "Dead End" sign. It turned right, onto the dirt road that mysteriously had received a thick coat of gravel from a parade of unmarked dump trucks only two days before. The road led into a densely wooded area marked for eventual development. Ten minutes later, the truck could be seen coming back out of the woods. It made more noise as it rolled by now, probably because it was empty....

This could be the beginning of a modern-day environmental horror story. It could easily be a true story. As landfills become fuller and fuller, and as individuals, businesses, and communities find it increasingly more difficult to dispose of their solid waste, several things are happening.

- Existing landfills and dumps are becoming overfilled or closing—forever.
- Cases of illegal dumping of solid and chemical waste are on the rise.
- Fierce battles are erupting in federal, state, and local governments about where to put solid, chemical, toxic, nuclear, and other kinds of waste.

- And many communities have banded together to do battle with state and federal governments who try to make those communities new sites for waste disposal.

This last phenomenon is often called the *NIMBY* syndrome. NIMBY stands for "Not-In-My-Back(-)Yard" and refers to individuals or communities who are opposed to having certain buildings or facilities located near their towns, villages, or cities. In this case, the "facilities" in question are for waste disposal. Most people who are NIMBYs with regard to waste disposal readily acknowledge that the world is facing a serious shortage of places to send and store all the waste that human activities produce. However, they are prepared to fight hard to force the waste to be placed somewhere else. They will argue that a waste disposal facility would not be fair or appropriate for a community filled with children, a community that pays a premium to live in the countryside, a community that keeps its own waste to a minimum, or a community that simply does not want to become a local big city's garbage dump.

Some people might call NIMBYs selfish or unrealistic. But think about it: would you really want to live near, say, a nuclear waste facility? Other people charge that businesses and wealthier, urban communities have plenty of money to "convince" poorer, suburban, or rural communities to take on their trash.

Still other people have suggested that we should simply place all of our waste where "no one" lives —like in the desert, or in space. Scientists from many disciplines remind us that it is not as simple as burying our trash in desert sands. In fact, the deserts of the world have extremely fragile ecosystems. And shooting trash into space would be ridiculously expensive (and besides, space is already full of junk!). As big as the world is, viable places for waste disposal are simply few and far between. Even the best-constructed landfills leak and can pollute the soil and groundwater.

What are your feelings and beliefs about NIMBYs? Are you a NIMBY? Why? Why not?

into the soil and its distribution was helped by a flood in December 1982, after which the Centers for Disease Control recommended that the town be evacuated. On January 3, 1983, President Ronald Reagan declared the entire town a federal disaster area. Today, the company whose waste dioxin caused this disaster has plans to clean up the town—then possibly use it as a toxic waste storage facility!

At Bhopal, India, a cloud of poison gas leaking from a nearby Union Carbide plant on December 3, 1984, formed around a 25-square-mile area. Although it appears that an alarm was signaled, some residents actually reacted by rushing toward the plant where relatives worked, only to breathe in more fatal gas, causing rapid swelling of moist lung tissue until victims literally drowned in their own fluids. Seventy funeral pyres burned throughout the day and night to handle the more than 2,000 dead bodies. Mass graves were overflowing, and hospitals, where more than 100,000 were treated, reported a death per minute. A nightmare had occurred—the worst chemical industry disaster in history.[9]

Pesticides and Herbicides

In 1958, a 50-year-old marine biologist named Rachel Carson started writing a book about the effects of deadly poisons on the living community. She would call this book *Silent Spring*, and its publication in 1962 would change the way a whole generation of people all over the world looked at pesticide use. Carson had spent most of her professional career working for the United States Fish and Wildlife Service. During that time, she and her colleagues had become alarmed at the increasing use of pesticides such as DDT and parathion (an organic phosphate). By the time she started work on *Silent Spring*, Carson was already a famous author, having published *The Sea Around Us* (1951) and *The Edge of the Sea* (1955). She had tried to interest various magazines in an article about the dangers of pesticide use. The *New Yorker* finally agreed to serialize parts of *Silent Spring*. Chemical companies attacked Rachel Carson brutally, labeling her a "hysterical" woman. However, President John F. Kennedy read the book and convened a special panel of his science advisory committee to investigate Carson's claims. This panel completely vindicated Carson's thesis that pesticides

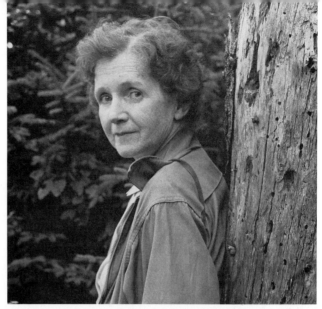

Rachel Carson was a quiet, thoughtful person who wrote a book called *Silent Spring*. The chemical industry attacked her with fury, but her book motivated an entire generation of people all over the world to become concerned about the use of pesticides.

were, in fact, causing great harm to human, animal, and plant populations in the United States and the world.

Today, pesticides and herbicides continue to pose a threat to the health of all living things and represent another kind of chemical "waste" pollution. Over three million pounds of pesticides are used in the United States each year (see Figure 21.9). Farmers use

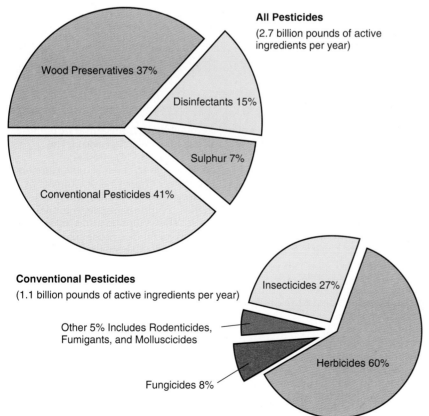

All Pesticides
(2.7 billion pounds of active ingredients per year)

Wood Preservatives 37%
Disinfectants 15%
Sulphur 7%
Conventional Pesticides 41%

Conventional Pesticides
(1.1 billion pounds of active ingredients per year)

Insecticides 27%
Other 5% Includes Rodenticides, Fumigants, and Molluscicides
Herbicides 60%
Fungicides 8%

FIGURE 21.9 • Pesticide Use in the United States (1986 Estimates)
Source: Office of Pesticide Programs, EPA

pesticides to improve crop yield through the control of weeds, insects, and plant diseases. Pesticides are also used by health officials to control the spread of disease by mosquitos and other insects. Unfortunately, any chemical capable of killing living organisms is also capable of causing serious damage to human life and the environment. Some pesticides survive for long periods of time and enter the food chain, eventually reaching the human diet. Others enter the soil and contaminate ground water. The EPA controls pesticide use through a registration process designed to evaluate and reduce health and environmental risks when used properly. The process involves a determination of whether the risks to health and the environment outweigh the benefits to society. Over 50,000 pesticide products are registered, many of which were used before their long-term health and environmental effects were understood. A 1972 amendment to the Federal Insecti-

cide, Fungicide, and Rodenticide Act (FIFRA) required existing pesticides to be reevaluated.[10]

The Food and Drug Administration sets allowable limits or "tolerance levels" for pesticide residues in food to protect human health. The EPA monitors the distribution and use of all pesticides and handles civil complaints and criminal penalties for violations of FIFRA regulations. Many uses of pesticides have been banned (see Table 21.4). As a result of EPA actions, levels of some pesticides have declined in humans and wildlife, and safer products have entered the market. Unfortunately, overall pesticide use is increasing and some insect pests seem to adapt and become resistant to their use. As a result, more and more deadly chemicals must be used to obtain the same effect, causing pesticide residues to continue to build up in our soil and enter the water supply.

Herbicides, such as the widely publicized Agent

A Question of Ethics

A Clean Environment: Who Pays?

In some countries, such as Switzerland and the Netherlands, the people expect and the government delivers clean air and water and undefiled land. Obviously, the technology needed to provide these benefits in the United States has long been available. The removal of environmental health hazards such as smog and air pollution would provide immediate relief to allergy sufferers and individuals with other breathing problems. The long-term benefits would translate into less disease and sickness and increased energy for millions of people.

Unfortunately, an all-out attack on pollution would involve substantial costs in the form of higher taxes and prices at a time when economic considerations receive higher priority than the quality of health and envi-

ronmental protection. Once again, it is argued, the nation's wealth seems more important than its health. Those who do emphasize individual health argue that a complete change in philosophy is needed. An economy based on consumption and waste is unsound. The public needs to become more aware of the causes of pollution and take action. Large corporations need to be forced into greater environmental responsibility. The creation of a clean, healthy environment must take priority over the profit motive. Some also feel that the individual citizen would not oppose increased taxation that translates into a cleaner, healthier environment. After all, industry has not created all pollution and should therefore not be burdened with all the cost. Individuals also pollute through smoking,

automobile use, unsanitary dumping, litter, and so forth, making the cleanup everyone's problem.

Opponents of strict environmental control argue that the impact of such policies on profits and taxes makes them impossible to implement. They point out that environmental standards cause too much economic displacement. Although the implementation of environmental control does increase the need for goods and services and create jobs, the economy suffers. An all-out attack on pollution can only occur with greatly increased taxation, which neither industry nor the private citizen is willing to accept.

What do you think? Are you willing to pay more taxes for a cleaner environment? Who should pay?

TABLE 21.4

A Number of Pesticides Have Been Taken Off the Market

Pesticides	Use	Concerns
Aldrin	Insecticide	Oncogenicity
Chlordane (Agricultural uses; termiticide uses suspended or cancelled)	Insecticide/Termites, Ants	Oncogenicity; reduction in non-target and endangered species
Compound 1080 (Livestock collar retained, rodenticide use under review)	Coyote control; Rodenticide	Reductions in non-target and endangered species; no known antidote
Dibromochloropropane (DBCP)	Soil Fumigant—Fruits and vegetables	Oncogenicity; mutagenicity; reproductive effects
DDT and related Compounds	Insecticide	Ecological (eggshell thinning); carcinogenicity
Dieldrin	Insecticide	Oncogenicity
Dinoseb (in hearings)	Herbicide/Crop dessicant	Fetotoxicity; reproductive effects; acute toxicity
Endrin (Avicide use retained)	Insecticide/Avicide	Oncogenicity; teratogenicity; reductions in non-target and endangered species
Ethylene Dibromide (EDB) (Very minor uses and use on citrus for export retained)	Insecticide/Fumigant	Oncogenicity; mutagenicity; reproductive effects
Heptachlor (Agricultural uses; termiticide uses suspended or cancelled)	Insecticide	Oncogenicity; reductions in non-target and endangered species
Kepone	Insecticide	Oncogenicity
Lindane (Indoor smoke bomb cancelled; some uses restricted)	Insecticide/Vaporizer	Oncogenicity; teratogenicity; reproductive effects; acute toxicity; other chronic effects
Mercury	Microbial Uses	Cumulative toxicant causing brain damage
Mirex	Insecticide/Fire Ant Control	Non-target species; potential oncogenicity
Silvex	Herbicide/Forestry, rights-of-way, weed control	Oncogenicity; teratogenicity; fetotoxicity
Strychnine (Rodenticide use and livestock collar retained)	Mammalian predator control; rodenticide	Reductions in non-target and endangered species
2,4,5-T	Herbicide/Forestry, rights-of-way, weed control	Oncogenicity; teratogenicity; fetotoxicity
Toxaphene (Livestock dip retained)	Insecticide—Cotton	Oncogenicity; reductions in non-target species; acute toxicity to aquatic organisms; chronic effects on wildlife

Oncogenicity—Causes tumors   Carcinogenicity—Causes cancer   Fetotoxicity—Causes toxicity to the unborn fetus
Mutagenicity—Causes mutation   Teratogenicity—Causes major birth defects

Source: Environmental Protection Agency, "Environmental Progress and Challenges: EPA's Update" (Washington, D.C.: Office of Policy Planning and Evaluation, 1988), p. 118.

Orange used by the U.S. military to clear jungles during the Vietnam War, are suspected of causing numerous health problems among Vietnam veterans and their offspring. The powerful Agent Orange was designed to clear away large areas of trees and other plant life to eliminate the enemy's ground cover. One of the ingredients of Agent Orange, dioxin, is highly poisonous and extremely toxic to human beings. There are now documented cases of thousands of veterans developing various disorders such as liver cancer, rashes, mood swings, memory problems, numbness, unexplained weight loss, and shortness of breath. In addition, wives of Vietnam veterans have experienced miscarriages and stillbirths, and offspring have been born with defects and abnormalities such as cleft palates, missing noses and eyes, blindness, deformities, and missing parts of the brain. More than 64,000 veterans attribute birth defects to Agent Orange exposure. Unfortunately, the Veterans Administration (VA) disagrees and continues to fight all such claims. In May 1989, a federal judge ordered the VA to reconsider the over 31,000 claims for health benefits made by veterans as a result of Agent Orange.

Dealing with Solid and Chemical Waste Pollution

The problem of toxic waste disposal is enormously difficult and will require concerted action by the federal and state governments. Severe penalties must be placed on industrial offenders who fail to comply with safe disposal techniques. At present, fines are not high enough to discourage inexpensive, hazardous methods of disposal. In addition, more government personnel are needed to enforce EPA regulations, visit industrial sites, and educate the business community on the least expensive and safest alternatives. New, inexpensive methods for safely disposing of chemical wastes must be found in the near future if the problem is to be solved. Industry should be provided with the financial incentive to conduct independent research in this area.

Congress has enacted a number of laws to regulate both the generation and the disposal of all hazardous wastes. The primary objectives of these laws are to ensure proper management and disposal of waste both now and in the future, to clean up sites where past practices are a threat to surrounding communities and the environment, to minimize the amount of waste, and to recycle materials. A number of important laws are also administered by the EPA to control major toxic chemicals (see Table 21.5).

The individual plays a vital role in minimizing solid waste pollution in the United States. Cooperative efforts in each household would produce significant results. A number of things are under your control:[11]

- **Reduce the amount of trash you discard.** Begin to purchase reusable items, such as coffee mugs instead of disposable cups, and cloth rags instead of paper towels; choose products with a minimum of packaging; and find other uses for packages whenever possible.
- **Focus on reusing and recycling instead of disposal.** Change your thinking from *disposal* as a first option to *reusing* and *recycling*. Think in terms of recycling instead of biodegradability. Products biodegrade very slowly if at all. Researchers have excavated from dumps newspapers that can still be read, and hot dogs, steaks, and vegetables that are relatively unchanged after 25 years. Recycling preserves natural resources, keeps valuable materials out of a landfill, lowers energy use, and is a constructive activity that does not hinder busy lives.

  Numerous materials can be recycled: glass, paper, metals (beverage and food cans, car battery metals), motor oil, rubber, plastics, yard waste (such as grass clippings and leaves), and furniture and appliances (refrigerators, chairs, and the like). Glass should be rinsed and separated by color; plastics and metals rinsed, flattened, and stored; motor oil stored in a clean, sealed container; newspapers stacked and tied in 8" to 12" bundles; and corrugated cardboard flattened, stacked, tied in bundles, and stored without staples. Once you have prepared and separated your recyclable materials, you can utilize a number of recycling systems, such as curbside collection, drop-off and buy-back centers, commercial pickup, service stations, retailers, charities, thrift stores, and shelters. You can even repair many items yourself. Find out how your community is handling recycling and get involved by sharing your enthusiasm, buying recycled goods, encouraging local officials, organ-

TABLE 21.5

Major Toxic Chemical Laws Administered by EPA

Statute	Provisions
Toxic Substances Control Act	Requires that EPA be notified of any new chemical prior to its manufacture and authorizes EPA to regulate production, use, or disposal of a chemical.
Federal Insecticide, Fungicide and Rodenticide Act	Authorizes EPA to register all pesticides and specify the terms and conditions of their use, and remove unreasonably hazardous pesticides from the marketplace.
Federal Food, Drug and Cosmetic Act	Authorizes EPA in cooperation with FDA to establish tolerance levels for pesticide residues on food and food products.
Resource Conservation and Recovery Act	Authorizes EPA to identify hazardous wastes and regulate their generation, transportation, treatment, storage, and disposal.
Comprehensive Environmental Response, Compensation and Liability Act	Requires EPA to designate hazardous substances that can present substantial danger and authorizes the cleanup of sites contaminated with such substances.
Clean Air Act	Authorizes EPA to set emission standards to limit the release of hazardous air pollutants.
Clean Water Act	Requires EPA to establish a list of toxic water pollutants and set standards.
Safe Drinking Water Act	Requires EPA to set drinking water standards to protect public health from hazardous substances.
Marine Protection Research and Sanctuaries Act	Regulates ocean dumping of toxic contaminants.
Asbestos School Hazard Act	Authorizes EPA to provide loans and grants to schools with financial need for abatement of severe asbestos hazards.
Asbestos Hazard Emergency Response Act	Requires EPA to establish a comprehensive regulatory framework for controlling asbestos hazards in schools.
Emergency Planning and Community Right-to-Know Act	Requires states to develop programs for responding to hazardous chemical releases and requires industries to report on the presence and release of certain hazardous substances.

Source: Environmental Protection Agency, "Environmental Progress and Challenges: EPA's Update" (Washington, D.C.: EPA, Office of Policy Planning and Evaluation, 1988), p. 113.

izing friends and neighbors, finding markets for various materials, avoiding extra packaging in your purchases, limiting your purchases, and starting a compost pile to recycle vegetable peels and lawn clippings.[12]

- **Recycle at home and at work.** Contact your local government to find out what recycling services are available in your community or call the Department of Waste Management's recycling hotline: 1-800-KEEP-ITT. Develop a system for delivery or pickup of newspaper, cardboard, aluminum, glass, paper, and plastics.

- **Purchase and use household chemical products wisely.** Read all labels carefully and follow directions for both use and disposal. Purchase nonhazardous alternatives whenever possible when buying paints, solvents, cleaners, and pesticides. Deliver your used motor oil to an Amoco gas station or other station that recycles oil; avoid pouring oil onto the ground or discarding it unsafely.

Nuclear Waste: In a Class by Itself

The problem of what to do with spent nuclear fuel and other radioactive materials has plagued the federal government since the first commercial nuclear power plant was built in 1957. To date, more than 10,000 metric tons of spent fuel have accumulated at nuclear power plants. This amount is expected to quadruple by the year 2000. The Nuclear Waste Policy Act of 1982 requires the Department of Energy (DOE) to select nine possible disposal sites and rank the top three. A number of sites are now being tested throughout the United States. Sites must be capable of storing at least 70,000 metric tons for 10,000 years (the time needed for the radioactivity to decay to harmless levels).

It is little wonder that states do not want to be selected and will resist federal moves to deliver and store these potentially dangerous wastes on their land. To date, the public has been given little reason to believe that its safety and health will be guaranteed.

Radiation

Humans have always been exposed to small amounts of radiation in nature. About 58 percent of our exposure comes from natural sources (radioactive gases released by soil and rock formations, cosmic rays, and radioactive agents in the atmosphere from sun flares), and about 41 percent comes from human-made sources (x-rays, luminous wristwatches, color television, radar, nuclear weapons testing, uranium mines, mills and fabrication plants, and various electronic devices). Nuclear power plants account for less than 0.15 percent of human-made radiation, and about 1 percent comes from nuclear fallout. The greatest single source of human-made radiation is medical x-rays. Radiation is beneficial in medical diagnosis, treatment, and research. Unfortunately, its use carries some health-risks to the patient, technician, and researchers.

Three types of radiation are harmful to health:

1. **Alpha particles** are potentially dangerous, but they cannot penetrate the skin or body except through inhalation or a cut.

2. **Beta particles** can penetrate the skin but not deeply enough to damage internal organs.

3. **Gamma rays** (similar to x-rays) pose the main threat to human health because they can easily penetrate the body and its major organs.

Even small amounts of radiation can cause damage to the genetic structure of cells. Low-level radiation is also suspected of causing skeletal abnormalities, bone marrow damage, eye damage (cataracts), leukemia, and other types of cancer. Exposure to large doses of radiation damages human tissue, affects white blood cells (reducing natural defenses against invading microorganisms), and results in radiation sickness (nausea, fatigue, sore throat, anemia, diarrhea, hair loss) and even death. There is also concern over potential damage to reproductive cells, alteration of genes, chromosome damage, and the possibility of mutations.

A recent study of Hiroshima bomb victims indicated that the long-term effects of radiation were underestimated. The risk of thyroid problems in those exposed to fallout, for example, were underestimated by 10 percent. Fallout-related abnormalities were also more widespread than originally predicted.

The Soviet Union's Chernobyl nuclear power plant disaster provides further insights into the effects of radiation. Early in the morning on Saturday, April 26, 1986, a series of explosions in the hall of reactor no. 4 spewed at least 50 tons of highly radioactive particles—more than ten times the fallout at Hiroshima—across a large portion of western Russia, including some of the most fertile and productive agricultural lands in the Soviet Union. In addition, radiation alarms sounded as far away as Sweden, and eventually farmers in Sweden, Lapland, Italy, Wales, and other countries to which winds carried radioactive particles from the Chernobyl site had to destroy livestock and produce that showed significant levels of radiation poisoning.

The immediate effects of the disaster were clear. Two workers at the plant died immediately in the explosions and fire, and a total of thirty-one other workers died of radiation sickness within ten weeks. The long-term effects are less certain. Scientists previously estimated that a radiation dose of 450 *rads* (for radiation-absorbed doses; one rad is equivalent to fifty chest x-rays) would be lethal to 50 percent of those exposed. More than 500 people—some of them exposed to more than 600 rads—were hospitalized with radiation sickness soon after the disaster. Although it seems heartening that 90 percent of these 500 people were doing well one year later, radiation is surely the culprit in the dozens of cases of thyroid cancer among children that were reported by 1991. In the United States, thyroid cancer is almost unknown in people under the age of 25. Approximately 600,000 people were involved in the cleanup at Chernobyl, and more than 200,000 people were evacuated from areas contaminated with radiation. Doctors remain concerned about the external doses of radiation people received soon after the disaster, but they are even more concerned about the internal doses people are still receiving by eating agricultural products tainted with radiation. Some experts fear that there may eventually be between 50,000 and 250,000 deaths in the Soviet Union from cancers attributable to the Chernobyl disaster, and that these numbers may be equaled in other countries where the radiation doses were lower but where the exposed population was much larger.[13]

Electromagnetic Radiation

The growing evidence that ordinary electricity may be a health hazard is frightening to both the power industry and those living near overhead power lines. Fields of electromagnetic sources spring from both household and industrial wire. Power lines, computers, and some household appliances are involved. Evidence is mounting to show that even ordinary electricity may be a serious health hazard. New sources of "electropollution" are being developed each year in the fields of modern medicine and nuclear energy. Studies have focused on radiation at frequencies below 300 hertz, or cycles per second. These low-frequency currents take in the 160-hertz alternating current supplying homes, offices, and factories.[14]

Public awareness and debates on regulation and protection are increasing. But conclusive evidence is lacking, and electromagnetic fields deserve additional study.

X-Rays

It is possible to protect yourself from certain types of radiation. Pregnant women, for example, should avoid x-rays during the first trimester of pregnancy and, ideally, throughout pregnancy. One should avoid having dental x-rays more than once a year. Annual chest x-rays are also questionable, due to radiation exposure.

Space Junk

Some experts feel that space is turning into a "celestial junkyard." Over 20,000 objects have entered space since 1957, when the Soviet Union launched the first successful Sputnik space probe. Today, less than 5 percent of these objects are operational. An estimated 3,000 tons of debris consisting of such items as spent rockets and old communications, weather, and military satellites orbit the earth and threaten not only future space missions but also life here on earth. Just how much damage can debris cause? In 1983, a grain of paint struck the space shuttle Challenger with enough force to require a front window to be replaced after the flight. The majority of debris objects in space are substantially larger than a grain of paint.

However, space debris does not always threaten only space missions. Occasionally an object will fall from orbit and reenter the earth's atmosphere. This can be especially dangerous when radioactive materials are involved. Many space launches have used nuclear power sources in the form of either a small nuclear reactor or a radioisotope power supply. Both types of power source convert heat to electric power. A reactor produces heat from the controlled fission of uranium fuel and a radioisotope thermoelectric generator, or RTG, culls heat from the decay of highly radioactive material. Both types of power source have also already been involved in accidents. In April 1964, an American RTG-powered craft failed to achieve orbit and its highly radioactive plutonium 238 power source disintegrated in the atmosphere. In January 1978, a Soviet nuclear reactor-powered satellite fell to the earth and spread radioactive debris over thousands of square miles of northwestern Canada. Although nuclear power sources have been used aboard several highly productive space missions, the peoples of the

earth face some serious choices about whether or not certain space objectives are worth the extremely high financial cost and the potential for vast environmental damage in the event of accidents.[15]

A Plan to Reduce Pollution

Important legislation has been passed in the areas of forestry, energy planning and conservation, coastal protection, smog, and auto emissions. The Environmental Protection Agency, established in 1970, has done much to protect health and the environment. Some states have also taken a leading role. Oregon, for example, received the first Citation for Excellence in Environmental Protection and Improvement for achieving federal water quality standards, passing an antilitter beverage container law, removing billboards, and funding the construction of bicycle paths. At present, more vigorous enforcement of the law is needed, and local efforts must gain momentum. A few suggestions follow.

What You Can Do

Study the Problem Joining an environmental group, such as the Sierra Club, Friends of the Earth, the Wilderness Society, or the Nature Conservancy, is a good way to keep informed about important environmental issues.

Call the Problem to the Attention of Those Who Can Help The editor of your newspaper, conservation groups, and city hall are sources you may want to contact. Be certain to point out that you are keeping a diary of all your efforts, including witnesses and photographs, in such cases as improper solid waste disposal. Keep in mind that authorities depend upon responsible citizens to combat pollution. Letter-writing campaigns to senators and representatives can be effective. If enough letters are written to a senator or

Year 2000 National Health Objective

In a comprehensive attempt to clean up the total environment, a national health objective seeks to reduce human exposure to toxic agents by confining total pounds released into the air, water, and soil each year to no more than 0.24 billion pounds of those agents listed as "carcinogens" (0.32 billion pounds were released in 1988) and 2.6 billion pounds of those agents listed as the "most toxic chemicals" (2.62 billion pounds were released in 1988).

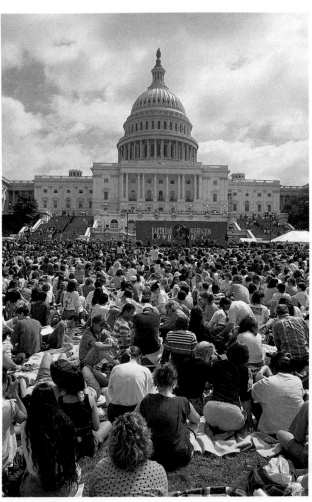

The environmental awareness and activism of the 1980s and 1990s should not be allowed to become merely a "fad." Our environment is in trouble. Your own involvement in local environmental issues and programs is absolutely necessary if we are to realize the goal of a healthy environment for the whole world.

representative, they can affect how he or she votes on particular bills or prompt an investigation into a situation the public is concerned about. Letter writing provides a permanent record and is preferable to a telephone call. A brief personal letter should be sent when the issue is hot; it should refer to the bill by name and number, point out how the bill affects the state or community, and list reasons for supporting or opposing the bill.

Consider Taking Legal Action Under the Federal Refuse Act of 1899, attorneys have the responsibility of prosecuting those who pollute. To make a citizen's arrest, you need merely identify the site of pollution and include supporting documents, such as photos or letters from a local conservation office. Action can be taken when either an individual or industry is violating the Refuse Act.

Exercise Your Voting Rights Groups that voice their intention to vote for leaders who will work to save the environment will receive attention. Legislators are apt to make some promises and compromises if there is a danger of losing votes.

Exercise Your Consumer Power When American consumers band together, things happen. If consumers purchased only environmentally safe products (reusable bottles, biodegradable cans and containers, recyclable packages, and so forth), industry would produce only these items. Widespread refusal to purchase from the known polluters in industry, as well as refusal to purchase energy-inefficient products and short-lived items, would bring about mass changes in manufacturing.

Learn about Local Land Use Find out how your county plans to use its land in the future. Attend meetings of the council, board of supervisors, and planning commission, and call your county planning department. Misuse of land has a major impact on environmental quality.

Promote Environmental Education Call high school principals or superintendents to find out about the environmental education programs in local school

Exploring Your Health 21.4

Taking Action

Think about the topics we've discussed in this chapter—the various dangers from environmental pollutants, radiation, and the like. Then select an issue that is of particular concern to you and compose a letter to the editor of your city newspaper. Outline your concerns and suggest what you think ought to be done. Be sure to do some research on the issue so you can back up your statements. Then send it off. You may be surprised to find that your letter is published!

---

districts. Suggest the use of programs such as Project WILD, Aquatic WILD, Project Learning Tree, and the National Wildlife Federation's CLASS PROJECT. Such programs show educators how to build environmental awareness into the curriculum.

Population and Health

Many environmental problems are closely related to the world's population growth. It wasn't until the year 1830 that world population reached 1 billion, yet 100 years later the population had doubled, and only 40 years after that, in 1970, it had grown to an estimated 3.5 billion. The population passed the 4 billion mark on April 1, 1975, reached 5 billion by the end of 1987, and climbed to over 5.2 billion by 1989, well ahead of population projections. At the present rate, it is projected that there will be 7 billion people on earth by the year 2000, with an additional billion added each subsequent five years.[16]

In the United States, population growth has been slowing as birth rates per family have dropped; however, the U.S. population grew by 2.5 million people each year from 1980 to 1985. The total population including armed forces overseas was approximately 248,800,000, up from 241,596,000 in 1986, and from the 227,061,000 in 1980.[17] The U.S. population is growing at a current rate of 0.7 percent per year. If it stays at this level, the U.S. population will double in about 100 years.

In most countries, birth rates continue to exceed death rates by more than 50 percent. Population growth in the developing countries of Latin America, Africa, and Asia has been nothing short of spectacular. In poorer countries, population has increased as fast or faster than food production, resulting in malnutrition and starvation.

Unchecked population growth affects health in several ways. The most serious, as already noted, is the hunger and starvation caused by food shortages. The American trend toward urbanization has brought its own problems. Today, more than 70 percent of the U.S. population lives on only 1 percent of the land. Urbanization is a prime contributor to environmental pollution of all types—air pollution from smog, water pollution, solid and chemical wastes—and to energy shortages. In addition, there is evidence that crowding, in combination with other factors, such as poverty, contributes to stress, disease, mental illness, and crime.

It is well known that, although Americans constitute only 6 percent of the earth's population, they consume 40 percent of its resources and produce more than 50 percent of the world's waste. Unless waste and overconsumption are checked, the result will be more despoiling of our resources and more health-related problems.

Dealing with Population Growth

An obvious approach to solving the problems related to population growth is to produce fewer offspring. Many countries are moving in this direction through education, legislation, or incentive programs. The distribution of condoms and birth control pills in many countries has had some impact. In China, the approach has been to institute strict government policy. The Chinese government issued a series of laws designed to reduce the birth rate by the year 2000. One law raised the minimum age for marriage; another provided that the monthly government family allowance for one child be cut off if the family had a second child; a third law gave preference to first children in admissions to nurseries, hospitals, and schools. Governments in some countries, such as South Korea, Taiwan, India, Pakistan, and Egypt, have initiated birth control programs that encourage the use of IUDs and vasectomies. The results have been mixed. In India, for example, there has been strong resistance to birth control by certain groups that traditionally regard large families as a measure of wealth and prestige.

Research is needed to determine how to motivate people from different cultural backgrounds to want fewer children. Some countries see population growth as essential to economic development because it adds workers to the labor force. Some Third World countries strongly oppose population policies, viewing them as a threat to their very survival. Nevertheless, a lowering of fertility rates is essential. The problem is how to break through centuries of tradition to convince individuals and countries to take action.[18]

Get Involved!

Working for a Healthier Environment

There is a great deal you can do to help clean the environment. Here are some suggestions:

1. Set a good example for others by being environmentally conscious in your daily life.

2. Organize a drop-off collection site for newspapers, aluminum cans, glass, scrap metal, plastics, and paper items on your university campus. Check with the recycling coordinator in your area to see what is being collected and how the university could get involved.

3. Organize a "plant a tree" day in your community to emphasize the value of plant life and the need to protect vegetation.

4. Meet with someone from the office of student activities in your university to see what is being done to protect hearing loss at university-sponsored rock concerts.

5. With a group of four or five, walk the entire outside area of your campus and identify the environmental problems that could be improved. Look for litter areas, the presence or absence of recycling centers, and so forth. Concentrate on recycling rather than disposal.

6. Start a letter-writing campaign to your senator or representative about a pressing environmental problem that is not receiving attention in your community. Prepare guideline letters for your friends to use when they write and continue your efforts until you receive a response.

7. Promote an environmental education day on your campus. Contact some of the special project coordinators mentioned in this chapter for assistance.

8. Leaves and grass clippings are much more useful in your yard than they are in a landfill. Yard waste makes up 20 percent of municipal waste. Start a compost pile for your land.

9. Each office worker generates one pound of paper each day. Find out how to recycle this valuable resource on your university campus by contacting the university's department of waste management.

10. Discourage littering in any fashion. Consider becoming a part of the "Adopt a Highway Program" and become part of a group that is responsible for keeping a section of the highway litter free. Groups can meet several times annually to collect trash along the road.

11. Reduce your use of an automobile to a strict minimum. Bicycle riding has gained popularity with American adults, who used to consider the bike a child's "toy." Get yourself a mountain bike or one of those new "hybrid" bikes (a cross between a mountain bike and a road racing bike) and use it for shopping and commuting. While at your bicycle dealer, ask about local bike clubs that bring casual and competitive riders together for evening and weekend rides and outings. Other, perhaps less fun alternatives to a car are walking and public transportation.

12. As a correlative of the activity above, encourage and support the creation of bicycle lanes and paths in your community. Many communities in Europe and Asia have long offered their bicyclists safe, well-kept roads that are often completely separate from automobile roads.

Conclusion

A clean environment is the responsibility of every human being. It starts with each person doing his or her part to avoid polluting the air, water, and land. It also involves insisting on a clean environment from industry, agriculture, and government; not contributing to the problem of overpopulation; and keeping pressure on the current political administration to legislate in favor of the environment. It is up to the consumer to maintain the proper balance between environmental and economic issues. We may hope that, with enough individual concern and pressure, salvaging and recycling will replace dumping as the primary means of disposing of waste.

Summary

1. Environmental pollution poses a serious threat to the human body, plant and animal life, and even mental health.

2. Air pollution in the atmosphere, home, and workplace imposes serious health risks on many individuals, causing a significant number of deaths each year.

3. Acid rain damages soil, surface water for aquatic life, forests, and agricultural products. Government, industrial, and personal efforts can significantly reduce acid rain. Recent 1990 legislation providing financial incentives to industry to reduce sulfur dioxide emissions, for example, should save billions of dollars annually and help reduce acid rain.

4. Global warming (the Greenhouse Effect) does not appear to be occurring as rapidly as projected. Nevertheless, current efforts should be stepped up to reduce global warming and prevent further depletion of the ozone layer.

5. Unsafe radon levels in the home and other buildings may be the leading cause of lung cancer among the nonsmoking population. Home test kits approved by the EPA provide fairly accurate readings at low cost. If levels are too high, steps can be taken to reduce radon exposure.

6. Noises exceeding 80 decibels, such as rock music, can result in permanent hearing loss.

7. Protection from waterborne infection is achieved through pollution prevention, purification of the water supply, or treatment of waste before it enters water bodies. In the future, much more emphasis must be placed on pollution prevention.

8. Contaminated drinking water is still too common in the United States. Individuals should have their water tested and take precautions to reduce contamination, or they should use an approved filtering system or bottled water for drinking and cooking.

9. Research is needed to uncover more effective means of handling solid wastes that do not contaminate the land, air, and water, or slowly use up our precious land.

10. The identification and removal of illegal dump sites (for chemical wastes) will take many years. The task of this generation is not just to locate and remove these sites but also to see that no new sites are created through indiscriminate, illegal dumping.

11. Individuals can make a difference in reducing air, water, solid waste, and noise pollution. A clean environment is the responsibility of the individual; if individuals follow sound environmental practices and police industry, agriculture, and others, improvement will take place. Existing legislation must be enforced. Consumers should exercise their voting and consumer power and even take legal action, if necessary, to eliminate contamination of the environment.

12. Although it appears that humans can survive much higher doses of radiation than originally projected, the long-term effects of exposure are much more severe and widespread than previously estimated.

13. The individual can greatly reduce radiation exposure by avoiding frequent dental and medical x-rays and using adequate protection when working near x-ray equipment.

14. Steps need to be taken immediately to eliminate potentially dangerous "space junk" and to prevent adding to the problem in all future space missions.

15. Population growth in the United States has been slowing considerably and is now less than 1.8 children per family. Some experts feel that this trend exposes the country to serious economic and political risks in the future.

16. Population growth is directly related to environmental pollution; each additional human being contributes to the problem of pollution.

Questions for Personal Growth

1. Analyze the quality of the air in your home, apartment, or dormitory, and in your workplace. What are the major sources of air pollution in these areas? How can you reduce your risk of exposure to these pollutants?

2. Acid rain, global warming, and ozone depletion are three serious problems in modern society. What is being done in your community to reverse the problem and prevent additional pollution? Are there organized efforts in your state? List five things you can personally do.

3. Visit several gas stations in your area. Inquire about their disposal of used motor oil and other auto fluids. Do they have a recycling system? Is their technique of disposal safe? Can you suggest any improvements for service stations?

4. Noise pollution appears to be getting worse. Evidence indicates that hearing loss is common due to loud sounds in our homes and in the workplace. Identify the major sources of noise pollution in your life. What can you do to protect your ears from permanent damage? Do you keep your stereo volume at safe levels? What special protection can you take at rock concerts and in close-quarter entertainment spots?

5. Analyze the drinking water supply in your home, apartment, or dormitory. Can you trace the water from its original source to your faucet? What is the greatest risk of contamination? How safe is your drinking water? Ask authorities to have your drinking water tested.

6. Examine the containers of food, chemicals, and other products in your dwelling. Are you choosing containers that can be recycled or used for other purposes instead of being discarded? Are you buying in large quantities to reduce the amount of disposal packages? What changes could you make in your purchasing habits to reduce the amount of household waste produced?

7. Visit your local supermarket and ask the manager to describe their recycling methods. Are they actively involved in community recycling of glass, aluminum, metal, paper, and other products? Do they avoid selling products in nonbiodegradable or unrecyclable containers? Is their major emphasis on disposal or recycling?

References

1. American Lung Association, "Facts About Air Pollution and Your Health" (1988).

2. Environmental Protection Agency, "Environmental Progress and Challenges: EPA's Update" (Washington, D.C.: EPA, Office of Policy Planning and Evaluation, 1988).

3. Ibid.

4. Environmental Protection Agency, "Environmental Progress and Challenges: EPA's Update."

5. Commonwealth of Virginia, Council on Environment, "25 Ways to Help Virginia's Environment" (1990).

6. Environmental Protection Agency, *EPA Journal: Agriculture and Environment* (Washington, D.C.: Office of Public Affairs, April 1988).

7. Ann Rucker, "Psychologist Questions Safety of Chemicals," *Virginia Commonwealth University Voice* (August 14, 1990), p. 2.

8. Ibid.

9. "India's Tragedy—A Warning Heard Around the World," *U.S. News and World Report* (December 17, 1984): 25–27.

10. Environmental Protection Agency, "Regulating Pesticides" (Washington, D.C.: Office of Public Affairs, 1988).

11. Environmental Protection Agency, "Environmental Progress and Challenges: EPA's Update; The Procter and Gamble Company, "Questions and Answers About Solid Waste" (1989); Water Pollution Control Federation, "Household Hazardous Waste: What You Should and Shouldn't Do."

12. "What You Should Know About Recycling" (South Deerfield, Mass.: Channing L. Bete Co., 1990).

13. Felicity Barringer, "Chernobyl Five Years Later: The Danger Persists," *The New York Times Magazine* (April 14, 1991): 28–36, 39, 74.

14. "An Electrifying New Hazard," *U.S. News and World Report* (March 30, 1987).

15. Aftergood, Steven, Hafemeister, David W., Prilutsky, Oleg F., Primack, Joel R., and Rodionov, Stanislav N., "Nuclear Power in Space," *Scientific American* (June 1991): 42–47.

16. Population Reference Bureau, *1989 World Population Data Sheet* (Washington, D.C.: Population Reference Bureau, 1989).

17. Ibid.

18. P. Henry, "Food and Population: Beyond Five Billion," *Population Bulletin* 43, 2 (Washington, D.C.: Population Reference Bureau, April 1988).

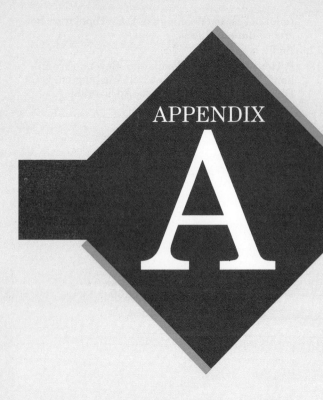

APPENDIX A

The Body Systems*

To make decisions related to your health, you must understand how your body functions. This appendix provides you with some basic information about the body systems. We don't expect you to become an expert; however, we do think some basic knowledge can help you understand some sections of the text. In addition, a greater familiarity with your body can help you know what to look for when you have a particular health problem.

The Skeletal System

Your skeleton (see Figure A.1) is composed of 206 bones. These bones have three basic functions: to support and protect the other body systems, to store minerals, and to produce cells for the circulatory system.

For your skeleton to support the other systems of the body, it must be strong enough physically to hold the other systems in position, and it must be light enough to permit movement with as much efficiency as possible. Therefore, most bones are composed of two types of tissue—a firm, compact external layer and a porous internal portion. Covering the bone is a layer of tissue called the *periosteum*. It aids bone growth (thickness or circumference) and provides tissue for the attachment of ligaments, tendons, muscles, and cartilage.

Protection of the other body systems is assured by the strong structure of the skeleton and the various cavities within or framed by the bones. The skull and vertebral column, for example, protect the brain and spinal cord; the pelvic girdle and rib cage help protect the intestines, heart, lungs, and other vital organs.

The bones of the skeletal system contain 95–98 percent of the body's calcium supply and approximately 80 percent of its phosphorus. These minerals are essential to life.

The skeleton produces the components of blood: red corpuscles, leukocytes, and platelets. *Red corpuscles* transport oxygen and carbon dioxide, *leukocytes* (white blood cells) fight infection, and *platelets* aid in blood clotting. The cavities within the bones are filled with either yellow marrow or red marrow. *Yellow marrow* is found in the shafts of the long bones; *red marrow* is found in the ends of the long bones, in short and flat bones, and in the vertebral bodies. Of particular importance is the red marrow, where the red corpuscles, leukocytes, and platelets are produced.

The Muscular System

The muscles of your body (see Figure A.2) are classified as striated or nonstriated. The *striated group* includes both skeletal and cardiac muscle. The *nonstriated group,* also called *smooth muscle,* includes the walls of the blood vessels and the tissues of the internal organs, particularly the gastrointestinal tract. All muscle tissue has

*Text contributed by Dr. Fred Browning.

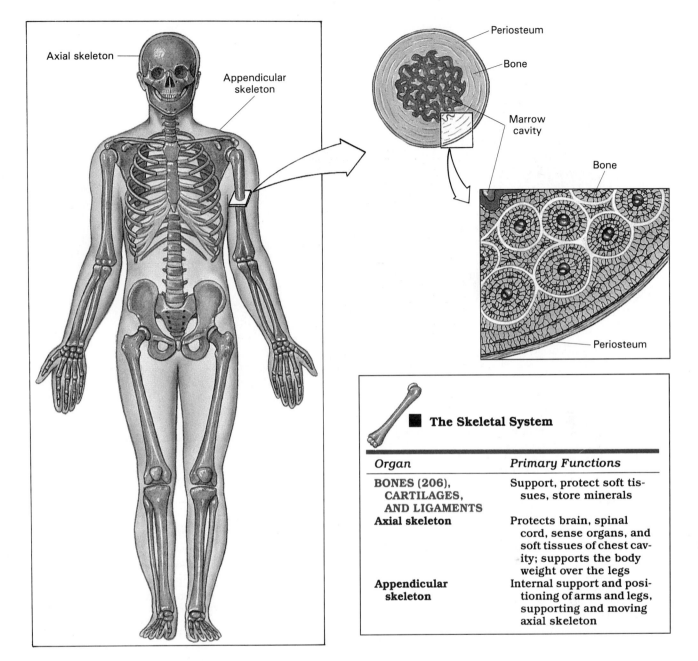

Axial skeleton

Appendicular skeleton

Periosteum

Bone

Marrow cavity

Bone

Periosteum

The Skeletal System

Organ	Primary Functions
BONES (206), CARTILAGES, AND LIGAMENTS	Support, protect soft tissues, store minerals
Axial skeleton	Protects brain, spinal cord, sense organs, and soft tissues of chest cavity; supports the body weight over the legs
Appendicular skeleton	Internal support and positioning of arms and legs, supporting and moving axial skeleton

FIGURE A.1 • The Skeletal System

the same function: to create force so that you can move.

Although most muscles attach to the skeletal system via tendinous tissue, several connect directly to the bone. These attachments allow two possibilities through muscle shortening: movement or stabilization of a joint or body segment. Thus it is possible to create force or perform work through movement of the body or body segments.

The Nervous System

The nervous system is as important to the body as the telephone system is to the life of a city. It receives and sends messages throughout the body, informing the

brain of the welfare of the total organism. *Interoceptors,* located within the tissue of the body, respond to internal stimuli; *exteroceptors,* located on or near the surface of the body, respond to external stimuli.

Exteroceptors consist of organs, such as the eyes, ears, taste buds, nose, and sensors of touch and temperature within the skin. Most of these organs receive stimuli from far and near: we hear loud sounds, we view objects, we smell distinct odors, we sense changes in temperature. Interoceptors receive stimuli from within the tissues (and skin) of the body and keep us informed of such things as pain, pressure, body position, movement of the body, and spatial orientation.

Anatomically, the nervous system consists of the cerebrum (two hemispheres housed within the skull), the midbrain stem (including the pons and the medulla), the cerebellum, the spinal cord, twelve pairs of

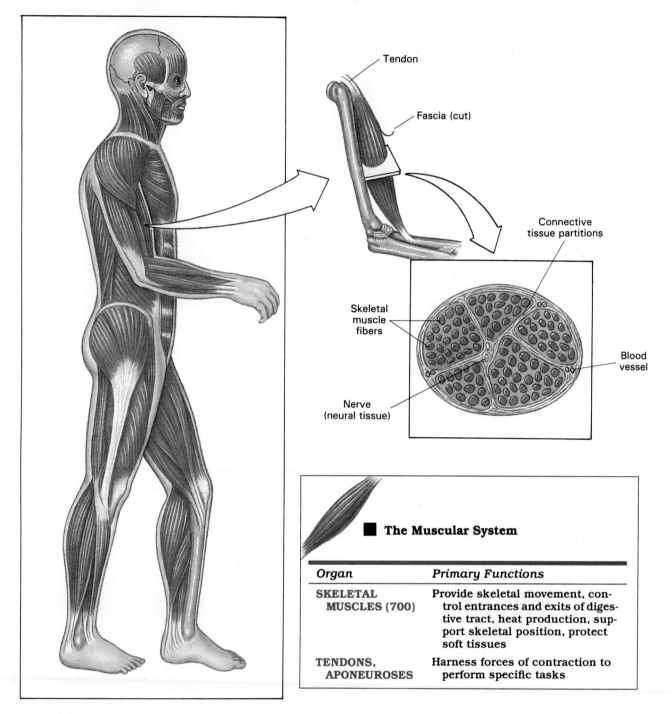

Labels on figure:
Tendon
Fascia (cut)
Connective tissue partitions
Skeletal muscle fibers
Blood vessel
Nerve (neural tissue)

▪ The Muscular System

Organ	Primary Functions
SKELETAL MUSCLES (700)	Provide skeletal movement, control entrances and exits of digestive tract, heat production, support skeletal position, protect soft tissues
TENDONS, APONEUROSES	Harness forces of contraction to perform specific tasks

FIGURE A.2 • The Muscular System

cranial nerves, and thirty pairs of spinal nerves (see Figure A.3). The brain and spinal cord are usually considered the *central nervous system,* and the pairs of cranial and spinal nerves are the *peripheral nervous system.* The central nervous system operates as a storage system (computer) and interprets the environment. Nerve cables extending from the brain and spinal cord convey electrical nerve impulses to and from every part of the body. The peripheral nervous system senses and responds to these impulses and works with the central nervous system as one unit to keep the organism alive and well.

The entire nervous system is composed of *neurons.* These neurons are similar to other cells and have the special property of conduction, which allows an impulse to be passed from one point to another, establishing a method of communication for the entire body. For example, if you step on a nail, the pain receptors in your foot send an impulse to the brain for further consideration, and the brain simultaneously sends an impulse to lower limbs, causing the injured foot to withdraw and the opposite lower limb to extend. In short, the nervous system keeps us in touch with our external environment and our internal needs.

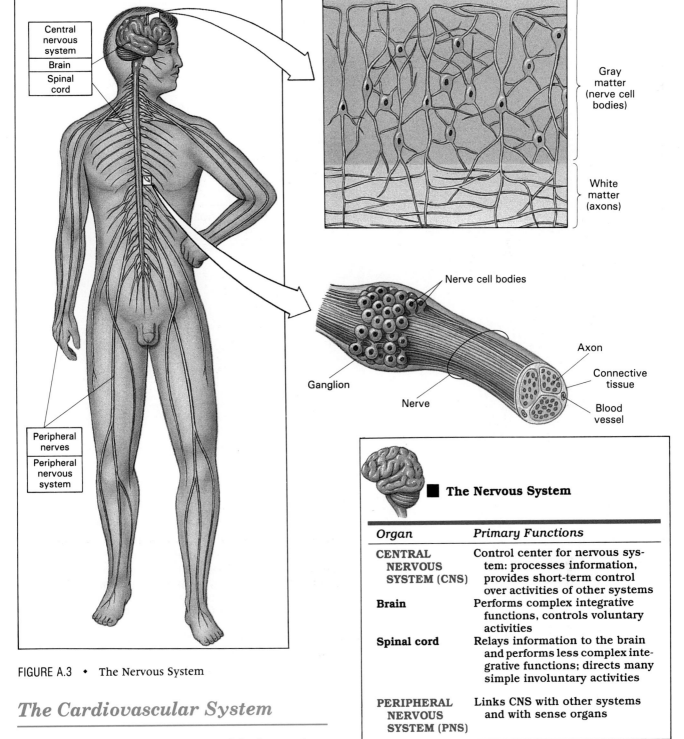

Gray matter (nerve cell bodies)

White matter (axons)

Nerve cell bodies

Axon

Connective tissue

Blood vessel

Ganglion

Nerve

FIGURE A.3 • The Nervous System

The Nervous System

Organ	Primary Functions
CENTRAL NERVOUS SYSTEM (CNS)	Control center for nervous system: processes information, provides short-term control over activities of other systems
Brain	Performs complex integrative functions, controls voluntary activities
Spinal cord	Relays information to the brain and performs less complex integrative functions; directs many simple involuntary activities
PERIPHERAL NERVOUS SYSTEM (PNS)	Links CNS with other systems and with sense organs

The Cardiovascular System

The cardiovascular system is a part of the larger circulatory system and consists of the heart, blood vessels, and blood (see Figure A.4). It is closely related to the lymphatic system—also a part of the circulatory system—which we will discuss next.

The heart is a muscular organ lying just beneath the breast bone in a diagonal plane. It is controlled largely by hormones and the autonomic nervous system and, to a lesser extent, by metabolism and bodily movements. The heart pumps the blood throughout the body, and the blood and lymph vessels keep it circulating. The heart is divided into right and left sides,

and the two sides function as two separate circulatory systems. In *pulmonary circulation* the right ventricle contracts, sending blood out via the pulmonary artery into the lungs. After passing from the lungs, the blood is returned to the left atrium of the heart via the pulmonary arteries.

Simultaneously, as the right ventricle contracts, the left ventricle also contracts, sending blood into the aorta and throughout the rest of the body. Blood leaving the left ventricle goes to the head, body, and limbs

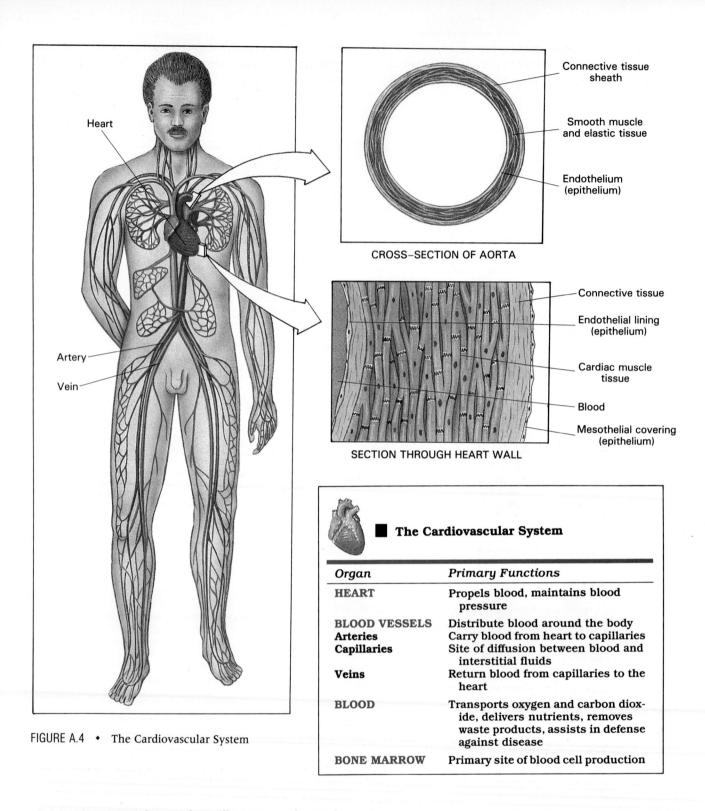

Heart

Artery

Vein

Connective tissue
sheath

Smooth muscle
and elastic tissue

Endothelium
(epithelium)

CROSS–SECTION OF AORTA

Connective tissue

Endothelial lining
(epithelium)

Cardiac muscle
tissue

Blood

Mesothelial covering
(epithelium)

SECTION THROUGH HEART WALL

■ **The Cardiovascular System**

Organ	Primary Functions
HEART	Propels blood, maintains blood pressure
BLOOD VESSELS	Distribute blood around the body
Arteries	Carry blood from heart to capillaries
Capillaries	Site of diffusion between blood and interstitial fluids
Veins	Return blood from capillaries to the heart
BLOOD	Transports oxygen and carbon dioxide, delivers nutrients, removes waste products, assists in defense against disease
BONE MARROW	Primary site of blood cell production

FIGURE A.4 ♦ The Cardiovascular System

via arteries, arterioles, and capillaries; venules and veins return the blood to the right atrium of the heart through the inferior and superior vena cava. This phase is called *systemic circulation.* The blood leaving the left ventricle goes through the aorta to the systems of the body. At the capillary level, fluids, nutrients, electrolytes, and minerals leave circulation and bathe all the cells of the body. The fluid is returned to the circulatory system by means of osmotic pressure within the blood and surrounding body tissues, and large vessels,

known as *veins,* carry the blood back to the right side of the heart.

The contraction of the atrium and ventricles of the heart is termed *systole;* the resting phase is termed *diastole.* The heart of an average adult beats approximately 70–75 times per minute. The amount of blood squeezed out of the ventricle on each beat is called the *stroke volume.* Heart rate (beats per minute) multiplied by stroke volume (amount of blood per beat) equals *cardiac output.* The blood makes up about one-thirteenth of the body weight, and at rest the heart pumps about the same quantity every minute. In an adult this is equivalent to between five and six liters of cardiac output.

The Lymphatic System

The lymphatic system is closely associated with the cardiovascular system because it comprises a vast network of vessels that deliver lymph to the circulatory system (see Figure A.5). The lymphatic system also contains *lymphatic organs* that produce or support a large number of disease-fighting cells such as lymphocytes and phagocytes (see Chapter 13), as well as

plasma cells. Lymphatic vessels normally lead to small, specialized organs called *lymph nodes* that contain cells sensitive to changes in the composition of lymph. Lymphatic organs significantly larger than lymph nodes include the thymus gland, the tonsils, and the spleen.

The lymphatic system defends the body from toxic substances and disease. Phagocytic cells patrol tissues throughout the body and attack pathogens. Macrophages (larger phagocytic cells) in lymph nodes attack damaged cells or pathogens that have escaped tissue defenses. Lymphocytes, like macrophages, circulate throughout the body and attack abnormal cells or intruding pathogens. Some lymphocytes convert to plasma cells, producing antibodies that provide biochemical defenses against disease.

FIGURE A.5 • The Lymphatic System

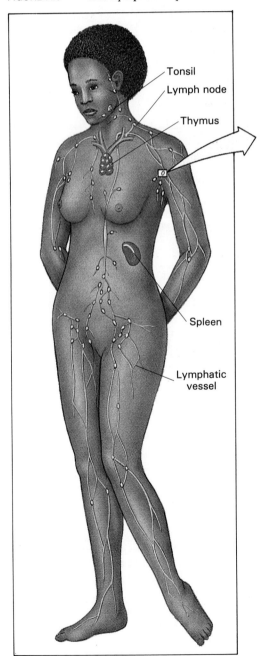

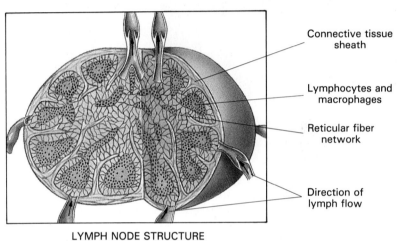

LYMPH NODE STRUCTURE

![lymphocyte icon] **The Lymphatic System**	
Organ	*Primary Functions*
LYMPHATIC VESSELS	Carry lymph from peripheral tissues to the veins of the cardiovascular system
LYMPH NODES	Monitor the composition of lymph, engulf pathogens, stimulate immune response
SPLEEN	Monitors circulating blood, engulfs pathogens, stimulates immune response
THYMUS	Controls development and maintenance of lymphocytes

The Respiratory System

Respiration is the process whereby oxygen is transported *to* the cells and carbon dioxide is transported *away* to be exhaled (see Figure A.6). Oxygen and carbon dioxide are exchanged in two locations. Oxygen is inhaled through the nose and the mouth and eventually enters the blood through the pulmonary membrane of the lungs and leaves the blood to enter the cells for metabolic use. Carbon dioxide takes the opposite path. It is produced by the cells, moves into the blood, and is transported to the lungs, where it passes through the pulmonary membrane to be exhaled.

FIGURE A.6 • The Respiratory System

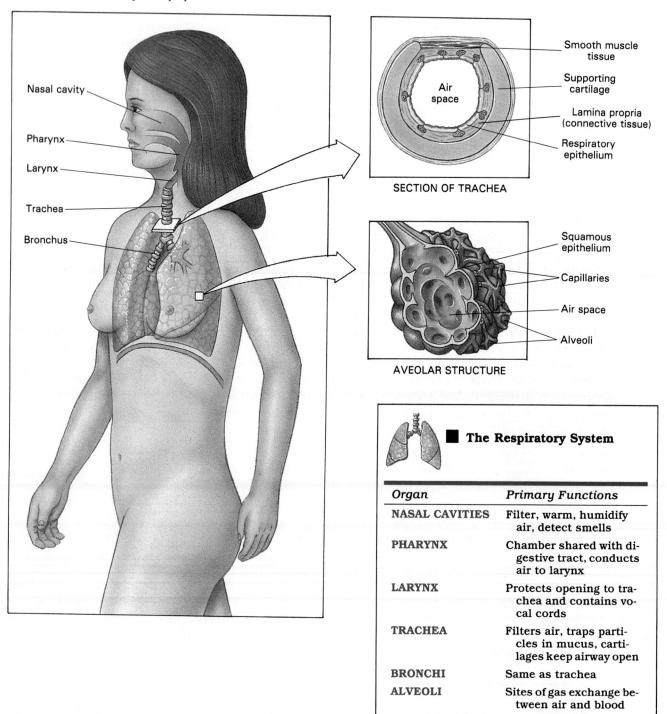

SECTION OF TRACHEA

AVEOLAR STRUCTURE

■ The Respiratory System

Organ	Primary Functions
NASAL CAVITIES	Filter, warm, humidify air, detect smells
PHARYNX	Chamber shared with digestive tract, conducts air to larynx
LARYNX	Protects opening to trachea and contains vocal cords
TRACHEA	Filters air, traps particles in mucus, cartilages keep airway open
BRONCHI	Same as trachea
ALVEOLI	Sites of gas exchange between air and blood

External respiration (ventilation) is a simple mechanical process similar to the functioning of a bellows. The ribs lift upward and outward or the diaphragm descends as it is contracted, creating a pressure that is negative relative to atmospheric pressure. Air rushes into the lungs. As the air comes in it is cleansed, moisturized, and warmed by the nasal and throat passages. In the lungs, it is exposed to the most important part of the pulmonary tissue, the membrane, before diffusing into the capillaries of the pulmonary circulation.

As the ribs fall downward and inward, the diaphragm relaxes and rises. This creates pressure slightly greater than the atmospheric pressure, and air is exhaled. In the young adult this process is repeated about twelve to twenty times per minute at rest and amounts to approximately 6 to 10 liters of ventilation. During strenuous activity, respiration may increase to about 50 breaths per minute and 150 liters of ventilation.

As oxygen diffuses through the pulmonary membrane, it is taken into the red blood cells and attached to molecules, called *hemoglobin,* that carry both oxygen and carbon dioxide. It remains attached until it reaches the metabolically active cells through the capillaries. At that point many of the molecules of oxygen will diffuse into the cells where they are used to produce energy units (ATP) from carbohydrates, fats, or proteins. One end product of this metabolic process is carbon dioxide, which then diffuses out of the cells into the blood, where it is transported back to the lungs to be exhaled. This process is termed *internal respiration.*

Respiration is automatically regulated, but it may be modified voluntarily for short periods of time. The control center of respiration is located in the medulla and lower pons of the brain. This center adjusts ventilation almost exactly to the demands of the body. Thus the relative pressure of oxygen and carbon dioxide remains fairly constant during rest and strenuous activity.

The Digestive System

The digestive system is a tubular structure (the digestive tract or alimentary canal) beginning at the mouth and ending at the anus (see Figure A.7). The digestive tract permits simple passage of food; storage of food or waste material (feces); digestion of food (carbohydrates, fats, and proteins); and absorption of all the end products of digestion, including minerals, vitamins, and water.

Let's follow some food down the digestive tract. First, the mouth and teeth grind food into smaller pieces, and then saliva softens and moisturizes it. Some other secretions help to initiate starch digestion, and mucus (a lubricant) is mixed with the food to facili-

tate its passage. Swallowing propels the food into the esophagus, which then moves the food through the system to the stomach.

The stomach has several functions. It acts as a temporary storage compartment, it further mixes the food until it becomes liquefied, it continues the digestion of carbohydrates (starches), and it initiates the digestion of protein and fat by secreting protein-splitting and lipid-splitting enzymes. As the food gradually becomes liquefied, it leaves the stomach and enters the small intestine (composed of the duodenum, jejunum, and ileum).

The food now is quite acidic, and almost immediately pancreatic secretions and bile (a fat emulsifier) from the gall bladder begin to enter the duodenum via the common bile duct to help neutralize the acid and to continue digestion of carbohydrates, protein, and fats.

The small intestine continues the movement of the liquefied food with wavelike movements. As the food passes through this segment of the gastrointestinal tract, it is exposed to a folded, irregular surface and small hairlike projections of the interior wall of the gut, called *villi.* The irregular surface and the villi increase the surface area of the small intestine and allow for greater absorption of the minute particles of food. During this passage from the stomach to the large intestine, the small intestine secretes more digestive enzymes to assist in further neutralizing the acid. On its passage through the small intestine, much of the food is absorbed as carbohydrates, proteins, fats, water, vitamins, and minerals.

Upon entering the large intestine, the remaining substance is lubricated with mucous secretions and more water, and most is absorbed. The remaining 100–150 ml of substance (now called *feces*) is stored in the distal portion of the large intestine (colon) until it is eliminated by defecation.

The Endocrine System

The *endocrine,* or *hormonal,* system is the chemical control mechanism for your bodily functions (see Figure A.8). *Hormones* are chemical substances secreted into the body fluids (blood, lymph, or cerebrospinal fluid) that exert physiological effects on all cells of the body. The nervous system acts as the messenger in situations needing quick response, and it helps to regulate hormonal secretions for long-term bodily functions. The endocrine system helps to maintain optimal internal conditions for the body by bringing messages to the vital centers of action.

Specific cells or groups of cells located throughout the body secrete certain hormones. These include the pituitary, adrenal, thymus, thyroid, and parathyroid

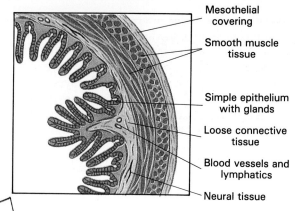

Mesothelial covering

Smooth muscle tissue

Simple epithelium with glands

Loose connective tissue

Blood vessels and lymphatics

Neural tissue

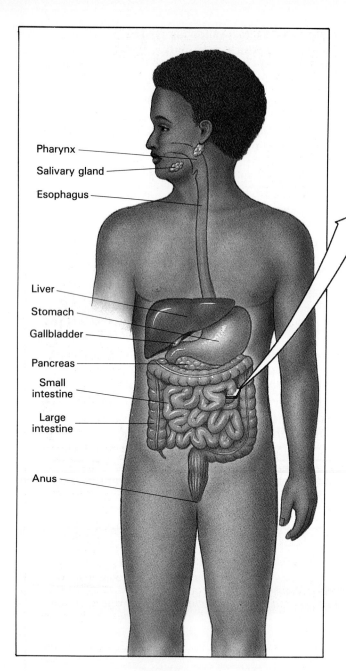

Pharynx

Salivary gland

Esophagus

Liver

Stomach

Gallbladder

Pancreas

Small intestine

Large intestine

Anus

FIGURE A.7 • The Digestive System

■ The Digestive System

Organ	Primary Functions
MOUTH	Mixes food with salivary secretions, taste, chewing
SALIVARY GLANDS	Produce buffers and enzymes that begin digestion
PHARYNX	Passageway shared with reproductive system, leads to esophagus
ESOPHAGUS	Delivers food to stomach
STOMACH	Secretes acids and digestive enzymes that break down proteins
SMALL INTESTINE	Absorbs nutrients
LIVER	Secretes bile (required for lipid digestion), regulates nutrient composition of blood, synthesizes blood proteins, stores lipid and carbohydrates reserves
GALLBLADDER	Stores bile for release into small intestine
PANCREAS	Secretes digestive enzymes and buffers into small intestine; contains endocrine cells
LARGE INTESTINE	Removes water from fecal material, stores wastes
ANUS	Opening to exterior for discharge of feces

glands, as well as the pancreas, ovaries, testes, kidneys, and pineal body. Table A.1 identifies the major hormones and their effects.

The Integumentary System

The body covering, or *integument,* is composed of three layers of flattened cells (see Figure A.9). The *epidermis* is the outside layer that people commonly think of as skin. Even though it continually sloughs off, it is tough, resistant to extreme temperature changes, and prevents excessive intake or loss of fluids.

The second layer, the *dermis,* supports and binds the epidermis to the underlying tissues. This layer is called the true skin; it contains blood vessels, nerve endings, oil and sweat glands, muscles, and hair follicles. The upper surface of the derma is rather irregularly shaped in conelike elevations called papillae. The *subcutaneous layer,* the deepest of the three layers of skin tissue, is supported by a thick layer of subcutaneous fatty tissue.

Because skin is living tissue, except for the epidermal layer, it must have a rich blood supply. Among its

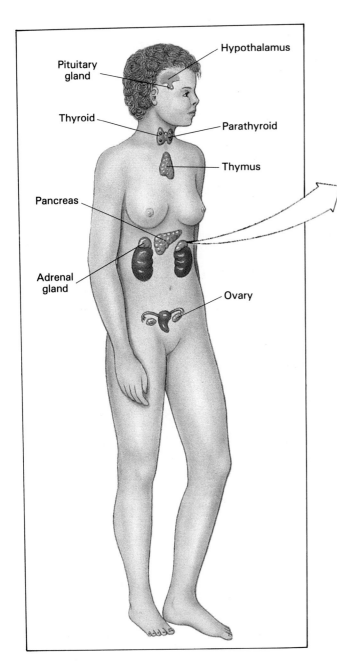

FIGURE A.8 • The Endocrine System

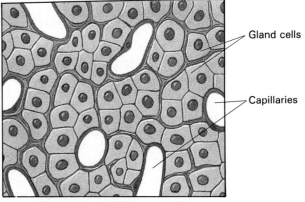

SECTION OF ENDOCRINE GLAND
(Adrenal medulla)

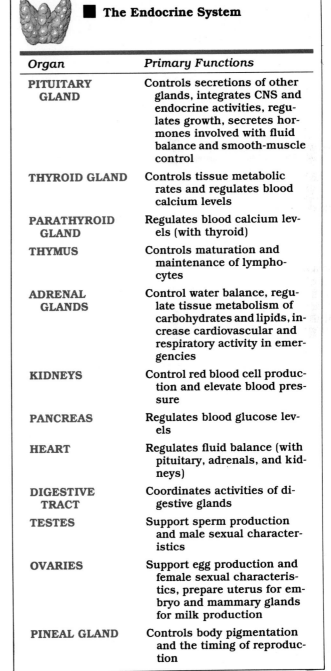

The Endocrine System

Organ	Primary Functions
PITUITARY GLAND	Controls secretions of other glands, integrates CNS and endocrine activities, regulates growth, secretes hormones involved with fluid balance and smooth-muscle control
THYROID GLAND	Controls tissue metabolic rates and regulates blood calcium levels
PARATHYROID GLAND	Regulates blood calcium levels (with thyroid)
THYMUS	Controls maturation and maintenance of lymphocytes
ADRENAL GLANDS	Control water balance, regulate tissue metabolism of carbohydrates and lipids, increase cardiovascular and respiratory activity in emergencies
KIDNEYS	Control red blood cell production and elevate blood pressure
PANCREAS	Regulates blood glucose levels
HEART	Regulates fluid balance (with pituitary, adrenals, and kidneys)
DIGESTIVE TRACT	Coordinates activities of digestive glands
TESTES	Support sperm production and male sexual characteristics
OVARIES	Support egg production and female sexual characteristics, prepare uterus for embryo and mammary glands for milk production
PINEAL GLAND	Controls body pigmentation and the timing of reproduction

many functions, it serves as a heat-dissipating organ. This requires the service of many blood vessels, so that in times of excessive internal heat buildup the blood can act as a heat transport mechanism. In extremely cold environments the fatty subcutaneous layer prevents excessive heat loss.

The integumentary system is important in protecting the body from the invasion of many types of bacteria, an excessive increase or decrease in body temperature, and excessive absorption or loss of water. It also helps the kidneys control blood urea through excretion and keeps the organism informed of environmental changes, skin damages, and excessive pressure.

To summarize, the skin covers the other systems of the body, protects them, and may prevent serious injuries.

Hormones and Their Effects

Hormone	Principal Effects	Secreted By
Adrenocorticotropic hormone (ACTH)	Stimulates the adrenal cortex	Pituitary
Thyrotropin (TSH)	Stimulates the thyroid gland	Pituitary
Follicle-stimulating hormone (FSH)	Stimulates production of egg cells by ovary and spermatozoa by testes	Pituitary
Luteinizing hormone (LH)	Helps maturation of egg-bearing follicles in ovary or stimulates production of testosterone (male hormone) in testes	Pituitary
Growth hormone	Governs normal growth and helps to regulate metabolism	Pituitary
Prolactin	Regulates breast development and milk production	Pituitary
Antidiuretichormone (ADH), or Vasopressin	Regulates absorption of water in the kidney	Neurohypophysis (part of the pituitary)
Oxytocin	Facilitates movement of sperm in Fallopian tube, stimulates uterine muscle in childbirth, stimulates secretion of milk by breasts	Neurohypophysis
Cortisol and similar hormones	Regulate metabolism of sugar, protein, fat, minerals, and water	Adrenal cortex (outer layer of adrenal gland)
Aldosterone and desoxycorticosterone	Regulate excretion and retention of minerals, particularly sodium and potassium, by kidneys	Adrenal cortex
Thyroid hormones	Regulate rate of body's metabolism	Thyroid
Estradiol 17-B ("Estrogen")	Regulates development of feminine characteristics and the menstrual-ovulatory cycle	Ovaries
Progesterone	Works with estrogen to regulate ovulation cycle and pregnancy, Estrogen-progesterone combinations, or similar agents, are the basis of birth-control pills	Ovaries
Testosterone	Regulates development of male characteristics and reproductive system	Testes
Insulin	Regulates utilization of sugar, proteins, and fats	Pancreas (Islets of Langerhans)
Glucagon	Helps to regulate utilization of sugar, antagonizes insulin	Pancreas (Islets of Langerhans)
Parathyroid hormone	Regulates calcium metabolism	Parathyroid glands
Thyrocalcitonin	Helps to regulate calcium metabolism	Thyroid
Adrenalin	Stimulates brain and heart rate, mobilizes sugar and fat	Adrenal medulla (inner layer of adrenal gland)
Noradrenalin	Increases force of heart contraction and constricts arterioles	Adrenal medulla
Releasing factors	Individual ones cause release of ACTH, TSH, LH, FSH, prolactin, and growth hormone by pituitary	Brain (hypothalamus)
Secretin	Stimulates pancreas to secrete chemicals needed for digestion of food	Lining of part of intestine
Cholecystokinin	Stimulates liver and pancreas to secrete chemicals for digestion of food	Lining of part of intestine
Gastrin	Stimulates stomach to secrete hydrocholoric acid	Lining of part of stomach and intestine

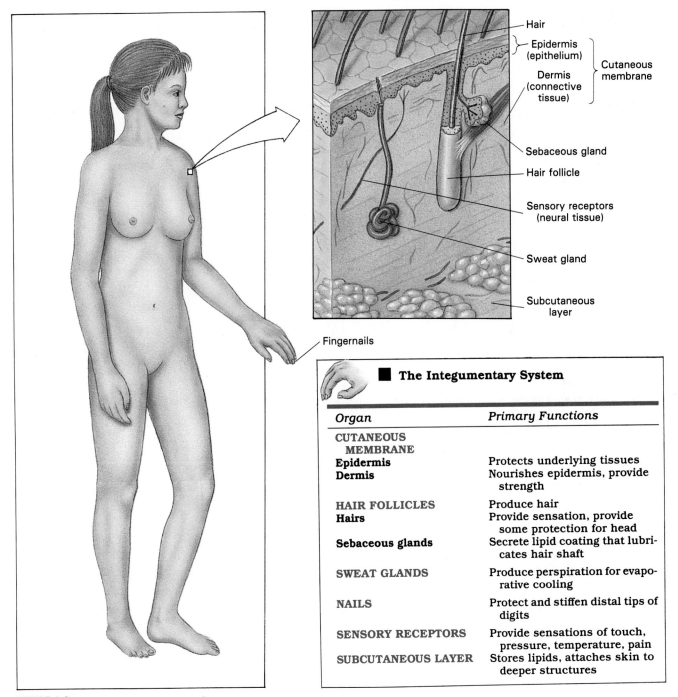

FIGURE A.9 • The Integumentary System

The Integumentary System

Organ	Primary Functions
CUTANEOUS MEMBRANE	
Epidermis	Protects underlying tissues
Dermis	Nourishes epidermis, provide strength
HAIR FOLLICLES	Produce hair
Hairs	Provide sensation, provide some protection for head
Sebaceous glands	Secrete lipid coating that lubricates hair shaft
SWEAT GLANDS	Produce perspiration for evaporative cooling
NAILS	Protect and stiffen distal tips of digits
SENSORY RECEPTORS	Provide sensations of touch, pressure, temperature, pain
SUBCUTANEOUS LAYER	Stores lipids, attaches skin to deeper structures

The Urinary System

The main function of the urinary system (see Figure A.10) is the elimination of waste products and acids that might alter the pH of body fluids. The urinary system also regulates the electrolyte and fluid composition of the blood. The urinary system consists of the *kidneys* (where urine is produced), the *ureters* (which carry urine to the urinary bladder for storage), and the *urethra* (the passageway for urine from the bladder to the outside of the body).

Urine production begins in the kidneys, where body fluids are filtered across the walls of special capillaries into *kidney tubules.* The filtered fluid passes along the tubules and eventually becomes urine, which is stored in the urinary bladder until it is eliminated through the process of *urination.*

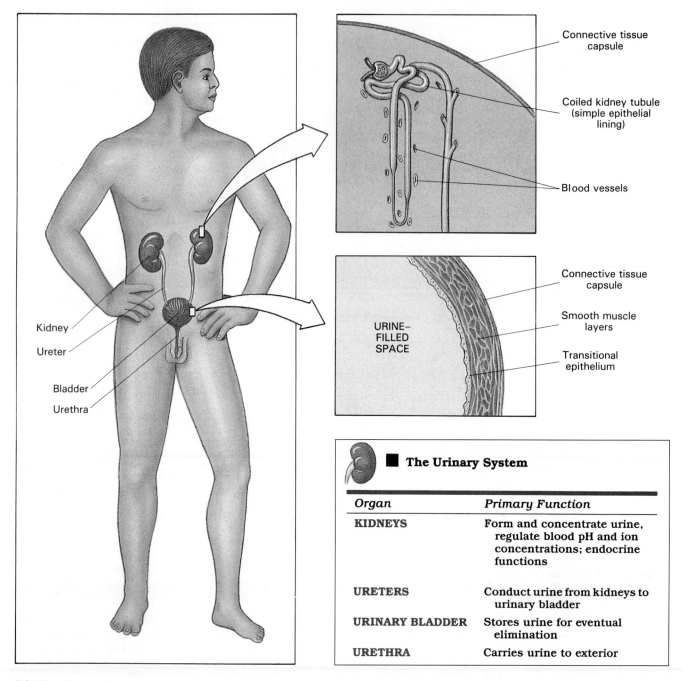

Connective tissue capsule

Coiled kidney tubule (simple epithelial lining)

Blood vessels

Connective tissue capsule

Smooth muscle layers

Transitional epithelium

URINE-FILLED SPACE

■ **The Urinary System**

Organ	Primary Function
KIDNEYS	Form and concentrate urine, regulate blood pH and ion concentrations; endocrine functions
URETERS	Conduct urine from kidneys to urinary bladder
URINARY BLADDER	Stores urine for eventual elimination
URETHRA	Carries urine to exterior

FIGURE A.10 • The Urinary System

The Reproductive System

As we saw in Chapters 5 and 6 on sexuality and fertility control, the reproductive system is responsible for producing future generations. The reproductive system also produces hormones that are vital for the maintenance and growth of many other body systems. Reproductive organs called the *gonads* produce *gametes* (reproductive cells), which travel to the exterior of the body through ducts that receive the secretions of accessory glands. The female gonads are the *ovaries,* which produce eggs. The male gonads are the *testes,* which produce sperm. The parts of reproductive anatomy that

are visible on the exterior of the body are called the *external genitalia.*

In the male (Figure A.11a), the sperm duct leaving each testis flows into the urethra. Within the sperm duct and urethra, secretions provided by the accessory glands nourish the sperm cells. The combination of sperm and accessory gland secretions forms *semen.* The *penis* and *scrotum* (a fleshy sac that holds the testes) comprise the male external genitalia.

In the female (Figure A.11b), eggs released by the ovaries travel into the *uterine tube* (or oviduct). The uterine tube flows into the *uterus,* which is connected to the exterior of the body by the *vagina.* The female

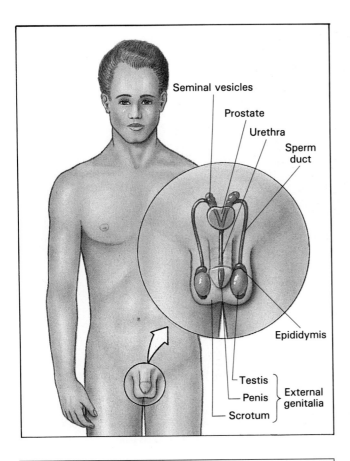

Labels on figure 1 (male):
- Seminal vesicles
- Prostate
- Urethra
- Sperm duct
- Epididymis
- Testis
- Penis
- Scrotum
- External genitalia

■ (a) The Reproductive System of the Male

Organ	Primary Functions
TESTES	Produce sperm
ACCESSORY ORGANS	
Epididymis	Site of sperm maturation
Ductus deferens (sperm duct)	Conducts sperm between epididymis and prostate
Seminal vesicles	Secrete fluid that makes up much of the volume of semen
Prostate	Secretes buffers and fluid
EXTERNAL GENITALIA	
Penis	Erectile organ used to deposit sperm in the vagina of a female
Scrotum	Surrounds the testes

FIGURE A.11a • The Male Reproductive System
FIGURE A.11 • The Reproductive System

external genitalia include the *labia majora, labia minora,* the *clitoris,* and the *vaginal opening.*

Fertilization of an egg by a sperm normally occurs in the uterine tube, and further growth occurs in the uterus. The female produces milk in the *mammary glands* of the breasts, and this milk provides the infant with nourishment for a variable period after birth.

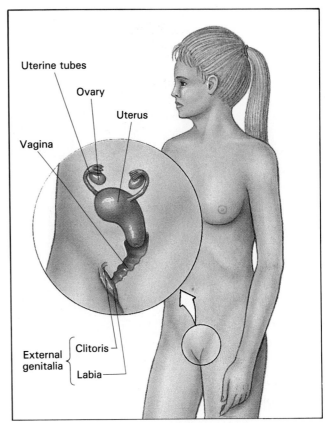

Labels on figure 2 (female):
- Uterine tubes
- Ovary
- Uterus
- Vagina
- External genitalia
- Clitoris
- Labia

■ (b) The Reproductive System of the Female

Organ	Primary Functions
OVARIES	Produce eggs
UTERINE TUBES	Deliver egg(s) or embryo(s) to uterus; site of normal fertilization
UTERUS	Site of embryonic development and diffusion between maternal and embryonic bloodstreams
VAGINA	Site of sperm deposition; birth canal at delivery; provides passage of fluids at menses
EXTERNAL GENITALIA	
Clitoris	Erectile organ, produces pleasurable sensations during sexual act
Labia	Contain glands that lubricate entrance to vagina
MAMMARY GLANDS	Produce milk that nourishes newborn infant

FIGURE A.11b • The Female Reproductive System

B

Health Emergencies, Accidents, and Safety—What You Can Do

In treating accident victims, actions of the first aider at the scene may be the difference between life and death or full recovery and permanent disability. The first aider is the initial link in a community chain or network of responsibility:

- Immediate and adequate first aid at the scene by the early responders, preferably trained in first aid and/or CPR.
- Prompt entry into the emergency medical services system—rescue squad, paramedic, or ambulance service.
- Accessible, well-staffed and well-equipped hospital emergency room.
- Follow-up medical treatment program.

Any delay or inadequacy in this chain could lessen one's chance for survival and increase one's chances for long-term disability. The most common weak link in the chain is the availability of a trained first aider for immediate action. It is obvious that if more of the general population receives first aid and CPR training, this will increase the odds of a trained individual being present when needed. It is an individual as well as community responsibility for every adult to be capable of practicing sound first aid principles in an emergency. Courses in first aid and CPR are readily available from local units of the American Red Cross and the American Heart Association.

Keep in mind that first aid is the immediate care given the victim of an accident or sudden illness. As the first responder and the first link in a survival chain, one of our primary jobs is to seek more advanced treatment for the victim. It is our responsibility to do only those procedures necessary to prevent death or further damage while comforting the victim, easing pain, and seeking medical help.

The American Red Cross suggests the following four emergency action principles for trained first aiders:

1. *Survey the scene.*
2. Do a *primary survey* of the victim to determine need for urgent care.
3. *Activate the Emergency Medical Service system:* phone 911.

4. Do a *secondary survey* of the victim to determine additional problems.

Survey the Scene

As you approach an accident scene, quick observations and questions may help determine the presence of hazards (such as fire, traffic, or electrical wires) for you and the victim, the nature of the injuries, the number of injured parties, what qualified help is available, and whether you are the most qualified to "take charge."

Primary Survey

A quick assessment of those areas which are life-threatening and may require immediate action include:

- Maintaining an open *airway*
- Restoring or maintaining *breathing*
- Restoring or maintaining *circulation*
- Stopping severe *bleeding*

Suspected poisoning and prevention of shock could be added factors.

Activation of the EMS System

As a vital link in the chances of survival, early contact with the EMS system is essential. In most localities the phone number to call for emergencies of all kinds is 911. The following is recommended information to give the EMS dispatcher in emergency calls:

- Location—street address, city or town, directions (cross streets, landmarks, and so on)
- Phone number from where call is being made
- Caller's name
- What happened
- How many injured
- Condition of victim(s)
- Help (first aid) being given

Note: Do not hang up first. Let the person you called hang up first.

Secondary Survey

A head-to-toe examination of the victim, asking questions and taking vital signs, is done to discover other problems that do not pose an immediate threat to life. Some of these problems may become life-threatening if uncorrected or may involve serious injury that may worsen if not handled with care. Examples include neck and spine injuries, head injuries, severe burns, and some broken bones.

The following pages will introduce some basic techniques that will enable you to administer help should the need arise. Seeking training and practice in a certifying course is highly recommended.

Rescue Breathing

Heart attack, toxic gas poisoning, electric shock, drug overdose, brain concussion, fracture of the skull, certain neck fractures, drowning, and choking are among the injuries and ailments that may stop respiration. When breathing stops, seconds count, and life can be saved providing that air enters the victim's lungs immediately. No more than fifteen seconds should elapse in determining the need for artificial respiration and in preparing the victim. The majority of cases of cessation of breathing will not require external heart massage (CPR); however, when the heart has stopped completely, CPR is indicated. Performing CPR properly requires complete training. We do not recommend trying it unless you have taken a CPR course offered at your university or through the Red Cross or American Heart Association.

Artificial Respiration

Figure B.1 illustrates the mouth-to-mouth method of artificial respiration, which is the most effective and rapid method of restoring breathing in adults, infants, and small children. When practicing with a real person as a victim, it is advisable to avoid both mouth-to-mouth contact and giving actual rescue breaths.

For Adults If you find a person lying on the ground, not moving, survey the scene to see if it is safe, and get some idea of what happened. Now begin doing a primary survey:

- **Check for Unresponsiveness.**
  Tap or gently shake the victim.
  Shout "Are you OK?"
  Shout "Help!" to alert bystanders.
- **Position the Victim.**
  Roll the victim onto his or her back, if necessary.
- **Open the Airway Using Head-Tilt/Chin-Lift Method.**
  Place one hand on the victim's forehead.
  Place the fingers of your other hand under the bony part of the lower jaw, near the chin.
  Tilt the victim's head and lift the jaw; avoid closing the victim's mouth.
- **Check for Breathlessness.**
  Maintain an open airway.
  Place your ear over the victim's mouth and nose.
  Look at the victim's chest, listen and feel for breathing for three to five seconds.
- **Give Two Full Breaths.**
  Maintain an open airway.
  Pinch the victim's nose shut.

Open your mouth wide, take a deep breath, and make a tight seal around the outside of the victim's mouth.

Give two full breaths at the rate of one to one and one-half seconds per breath.

Observe the victim's chest rise and fall; listen and feel for escaping air.

- **Check for the Victim's Pulse.**

  Maintain head tilt with one hand on the forehead.

  Locate the victim's Adam's apple with the middle and index fingers of your hand closest to the victim's feet.

  Slide your fingers down into the groove of the victim' neck on the side closest to you.

  Feel for carotid pulse for five to ten seconds.

- **Phone the EMST System for Help**

  Tell someone to call for an ambulance.

  Say "No breathing, has a pulse, call _____ (Local emergency number or operator)."

- **Begin Rescue Breathing.**

  Maintain an open airway.

  Pinch the victim's nose shut.

  Open your mouth wide, take a deep breath, and make a tight seal around the victim's mouth.

  Give one breath every five seconds at the rate of one to one and one-half seconds per breath.

  Observe the victim's chest rise and fall; listen and feel for escaping air and the return of breathing.

  Continue for one minute—about twelve breaths.

- **Recheck Pulse.**

  Tilt the victim's head.

  Locate his or her carotid pulse and feel for five seconds.

  Look, listen, and feel for breathing for three to five seconds.

- **Continue Rescue Breathing.**

  Maintain an open airway.

  Give one breath every five seconds at the rate of one to one and one-half seconds per breath.

  Recheck pulse every minute.

For Infants and Small Children

Basic life support for infants and small children is similar to that for adults. A few important differences to remember are given below.

- **Airway**

  Be careful when handling an infant what you do not exaggerate the backward position of the head tilt. An infant's neck is so pliable that forceful backward tilting might block breathing passages instead of opening them.

- **Breathing**

  Don't try to pinch off the nose. Cover both the mouth and nose of an infant or small child who is not breathing. Use small breaths with less volume to inflate the lungs. Give one small breath every three seconds.

Choking

Many experts believe that the quickest and most effective method (some say the only method) of first aid for choking is the *Heimlich maneuver* (see Figure B.2). The victim is grasped from behind in the "bear hug" position, with the fist of one hand placed just above the umbilicus and below the rib cage and covered by the other hand. A sharp, hard upward squeeze is given, forcing the diaphragm upward to compress the lungs. The air in the lungs will create an upward draft or pressure so great that the obstruction will often be spewed several feet. If the first attempt is unsuccessful, the

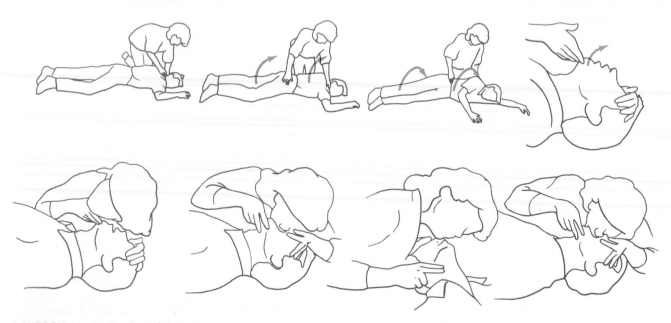

FIGURE B.1 • Rescue breathing

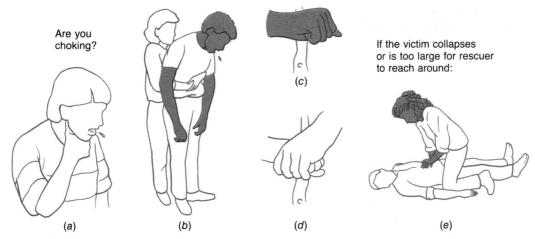

Are you choking?

(a)

(b)

(c)

(d)

If the victim collapses
or is too large for rescuer
to reach around:

(e)

FIGURE B.2 ◆ The Heimlich Maneuver. (a) The universal sign for choking—learn it! Recognize it! The choking victim cannot cough, speak, or breathe. (b-e) Positions to assume while performing the Heimlich maneuver.
Source: Health Thyself®, Blue Cross/Blue Shield of Massachusetts.

squeeze is repeated until the obstruction is expelled. After the object is removed, mouth-to-mouth resuscitation is initiated if normal breathing does not occur.

Steps in performing the Heimlich maneuver are:

- Have the victim stand. Standing behind the victim, place your arms around his or her waist.
- Make a fist. Place the thumb side against the victim's abdomen below the ribcage and just above the belly button (Figure B.2c).
- Cover your fist with your other hand and pull into the victim's abdomen with a *strong, quick upward thrust* (Figure B.2d).
- Avoid squeezing the victim's sides by keeping your elbows out.
- Object should pop out of the victim's mouth . . . if it doesn't, *repeat maneuver immediately.*
- The victim should see a doctor as soon as possible.

If victim is sitting, have him stand immediately and apply maneuver as described above. If the victim collapses or is too large for rescuer to reach around:

- Place the victim on the floor on his or her back, face up, head to one side. Open the mouth if the victim is unconscious.
- Facing the victim, straddle the hips.
- Place the heel of one hand against the victim's abdomen below the ribcage and just above the belly button (See Figure B.2e).
- Place your second hand directly on top of the other hand.
- Press into the victim's abdomen with a *strong, quick upward thrust.* Then check the mouth for the expelled object and remove it.
- The object should pop out of victim's mouth; if it doesn't, *repeat maneuver immediately.*
- The victim should see a doctor as soon as possible.

Hyperventilation

Under some circumstances an individual feels unable to get enough air to breathe. Chest pain or constriction may or may not accompany this feeling. The victim tries to compensate by overbreathing, which lowers carbon dioxide levels in the blood, leading to numbness and tingling in the hands and dizziness. This hyperventilation syndrome is most likely to occur when the individual is under stress or under the influence of alcohol. Symptoms are a direct result of the loss of additional carbon dioxide to the atmosphere from overbreathing. If the victim can remain calm enough and breathe into a paper bag for five to fifteen minutes (holding the bag over both nose and mouth), the symptoms will disappear as carbon dioxide levels are elevated. If in doubt, the victim should be taken to a physician's office.

Control of Hemorrhage

Bleeding is classified according to the three main sources from which it occurs—arteries, veins, and capillaries.

1. *Arterial bleeding.* Bright red blood may spurt from a wound; however, death is unlikely to occur unless a large artery is involved. Bleeding from the carotid (neck), axillary (armpit), brachial (inside of upper arm), or femoral (groin area) artery can cause death in three minutes or less. Arterial bleeding is extremely dangerous, because the force of blood flow through the arterial opening is so strong that the blood will not clot.

2. *Venous bleeding.* A steady flow of dark red blood, profuse at times, suggests that the source is a vein. Although it is easier to control venous bleeding than arterial bleeding, there is the

danger of an air bubble or air embolism, particularly if a large vein is affected. Because the blood is being sucked toward the heart, air could enter the opening and interfere with the ability of the heart to pump blood.

3. *Capillary bleeding.* A general oozing of blood from tissue is not serious, and such bleeding is easily controlled.

Controlling External Bleeding

When severe external bleeding occurs, the first step is to elevate the area of the body that is bleeding above the heart level. Once this is done, there are four basic methods of controlling hemorrhage: direct pressure, pressure dressing, pressure points, and tourniquet, in that order; only as a last resort and under certain unique circumstances is a tourniquet ever applied. Although direct pressure is a first step in most wounds, never apply direct pressure to a head injury because of the risk of pushing contaminants into the brain. Instead, apply a bandage and very light direct pressure, and use the pressure points.

1. *Direct pressure.* Place a heavy, sterile gauze over the wound, with the injured part flat against the floor or table. The edges of the wound should be placed tightly together (use adhesive or butterfly strips) before the compress is in place. Use the heel of the hand to apply just enough steady pressure to stop the bleeding.

2. *Pressure dressing.* After bleeding has been stopped by other means, a pressure dressing is effective in controlling capillary hemorrhage, mild venous bleeding, and arterial bleeding. Edges of the wound are held together with the fingers or strips of clean adhesive before covering with a thick sterile gauze compress or clean fabric. The compress is now firmly bandaged in place (with a roller bandage, conforming bandage, or cravat). Only enough pressure is applied to stop the bleeding. If a pulse cannot be felt below the point of the dressing, it must be loosened until a pulse is felt. If the wound begins to bleed again, it is an indication that it may not be controllable with a pressure dressing.

3. *Pressure points.* When a pressure dressing fails, bleeding can usually be controlled by strong finger pressure on the main artery of blood supply to the wounded part. Of the twenty-two pressure points (eleven on each side), six are used to control external bleeding (see Figure B.3). Pressure points represent the method of choice to control bleeding body parts.

4. *Tourniquet.* A tourniquet is some material—a belt or cord, for example—that can be tightened over an artery to stop the flow of blood. Keep in mind that a tourniquet is a last resort and is rarely needed. Only in the case of a partially torn vessel is a tourniquet indicated, and even then it would

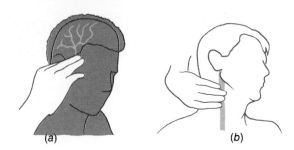

(a) Scalp bleeding: pressure on the temporary artery just in front of the ear.

(b) Head and neck bleeding: pressure on the common carotid artery through constriction against the vertebrae of the neck.

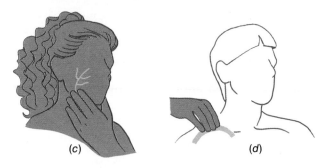

(c) Facial bleeding: pressure on the facial artery against the jawbone; may require pressure on both sides simultaneously.

(d) Armpit and chest wall bleeding: pressure on the subclavian artery as it passes behind the collarbone, downward with the thumb to press the artery against the first rib.

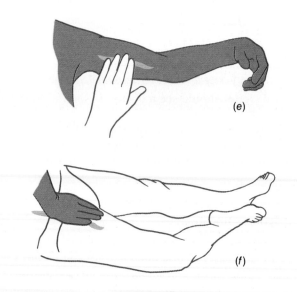

(e) Arm: pressure on the brachial artery against the bone midway between the shoulder and elbow.

(f) Leg: deep pressure on the femoral artery in the groin.

FIGURE B.3 • Pressure Points

have to be applied immediately to prevent fatal bleeding. The use of a tourniquet is controversial; many physicians suggest that lay persons not be instructed in its use. It has been used too often with harmful effects when firm, direct pressure on the pressure points could have controlled bleeding. For that reason, we will not describe it here, but recommend a first aid course for those who wish instruction.

Recognizing Internal Bleeding

Severe internal hemorrhage can result in death as rapidly as external bleeding. Common signs of internal bleeding are thirst, faintness, dizziness, cold and clammy skin, dilated pupils, shallow or irregular breathing, coughing up blood, and rapid, weak, and irregular pulse—symptoms similar to shock. Internal bleeding from an artery, vein, or capillary involves blood loss into the chest, abdominal, or pelvic cavities or into any organ contained therein. A tearing or bruising force, typical of automobile accidents or falls, often causes internal damage.

The color of the blood provides an indication of the injured site:

- Lungs: Coughed-up blood is bright red and frothy.
- Stomach: Vomited blood is bright red; if chronic over a longer period of time, blood may resemble coffee grounds.
- Intestinal tract above the sigmoid colon: Stools are jet black.
- Low in intestinal tract and recent: Blood in stools is bright red.
- Bladder: Blood in the urine.

Intra-abdominal bleeding is characterized by vomiting, tenderness, and rigidity of the stomach muscles. Severe internal bleeding can be controlled only by surgery. Blood transfusions may be necessary at the hospital while surgery is arranged. Until medical assistance arrives, the victim must be kept still in a slightly reclined position or transported to a nearby hospital.

Shock

Shock is one of the body's strongest natural reactions to disease and injury. It slows blood flow, acts as a natural tourniquet until the wound clots, and in a serious injury reduces pain and eases the body's agony when approaching death. The basic types of shock are *traumatic* (injury or loss of blood), *septic* (infection induced), and *cardiogenic* (from a heart attack). All three types can kill and represent one of the greatest dangers for accident and heart attack victims, the severely burned, and those with broken or crushed bones, infection, and insect stings.

The body maintains a delicate balance between blood volume and the space the blood fills. When this balance is upset (as when an artery is severed, resulting in the loss of blood, or in the case of burns, where damaged tissue swells, space expands, and fluids are soaked up from the blood), shock may occur. When the heart or the circulatory system is affected the shock mechanism may be triggered. The chain of events goes something like this:

1. Injury causes a reaction in the adrenal glands, which inject epinephrine into the blood stream and the sympathetic nervous system.
2. Blood vessels constrict, reducing the blood supply to body tissues through the capillaries.
3. Breathing quickens and the heart rate increases in an attempt to pump more oxygen via the blood to the tissues.
4. Inadequate oxygen is available to vital organs, such as the brain, liver, heart, lungs, and kidneys.
5. Tissue dies, the organ ceases functioning, and death occurs (see Figure B.4).

Shock is much easier to prevent than to treat. Careful splinting of broken bones, careful handling, stopping a hemorrhage, and keeping the patient warm all go a long way toward prevention.

First Aid for Shock

Cold and clammy hands, weak and rapid pulse, low blood pressure, and shallow breathing are common signs of shock. Treatment for shock has changed in recent years. No longer is it recommended to lower the victim's head and elevate the feet. Until medical help arrives, the recommended first aid treatment is to stop all bleeding, clear the mouth of vomit, keep the victim lying down, and cover the victim only enough to prevent loss of body heat.

Fractures

Splints can be applied to a leg by laying a board two feet longer than the leg along the side of the leg with its end butted against the groin. A bandage around the ankle and board completes a gentle traction, which will aid in preventing shock for a fractured thigh. Pillows and boards also make excellent splints for legs and knees. It is possible to bind the upper extremity to the body after using boards or magazines as splints for forearms or to bind the legs together for fractures of the thigh, if boards are available. Figure B.5 demonstrates fixation splinting for the lower leg, lower arm, or wrist.

Great emphasis is placed on care of handling. If the victim is in no immediate danger, it is better to await medical personnel or others skilled in moving the injured. A patient should not be lifted by the knees

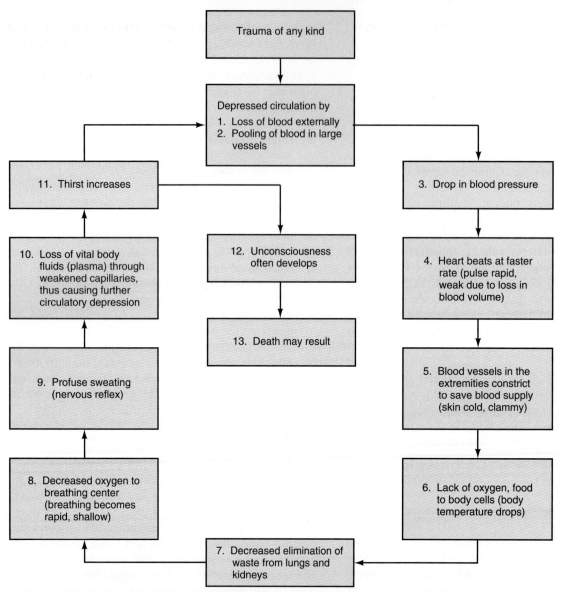

FIGURE B.4 • Continuous cycle of traumatic shock

The flowchart contains the following boxes:

- Trauma of any kind
- Depressed circulation by
  1. Loss of blood externally
  2. Pooling of blood in large vessels
- 11. Thirst increases
- 3. Drop in blood pressure
- 10. Loss of vital body fluids (plasma) through weakened capillaries, thus causing further circulatory depression
- 12. Unconsciousness often develops
- 4. Heart beats at faster rate (pulse rapid, weak due to loss in blood volume)
- 13. Death may result
- 9. Profuse sweating (nervous reflex)
- 5. Blood vessels in the extremities constrict to save blood supply (skin cold, clammy)
- 8. Decreased oxygen to breathing center (breathing becomes rapid, shallow)
- 6. Lack of oxygen, food to body cells (body temperature drops)
- 7. Decreased elimination of waste from lungs and kidneys

FIGURE B.5 • Fixation splinting for the lower leg, lower arm, or wrist

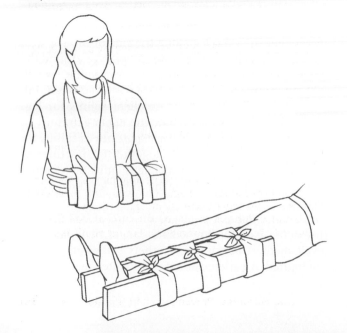

and shoulders, allowing the spine to double. A blanket or five-person carry (four people lifting the patient by holding his or her clothes, while the fifth supports the head and neck) can be used to move the victim if absolutely necessary.

Oral Poisoning: Prevention and First Aid

If medications, insecticides, caustic cleaners, and organic solvents were stored out of the reach of young children, the majority of household poisonings would be prevented. The most common involve strong alkali solutions used in drain cleaners that are capable of destroying tissue on contact. Additional precautionary measures to consider are:

1. Properly labeling all medical and chemical preparations
2. Avoiding the storage of chemicals in food containers
3. Avoiding taking medicine in the dark
4. Listing the purpose and dosage of medicines on the label
5. Washing the hands thoroughly after handling poisons
6. Discarding prescription drugs after they have served their purpose.

Poisons enter the system by way of the mouth (most common), inhalation (for example, vapors or fumes from insecticides, leaky gas appliances, or exhaust systems on autos), injection (from insects), and absorption (directly through the skin). Poisons act in different ways once absorbed into the system: Acids and alkalis burn and corrode tissue, sleeping pills and alcohol depress the central nervous system, insecticides produce extreme stimulation of the central nervous system, and cyanide and carbon monoxide prevent oxygen from being carried to tissues and cause an asphyxial death. Each type requires a different kind of emergency treatment. Table B.1 lists emergency procedures for various oral poisonings.

If you are confronted with a case of oral poisoning, do not panic. Quickly identify the ingested substance, then call the poison control center for advice. Do not start treatment before the substance is identified. If a hospital is nearby, you can bring the substance along to the emergency room. Two types of first aid are indicated: inducing vomiting and diluting or neutralizing the substance. It is essential to find out which treatment is appropriate for the particular kind of poison before proceeding. Vomiting can be induced by stimulating the back of the throat with a finger or using syrup of ipecac followed by water.

TABLE B.1

First Aid for Oral Poisoning

Emergency Situation	Emergency First Aid
No knowledge of poison swallowed	Dilute with several ounces of milk; if not available, use water. Milk of magnesia may neutralize acids and induce catharsis. Search for original container, call poison control center (PCC) to report symptoms and secure advice, transport to hospital.
Knowledge that strong acid alkali or petroleum product was *not* swallowed, but container cannot be found	Dilute with water or milk, induce vomiting (tickling back of throat with index finger or administer syrup of ipecac or mustard and water), call PCC, transport to medical help.
No knowledge of poison swallowed, presence of some of these symptoms: burns around lips and mouth, breath odor (petroleum), unconsciousness, convulsions, exhaustion	Follow suggestions for item 1; avoid administering anything orally to unconscious victim. Keep warm and seek medical help.
Acids	Dilute ingested acid a hundredfold with water or milk or neutralize with milk of magnesia or weak alkali in water (1–2 glasses for children, 3–4 for adults); use milk, olive oil, or egg white as a demulcent without inducing vomiting. Avoid sodium bicarbonate.
Petroleum product (such as kerosene, gasoline, or furniture polish)	Vegetable oil and a saline cathartic will decrease absorption; avoid use of a neutralizing fluid or demulcent; prevent aspiration; call PCC, transport victim.
Alkalis	Dilute ingested alkali with large amounts of water or milk; neutralize with vinegar or lemon juice mixed with water and use milk, olive oil, or egg white as a demulcent. The volume of liquid should exceed the ingested alkali one hundredfold. Permit vomiting.

Emergency Situation	Emergency First Aid
Inhaled poison gases (carbon monoxide)	Hold your breath before entering closed garage or room. Move victim into fresh air; maintain an open airway; administer artificial respiration; call emergency rescue squad.
Unconscious victim	Keep airway open; administer artificial respiration, transport to medical help; deliver poison container.
Alcohol intoxication	Not needed if victim is breathing normally and has regular pulse. With signs of shock, irregular breathing, lack of response, maintain open airway, administer artificial respiration, keep warm, and transport.
Barbiturate (depressant) overdose—opium and morphine substances	Arouse with light slapping or cold compress; maintain open airway; administer artificial respiration if breathing ceases; keep warm, transport to hospital.
Hallucinogenic reaction (LSD, mescaline, psilocybin, morning glory seeds, and synthetic substances)	Protect from bodily harm; move to safe, quiet surroundings; transport to hospital.
Inhalant overdose (glue sniffing, paints and lacquers, gasoline, kerosene, nail polish, nail polish remover)	Administer artificial respiration if breathing stops; transport to hospital.
Stimulant overdose (Benzedrine, Dexedrine, Methedrine, ritalin)	Protect against injury; maintain open airway; administer artifical respiration if breathing stops; keep warm; transport to hospital.

Common Injuries and Their Treatment

Many emergencies can be adequately and safely handled at home without the aid of a physician. Every adult should learn the proper treatment of minor ailments and injuries and be able to determine if and when a physician should be seen. Table B.2 provides some guidelines for the treatment of several common emergencies.

Common Injuries and Their Treatment

Injury	Emergency Home Treatment	Need for a Physician
Abrasion (with skin or layers scraped off)	Clean thoroughly with soap and warm water or hydrogen peroxide. Use bandage if wound oozes blood. Remove loose skin flaps with scissors if they are dirty; allow to remain if clean.	If all dirt and foreign matter cannot be removed If signs of infection occur
Animal bite	Catch the animal and arrange to have it observed for fifteen days to be certain it does not develop rabies. Treat as a cut or puncture wound.	If a wild animal is involved If the animal's immunizations are not current If the observed animal develops rabies If the wound needs a physician's care
Ankle or knee sprain	Stop activity, apply ice pack immediately. Continue ice three times daily for 48 hours before switching to heat. Use crutches for two to three days if pain is severe when walking. Recovery should take this course: swelling and pain for 24–72 hours, decreasing symptoms for six to ten days, full return to normal in six to eight weeks.	If swelling and severe pain continue for more than three days If pain prevents any weight-bearing If there is knee injury other than contusion If there is ligament or tendon damage

Injury	Emergency Home Treatment	Need for a Physician
Broken bone	Look for evidence of a broken bone. Apply ice packs. Protect and rest the injured part for 72 hours. No additional damage is likely to occur if proper rest and protection are provided. Immobilize, call rescue squad, and transport to emergency room.	If the limb is cold, blue, or numb If the pelvis or thigh is involved If the limb is crooked, unusable If there is considerable bleeding and bruising If shock symptoms are present If pain lasts more than 72 hours
Burn	Diagnose the depth of the burn; first degree—superficial; second degree—deeper burns resulting in splitting of layers or blistering from scalding, sunburn, and the like; and third degree—destruction of all layers with damage to the deeper tissues. Apply cold compress for five to ten minutes to reduce skin damage and pain; avoid rupturing blisters. Aspirin may be used for pain.	For all third-degree burns For second-degree burns involving an area greater than 25–35 sq. in. If pain continues for more than two days
Dental injury	Chipped tooth—avoid hot and cold drinks; swelling of face due to abscessed tooth—apply ice pack; excessive bleeding of tooth socket after extraction—place gauze over socket and bite down, maintaining pressure; toothache—ice packs may be used.	If victim has a chipped tooth, an abscessed tooth, excessive bleeding of socket, or a toothache
Fainting and dizziness	Lack of blood flow to the brain commonly occurs with increasing age and may result in a temporary loss of vision or lightheadedness. Avoid sudden changes in posture, reduce anxiety level.	If loss of consciousness occurs If room appears to be spinning If dizziness occurs frequently
Frostbite	Thaw rapidly in a warm water bath. Avoid rubbing frostbite with snow. Water should be comfortable to a normal, unfrozen hand (not over 104°F). When a flush reaches the fingers, remove the frostbitten part immediately. For an ear or nose, use cloths soaked in warm water.	Always see a doctor
Head injury	Apply ice bag to bruised area. Observe patient every two hours for the next 72 hours for alertness (unresponsiveness, deep sleep), unequal pupil size (one-fourth of population have unequal size all the time), and severe vomiting. Pressure inside skull may develop over a 72-hour period.	If there is bleeding from ears, eyes, or mouth If the victim has black eyes If there is unconsciousness, unequal pupil size, lethargy, or severe vomiting
Infected wound (blood poisoning)	Bacterial infection in the bloodstream, or septicemia. Keep area clean, changing the bandage twice daily. Soak and clean in warm water several times daily. Have patience—up to ten to twelve days may be needed for normal healing.	If there is fever above 99.6°F If there is thick pus, swelling since the second day
Insect bite/sting	Apply cold compress, use aspirin or other pain relievers. Identify the insect—black widow spiders have a glossy black body about one-half inch in diameter, red "hour glass" on abdomen. Bite produces sharp pain at the site; cramps appear within an hour and may involve the extremities and trunk. Breathing becomes difficult; nausea, vomiting, twitching, tingling sensations of the hand may occur.	If there is evidence of wheezing, difficulty in breathing, fainting, or hives or skin rash For bite from a black widow spider For severe local reaction

Common Injuries and Their Treatment • 583

Injury	Emergency Home Treatment	Need for a Physician
Minor cut	Clean the wound vigorously with soap and water or hydrogen peroxide, removing all dirt and foreign matter. Use a butterfly bandaid or steristrip to bring the edges of the wound tightly together without trapping the fat or rolling the skin under. Avoid antiseptics: they may destroy tissue and retard healing and do not kill and wash away bacteria as effectively as soap and water.	For cuts on trunk or face, or deep cuts that may involve tendons, ligaments, blood vessels, or nerves For blood pumping from a wound For tingling or limb weakness If signs of infection exist For cuts that cannot be pulled together without trapping the fat
Nosebleed	Squeeze the nose between the thumb and forefinger just below the hard portion for five to ten minutes while seated with the head back. Do not lie down. Apply cold compresses to the bridge of the nose and avoid blowing.	If it occurs frequently and is associated with a cold If victim has a history of high blood pressure
Object in eye	Avoid rubbing—you could scratch the cornea. Close both eyes for several minutes to allow tears to wash out the foreign body. Grasp the lashes of the upper lid and draw out and down over the lower lid. If it feels like the foreign object is present but it is not, cornea scrape probably occurred and will heal in 24–48 hours. Using medicine dropper, flush eye with plain water. If speck is visible, touch lightly with moistened corner of hankerchief. If chemical was splashed in eye, dilute immediately by placing face under lukewarm shower with thick spray.	If the foreign object is on the eye itself If it remains after washing If the object could have penetrated the globe of the eye If blood is visible in eye If vision is impaired If pain is present after 48 hours
Poison ivy and oak	After initial exposure, 12–48 hours may pass before a rash appears. If plant oil is removed from the skin with vigorous washing (two to three times) a rash may be prevented. Apply cool compresses of Burrow's Solution. Cleanse the skin thoroughly. A hot bath will release histamine and cause intense itching; however, the cells of histamine will eventually be depleted and six to eight hours of relief will follow.	If rash occurs without itching, redness or exposure to oak or ivy Contact may be from pets, clothing, or smoke from burning *Rhus* plants
Puncture wound	Let wound bleed as much as possible. Clean thoroughly with soap and water or hydrogen peroxide diluted to 3 percent. Soak the wound at least twice daily in warm water for three to four days to keep the skin puncture open and allow germs and foreign matter to drain.	If the wound is in the head, abdomen, or chest; danger of internal damage If the object is still inside the wound If the wound is deep, cannot be cleaned thoroughly, or a tetanus shot is needed
Sunburn	Apply cool compress using Aveeno or one-half cup baking soda in a tub of water. Avoid Vaseline and other lubricants the first day.	If there are abdominal cramps, dizziness, or second-degree burns

Medic Alert

Approximately one in five persons has special medical conditions or is allergic to particular medications. If such an individual is unable to speak, due to unconsciousness, shock, delirium, hysteria, or injury, then rapid diagnosis and treatment, even by a physician, is not always possible. A diabetic could be diagnosed as intoxicated and go untreated, a shot of penicillin could kill an allergic victim, and those dependent on life-saving medication could mistakenly be given improper doses or incorrect drugs. These and other individuals should wear a Medic Alert bracelet or necklace (see Figure B.6). The Medic Alert symbol is recognized the world over. The bracelet or necklace contains the following vital information: the medical problem, file number, and telephone number of Medic Alert's central file. Information about a medical condition can be obtained in minutes via a collect telephone call twenty-four hours a day.

The fourteen most common medical conditions that may require Medic Alert are asthma, diabetes, heart condition, taking anticoagulants, epilepsy, contact lenses, glaucoma, neck breather, implanted pacemaker, and allergy to penicillin, insect stings, sulfa, codeine, or tetanus antitoxin.

Medic Alert is a charitable, nonprofit organization. It was founded in 1956 by Marion C. Collins, M.D., and is currently endorsed by more than 100 organizations, including the American Academy of Family Physicians, the International Associations of Fire Chiefs and Police Chiefs, the National Sheriffs' Association, and the National Association of Life Underwriters. The cost for a Medic Alert bracelet or necklace is as low as $10.00. For further information, write to Medic Alert Foundation International, Turlock, California 95380.

FIGURE B.6 • Medic Alert Symbol: The two sides of the Medic Alert bracelet
Source: Medic Alert Foundation International

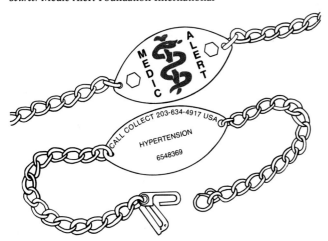

Accidents and Safety

Although accident rates have declined slightly over the past forty years, accidents remain a leading cause of death in the United States. In the general population accidents are the fourth leading cause of death, behind heart disease, cancer, and stroke. In the one-to-twenty-four age group accidents are the leading cause of death, and the accident rate for men is more than twice the rate for women.

Approximately one accidental death occurs every four minutes, with an accidental injury taking place every three or four seconds. Motor vehicle accidents are the major cause of death at all age levels, followed by falls, drowning, fires and burns, ingestion of food and other small objects, poisoning, firearm accidents, and poisoning by gas. Each year approximately 50,000 deaths and millions of injuries are caused by motor vehicle accidents; about one person in two can be expected to be killed or injured in an auto accident during his or her lifetime. Home accidents cause the greatest number of injuries.

Factors Contributing to Accidents

Accidents are caused by the interaction of several factors and may not have a single cause. Although the layperson may view accidents as "acts of God," "fate," or simply "bad luck," only a small percentage of accidents can be attributed to chance. Most often, accidents are caused by a combination of factors, such as individual neglect, attitude, psychological/emotional factors, personality, cultural factors, and environmental factors.

Various personality traits have been associated with high accident rates. Poor judgment, impulsiveness, overconfidence in one's ability, lack of patience, and an exaggerated opinion of one's importance may contribute to vehicle accidents, particularly in the sixteen-to-twenty-four age group. Similar associations have been established for the accident-prone individual.

Cultural factors also contribute to accidents in the United States. As our society grows increasingly complex and competitive, the individual experiences more tension and strain. Divorce, inadequate parental guidance, widespread use of drugs and pills, and the worship of the automobile and of speed (auto races, boat races, airplane races, bicycle races, and so forth) all contribute to the accident rate in this country.

Physiological factors, such as poor coordination and motor skill, poor sight and hearing, or other physical handicaps, have little to do with the cause of accidents. Fatigue, however, does reduce reaction time and thus contributes to accidents of all types. In addition, those who have certain diseases (epilepsy, heart disease, and so forth) are somewhat more likely to be involved in an accident. Many over-the-counter and prescription drugs can cause drowsiness, and stimulants, depressants, and hallucinogens also drastically reduce performance, making the user more susceptible to all types of accidents. Even a low level of physical fitness is a contributing factor, particularly late in the day, when fatigue become evident. Perhaps the major drug contributing to accidents is alcohol, which is responsible for a large percentage of both automobile and occupational accidents. Among teenagers, use of alcohol and other drugs, such as quaaludes, frequently leads to automobile accidents.

Accident Prevention

Home and motor vehicle accidents don't always happen to other people. Unless you take some precautions, you too are likely to become involved before too long in a major accident of some type. The following suggestions may help avoid such an occurrence.

Preventing Home Accidents

Fires

1. Avoid smoking in bed or near flammable material.
2. Avoid overloading electrical outlets.
3. Check electrical equipment regularly, looking for frayed wires, unplugging appliances not in use, and making certain proper fuses are being used.
4. Install a smoke alarm system in your home.
5. Avoid keeping flammable liquids, such as paint and fuel, in your home.
6. Wipe grease spills immediately and water down the area.
7. Store matches, cigarette lighters, and heating and cooking appliances out of the reach of children.
8. Inspect attics, garages, and cellars carefully for potential firetraps.
9. Develop and rehearse a plan of action in case of a fire that requires leaving the home through an exit other than the doors; go through the procedure with the entire family.
10. Keep emergency fire numbers and a fire extinguisher accessible.

Poisoning

See the section on ''Oral Poisoning,'' above

Falls

1. Keep a close watch on infants at all times.

2. Keep floors uncluttered and well lit. Check handrails near stairs for sturdiness.
3. Check ladders carefully before each use; place them carefully and avoid climbing beyond the third rung from the top under any condition.
4. Clean ice and snow from porches and steps.
5. Consider use of rubber matting to avoid slipping in hallways, on porches, and in bathtubs.

Suffocation

1. Do not allow infants to sleep on pillows.
2. Discard plastic bags (such as those accompanying clothes from the cleaners) immediately.
3. Remove doors and lids from all discarded large objects (refrigerators, coolers, trunks).
4. Inspect toys carefully and throw away items with loose objects or stuffing that could result in choking if swallowed.
5. Practice the proper first aid procedure (Heimlich maneuver) for choking with the entire family.

Drowning

1. Learn to swim in one of the many programs available to the public (YMCA and YWCA clubs, American Red Cross, youth centers, and so forth).
2. Learn proper boat safety and exercise caution at all times. If your boat capsizes, cling to it rather than trying to swim to shore.
3. Don't swim alone in unattended areas and don't swim at night. Don't leave a child alone in a children's pool, no matter how shallow.
4. Swim near the shore.
5. Be certain the water is deep enough before diving.
6. Before entering the water to rescue a victim in difficulty, throw out a life preserver or rope.

Gun Accidents

1. Avoid storing loaded weapons in the house; keep under lock and key and hidden from children.
2. Unload your weapon while cleaning; avoid showing off with guns.
3. If you must have a gun in your home, learn how to use it properly. Practice in a safe area until you feel comfortable with the weapon.
4. Never point a gun at another person.

Preventing Motor Vehicle Accidents

Automobiles, Trucks, and Buses

1. The automobile is slowly becoming a safer vehicle, although it remains a deadly weapon at high speeds. Several changes in safety standards

and design either have already taken place or will eventually occur to improve the safety of the automobile: elimination of sharp parts on the dashboard and other interior parts, seat and shoulder belts, strategic location of rupture-resistant gas tanks, energy-absorbing bumpers, collapsible steering columns, padded interiors, air bags, outside review mirrors, larger and sturdier tires, door safety catches, removal of protruding hub-cap ornaments, emergency brake systems, energy-absorbing frames, engines that deflect downward rather than into the driver in a head-on collision, and roll bars to prevent the roof from collapsing during a roll-over. Additional changes are needed.

2. Don't drive while under the influence of alcohol or any other drug.

3. Have your car inspected periodically; check brakes, lights, and engine between inspection dates.

4. Buckle up, even if you are only going ''up the street.'' Insist that all passengers in your car use seat and shoulder belts.

5. Obey speed limits; avoid driving too fast or too slow.

6. Keep a safe distance from the car ahead of you (one car length for every 10 mph of speed).

7. Leave for your destination in plenty of time to avoid rushing and tension.

8. Use the proper lane before turning; signal your intentions.

9. Yield to other drivers.

10. Stay in the right lane except to pass.

11. Don't drive when emotionally upset.

12. Learn and follow good seeing habits: Aim high in steering by looking far ahead of the path your car will follow; keep your eyes moving, get the big picture by scanning in front, to the sides and behind you; make sure others see you by communicating with your brake light, headlights, horn, car position, and turn signals, and always leave yourself an out or escape path.

Motorcycles

1. Follow the suggestions listed under automobiles, trucks, and buses.

2. Use an approved helmet and eye protection device, and insist on all passengers wearing the same.

3. Inspect your motorcycle regularly and keep the rearview mirror clean and properly positioned.

4. Practice riding your motorcycle in a field or desolate area before entering a highway.

5. Don't borrow a motorcycle you are not used to. Habits are difficult to break, and mechanical handling varies from one motorcycle to another.

6. Wear long pants and a leather jacket to reduce injury in case of a fall.

7. Keep headlights on at all times to aid other motorists in seeing you.

8. Use a proper muffler to keep the noise level low and unalarming to other motorists.

9. Avoid changing lanes unless absolutely necessary; remember, you are difficult for the motorist to see.

10. Avoid riding in a driver's blind spot (at the right or left rear of the car).

11. Avoid riding between the lines of moving cars.

12. Ride in the left car-wheel track of a lane.

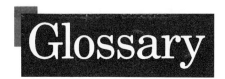
Glossary

abortifacients Chemical substances that cause abortion or terminate pregnancy.

abortion The termination of a pregnancy.

abstinence Abstaining from sexual intercourse.

abstinence syndrome A medical condition experienced by many people who try to give up an addiction to nicotine or any other psychoactive drug. Symptoms include restlessness, changes in heart rate and blood pressure, and a craving for nicotine.

acid rain Rain that is more acidic than rain usually is or should be; a health hazard in all areas of the industrialized world.

acne Skin blemishes, such as pimples and blackheads, caused by excessively oily skin; a common complaint of the adolescent and young adult years.

acquaintance rape Forcible sexual intercourse by anyone known to the victim.

acquired immune deficiency syndrome (AIDS) An STD that weakens the human immune system leading to serious opportunistic diseases; usually fatal in the long run.

active euthanasia Actions that hasten or cause the death of someone who is terminally ill and without hope of recovery; also called "mercy killing."

active immunity When a body can produce antibodies against a specific antigen, causing a long-term immune response to that antigen and its associated disease.

acupuncture A method of medical treatment that uses needles inserted at specific points on the body to relieve pain and to bring about a treatment or cure for disease.

acute bronchitis A short-term severe inflammation of the bronchial tubes.

aerobic Aerobic means "with oxygen" and describes extended vigorous exercise that stimulates heart-lung activity and conditioning.

affective disorders Mental disturbances in which people act inappropriately joyful, sad, or both.

ageism A negative attitude toward growing old and toward old people; a common prejudice against older people (senior citizens), as reflected in stereotypes and derogatory language about older people.

AIDS-related complex (ARC) A medical condition which is an STD, wherein the HIV virus that causes AIDS is contracted by the patient, but the patient does not develop a full-blown case of AIDS, although the immune system is weakened.

alcohol abuser A person who frequently drinks alcoholic beverages to excess, who suffers from psychological and physical problems from drinking alcohol, but who is not yet dependent on alcohol.

alcohol dependent person A person who drinks alcoholic beverages excessively to the point of dependence upon alcohol, and who suffers from chronic alcohol-related psychological and physical problems. These people are commonly called "alcoholics."

alcoholic The term commonly used to indicate an alcohol dependent person.

Alcoholics Anonymous A worldwide organization dedicated to the rehabilitation of the alcoholic and to the prevention of alcoholism.

alienation The feeling of being separated from the society in which one lives.

allergens Substances that induce an allergic reaction.

allergy A hypersensitivity to a specific substance (such as food, pollen, or dust) or condition (such as cold or heat) that in similar amounts would appear to be harmless to most people.

Alzheimer's disease A brain disorder, affecting 6 to 8 percent of the older population over 65; it is characterized by memory loss, and gradually leads to a generalized inability to function independently.

amniocentesis A medical test in which amniotic fluid is drawn from the uterus of a pregnant woman to determine the health of the unborn fetus.

amphetamines A powerful stimulant drug with dangerous side effects and addictive qualities; found in pharmaceuticals and in illegal drug compounds.

anaerobic Anaerobic means "without oxygen" and describes short, all-out exercise efforts.

androgyny The blending of (stereotypically) "masculine" and "feminine" characteristics in one person.

angina pectoris A common symptom of heart disease, angina pectoris is chest pain caused by ischemia, a reduced blood supply to the heart.

anorexia nervosa An eating disorder, found most often in women, that involves lack of appetite to the point of self-starvation and dangerous weight loss.

antabuse A drug that causes nausea when alcohol is ingested. It is sometimes used to treat alcoholism.

antibiotic A pharmaceutical, such as penicillin, which will destroy bacteria and other microbes that cause disease.

antibody Specific protein complexes that are produced by a body to defend against, destroy, or neutralize antigens.

antigen A specific outside agent that upon entering the body promotes antibody formation.

anxiety Feelings of apprehension that may stem from either real or imagined concerns or situations.

anxiety disorders Mental disturbances in which individuals experience high levels of anxiety, including phobic disorders and obsessive-compulsive disorders.

aphasia Speech and language difficulties, often occurring with left-sided hemiplegia, a common finding in cases of stroke.

arteriosclerosis The thickening and hardening of the arteries, a process that normally occurs as a person ages.

arthritis A disease in which there is a degeneration of the joints and connective tissues, leading to inflammation and pain.

artificial insemination The impregnation of a woman with the aid of medical techniques, using semen gathered from her husband or from another donor if the husband is sterile.

asymptomatic An asymptomatic medical condition has no visible symptoms and may, therefore, be unknown to the individual.

atherosclerosis The buildup of plaque on the inner lining of arteries; a major cause of cardiovascular disease.

aura A certain feeling which to an epileptic is a warning that a seizure is impending.

autogenic training A means of learning general body relaxation through the use of imagery and the feeling of heaviness and warmth in the body's limbs.

autoinoculation The spread of a disease from one part of the body to another because of poor hygiene habits.

autonomous stage In Piaget's theory of the personality, at this stage the personality is less dependent on external authority as a guide to behavior.

azidothymidine (AZT) An AIDS-fighting pharmaceutical approved by the FDA in March 1987.

bacteria Microscopic, single-cell organisms; plantlike in some characteristics. Some bacteria cause disease; others are beneficial. They are often classified by shape.

barbiturate A common depressant-type drug, found in pharmaceuticals and in illegal forms.

basal body temperature (BBT) The body's core temperature; in women, it usually decreases before ovulation and increases during ovulation.

basal metabolism or metabolic rate The number of calories burned by a person while at rest but not while sleeping.

battered spouse In situations of spouse abuse, the assaulted or physically abused marriage partner is called the "battered spouse."

behaviorism A psychological theory that postulates that behavior is caused, or conditioned, by dynamics and stimuli that are external to the individual.

behavior therapy A treatment program for mental illness that emphasizes behavior modification.

bereavement The time period during which one mourns the death of a loved one.

binuclear family A family arrangement in which a man and a woman no longer married, and living in separate households, still share in the care of their children, providing space in each household for the children.

biofeedback The monitoring of the physiological events of the body and the instantaneous reporting of these events to the individual so that relaxation techniques may be employed.

birth control pill Any of a variety of hormone-containing pills that women ingest on specific schedules in order to prevent conception.

bisexual Describes persons who engage in sexual behavior with males on some occasions and with females on other occasions.

blackout The loss of memory of what occurred during a bout of heavy drinking; this is an early symptom of alcoholism.

blood alcohol level (BAL) A measure of the amount of alcohol present in the total blood of an individual, presented as a percentage of the total blood volume.

blood pressure The pressure of the blood as it flows through and presses against the arterial walls of the body; an important measure of cardiovascular and general health.

bonding The attachment that develops between mother and newborn soon after birth.

botulism A serious food-poisoning disease caused by the botulism bacteria.

brain death A medical definition of death that includes the criteria of unresponsiveness, unreceptiveness, lack of movement, lack of breathing, lack of reflex, and a total lack of brain wave (EEG) activity.

bulimia An eating disorder, found most often in women, that involves eating binges followed by self-induced vomiting or the use of laxatives to expel the unwanted food.

burnout A syndrome that includes feelings of physical and mental exhaustion caused by excessive work and stress.

caffeine A common stimulant drug found in many foods, drinks, and medications, including coffee, tea, soft drinks, and over-the-counter drugs.

calculus (tartar) The hardened mineralized deposit made up of plaque that has not been properly removed from the teeth.

caloric balance When caloric intake per day equals caloric expenditures per day, at which point no weight loss or gain occurs.

calories A unit of measurement indicating the amount of energy contained in a given amount of food.

cancer Not a single disease, but a group of more than 100 diseases that are characterized by abnormal cell growth.

carbohydrate loading A special diet used by athletes in the seven days before competition to help improve their performance.

carbon monoxide A poisonous gas found in tobacco smoke. It displaces oxygen in the bloodstream, causing a lack of oxygen in the body.

carcinogen Any substance that acts as a cancer-causing agent.

carcinomas Cancers that begin in the epithelial cells (the linings) of the lungs, digestive organs, reproductive organs, mouth, and other body cavities.

cardiovascular disease A general term used to describe heart disease, stroke, high blood pressure, and other diseases of the circulatory system.

carotid pulse The pulse as taken by placing the index and middle fingers in the hollow of the neck under the jaw bone in order to palpate the carotid artery.

cellulite The name commonly given to fat that accumulates on the legs and buttocks in overweight individuals; medically speaking, it is no different from fat in other parts of the body.

cerebral palsy A disease of the central nervous system characterized by uncontrolled muscular contractions.

cerebrovascular accident (CVA) The severe reduction of blood flow to a portion of the brain, often caused by a blood clot, causing a part of the brain to be damaged; commonly called a stroke.

cervical cap A rubber, plastic, or metal cap that covers the cervix, creating a barrier to sperm; unlike the diaphragm, it may remain in place for two days.

cesarean section (C-section) A fetal delivery procedure that involves cutting through the abdominal wall into the uterus, performed when a vaginal delivery would place the mother or the baby at risk.

chancre A painless sore on the penis, mouth, anus, or in the vagina where the spirochete that causes syphilis has entered the body.

chancroid An STD that results in sores very similar to the chancre sores of syphilis.

chemotherapy The treatment of mental illness through the use of medications, such as tranquilizers and antidepressants.

chiropractic A method of medical treatment originated in 1895 by David Palmer, chiropractic medicine relies on manipulation of the vertebrae and other body parts to bring about efficacious medical treatment.

chlamydia A common STD caused by a viruslike bacterium; can lead to sterility, inflammation in the reproductive and urinary tracts, and pelvic inflammatory disease. Treated with antibiotics.

cholesterol One of the sterols or fatlike chemical substances manufactured by the body and also consumed in foods of animal origin. Excess cholesterol is associated with coronary heart and artery disease.

chronic bronchitis A long-term inflammation of the bronchial tubes resulting in a constant cough, phlegm production, expectorating of mucus, and labored breathing; aggravated by smoking.

cirrhosis The final stage of a liver disease directly related to alcohol abuse. At this stage, liver cells are dying and damage to the liver is permanent.

client-centered therapy A treatment program for mental illness developed by Carl Rogers that focuses on the positive acceptance of the patient by himself or herself.

coalcoholic A term used to describe the family members that are affected by the alcoholic's problems.

coastal waters Those waters from the coast to the head of tide, the farthest point inland where the influence of the tide on water levels is detected.

cocaine A highly dangerous and illegal stimulant-type drug with serious side effects and addictive properties. It has been a very commonly used drug in the past decade and is found in various forms with various street names.

cohabitation Living together in a sexual relationship without being married.

coinsurance clause A statement indicating that a specified percentage of insurance-covered cost must be paid by the insured after the deductible amount is subtracted.

coitus Sexual intercourse, specifically penile-vaginal intercourse.

coitus interruptus During coitus, the withdrawal of the penis from the vagina prior to ejaculation; a method of contraception, but not very effective.

collateral circulation The development of small arteries called arterioles that bypass a blockage in a main artery.

Comprehensive Smokeless Tobacco Health Education Act An Act of Congress enacted in 1986 that seeks to discourage the use of chewing tobacco and snuff because of the health hazards associated with those products.

Comprehensive Smoking Education Act An Act of Congress enacted in 1984 that calls for various measures to discourage the use of cigarettes, cigars, and pipe tobacco because of the health hazards connected with those products.

condom A sheath of latex rubber or animal skin placed on the erect penis to prevent sperm from entering the vagina.

confirmation The type of feedback that partners give each other in an intimate relationship.

congestive heart failure A condition in which the heart is not strong enough to keep the blood circulating properly, causing the blood to back up as it returns to the heart.

conjunctivitis An infection of the mucous membranes (conjunctiva) lining the inner surface of the eyelids and covering the surface of the whites of the eyes; also called "pinkeye."

contraception The prevention of fertilization of the ovum by the sperm.

coronary occlusion A complete blockage of the coronary artery caused by a blood clot.

coronary thrombosis A blood clot in the coronary artery, frequently the cause of myocardial infarction.

covert modeling Vividly imagining someone else performing a desired behavior and then substituting yourself for that person.

covert rehearsal Vividly imagining yourself performing some desired behavior.

covert reinforcement Rewarding yourself for being able to imagine yourself performing some desired behavior.

crank The street name for the pill form of a common methamphetamine.

cremation The incineration of a corpse in a special oven at a very high temperature.

cryosurgery Freezing the skin or other tissue with liquid nitrogen; sometimes used as a treatment for age spots.

cunnilingus The act of sucking or licking the vulva.

dandruff A combination of sebum and dead skin that forms on the scalp and is then sloughed off in small flakes; treatment is obtained through the use of special shampoos.

date rape Forcible sexual intercourse by one's date.

decibel A measure of sound based on the pressure of sound on the human ear; 1 decibel is the faintest sound a person can hear; 120 decibels will produce physical pain in the ears.

deductible The initial portion of an insurance claim that is paid by the insured; the higher the deductible, the lower the premium.

defense mechanism The attempt by an individual to manage anxiety-provoking situations by unconsciously distorting reality.

dementia A term used to describe both Alzheimer's disease and a nonspecific progressive mental impairment found in some older people.

dental caries Tooth decay or cavities, usually occurring on tooth surfaces that are in contact with other teeth.

depression A psychological condition or illness characterized by feelings of sadness, despair, and lack of self-esteem.

DES DES (Diethylstilbestrol) is a synthetic estrogen used in emergency cases of rape or incest to terminate pregnancies.

DESC An acronym that expresses an effective way to assert oneself verbally: Describe, Express, Specify, Choose.

diabetes A disease of the metabolic system caused by an insufficient amount of the hormone insulin, which is produced by the pancreas.

diaphragm A latex rubber cap around a collapsible metal ring, designed to fit over the cervix and prevent sperm from entering the uterus; best used in conjunction with a spermicidal cream or jelly.

dietary fiber The undigested portion of complex carbohydrates, a nonnutritive substance that comes from plant sources.

disability insurance Private health insurance designed to provide income during periods of sickness or injury.

disease The destructive processes found during an illness that lead to noticeable symptoms of pain and discomfort.

dosage The specific amount of a specific drug needed to produce a pharmacological effect.

Down's syndrome A genetically transmitted disease that results in some facial and body abnormalities and in mild to severe mental retardation.

drug Any substance that by its chemical nature alters the structure or function in a living organism.

drug abuse When the use of drugs for either medical or recreational purposes results in physiological or psychological harm to the users or to others.

drug misuse The inappropriate and excessive use of pharmaceuticals and over-the-counter drugs in ways or in dosages not originally intended.

Durable Power of Attorney Often written in conjunction with a Living Will, a Durable Power of Attorney is legally binding and instructs a person to act as agent or attorney for another person who is incapacitated by illness or accident.

dyathanasia A term that is synonymous with passive euthanasia.

dying The process by which living matter arrives at death.

dyspareunia Painful sexual intercourse.

early pregnancy tests (EPTs) Do-it-yourself kits of varying accuracy that women can use on their own for determining pregnancy.

edentulism The loss of the natural teeth; hastened by smoking.

ego In Freudian psychology, the part of our personality that is in touch with reality.

ejaculatory incompetence The inability of a man to ejaculate into the vagina during coitus.

electroencephalogram (EEG) A medical measure of the electrical impulses within the brain (brain wave activity).

electrolysis The permanent removal of unwanted body hair through the use of an electrical current administered by the injection of a needle into the hair follicle.

embalming The replacement of the blood in a corpse with various fluids to make the body more presentable for a funeral, to prepare the body for transport, or to preserve the body if refrigeration is not available.

embolus A stroke caused by a blood clot that travels from another part of the body to the brain; only about 10 percent of strokes occur in this way.

emotional health The ability to deal constructively with reality, regardless of whether the actual situation is good or bad.

emphysema A chronic lung disease characterized by coughing, shortness of breath, and extreme weakness, eventually resulting in debilitation and death; thirteen times more prevalent among cigarette smokers than among nonsmokers.

encephalitis An inflammation of the brain. Encephalitis is sometimes a complication of measles.

epilepsy A disease of the central nervous system that causes seizures; various causes exist.

erectile dysfunction The correct term for describing difficulty in achieving and maintaining a penile erection; popularly known as "impotence."

essential amino acids Those amino acids that cannot be manufactured by the body and must be obtained from food.

estrogen replacement therapy (ERT) Through medication, the artificial replacement of estrogen in menopausal women in order to alleviate the unpleasant symptoms of menopause.

expectorant A medication that causes an increase in the flow of respiratory tract secretions and facilitates the removal of irritating substances that cause coughing.

external genitalia Those parts of the female genitalia that can be clearly seen.

family therapy Treatment for mental illness that focuses not only on the disturbed client but also on his or her family.

fat-soluble vitamins Those vitamins that are dissolved in fatty acids and are stored in the body, such as vitamins A, D, E, and K.

fellatio The act of sucking or licking the penis or scrotum.

fetal alcohol effect (FAE) A condition found in babies whose mothers were heavy users of alcohol during pregnancy; the condition is characterized by low birth weight, growth deficiencies, central nervous system dysfunctions, and serious developmental problems.

fetal alcohol syndrome (FAS) A condition found in babies whose mothers were heavy users of alcohol during pregnancy; the condition is characterized by low birth weight, growth deficiencies, central nervous system dysfunctions, and serious developmental problems.

flashback A hallucination that occurs sometime *after* the use of a psychedelic or hallucinogenic drug, indicating that the drug has some sort of retroactive effect on the user.

functional heart murmur A murmur occurring in a normal heart.

fungi Plantlike organisms that obtain nutrition by growing on the tissue of other organisms. Fungi cause some diseases in humans.

gender Gender refers to how you were born, male or female.

gender identity The conviction about and the acceptance of being a male or a female that an individual develops as he or she matures.

gender roles A society's set of rules or norms that govern male and female behaviors.

generic drug A pharmaceutical drug that is produced after the patent has expired on the original brand-name drug; generic drugs have the same formulation, safety, and effectiveness as brand-name drugs, but they are indicated by their chemical names and usually cost less than their brand-name counterparts.

genital herpes An STD that is caused by the herpes simplex, type 2 virus. The disease is incurable. Carefully treated it is not a serious disease, but its spread to the rest of the body can result in serious complications. It has been linked to the onset of cervical cancer.

genital warts An STD of the genital and perineal areas of both men and women caused by a virus; linked to an increased incidence of cancer.

gerontology The study of aging as a scientific discipline; *geriatrics* is the medical treatment of older people.

gestation The period of time from conception to birth.

gingivitis A gum inflammation resulting in bleeding gums, pain, and foul mouth odor; aggravated by smoking.

glaucoma An eye disorder characterized by increased pressure within the eye; a serious disease causing blindness if not treated, but easily controlled with medication.

global warming The long-term warming of the earth's climate due to excessive amounts of carbon dioxide, a by-product of fossil fuel use.

gonorrhea An STD that is caused by a bacterium. Although the disease can be treated with antibiotics, if left untreated it can lead to serious complications, including bladder and kidney disease and diseases of the pelvic and genital areas.

Gossypol A substance derived from cottonseed oil that shows promise as an oral contraceptive for males, though there are some side effects.

granuloma inguinale An STD, usually of tropical areas, which exhibits painful sores and blisters on the genitalia.

greenhouse effect Warming of the earth's atmosphere and surface produced when the sun's heat is trapped by layers of carbon dioxide and other gases.

grief The emotions of anger and sadness and the sense of loss that follow after the death of a loved one.

group practice Three or more physicians working together in their various specialties.

group therapy A treatment program for mental illness where one therapist works with several clients at the same time.

habituation The process of becoming used to a stimulus after experiencing it repeatedly.

hallucinogens A term used interchangeably with the term "psychedelics" to describe drugs that alter mood, behavior, and perception, and which sometimes cause hallucinations.

hardiness Behavior that responds to stress positively, viewing stressful events as challenges rather than as threats; and being committed and exercising control over the event.

hay fever Also called *allergic rhinitis,* hay fever is a commonly found allergic hypersensitivity reaction to house dust, pollen, mold, or spores.

health maintenance organization (HMO) A comprehensive medical insurance plan that covers both treatment and prevention for a fixed, prepaid monthly fee.

heart murmur A sound audible on listening to the heart.

hemiplegia A paralysis on one side of the body; a classic finding in cases of stroke.

heroin A common, illegal, dangerous, and addictive opiate. Often injected by syringe, its use has contributed to the spread of AIDS and hepatitis.

heteronomous stage In Piaget's theory of the personality, at this stage of development the individual relies upon rigid and authoritarian rules for behavioral guidance.

high-density lipoproteins (HDL) A type of cholesterol that is considered beneficial in certain amounts because it lubricates the inner linings of arteries.

homophobia An irrational fear of homosexuality.

hospice A special facility or service that provides for the care of dying patients at their home or in a homelike setting.

hot flashes Commonly experienced symptoms of menopause, hot flashes are sensations of heat caused by the irregular dilation of blood vessels, often in the face.

hyperpigmentation An excessive darkening of the skin, usually in certain areas, caused by too much exposure to the sun, disease, oral contraceptives, and pregnancy.

hypertension Abnormally high blood pressure; associated with stress, hypertension is often a cause of coronary heart disease and stroke.

hypervitaminosis The name given to the serious toxic side effects that result from the overconsumption of vitamins.

hyposensitization A treatment of allergies that employs small doses of the allergen over a period of time in order to desensitize the patient to the allergen and thereby to lessen the allergic reaction.

ice A highly addictive methamphetamine that is even more potent than crank.

id In Freudian psychology, the part of our personality that seeks pleasure and gratification.

immunity The ability of the human body, or another organism's body, to recognize and defend itself against specific infectious agents.

immunotherapy A cancer treatment involving the stimulation of the body's own disease-fighting systems to combat cancer; also, a term used synonymously with *hyposensitization* to describe a therapy which desensitizes a patient to a particular allergen.

impotence The inability of the male to maintain an erection long enough to have sexual intercourse.

incest Sexual intercourse or coercive sexual contact between close blood relatives.

infectious hepatitis (type A hepatitis) A common disease characterized by an inflammation of the liver, caused by a virus. Contracted usually through fecal contamination of food; usually not a severe disease.

infectious mononucleosis A viral infection like the common cold, but lasting much longer; occasionally there are serious complications.

infertility Generally defined as the inability to conceive after a year or more of sexual relations without contraception.

influenza (flu) A viral infection of the upper respiratory tract causing severe coldlike symptoms. There are several strains of flu and various vaccines are manufactured to combat them. Influenza can lead to pneumonia or death in weak or aged people.

inhibited sexual desire (ISD) A lack of sexual appetite or a disinterest in sexual activity.

insulin A hormone produced by the pancreas that is used by the body to metabolize glucose to provide energy for bodily functions. It may be administered as a medication to treat diabetes.

insulin shock A medical condition in a diabetic individual who is suffering from low blood sugar due to excessive insulin administration. The condition can be relieved by giving the person something sweet to eat or drink.

interferon A protein released by body cells infected with a virus that works with body membranes to prevent and fight viral infection.

internal genitalia Those parts of the genitalia that are within the body and are not directly observable.

intimacy The ability to form close and lasting relationships.

intrauterine device (IUD) A small object of metal or plastic that is placed into the uterus to prevent conception.

in vitro fertilization The fertilization of a human egg (ovum) by a sperm cell outside the body in a sterile, medically controlled environment. The fertilized egg is then placed within the mother-to-be's body for gestation and eventual birth.

iron deficiency anemia A major health problem in the United States among certain population groups, iron deficiency anemia is caused by a lack of iron in the diet, resulting in a low hemoglobin level in the blood.

iron overload The ingestion of too much iron in the diet, resulting in constipation and possible liver damage.

irritable bowel syndrome Constipation or diarrhea caused by intestinal spasms, usually related to worry, fear, and anxiety.

jaundice A yellowing of the skin and the whites of the eyes, caused by an inflammation of the liver.

labor The birth process.

latchkey children In dual-career families, children of school age who are literally given a house key so that they can come home and care for themselves.

laxatives Substances that loosen feces in the bowels and relieve constipation.

lead poisoning (plumbism) A serious disease resulting from the ingestion or inhalation of lead; findings include weakness, anemia, brain damage, and mental retardation. Lead has been a serious pollutant of water, soil, and air.

leukemia Cancers that form in the blood-forming parts of the body, the bone marrow and the spleen. These nonsolid tumors are characterized by an abnormally high number of white blood cells.

Living Will A written statement, legally binding, that instructs doctors and others on the medical procedures to be used in case of catastrophic illness or accident because of which the writer of the will is incapable of making or communicating decisions. The will applies in situations in which the writer cannot regain a normal life or is terminally ill.

low-density lipoproteins (LDL) A type of cholesterol that is considered harmful because it promotes fatty deposits on the inner lining of arteries.

Lyme disease A disease caused by a vector-borne bacteria; it resembles arthritis. Effectively treated with antibiotics; transmitted by deer ticks.

lymphocytes White blood cells formed in the bone marrow that produce antibodies to battle specific disease-causing agents.

lymphogranuloma venereum (LGV) An STD, usually of tropical areas, which exhibits pimplelike sores on the genitalia.

lymphomas Cancers that begin in the infection-fighting regions of the body—principally the lymphatic system.

macrominerals Those minerals needed in large amounts by the body.

mammography A radiological medical test to diagnose cancer of the breast.

marijuana The crushed leaves of the *cannabis sativa* or hemp plant, which contain the chemical tetrahydrocannabinol (THC), a depressant drug.

maximum oxygen uptake The maximum amount of oxygen breathed in and then used at the tissue level.

measles A highly infectious disease caused by the measles virus.

meditation A relaxation technique that focuses the individual's attention on something that is repetitive or unchanging.

megavitamin approach The practice, advocated by some, of taking large doses of vitamins to enhance health.

melanoma Skin cancers, often related to overexposure to the sun, that may spread to other parts of the body.

memorial service A ceremonial gathering of the family and friends of a deceased person to remember that person; often done in lieu of a funeral or when there is no corpse.

menarche The advent of menstruation in women, normally occurring between the ages of 9 and 14.

menopause The cessation in menstruation, normally occurring between the ages of 45 and 55.

menses The proper term for the monthly "period" of menstruation.

menstruation The "monthly" discharge of the endometrium and unfertilized ovum through the vagina.

metastasis The spread of cancer cells through the circulatory and lymphatic systems to other parts of the body, causing cancer in new areas of the body.

methadone A synthetic drug developed during World War II that is used to treat heroin addiction.

mid-life crisis A period of confusion, doubt, depression, and anxiety experienced by many middle-aged men and women; it is related to growing older and to the psychological and physical changes inherent in that process.

minerals Basic substances found in foods that are the key components of various hormones, enzymes, and other substances that aid in cell chemistry.

moniliasis A common form of vaginitis caused by the fungus *candida albicans;* not necessarily an STD.

morbid obesity Usually refers to extreme cases of obesity that are obviously life-threatening; however, all obesity is potentially life-threatening.

morning drinking A technique used by alcohol dependent persons to alleviate the after-effects or "hangover" resulting from excessive alcohol use.

mourning The manner in which grief is manifested.

multiple sclerosis (MS) A disease of unknown origin, possibly caused by a virus, that attacks the myelin sheaths of nerves. MS can lead to difficulty with motor control of the body and to paralysis.

muscular dystrophy A genetically transmitted disease that disables the muscles.

muscular endurance The maximum number of times (repetitions) a particular amount of weight can be moved through a complete range of motion by a muscle or a muscle group.

myocardial infarction (MI) Commonly called a "heart attack," myocardial infarction occurs when a restricted blood flow to the heart (ischemia) causes tissue death in a part of the heart.

narcotics A term originally used to indicate several of the opiate or opiate-like drugs, including morphine, heroin, and codeine. The term ''narcotic'' is now used to indicate a wide variety of illegal drugs.

nicotine A colorless, odorless chemical compound found in the tobacco leaf. It is an addictive drug, acting first as a stimulant and then as a tranquilizer.

nonessential amino acids Those amino acids that can be manufactured by the body if not obtained from the diet.

nongonococcal urethritis (NGU) An STD caused by some organism other than the *Gonococcus* bacterium and which causes urethritis.

noninfectious diseases Chronic and degenerative diseases.

Norplant The brand name of a new contraceptive implant which is placed just under the skin of a woman's upper arm and is effective for up to five years.

obesity An overweight condition in which there is an abnormally high proportion of body fat, usually 25 to 30 percent or more of total body weight.

oncogenes Genes found in tumor cells whose activation is associated with the transformation of normal cells into cancer cells.

opiates Those drugs derived from opium, which comes from the opium poppy.

orgasmic dysfunction Inability to achieve orgasm.

osteoporosis The weakening of bones as a result of decalcification; often considered a normal part of aging.

over-the-counter (OTC) drugs Drugs that can be purchased at a pharmacy without a prescription.

ovulation The release of one egg by an ovary, occurring in most women about once a month.

ovulation method A contraceptive method that involves determining the onset of a woman's ovulation by interpreting her cervical mucus pattern.

ozone layer The ozone gas in the atmosphere of the earth that protects the earth from the ultraviolet radiation of the sun; the ozone layer is damaged by air pollution.

Pap test A simple test used to diagnose precancerous and cancerous conditions of the cervix and uterus.

parasitic worms Multicelled animals that live in or on other organisms, sometimes causing disease.

passive euthanasia The withholding of life-supporting treatment or other measures that would prolong the life of a person who would certainly die otherwise.

passive immunity The injection or ingestion of pharmaceutically produced antibodies against a specific antigen in order to boost the immune system and provide short-term immunity to a disease.

passive smoking Inhaling tobacco smoke that comes from the cigarettes, cigars, and pipes of other people. The smoke from these sources is known as secondhand smoke.

pathogen Any disease-causing agent, such as a bacteria, a virus, or a toxin.

pelvic inflammatory disease (PID) A dangerous and difficult to diagnose disease that afflicts women; not necessarily an STD.

periodontal disease A disease of the gums; aggravated by smoking.

periodontitis (pyorrhea) The most common form of periodontal disease in which the gums gradually become detached from the teeth.

periodontosis A rare form of periodontal disease in which some of the bone around the roots of molar and upper incisor teeth has been destroyed; afflicts adolescents and young adults and has few symptoms.

personality disorders Mental disturbances in which individuals exhibit a set of inflexible behaviors or personality traits that impair their social functioning, including antisocial personality and paranoid personality.

phencyclidine (PCP) An illegal depressant drug that can act as a psychedelic with highly unpredictable and dangerous effects. It is sometimes falsely sold as THC, the active ingredient in marijuana, to unsuspecting users.

physical dependence Physiological changes in an individual that result in a physical need for a particular drug.

physical health Those aspects of health that concern the physical body alone and do not directly concern the social, mental, emotional, or spiritual health of the individual.

plaque Fatty deposits that build up on the walls of arteries, causing coronary heart disease; also refers to a sticky, colorless layer of harmful bacteria that builds up on the teeth.

pneumoconiosis Usually an occupational or environmental lung disease caused by deposition of particulate matter in the lungs, such as black lung or asbestosis.

pneumonia An acute inflammation of the lungs; pneumonia can be caused by a variety of agents, such as bacteria, viruses, fungi, or inorganic chemicals.

postexercise peril The physiological factors that occur immediately after strenuous exercise that can lead to illness or sudden death.

potency A measure of a drug's pharmacological strength. The greater the potency, the smaller the dosage needed to produce an effect.

preferred provider organization (PPO) A comprehensive medical insurance plan, similar to an HMO except that consumers may choose to select a health care facility that is not ''preferred'' by the plan.

premature ejaculation The inability to control the timing of ejaculation by the male during coitus, often resulting in a lack of sexual satisfaction on the part of the female.

premium The amount of money paid for an insurance policy.

primary aging The basic and inevitable process of aging, which is rooted in biological and genetic factors, regardless of health factors and lifestyle.

primary care physician A physician who serves as the patient's first and regular contact with medical treatment; these doctors are usually specialists in family medicine or in internal medicine.

prodrome An itching or tingling sensation that develops near the site where the herpes simplex, type 2 virus enters the body.

progressive relaxation A relaxation technique that employs the tensing and then the relaxing of muscles and muscle groups.

protozoa Single-cell animals that live in or on other organisms, sometimes causing disease.

psychedelics A broad group of drugs that produce extreme changes in mood, behavior, and perception, sometimes causing hallucinations and other symptoms associated with mental illness.

psychological dependence The habit, or keenly felt need, for a particular drug, without necessarily the physical dependence on it.

psychosomatic illness A physical disorder that has its origin in, or is worsened by, psychological or emotional processes.

psychotherapy As promoted by Freud, psychotherapy is the long-term treatment of mental illness through the gradual discovery by the patient of unconscious, repressed material that affects behavior.

pubic lice A parasite that prefers to live in the genital areas of both men and women, often (but not always) transmitted through sexual contact.

quacks People who used false advertising and other inducements to entice consumers to purchase and use bogus medical procedures, medicines, and health-care products.

radial pulse The pulse (heart beats per minute) as taken at the artery that runs under the hollow of the wrist at the base of each thumb.

rape The sexual penetration of an individual (usually female) against that individual's will.

rebound congestion The tendency of nasal passages to become more inflamed and swollen after a topical decongestant, which has been applied to relieve nasal stuffiness, has ceased to work.

relabeling A deliberate change in the value or description of something in order to better cope with an anxiety-producing situation.

remission A situation in which cancer remains asymptomatic, when it ceases to grow or to spread, or when it disappears.

responsible drug use The wise and prudent use of pharmaceuticals and over-the-counter medications with a conscientious regard for the physiological, psychological, social, and legal factors and effects of their use.

resting metabolic rate Calories used while an individual is at rest, but not while sleeping.

rhythm method The timing of coitus so that it does not occur during the time of the month when the woman is most likely to conceive; only partially effective as a contraceptive method.

rickettsia Now believed to be a very small form of bacteria, rickettsia cause the diseases of typhus and Rocky Mountain spotted fever in humans.

RU 486 A French-manufactured pharmaceutical used to terminate unwanted pregnancies.

sarcomas Cancers that arise in the mesodermal or middle layers of the tissues that form the bones, muscles, and connective tissues.

scabies A parasite of the genital and other areas often (but not always) transmitted through sexual contact.

scalp reduction The reduction of bald spots by surgery, with the unwanted bald skin being removed.

schizophrenic disorders Mental disturbances characterized by dramatic breaks from reality and severe distortion in thought and perception, including disorganized schizophrenia and paranoid schizophrenia.

secondary aging The disabilities arising from degenerative diseases, such as arthritis and atherosclerosis; often such diseases can be delayed, prevented, or cured through medicine and good health habits.

self-actualization In Abraham Maslow's "Hierarchy of Needs" system, self-actualization is the need for the individual to achieve his or her fullest potential as a human being. It can be addressed only after all other needs have been met.

self-care When an individual takes responsibility for the monitoring of his or her own health, determining when to use self-treatment and when to seek the help of health-care specialists.

self-disclosure The revealing of personal information about oneself—one's thoughts and feelings—in an intimate relationship.

self-talk As an aid to overcoming anxiety, self-talk is dialogue with oneself, where problems are talked about in an imaginary conversation.

serum hepatitis (type B hepatitis) A serious disease characterized by an inflammation of the liver, caused by a virus. Transmitted through the blood, semen, and saliva of infected people; it is much less common than infectious hepatitis.

set point theory A theory that postulates that each individual has an ideal weight (the set point), and that the body will attempt to maintain this weight against pressures to change it.

sex Sex refers to something you do; your lovemaking habits.

sex-role or gender-role stereotyping The expectation by society that an individual should behave in particular ways because he or she is male or female.

sexual harassment The threatening sexual advances made by someone in authority or in a position of power toward subordinates.

sexuality In terms of psychology, sexuality refers to an individual's socially and culturally determined gender-related behaviors.

sexually transmitted diseases (STDs) Bacterial, viral, and parasitic diseases that are transmitted through sexual contact, which usually affect the genital areas and may cause serious disease complications throughout the body.

sexual unresponsiveness The inability of a woman to experience erotic pleasure from sexual contact, popularly known as "frigidity."

sickle-cell anemia A genetically transmitted blood disease that becomes manifest in one out of every four hundred African-American people.

silt The soil that is eroded and washed away from the earth's surface by the runoff of precipitation.

situational adaptability The flexibility needed in a relationship to ensure effective communication in different situations.

skinfold measurement An accurate method of determining body fat (adipose tissue) and ideal body weight.

socialization The influences of our home life, our experiences at school, and our interactions with other people that help determine the type of individual we become.

sociobiology The study of the biological basis of social behavior.

solubility A measure of the amount of a substance that can be dissolved in a given solvent under certain conditions.

somatoform disorders Mental disturbances in which individuals experience physical symptoms that have no known organic cause.

spermicide Any of several contraceptive foams, creams, jellies, or other medications that immobilize and kill or block sperm from entering the cervix.

spouse abuse When one marriage partner physically or psychologically assaults his or her spouse.

statutory rape Unlawful sexual intercourse with a minor.

strength Physiologically speaking, strength is the total amount of force a person can apply with a particular muscle or group of muscles at one time.

stress The nonspecific response of the body to any change and to the demands caused by that change.

stressor Any stimulus that causes stress.

successful aging A life characterized by satisfaction and high morale in old age, usually the result of high activity and engagement of the older person in his or her society and environment.

sudden cardiac death A sudden malfunctioning of the heart that causes it to behave chaotically and finally stop beating, causing death.

superego In Freudian psychology, our conscience; our sense of right and wrong.

syphilis A serious STD caused by a spirochete; untreated syphilis has very serious complications and is eventually fatal. Treatment includes the use of antibiotics, but some strains of syphilis are resistant to treatment.

systematic desensitization Arranging anxiety-producing stimuli in a hierarchy or sequence according to the amount of fear they produce, after which the individual deals with each stimulus systematically to overcome the fears and anxiety.

tachycardia A very rapid beating of the heart.

tar A dark, thick, sticky by-product of burned tobacco leaves; it is poisonous and carcinogenic.

target heart rate The heart rate, measured as pulse per minute, needed to be attained and maintained during exercise to produce a training or conditioning effect.

Tay-Sachs disease A serious genetically transmitted disease that is found primarily in Jewish families from Eastern Europe.

teaching hospitals Hospitals that are associated with medical schools and serve as on-the-job training centers for doctors and nurses; the hospital staff serves as the faculty, the students are medical students, interns, residents, and student nurses.

tetanus A serious blood-poisoning disease caused by the tetanus bacteria.

thanatologist Someone who studies or who is an expert on death and dying.

Therapeutic Index A measure of a drug's safety as based on testing to determine its lethal dosage and its effective dosage.

tolerance A measure of the tendency of an individual to need more and more of a drug, that is, a higher dose, to achieve a given effect.

toxin A poison formed by antigens; toxins stimulate an immune response in the body, causing antibodies to the toxin to be formed.

trace minerals Those minerals needed in small amounts by the body.

transaction management The establishing of rules in a relationship to enhance communication and work toward common goals.

transitory ischemic attack (TIA) A mild stroke caused by a temporarily inadequate supply of blood to the brain; although permanent damage may not result, it is a sign of serious cardiovascular disease.

trichomoniasis A disease that invades the vagina, causing vaginitis and other complications; not necessarily an STD.

tuberculosis (TB) A highly contagious disease most commonly affecting the lungs. Serious complications can lead to death if the disease is untreated.

type A behavior pattern Behavior that is excessively competitive, with free-floating hostility, aggressiveness, and impatience.

type B behavior pattern Behavior that is patient, relaxed, and noncompetitive.

urethritis An infection of the urethra.

U.S. RDA A simplified recommended dietary allowance listing that is printed on food package labels, showing the percentage of each nutrient's RDA per day provided by one serving of the food in the package.

vaccination The injection or ingestion of a vaccine in order to stimulate an immune response to a specific antigen.

vaccine A pharmaceutical preparation made from specific antigens that, when injected or ingested by an individual, stimulates the production of antibodies against that antigen, causing either a partial or complete immune response to that antigen.

vaginismus The involuntary tightening of the muscles of the vagina so that the penis cannot enter or so that dyspareunia results.

vaginitis A disease that causes inflammation in the vagina; not necessarily an STD.

values Those thoughts and feelings about life that the individual most strongly regards as being true.

valvular or rheumatic heart disease Damage to the valves of the heart caused by a bacterial infection, commonly a streptococcal infection that begins in the throat or tonsils and leads to rheumatic fever.

varicose veins Permanently distended veins resulting from an improper functioning of valves within the veins.

vasectomy The most effective method of contraception for males, vasectomy involves minor surgery that severs the vas deferens.

vector An organism or some other object that carries a disease-causing agent from one organism to another.

veins The vessels through which the blood returns to the heart from other parts of the body.

viruses Minute parasitic agents that live and reproduce inside living cells; viruses cause many diseases, including the common cold and serious, often fatal, illnesses.

water-soluble vitamins Those vitamins that are dissolved in water and are not stored in the body, such as vitamin C and the B complex vitamins.

wellness Wellness is the harmonious integration of all aspects of health, physical and otherwise, by the individual at any level of that individual's own health or illness.

wetlands Those lands that are adjacent to bodies of water and which are covered with water at certain times of the year; wetlands are very important resources of food and habitat for many organisms.

withdrawal syndrome Physiological changes that occur when the physical need (physical dependence) for a particular drug is denied.

work hypertrophy A physiological process whereby there is a temporary decline in conditioning level following a strenuous workout, followed by the development of a higher level of conditioning after recovery.

zidovudine A new name for the AIDS-fighting pharmaceutical azidothymidine (AZT).

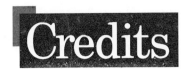

Credits

Exploring Your Health 2.1   From M. Rosenberg, *Society and the Adolescent Self-Image.* Copyright © 1965 Princeton University Press. Self-Esteem Scale reprinted with permission of Princeton University Press.

p. 35, "Steps for Overcoming Shyness."   Philip G. Zimbardo, *Shyness: What It Is and What to Do About It.* © 1990 by Addison-Wesley Publishing Company. Reprinted by permission of Addison-Wesley Publishing Co., Inc., Reading, MA.

p. 50   Excerpt from *Stress Without Distress* by Hans Selye, M.D. Copyright © 1974 by Hans Selye, M.D. Reprinted by permission of HarperCollins Publishers.

Table 3.1   Thomas H. Holmes and Richard H. Rahe, "The Social Readjustment Rating Scale," *Journal of Psychosomatic Research.* Copyright © 1967, Pergamon Press plc. Reprinted by permission of Pergamon Press plc.

Table 6.1   Robin Sawyer and Kenneth H. Beck, "Predicting Pregnancy and Contraceptive Usage Among College Women," *Health Education* 19 (1988): 42–47. Reprinted with permission of the Association for the Advancement of Health Education.

Table 8.1   Basic data from *1979 Build Study,* Society of Actuaries and Association of Life Insurance Medical Directors of America, 1980. Courtesy *Statistical Bulletin,* Metropolitan Life Insurance Company.

Table 8.2   Courtesy *Statistical Bulletin,* Metropolitan Life Insurance Company.

Table 8.3   Adapted from A. R. Frisancho, "New norms of upper limb fat and muscle areas for assessment of nutritional status," *American Journal of Clinical Nutrition* 34 (1981): 2540–2545. © American Journal of Clinical Nutrition, American Society for Clinical Nutrition. Reprinted with permission.

Figure 8.3   Adapted from T. W. Castonguay and coauthors, "Hunger and Appetite: Old Concepts/New Distinctions," *Nutrition Reviews* 41, April 1983, pp. 101–110. © ILSI-Nutrition Foundation. Used with permission.

Figure 12.2   Courtesy of the American Cancer Society.

Figure 16.2   Data from the American Cancer Society, *Cancer Facts and Figures* (1990). Courtesy of the American Cancer Society.

Table 16.2   Courtesy of the American Cancer Society.

Table 16.3   Courtesy of the American Cancer Society.

Exploring Your Health 16.2   Courtesy of the American Cancer Society.

Exploring Your Health 16.4   Courtesy of the American Cancer Society.

Table 18.3   Federated Funeral Directors, cited in "Getting the Best Value for a Funeral," *USA Today,* February 20, 1989, p. 3B.

Table 19.1   Donald M. Vickery and James F. Fries, *Take Care of Yourself: A Consumer's Guide to Medical Care.* © 1990 by Addison-Wesley Publishing Company. Reprinted by permission of Addison-Wesley Publishing Co., Inc., Reading, MA.

Photographs

Chapter 1:   *1*   John Blaustein/Woodfin Camp & Associates   *6* (left)   National Institute on Aging   *6* (right)   Stacy Pick/Stock Boston   *7*   Alon Reininger/Contact Press 1990   *10*   Laima Druskis

Chapter 2:   *19*   Daemmrich/Stock Boston   *20*   Dave Schaefer/Monkmeyer Press   *25*   Laima Druskis   *37*   Mimi Forsyth/Monkmeyer Press   *40*   Richard Pasley/Stock Boston

Chapter 3:   *47*   Bob Daemmrich/The Image Works   *50*   Daemmrich/Stock Boston   *56*   Willie Hill, Jr./The Image Works   *62*   Rafael Macia/Photo Researchers Inc.

Chapter 4:   *67*   Julie Houck/Stock Boston   *68*   Cary Wolinsky/Stock Boston   *69*   Bob Daemmrich/The Image Works   *74*   Rainer Drexel/Bilderberg/The Stock Market   *85*   Lawrence Migdale/Stock Boston   *92*   Deborah Davis/PhotoEdit

Chapter 5:   *97*   Robert Brenner/PhotoEdit   *104* (left)   Bettmann Newsphotos   *104* (right)   L. Druskis/Stock Boston   *109*   Matthew McVay/Stock Boston   *114*   Paul Conklin/PhotoEdit   *115*   Rick Kopstein/Monkmeyer

Chapter 6:   *125*   Michel Tcherevkoff/The Image Bank   *129*   Rhoda Sidney/Monkmeyer Press   *142*   Joe Sohm/Image Works   *148*   S.I.U. School of Medicine/Science Source/Photo Researchers   *149*   Robert Brenner/PhotoEdit

Chapter 7:   *157*   David Parker/Science Photo Library/Photo Researchers Inc.   *158*   Stephen Frisch/Stock Boston   *161*   Stephen McBrady/PhotoEdit   *165*   Richard Hutchings/Photo   Researchers   *178*   Arlene   Collins/Monkmeyer   Press   *181* Daemmrich/Stock Boston

Chapter 8:   *191*   Eric Neurath/PhotoEdit   *196*   Elizabeth Zuckerman/PhotoEdit   *202*   CNRI/Phototake   *206*   Robert Brenner/PhotoEdit   *209* (left)   AP/Wide World Photos   *209* (right)   AP/Wide World Photos   *210*   C. M. Brown

Chapter 9:   *217*   Bill Gallery/Stock Boston   *223*   Dan Budnik/Woodfin Camp & Associates   *226*   Richard Hutchings/Photo Researchers Inc.   *232* (top)   Matthew McVay/Stock Boston   *232* (bottom)   Jim Harrison/Stock Boston   *240*   Robert Brenner/PhotoEdit

Chapter 10:   *245*   A.G.E. Fotostock/FPG   *247*   Richard Hutchings/Photo Researchers Inc.   *253*   Daemmrich/Stock Boston   *257*   AP/Wide World Photos   *259*   Arlene Collins/Monkmeyer Press   *264*   Michael Edrington/The Image Works   *265*   Mark Antman/The Image Works

Chapter 11:   *271*   Hugh Rogers/Monkmeyer Press   *275* (left)   Spencer Grant/Monkmeyer Press   *275* (middle)   Michael Weisbrot/Stock Boston   *275* (right)   Larry Kolvoord/The Image Works   *281*   From *Journal of the American Medical Association* vol. 235 (1976): 1458–60. Courtesy of James W. Hanson, M.D.   *288*   M. Siluk/The Image Works   *294*   David York/Medichrome/The Stock Shop

Chapter 12:   *301*   Jim Anderson/Woodfin Camp & Associates   *302*   R. Erodoes   *303*   Richard Hutchings/InfoEdit   *308*   Michael Edrington/The Image Works   *311* (left)   Susan Leavines/Photo Researchers   *311* (right)   WHO/Photo   *319*   Elena Rooraid/PhotoEdit

Chapter 13:   *331*   Bettmann Archive   *338*   John Griffin/Medichrome/The Stock Shop   *344* (top)   Hank Morgan/Science Source/Photo Researchers   *344* (bottom)   Centers for Disease Control   *348*   Chris Priest & Mark Clarke/Science Photo Library   *351*   The Bettmann Archive   *359*   BioPhoto Associates/Science Source/Photo Researchers

Chapter 14:   *365*   Rob Nelson/Picture Group   *367*   The Image Works Archives   *368*   Centers for Disease Control, Atlanta, Ga.   *369*   Centers for Disease Control, Atlanta, Ga.   *371*   Centers for Disease Control, Atlanta, Ga.   *374*   Centers for Disease Control, Atlanta, Ga.   *383*   Timothy Eagan/Woodfin Camp & Associates

Chapter 15:   *389*   Howard Sochurek/Medical Images   *396*   Joseph Daniels/Photo Researchers Inc.   *399* (left)   Leonard Kamsler/Medichrome/The Stock Shop   *399* (right)   Stacy Pick/Stock Boston   *402*   Janeart LTD/The Image Bank

Chapter 16:   *411*   Will & Deni McIntyre/Photo Researchers   *414*   C. Blankenhorn/Black Star   *421*   National Cancer Institute   *428*   Elizabeth Zuckerman/PhotoEdit   *431*   Paul Shambroom/Science Source/Photo Researchers

Chapter 17:   *437*   Luis Villota/The Stock Market   *440*   Tony Freeman/PhotoEdit   *441*   Grant LeDuc/Monkmeyer Press   *447*   Page Poore   *449*   Julie Marcotte/Stock Boston   *454*   Paul Conklin/Monkmeyer Press

Chapter 18:   *459*   Suzanne Goldstein/Photo Researchers   *462*   James D. Wilson/Woodfin Camp & Associates   *466*   Tony Freeman/PhotoEdit   *471*   Hank Morgan/Photo Researchers   *472*   AP/Wide World   *476*   Christine Osborne/Photo Researchers Inc.

Chapter 19:   *483*   Doug Plummer/Photo Researchers   *491*   The Granger Collection   *493* (left)   Honeywell   *493* (right)   Sybil Shackman/Monkmeyer Press   *496*   Len Barbiero/The Stock Shop

Chapter 20:   *507*   Blair Seitz/Photo Researchers   *510*   Stephen Frisch/Stock Boston   *511*   Larry Mulvehill/Science Source/Photo Researchers   *513*   Paul Biddle & Tim Malyon/Science Source/Photo Researchers   *517*   Bill Aron/PhotoEdit   *523*   Guy Gillette/Photo Researchers Inc.

Chapter 21:   *529*   Gary Retherford/Photo Researchers   *536*   Daemmrich/The Image Works   *542*   Paul Conklin/Monkmeyer Press   *547*   Photograph by Erich Hartmann, © 1961, used by permission of Rachel Carson, Inc.   *554*   Paul Conklin/Monkmeyer Press

Appendix A: All art is from *Fundamentals of Anatomy and Physiology,* 2/E, by Frederic Martini. Copyright © 1992 by Prentice Hall, Englewood Cliffs, N.J. Reproduced by permission of Prentice Hall.

Index

A

Abnormal behavior, 41
Abortifacients, 141
Abortion, 140-43, 349
Abrasion, treatment of, 582
Abscess, 337
Abstinence, 130, 131-32, 378
Abstinence syndrome, 310
Abuse
   child, 82-84
      incest and, 84, 116, 117-19
      sexual, 84-85, 89
   spouse, 84, 85
Acanthamoeba keratitis, 487
Acceptance of death, 464, 465
Access
   to medical care, changes in, 520, 521
   to preventive health services, 6-7
Accidental contamination with AIDS virus, 380
Accidents, 574
   lifestyle risk factors in, 442
   safety and, 585-87
   surveying scene of, 575
   See also Emergencies, first aid in
Accreditation status of hospitals, 511
Accumulation of deleterious material theory of
   aging, 441
ACE inhibitors, 401
Acetaminophen, 254, 488, 489
Acetylsalicylic acid. *See* Aspirin
Acid, oral poisoning with, 581
Acid imbalance, stomach cancer and, 429
Acid indigestion, 489
Acid rain, 532-33, 535
Acne, 493
Acne preparations, 493-95
Acquaintance rape, 116
Acquired immune deficiency syndrome (AIDS),
   14, 92, 114, 116, 118, 119, 134, 138, 332,
   376, 378-84
   AIDS-related complex (ARC), 378
   dementia and, 449
   drug abuse and, 259
   dying from, 462
   homosexuality and, 378, 380, 383-84
   incidence in America, 378-79, 380
   social and political implications of, 383-84
   spread of, 379-81
   testing for, 120, 383
   treating AIDS patients, 381-83
ACTH, 58, 570
Active euthanasia, 472
Active immunity, 338-40
Activity theory of aging, 449-50
Acupuncture, 512, 513
Acute bronchitis, 354
Acute necrotizing gingivitis, 359-60
Adaptability, situational, 77
Adaptation syndrome, general, 50
Addiction
   alcohol (alcoholism), 287-97
   drug, treating, 265-67
   tobacco, 310
      kicking the habit, 319-22
Additives, food, 179-81, 185
Adenosine triphosphate (ATP), 235
Adenovirus, 339
ADH, 570
Adipose tissue, 210; *See also* Body fat; Fat cells
Adjustment, aging and social, 449-53
Adjustment theory, 11-12
Adkins, Janet, 472
Adrenal glands, 58, 441

Adrenaline, 58, 570
Adrenocorticotropic hormone (ACTH), 58, 570
Adulthood, stages of, 21-23; *See also* Aging
Adult modeling, drug abuse and, 264
Advertising
   alcohol use and, 276, 277
   by drug manufacturers, 246-47
   learning to judge, 503
   mail-order health, 490-91
   tobacco use and, 302, 303, 307, 315
Aerobic dance, 232, 233
Aerobic exercise, 230, 443
   metabolic rates and, 200, 201
   prevention of cardiovascular disease and, 401,
      405-6
   programs, 231-34
Aerosal pentamidine, 382
Aerosols, CFC use in, 535
Affection, 73
Affective disorders, 38
African-Americans. *See* Blacks
"After-burn," 200, 219
Age
   alcohol use and, 290-91
   at marriage, 75-76
   noninfectious diseases and, 346
   overweight and, 201
Ageism, 438-40, 454
Agent Orange, 548-50
Age spots, 494-95
Aggressive behavior, 29, 30, 33
Aging, 436-57
   cognitive functioning and, 447-49
   economics and, 453-54
   in the future, 454-55
   lifestyle change to alter process of, 441-43
   physical health and, 443-47
   premature skin, 426
   primary, 440
   products to slow down, 448
   programs available to older people, 451-53
   secondary, 440
   social adjustment and, 449-53
   successful, 448, 449-50
   suicide rate among older people, 38
   theories of, 440-41, 449-50
Aging hits theory, 441
Agricultural waste, 542
AIDS. *See* Acquired immune deficiency syndrome
   (AIDS)
AIDS-related complex (ARC), 378
Air pollution, 530-36
Airways, opening accident victim's, 575
Alarm stage of general adaptation syndrome, 50
Alaska Natives, alcohol use by, 291, 292
Albrecht, Stan L., 80
Alcohol abuser, 274
Alcohol dependent persons, 274-75
Alcoholic(s), 288
   children of, 290, 294-95
   likelihood of becoming, 289
Alcoholics Anonymous (AA), 294, 296-97
Alcohol intoxication, 582
Alcohol use and abuse, 2-3, 270-99
   absorption and metabolism of alcohol, 277-80
   alcoholism, 287-97
      basic factors contributing to, 288-90
      family and, 290, 294-95
      signs of, 295
      sociocultural correlates of, 273, 290-93
      stages in development of, 293-94
      treatment of, 295-97
   in American society, 272-76
   as cancer risk factor, 281, 418
   dependence on, 274-75, 293

determining alcohol content in body, 276-79
fetal alcohol syndrome and, 144, 145, 280,
   281-83
interaction with other drugs, 281, 282-83
psychological and physiological effects of,
   280-83, 286
research data on, 272-73
responsible use, 283-87, 296
reverse tolerance of, 252
trends in, 248
Aldosterone, 570
Alienation, 25-26, 263
Alienation scale, 26, 28-29
Alimentary canal, 567
Alkalis, oral poisoning with, 581
Allergens, 354, 355, 356
Allergic hypersensitivity reaction, 354, 355
Allergic rhinitis, 356
Allergies, 59, 354, 355-57
Alpha-1-antitrypsin deficiency, 354
Alpha particles, 552
Alzheimer's disease, 448-49, 472
Ambiguity, role, 55
Amenorrhea, 205
American Academy of Pediatrics, 150
American Alliance of Health, Physical Education,
   Recreation and Dance, 218
American Association for Marriage and Family
   Therapy, 77
American Association of Retired Persons, 439-40
American Cancer Society, 310, 319, 326, 417
   Cancer Prevention Study II, 418
American College of Nutrition, 499
American College of Obstetricians and
   Gynecologists, 136
American Heart Association, 165, 166, 326, 575
American Hospital Association, 512
   Blue Cross Commission, 516
American Lung Association, 318, 326
American Medical Association (AMA), 173, 208,
   513, 520, 523, 525
American Psychiatric Association, 115
American Red Cross emergency action principles,
   574-75
American Schizophrenia Association, 40
Amino acids, 164-65
Amino acid supplements, 201
Amniocentesis, 353
Amotivational syndrome, 260
Amphetamine analogs, 261
Amphetamines, 250, 256-58
Ampulla, 98, 99
Anabolic steroids, 201, 235, 262-63
Anaerobics, 233, 234-35
Analgesics, alcohol's interaction with, 282, 283
Anal intercourse, 114, 380
Anal stage, 22
Android (upper body) obesity, 200
Anemia
   iron deficiency, 174
   sickle-cell, 352
Anesthesia, acupuncture, 513
Anger
   coping with, 36
   coping with sexually transmitted diseases and,
     376
Anger stage of dying, 464, 465
Angina pectoris, 394
Angioplasty, coronary, 407
Angiotensin, 401
Animal bite, treatment of, 582
Animal parasites, 334-35
Animal protein, 165
Anorexia, 200, 201-3
Anoxia, 352

M

McDonald, G.W., 149
Macklin, Eleanor, 90-91
Macrominerals, 170-71
Macrophages, 336, 337, 565, 566
Magnesium, 171
Magnetic resonance imaging (MRI), 431
Mail-order quacks, 490-91
Mainstream smoke, 316
Maintenance, training for, 231
Major tranquilizers, 258
Male anorexics, 202
Male climacteric, 129
Male contraceptives, 139
Male reproductive system, 98-100, 101, 573
Males
  infertility in, 150
  sexual problems in, 109-11
Malignant tumors, 412; See also Cancer
Malpractice, 523-25
Mammary glands, 149, 573
Mammography, 420, 421
Managed health care programs, 516-17
Manganese, 172
Manic-depressive disorders, 38
Mantra, 62, 63
Marijuana, 145, 247, 248, 250, 252, 259-61
Marine Protection Research and Sanctuaries Act, 551
Marriage, 74-81
  alternatives to, 89-93, 450-51
  attractions of, 75
  choosing partner in, 76
  communication in, 76-77
  divorce and, 74, 78-80, 88, 294
  factors contributing to success in, 75-76
  having children and satisfaction in, 81
  reasons for failure of first, 80
  remarriage, 450-51
  types of, 74, 75
  See also Family relationships
Marrow, bone, 560
Maslow, Abraham, 10, 11
Mastectomy, 421, 430
Masters, William, 104, 105, 109, 110
Masturbation, 107
Maturity, marital success and emotional, 75
Maximum oxygen uptake, 218, 219
MDMA, 261-62
Meal programs for the elderly, 453
Measles, 339, 342
Meat, consumption of, 166
Mediators, chemical, 355-56
Medical agencies, 502
Medical care, 508-13
  changes in access to, 520, 521
  choosing, 524
  community health care, 512-13
  dentist, selecting, 508
  hospital, selecting, 510-12
  patients' bill of rights, 512
  physicians and, 508-10, 520-21
  prevention of cardiovascular disease and, 403-5
  therapy for drug addiction combined with, 265-66
Medic Alert bracelets or necklaces, 585
Medical history, exercise program and, 235
Medical school, hospital affiliation with, 511-12
Medical tests, home, 487-88
Medical x-rays, 416, 551-52, 553
Medicare and Medicaid, 453, 517
Medicine, defensive, 522-23; See also Health care
Meditation, 61-62
Megavitamin approach, 166, 167
Melanoma, 416, 427
Memorial services, 478-79
Menarche, 126
Menopause, 126, 127-28, 447
Menses, 126
Menstrual cycle, 126-27, 202
Menstruation, 126, 129
  sexual intercourse during, 107
Mental health, 18-45
  characteristics of emotional health, 20-21
  of children of divorce, 80

coping and, 31-37
  with common problems, 34-37
  modes of, 31-34
defined, 8
exercise and, 219
of homosexuals, 115
mental disorders, 37-39, 42-43
personality development and, 21-25
psychosocial influences on health behavior and, 25-31
seeking help for, 39-43
Mental health resources, 40
Mental illness
  debate over existence of, 41
  stress-related, 60
Meperidine, 250, 261
Mercury, 533, 543-44
Mercy killing, 472
Meredith, Dennis, 90
Mesoderm, 146
Metabolism, 158, 198
  age and, 201
  of alcohol, 277-80
  anaerobic, 235
  basal, 160, 161
  overweight and, 200
  resting, 218, 219
Metastasis, 412, 433
Methadone, 250, 266
Methamphetamine, 250, 256-58
Methamphetamine analogs, 261
3,4-Methylenedioxymetham-phetamine (MDMA), 261-62
Metronidazole, 373
Metropolitan Life Insurance Company, 199
Middle adulthood, 22, 447
Mid-life crisis, 129, 450
Migraine headache, 59, 486
Milk in diet, 179, 183, 185
Mind-body relationship, 48; See also Stress
Minerals, 170-74, 560
Minilaparotomy, 139
"Minipill," 136
Minors with sexually transmitted diseases, treatment of, 371
Minor tranquilizers, 258
Minoxidil, 496
Miscarriages (spontaneous abortions), 140, 141
Misuse of drugs, 248, 263
Modeling
  covert, 12, 13
  drug abuse and adult, 264
Modified mastectomy, 430
Moisturizer, 494
Moniliasis, 373-74
Monoclonal antibodies, 431
Monogamy, 74, 75, 118
Mononucleosis, 342-43
Monounsaturated fats, 162
Mons veneris (mons pubis), 100, 101
Mood alteration, drug abuse and, 264
Moral development, 23-25
Morality, education about sexually transmitted diseases and, 377
Morning-after pills, 141
Morning drinking, 274
Morphine, 250, 258-59
Mothering, surrogate, 152
Motility, sperm, 150
Motorcycles, preventing accidents with, 587
Motor vehicle accidents
  drinking and, 285-88
  preventing, 586-87
Mourning, 472, 473-75
Mouth, pH in, 360, 497
Mouthwashes, 497
MPPP, 261
MRI, 431
Mucus, cervical, 133
Mullen, Kathy, 113
Multifactorial inheritance, 352
Multiple orgasms, 105
Multiple sclerosis (MS), 350-51
Mumps, 339, 342
Murmur, heart, 396-97
Muscle tension as sexual response, 104, 105
Muscle weight gain, 201, 235

Muscular dystrophy, 353
Muscular endurance, 226
Muscular system, 560-61, 562
Mycostatin, 374
Myocardial infarction (M.I.), 393
Myocarditis, 398
Myocardium, 393
Myometrium, 102, 103
Myotonia, 104, 105

N

Nagele's rule, 145
Naltrexone, 267
Narcotics, 145, 258-59
Nasal decongestants, 255, 488
Nass, Gilbert D., 117, 149
National Academy of Sciences, 177, 544
  National Research Council, Food and Nutritional Board of, 158
National Alliance for the Mentally Ill, 40
National Association of Elementary School Principals, 87
National Center for Health Statistics, 6, 109
  National Fetal Mortality Survey (1980), 145
  National Natality Survey (1980), 145
National Center on Child Abuse and Neglect (NCCAN), 84
National Committee for Prevention of Child Abuse, 83
National Criminal Justice Reference Service, 83
National Easter Seal Society, 396
National health, objectives for, 5-7
National health insurance, 453, 523
National Heart, Lung, and Blood Institute, 6
National High Blood Pressure Coordinating Committee, 400-401
National Highway Safety Administration, 285
National Institute of Education, 90
National Institute of Mental Health (NIMH), 84
National Institute of Occupational Safety and Health, 543
National Institute on Aging (NIA), 452-53
National Institute on Drug Abuse Warning Network, 257
National Institutes of Health, 6
National Institution on Alcohol Abuse and Alcoholism (NIAAA), 272, 274
National Organization of Women (NOW), 89
National Self-Health Association, 40
National Self-Help Clearinghouse, 40
National Study of the Incidence and Severity of Child Abuse and Neglect (1980), 84
Native Americans
  alcohol consumption rates of, 273, 291, 292
  fetal alcohol syndrome among, 281-83
  life span of, 6
  tobacco use by, 302, 306
Natural disaster, 530
Natural foods, 184-85
Naturopathy, 513-14
Necrophilia, 115
Needs, hierarchy of, 10, 11
Neglect, child, 82
Neisseria gonorrhoeae bacteria, 368
Nerve cells in brain, theory of aging based on loss of, 441
Nerve-sparing radical retropubic prostatectomy, 425
Nervous system, 561-62, 563
  disorders of, 350-52
  stress and, 57
Neurons, 562
Newborns, bonding with, 149; See also Childbirth
New England Journal of Medicine, 253
Niacin (nicotinic acid), 167
Nickel carbonyl, 415
Nicotine, 306, 307, 308-10, 312, 322
Nicotine substitutes and gums, 322
NIMBYs, 546
Nipples, erection of, 104, 105
Nitrites and nitrates, 179
"No-fault" divorce, 79
Noise pollution, 536-38

Planned Parenthood/World Population, 130
Planning
    for death, 466-73
    environmental, 34
Plant protein, 165
Plaque
    arterial, 218, 219, 390, 391, 399
    dental, 360
Plasma, 565
Plasmodium protozoan parasite, 334-35
Plastic trash dangers, 541
Plateau phase in sexual response cycle, 103
Platelets, 560
Plumbism, 544
Pneumoconiosis, 354
Pneumonia, 344, 345, 442
Podophyllin, 375
Poison control centers, 581
Poisoning
    food, minimizing risks of, 497-99
    lead, 544
    oral, first aid for, 580-82
    self-medication for, 489
Poison ivy or oak, treatment of, 584
Poison Prevention Packaging Act, 501
Poliomyelitis, 339
Political implications of AIDS, 383-84
Pollutants
    air, health effects of regulated, 531
    home, 533
    sources of, 541
Pollution, 530-51
    air, 530-36
    cancer and environmental, 413, 415-16
    noise, 536-38
    plan to reduce, 553-55
    solid and chemical waste, 542-51
    water, 538-42
Polygamy, 74
Polygenic (multifactorial) inheritance, 352
Polyunsaturated fats, 162
Population
    age 65 and over in U.S. (1900-1986), 438
    environment and growth of, 555-56
Population pyramids, 439
Postconventional level of moral development, 25
Postexercise peril, 224
Potassium, 171
Potency of drug, 248, 249
Powerlessness, alienation and, 25, 26
Power of Attorney, 469-71
PPO, 516, 517
Prealcoholic phase, 293
Precancerous conditions, 417
Preconventional level of moral development, 25
Preejaculatory fluid, 99, 132
Pre-event meal for athlete, 186
Preferred provider organizations (PPO), 516, 517
Pregnancy, 126, 143-47
    abortion to terminate, 140-43, 349
    avoidance of x-rays during, 553
    determining due date, 145
    genetic counseling and, 349
    genital herpes and, 372
    gestation period, 145-47
    IUD and, 137
    prenatal care and, 144-45
    preventing epilepsy from developing in children
        during, 350
    rubella infection during, 342, 352
    smoking during, 145, 308, 313-14
    teenage, 129, 130-31
    transmission of syphilis during, 369, 370
    tubal, 373
Pregnancy Discrimination Act of 1978, 89
Pregnancy testing, 487
Premature birth, 146, 149
Premature deaths, reducing number of, 15
Premature ejaculation, 108, 109-10
Premature skin aging, 426
Premiums, health insurance, 514, 515
Prenatal care, 144-45
Prepared childbirth, 149
Prepuce, 98, 99
Prescription drugs, misuse of, 248
President's Commission for the Study of Ethical

Problems in Medicine and Biomedical and
    Behavioral Research, 461
Pressure dressing, 578
Pressure points, 578
Prestige, date selection and, 73
Preventive health care, 484-90, 515
    access to, 6-7
    consumer and, 484-90, 500
Preventive services priorities, 7
Primary aging, 440
Primary care physician, 508
Primary ejaculatory incompetence, 111
Primary erectile dysfunction, 110
Pritchard, J.A., 145
Private agencies, protection of consumer by,
    501-2
Private hospital, 510-11
Processed food, 183, 185
''Pro-choice'' groups, 142
Prodrome, 370, 372
Product labeling, 499
Product safety, 501
Professional help to change health behavior,
    12-13
Progesterone, 126, 127, 570
Progestins, 128, 135
Progressive overload principle, 226, 237
Progressive relaxation, 62-63
Projection, 32
Prolactin, 149, 570
''Pro-life'' groups, 142
Proof (alcohol content), 276
Prostaglandins, 253, 254, 405
Prostate, 98, 99, 129
Prostate cancer, 424-25
Protein, 164-66
    complementary, 166
    exercise and intake of, 186, 210
    on food labels, 183
    recommended for American diet, 176
Protozoa, 334-35
Proxy Designations Clause in living will, 468
Psychedelics, 260, 261
Psychoactive drugs, 256-63
    anabolic steroids, 201, 235, 262-63
    depressants, 258-59, 582
    designer drugs, 261-62
    marijuana, 145, 247, 248, 250, 252, 259-61
    psychedelics and hallucinogens, 260, 261
    stimulants, 250, 256-58, 283, 492
Psychodrama, 43
Psychological dependence, 252
Psychological withdrawal, 93
Psychomotor attacks, 350
Psychosexual development, Freud's analysis of,
    21, 22
Psychosocial influences on health behavior, 25-31
Psychosomatic illness, 59-61
Psychotherapy, 40, 41
Psychotropics, alcohol's interaction with, 283
Puberty, 22, 126
Pubic lice, 375
Public transportation, 535
Pulmonary arteries, 563
Pulmonary circulation, 565, 567
Pulmonary disease, chronic obstructive, 442
Pulse
    carotid, 484, 485-86
    radial, 234, 484, 485
    taking a, 484, 485-86, 576
Puncture wound, treatment of, 584
Purinegic theory of hunger regulation, 203
Pus, 337
Pyorrhea, 312, 358, 359
Pyridoxine, 168

Q

Q-Day, setting, 325, 326
Quacks and quackery, 490-91
Questionnaire, health behavior, 2-5
Quickening, 146
Quinlan, Karen Ann, 467
Quit list for smokers, 323-25

R

Rabies, 339
Race
    alcohol consumption and, 273, 281-83, 291,
        292
    divorce rate and, 79
    fetal alcohol syndrome and, 281-83
    single-parent families and, 85-87
Radial pulse, 234, 484, 485
Radiation, 416, 532, 551-53
Radiation therapy, 429; *See also* Cancer
Radical mastectomy, 421, 430
Radioactive dusts, 415
Radon, 416, 533, 534
Rahe, Richard H., 51, 53
Rape, 114, 115-17
Rational emotive therapy, 43
Rationalization, 32
Reaction formation, 32
Reagan, Ronald, 314, 546
Reasoning, moral, 24-25
Rebound congestion, 488, 489
Recessive inheritance, 352
Recommended dietary allowances (RDAs), 158,
    159, 166, 183, 499
Recovery, Inc., 40
Rectum cancer, 422
Recycling, 550-51
Red blood cells (erythrocytes), 560, 565
Redbook magazine survey on sex, 109
Red marrow, 560
Reflective listening, 77, 78
Refrigerator Door Safety Act, 501
Regression, 32
Rehearsal, covert, 12, 13
Reinforcement, covert, 12, 13
Rejuvenation products, skin, 493-94
Relabeling, 34
Relationships. See Family relationships; Intimate
    relationships
Relaxation response, 62
Relaxation techniques for stress management,
    61-63
Releasing factors, 570
Religion
    contraception and, 130
    stress management with, 64
Remarriage, 450-51
Reminder systems, 12
Remission, 412
Remodeling of bone, 445
Repression, 32
Reproduction, marriage to legitimize, 75
Reproductive systems, 98-102, 103, 106, 572-73
    female, 100-102, 103, 573
    male, 99-100, 101, 573
R-erythroporetin, 382
Rescue breathing, 575-77
Research
    air pollution, 534-35
    on alcohol use and abuse, 272-73
    cancer, 432-33
Resistance stage of general adaptation syndrome,
    50
Resolution phase of sexual response cycle, 104
Resource Conservation and Recovery Act, 551
Resources, mental health, 40
Respect, love and, 73
Respiration, 227, 566-67
    artificial, 575-76
    circulation and, 565
Respiratory disease, 353-57
Respiratory distress syndrome, 353
Respiratory system, 566-67
Respiratory tract, infections of, 341
Responsibility, sexual, 119
Responsible alcohol use, 283-87, 296
Responsible drug use, 246, 247
Responsive Parent, 82
Resting metabolic rate, 218, 219
Retarded ejaculation, 111
Reticular fiber network, 565
Retin A, 448, 494
Retinoblastoma, 416